# Understanding Pharmacology

## Essentials for Medication Safety

**M. Linda Workman**, PhD, RN, FAAN

**Linda LaCharity**, PhD, RN

**Susan C. Kruchko**, MS, RN

*With*

**Jennifer Ponto**, RN, BSN
Instructor
Department of Vocational Nursing
South Plains College
Levelland, Texas

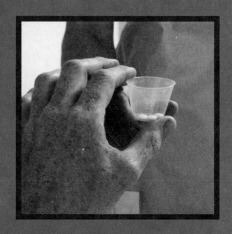

ELSEVIER
SAUNDERS

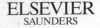

3251 Riverport Lane
St. Louis, Missouri 63043

UNDERSTANDING PHARMACOLOGY: ESSENTIALS FOR                    ISBN: 978-1-4160-2917-5
MEDICATION SAFETY

**Copyright © 2011 by Saunders, an imprint of Elsevier Inc.**

---

**Notices**

Knowledge and best practice in this field are constantly changing. As new research and experience broaden our understanding, changes in research methods, professional practices, or medical treatment may become necessary.

   Practitioners and researchers must always rely on their own experience and knowledge in evaluating and using any information, methods, compounds, or experiments described herein. In using such information or methods they should be mindful of their own safety and the safety of others, including parties for whom they have a professional responsibility.

   With respect to any drug or pharmaceutical products identified, readers are advised to check the most current information provided (i) on procedures featured or (ii) by the manufacturer of each product to be administered, to verify the recommended dose or formula, the method and duration of administration, and contraindications. It is the responsibility of practitioners, relying on their own experience and knowledge of their patients, to make diagnoses, to determine dosages and the best treatment for each individual patient, and to take all appropriate safety precautions.

   To the fullest extent of the law, neither the Publisher nor the authors, contributors, or editors assume any liability for any injury and/or damage to persons or property as a matter of products liability, negligence or otherwise, or from any use or operation of any methods, products, instructions, or ideas contained in the material herein.

---

**Library of Congress Cataloging-in-Publication Data**
Workman, M. Linda.
   Understanding pharmacology : essentials for medication safety / M. Linda Workman,
Linda LaCharity, Susan C. Kruchko; with Jennifer Ponto.
       p. ; cm.
   Includes bibliographical references and index.
   ISBN 978-1-4160-2917-5 (pbk. : alk. paper) 1. Pharmacology. 2. Drugs—
Administration. 3. Medication errors—Prevention. 4. Nursing. I. LaCharity, Linda A.
II. Kruchko, Susan C. III. Title.
   [DNLM: 1. Drug Therapy—nursing. 2. Pharmacological Phenomena. 3. Safety Management.
WY 100.1 W926u 2011]
   RM300.W675 2011
   615'.1—dc22

                                                                2010025796

*Senior Editor:* Lee Henderson
*Senior Developmental Editor:* Rae L. Robertson
*Publishing Services Manager:* Deborah L. Vogel
*Senior Project Manager:* Jodi M. Willard
*Design Direction:* Teresa McBryan

Printed in the United States of America.

Last digit is the print number:  9  8  7  6  5  4

# Understanding Pharmacology

## Essentials for Medication Safety

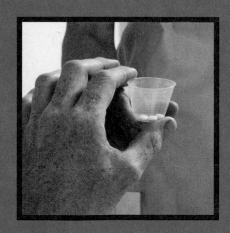

# About the Authors

**M. Linda Workman**, a native of Canada, received her BSN from the University of Cincinnati College of Nursing and Health. She later earned her MSN and a PhD in Developmental Biology from the University of Cincinnati. Linda's 30 years of academic experience include teaching at the diploma, associate degree, baccalaureate, and master's levels. Her areas of teaching expertise include medical-surgical nursing, pharmacology, physiology, and pathophysiology. Linda has been called the "Mr. Rogers" of nursing education for her ability to creatively present complex physiologic concepts in a manner that promotes student retention of the information. She has been recognized nationally for her teaching expertise and received Excellence in Teaching awards from Raymond Walters College, the University of Cincinnati, and Case Western Reserve University. Currently she is Senior Volunteer Faculty at the College of Nursing, University of Cincinnati.

**Linda LaCharity** received her BSN from Kent State University's College of Nursing. During her career in the U.S. Army Nurse Corps, she earned an MN from the University of Washington in Seattle. She worked as a staff nurse and nurse manager in adult medical-surgical and critical care settings supervising RNs, LPN/LVNs, and nursing assistant staff. Linda's academic experience includes teaching EMTs and critical care nurses for the military and across the curriculum at the University of Cincinnati (BSN, MSN, Accelerated BSN/MSN, and PhD). Her area of teaching expertise in both classroom and patient care settings is adult health. She is currently director of the Accelerated Program and an Assistant Professor in the College of Nursing at the University of Cincinnati in Cincinnati, Ohio.

**Susan C. Kruchko** earned her BSN at the University of Cincinnati and her MS in nursing at the University of Maryland. She was a founding coordinator of the practical nursing program at Lafayette High School in Williamsburg, Virginia, and was an instructor in the Practical Nursing Programs at Eastern Vocational-Technical High School in Baltimore, Maryland and at Presbyterian Hospital in Philadelphia, Pennsylvania. Her favorite teaching topics were math for meds and pharmacology. She was best known as an educator who instilled confidence in nontraditional students to help them believe in themselves and achieve their dreams.

To the late Susan Clendaniel Kruchko

An extraordinary teacher and friend whose teaching style

and vision were instrumental in shaping the format

and content of this textbook.

# Reviewers

Hilaree E. Alexander, BSN, RN
Northeast Iowa Community College–Calmar
Calmar, Iowa

Maija R. Anderson, RN, DNP
Sojourner-Douglass College
Baltimore, Maryland

Yolanda M. Arreola, BSN, RN
Anamarc Educational Institute
El Paso, Texas;
Santa Teresa, New Mexico

Christopher Bridgers, PharmD
Saint Joseph's Hospital
Atlanta, Georgia

Patricia A. Bumby, RN, BSPA
Intercoast Career Institute
South Portland, Maine

Laura Higgs, MSN, RN, BC, MdED
Chesapeake College
Wye Mills, Maryland

Tracy K. Justice, BSN, RN
Mercy Hospital
Fairfield, Ohio

Susan Kenna, MS, RN
NHTI–Concord's Community College
Concord, New Hampshire

T. Camille Killough, BSN, RN
Pearl River Community College,
   Forrest County Campus
Hattiesburg, Mississippi

Linda G. Locke, BS
Cherokee High School
Marlton, New Jersey

Cathy L.S. Maddry, MSN, RN
Northwest Louisiana Technical College
Minden, Louisiana

Phyllis M. Magaletto, MS, RN, BC
Cochran School of Nursing
Yonkers, New York

Michael McGlynn, MSN, CFNP
Jackson Community College
Jackson, Michigan

Laura M. Moskaluk, BSN, RN
Somerset County Technology Institute
Bridgewater, New Jersey

Sallie Noto, MS, MSN, RN
Career Technology Center of Lackawanna County
Scranton, Pennsylvania

Susan Seiboldt, MSN, RN, CNE
Carl Sandburg College
Galesburg, Illinois

Stephen M. Setter, PharmD, CDE, CGP, DVM
Washington State University–Spokane
Spokane, Washington

Karen Snipe, CPhT, MEd
Trident Technical College
Charleston, South Carolina

Rebecca S. Utz, BSN, RN
University of Arkansas Community College
   at Batesville
Batesville, Arkansas

Linda P. Walton, BSN, RN
Blue Ridge Job Corps
Marion, Virginia

## STUDENT REVIEWERS

Vionnette Astrinos
Van Alstyne, Texas

Dana M. Brown
Lewiston, Idaho;
Missoula, Montana

Brandy G. Casey
Riverside, California

Millicent Fila
Las Vegas, Nevada

Vernlinciea Harris
Sherman, Texas

**Patricia L. Jensen**
Batesville, Arkansas

**Heather E. Kesinger**
Edmond, Oklahoma

**Natalie Kulkarni**
Bottineau, North Dakota

**Abiodun Oladimeji**
Garland, Texas

**Kristin J. Wainwright**
Greenville, North Carolina

**Lindsay L. Wilson**
Van Alstyne, Texas

# Advisory Board

**M. Gie Archer, MS, RN, C, WHCNP**
Dean of Health Sciences
LVN Program Coordinator
North Central Texas College
Gainesville, Texas

**Mary Brothers, MEd, RN**
Coordinator,
Garnet Career Center School of Practical Nursing
Charleston, West Virginia

**Patricia A. Castaldi, RN, BSN, MSN**
Union County College
Plainfield, New Jersey

**Dolores Ann Cotton, RN, BSN, MS**
Meridian Technology Center
Stillwater, Oklahoma

**Lora Lee Crawford, RN, BSN**
Emanuel Turlock Vocational Nursing Program
Turlock, California

**Ruth Ann Eckenstein, RN, BS, MEd**
Oklahoma Department of Career and
   Technology Education
Stillwater, Oklahoma

**Gail Ann Hamilton Finney, RN, MSN**
Nursing Education Specialist
Concorde Career Colleges, Inc.
Mission, Kansas

**Pam Hinckley, RN, MSN**
Redlands Adult School
Redlands, California

**Deborah W. Keller, RN, BSN, MSN**
Erie Huron Ottawa Vocational Education School of
   Practical Nursing
Milan, Ohio

**Patty Knecht, MSN, RN**
Nursing Program Director
Center for Arts & Technology
Brandywine Campus
Coatesville, Pennsylvania

**Lt Col (Ret) Teresa Y. McPherson, RN, BSN, MSN**
Adjunct Instructor
St. Philip's College LVN/AND Nursing Program
San Antonio, Texas

**Frances Neu Shull, RN, MS, BSN**
Miami Valley Career Technology Center
Clayton, Ohio

**Beverley Turner, MA, RN**
Director, Vocational Nursing Department
Maric College, San Diego Campus
San Diego, California

**Sister Ann Wiesen, RN, MRa**
Erwin Technical Center
Tampa, Florida

# Preface

The authors of this text are nurses and educators with many decades of clinical and teaching experience. Our concept of what is needed in a pharmacology textbook is derived from the desire to create a book that will help students identify the most important content areas for safe drug administration and patient teaching. With this goal in mind, we developed a unique format based on four focus areas:

- Why specific drugs are prescribed as therapy for health problems
- How different drugs work to induce their intended responses
- What critical actions and assessments to perform before and after administering drugs
- Which points are most important to teach patients about their drug therapy

Using these focus areas, we present pharmacology content in a framework that promotes in-depth learning versus rote memorization, which is truly essential in understanding the principles of pharmacology and safe drug administration.

## CHAPTER ORGANIZATION

Our presentation style for the content of this text is direct, active, and clear. Health care terms and related physiological mechanisms are explained in clear, straightforward, everyday language to promote better student understanding and application of the content in the clinical setting. Photographs and other illustrations have been selected and developed to better explain drug administration techniques, drug actions, and appropriate health care interventions.

Chapter **Objectives** presented at the beginning of each chapter focus the student on "need to know" information, clarifying which issues have the highest priority for safe drug administration. A list of **Key Terms** includes phonetic pronunciations, definitions, and page numbers where each term is first used.

The **mathematics review chapters** (Chapters 4, 5, and 6) are written in a self-paced, guided-study format and contain easy-to-understand explanations and examples. **Try This!** boxes provide a total of more than 150 practice questions within these chapters, in addition to the end-of-chapter review material. Answers to these exercises are found at the ends of the chapters.

In-text **drug tables** outline the most common drugs used to treat highlighted disorders and diseases. Generic and trade names and common dosage ranges for adults and children are included, and a special

icon 🔲 designates those drugs that are among the top 100 prescribed drugs in the United States.

Discussion sections on **"What To Do Before," "What To Do After,"** and **"What To Teach Patients"** about each highlighted drug or drug category emphasize the important aspects of drug administration, monitoring, follow-up, and patient teaching.

**Life Span Considerations** sections receive particular attention in most chapters. Differences in actions, the risks for side effects, precautions, or dosing for pediatric patients, pregnant or breastfeeding patients, or older adults are presented as appropriate for each drug class.

A **Get Ready for Practice!** section at the end of each chapter features Key Points, Additional Learning Resources, Review Questions, and Critical Thinking Activities.

- **Key Points** emphasize selected need-to-know content from the chapter to help students study for tests and certification/licensure exams.
- **Additional Learning Resources** sections refer students to related review material in the accompanying Study Guide and on the Evolve website at http://evolve.elsevier.com/Workman/pharmacology/.
- **Review Questions** correspond item-by-item with the Objectives at the beginning of the chapter. Drug calculation questions are also included in this section. Answers to the Review Questions are located on the inside back cover.
- **Critical Thinking Activities** are true-to-practice case studies that present issues and problems requiring clinical decision making related to individual patients receiving pharmacologic therapy. Answer guidelines to the questions are available to instructors only on the secure Evolve instructor website at http://evolve.elsevier.com/Workman/pharmacology/.

## LEARNER-FRIENDLY INSTRUCTIONAL DESIGN

One of the most innovative features of this text is its unique instructional design. A single column presents the narrative, and a wide margin is used to reinforce important concepts and prevent medication errors with special boxed features. This wide margin also allows generous space for note-taking. Special learning features found in the wide margin include the following:

- **Drug Alert!** boxes help reinforce crucial actions or interventions, teaching, and drug administration information. Each of these boxes is classified into one of five categories: Teaching, Interaction, Administration, Dosage, or Action/Intervention.

- **Memory Jogger** boxes highlight and summarize essential information, including major categories of drugs and the diseases they are used to treat.
- **Clinical Pitfall** boxes focus on information vital for safe practice and medication administration.
- **Common Side Effects** boxes focus on individual drug groups and feature unique icons that promote rapid recognition.
- **Do Not Confuse** boxes highlight lookalike/soundalike drug names.
- **Did You Know?** boxes help students link pharmacology content to the world around them.
- **Cultural Awareness** boxes emphasize important cultural considerations related to pharmacology.

We believe you'll find that the authors and publisher have crafted a balance of these features to minimize wasted space and at the same time promote in-depth learning versus rote memorization.

## TEACHING AND LEARNING PACKAGE

### FOR STUDENTS

A companion **Study Guide**, available for purchase at elsevierhealth.com, features a variety of engaging learning activities that complement those in the textbook. Clinically focused Medication Safety Practice questions and a Practice Quiz are provided in each chapter, along with a variety of other Learning Activities that promote an understanding of pharmacology and safe drug administration.

The **Evolve website** at http://evolve.elsevier.com/Workman/pharmacology/ provides free student learning resources that include the following:

- **eLearning Activities** keyed to callouts in the text help reinforce content that has just been learned.
- Over 390 **Interactive Review Questions** in multiple-choice and alternate item formats, with rationales for correct and incorrect answers, help students review important chapter material.
- **Audio Key Points** provide point-by-point highlights from each chapter, along with integrated quiz questions, and are provided in both print and downloadable MP3 audio files for audio CDs and MP3 players.
- A **Key Terms Audio Glossary** provides the definitions for all Key Terms in the book along with audio pronunciations for each term.
- **Animations and Video Clips** explain important concepts from anatomy and physiology to drug administration and are keyed to the text by distinctive icons.
- Twelve interactive **Drug Dosage Calculators** offer a quick way to calculate IV dosages, body surface area, oral doses, and more.

- An extensive **Spanish/English Audio Glossary** provides a vast array of health care–related terms and their definitions, with audio, in both English and Spanish.
- A collection of **Essential Drug Patient Teaching Handouts** can be used to provide patients with information on almost any available drug in both English and Spanish.

### FOR INSTRUCTORS

The comprehensive *Evolve Resources with TEACH Instructor Resource* provides everything a new or seasoned instructor will need to teach the content, including the following:

- **TEACH Lesson Plans** with **Lecture Outlines,** based on textbook Objectives, tie together the text and all other learning resources in ready-to-use, customizable lessons.
- A high-quality **Test Bank,** delivered in ExamView, RTF, and ParTest formats, as well as within the Assessment area of Evolve, contains more than 700 new test items created by the authors. Approximately 75% of these items are written at the Applying or higher cognitive level of the new Bloom's taxonomy. Each question includes the correct answer, rationale, step of the Nursing Process, and NCLEX Client Needs Category (for nursing programs), as well as corresponding textbook page numbers, where appropriate (page numbers are not appropriate for questions at the Applying level or above because they draw on multiple sources of information).
- A new collection of **Audience Response System Questions** (5 questions per chapter)—discussion-oriented questions with correct answers and rationales—is provided in PowerPoint format for use with iClicker and other audience response systems.
- An **Image Collection** contains every reproducible image from the text. Images are suitable for incorporation into classroom lectures, PowerPoint presentations, or distance-learning applications.
- A collection of **PowerPoint Lecture Slides** highlight key concepts and discussion in the text.
- **Answer Keys** are provided for the Critical Thinking Activities in the text and for the Study Guide.

*Understanding Pharmacology: Essentials for Medication Safety*, together with its fully integrated multimedia ancillary package, provides the tools needed to fully understand pharmacology principles and how to apply them effectively and safely in today's health care environment. For more information on any of these innovative companion publications, or if you simply wish to provide us feedback, please contact your Elsevier sales representative, visit us at http://www.us.elsevierhealth.com/, or contact Elsevier Faculty Support at 1-800-222-9570 or sales.inquiry@elsevier.com.

# Acknowledgments

Many talented people are needed to make any textbook a success. The authors wish to acknowledge the following individuals and groups for their guidance, dedication, hard work, constructive criticism, and creative input that were so important to this project: Lee Henderson, Rae Robertson, Jodi Willard, Jennifer Ponto, Sandra Cooper, Catherine Harold, all of the faculty reviewers, all of the student reviewers, and Yvonne LaCharity and Gregory Workman—our very own math experts.

# Special Features

*Understanding Pharmacology: Essentials for Medication Safety* focuses on promoting an *understanding* of pharmacology principles and safety of drug administration by using clear, everyday language. Full-color illustrations and a unique, user-friendly design accompany practical, understandable discussions of important drugs and drug classes, which are presented by body system.

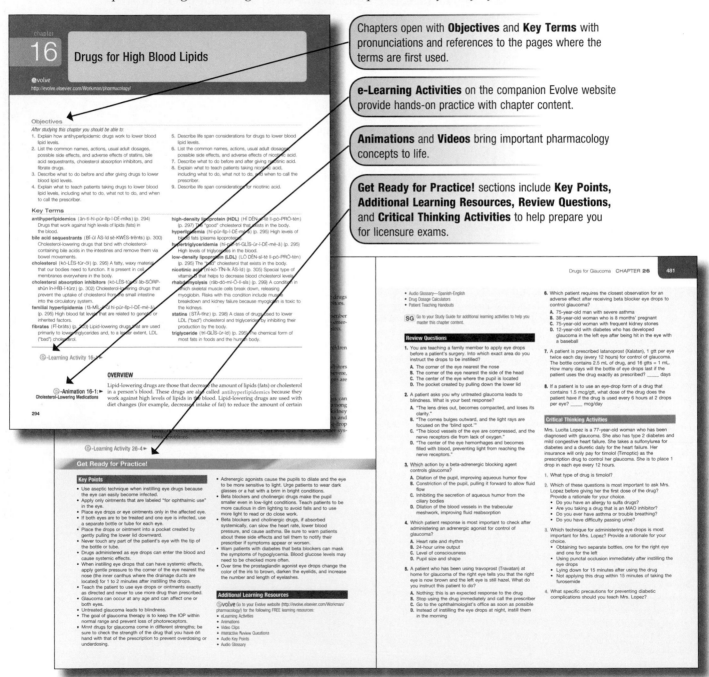

Chapters open with **Objectives** and **Key Terms** with pronunciations and references to the pages where the terms are first used.

**e-Learning Activities** on the companion Evolve website provide hands-on practice with chapter content.

**Animations** and **Videos** bring important pharmacology concepts to life.

**Get Ready for Practice!** sections include **Key Points**, **Additional Learning Resources**, **Review Questions**, and **Critical Thinking Activities** to help prepare you for licensure exams.

**STUDY GUIDE** (sold separately) Includes *Learning Activities*, a *Medication Safety Practice* section, and a *Practice Quiz* for each textbook chapter. Answers are available to instructors.

**Try This!** boxes in the math chapters let you practice math and dosage calculation concepts as you learn them. Answers are found at the end of the chapter.

**Did You Know?** boxes relate pharmacology content to everyday life.

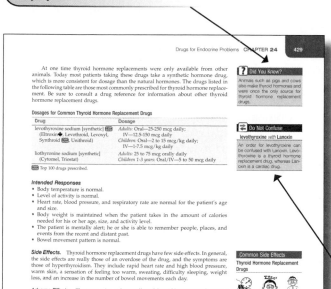

**Drug Alert!** boxes and **Memory Jogger** boxes highlight important tips for safe medication administration.

**Do Not Confuse** boxes highlight lookalike/soundalike drugs to help you avoid drug errors.

**Common Side Effects** boxes use memorable, easy-to-recognize icons to emphasize common side effects of drugs.

**Clinical Pitfall** boxes highlight critically important clinical situations to avoid.

**Full-color illustrations** explain key pathophysiology and pharmacology concepts.

**Wide margins** provide plenty of room for note-taking.

**Drug tables** provide generic drug names, brand names, and typical dosage ranges.

**Top 100 Drugs Prescribed** icons identify the most commonly prescribed drugs.

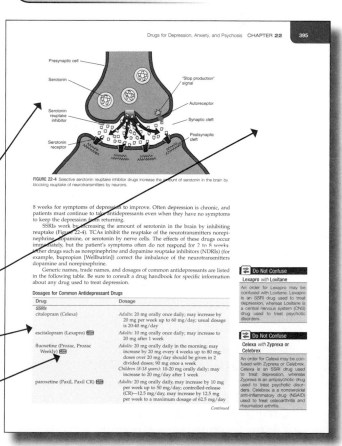

# Contents

# Drug Actions and Body Responses

## Objectives

*After studying this chapter you should be able to:*

1. Define the common terms associated with drug therapy.
2. Explain the roles of different health care professionals in drug therapy.
3. Explain the differences of a drug therapeutic effect (intended action), a drug side effect, and an adverse drug effect.
4. Identify substances that are intrinsic drugs and substances that are extrinsic drugs.
5. Compare the activity of a cell when an agonist drug binds to the receptor and when an antagonist drug binds to the receptor.
6. Explain the similarities and differences between allergic responses and personal responses to drugs.
7. Explain the purposes, advantages, and disadvantages of the different routes of drug administration.

8. Describe the processes and organs involved in drug metabolism and elimination.
9. Explain the influence of drug half-life, peak blood level, and trough of blood level on drug activity.
10. Describe the ways in which drug therapy for children differs from drug therapy for adults.
11. Describe two changes in older adults that make drug action, drug metabolism, and drug elimination different than for younger adults.
12. Explain how pregnancy and breastfeeding should be taken into consideration with drug therapy.
13. List two common drug interactions and their significance.

## Key Terms

**absorption** (ăb-SŌRP-shŭn) (p. 12) Movement of a drug from the outside of the body into the bloodstream.

**adverse drug reaction (ADR)** (ĂD-vŭrs DRŬG rē-ĂK-shŭn) (p. 9) Same as adverse effect.

**adverse effect** (ĂD-vŭrs ĕf-FĔKT) (p. 9) A drug effect that is more severe than expected and has the potential to damage tissue or cause serious health problems. It may also be called a *toxic effect* or *toxicity* and usually requires intervention by the prescriber.

**agonist** (ĂG-ŏn-ĭst) (p. 7) An extrinsic drug that activates the receptor site of a cell and mimics the actions of naturally occurring drugs (intrinsic drugs).

**allergic response** (ă-LŬR-jĭk rē-SPŎNS) (p. 10) Type of adverse effect in which the presence of the drug stimulates the release of histamine and other body chemicals that cause inflammatory reactions. The response may be as mild as a rash or as severe and life threatening as anaphylaxis.

**antagonist** (ăn-TĂG-ŏn-ĭst) (p. 7) An extrinsic drug that blocks the receptor site of a cell, preventing the naturally occurring substance from binding to the receptor.

**bioavailability** (bī-ō-ă-văl-ă-BĬL-ĭ-tē) (p. 12) The percentage of a drug dose that actually reaches the blood.

**black box warning** (BLĂK BŎKS WŌR-nĭng) (p. 10) A notice that a drug may produce serious or even life-threatening effects in some people in addition to its beneficial effects.

**brand name** (BRĂND NĀM) (p. 4) A manufacturer-owned name of a generic drug; also called "trade name" or "proprietary name."

**cytotoxic** (sī-tō-TŎKS-ĭk) (p. 8) Drug action that is intended to kill a cell or an organism.

**distribution** (dĭs-trĭ-BYŪ-shŭn) (p. 14) (drug distribution) The extent that a drug absorbed into the bloodstream spreads into the three body water compartments.

**drug** (DRŬG) (p. 2) Any small molecule that changes any body function by working at the chemical and cell levels.

**drug therapy** (DRŬG THĂR-ă-pē) (p. 3) The planned use of a drug to prevent or improve a health problem.

**duration of action** (dū-RĂ-shŭn of ĂK-shŭn) (p. 11) The length of time a drug is present in the blood at or above the level needed to produce an effect or response.

**elimination** (ē-lĭm-ĭ-NĀ-shŭn) (p. 16) The inactivation or removal of drugs from the body accomplished by certain body systems.

**enteral route** (ĔN-tĕr-ŭl ROWT) (p. 12) Movement of drugs from the outside of the body to the inside using the gastrointestinal tract.

**extrinsic drugs** (ĕks-TRĬN-sĭk DRŬGZ) (p. 3) Drugs that are man-made (synthetic) or derived from another species; not made by the human body.

**first-pass loss** (FŬRST PĂS LŎS) (p. 16) Rapid inactivation or elimination of oral drugs as a result of liver metabolism.

**generic name** ( jĕn-ĂR-ĭk NĀM) (p. 4) National and international public drug name created by the United States Adopted Names (USAN) Council to indicate the usual use or chemical composition of a drug.

**half-life** (HĂF LĪF) (p. 17) Time span needed for one half of a drug dose to be eliminated.

**herbals** (ŬR-bŭlz) (p. 5) Natural products made from plants that cause a response in the body similar to that of a drug; also called *botanicals*.

**high-alert drug** (HĪ ă-LŬRT DRŬG) (p. 5) A drug that has an increased risk of causing patient harm if it is used in error.

**intended action** (ĭn-TĔN-dĕd ĂK-shŭn) (p. 3) Desired effect (main effect) of a drug on specific body cells or tissues; same as therapeutic response.

**intrinsic drugs** (ĭn-TRĬN-sĭk DRŬGZ) (p. 3) Hormones, enzymes, growth factors, and other chemicals made by the body that change the activity of cells.

**loading dose** (LŌ-dĭng DŌS) (p. 17) The first dose of a drug that is larger than all subsequent doses of the same drug; used when it takes more drug to reach steady state than it does to maintain it.

**mechanism of action** (MĔK-ă-nĭz-ŭm of ĂK-shŭn) (p. 6) Exactly how, at the cellular level, a drug changes the activity of a cell.

**medication** (mĕ-dĭ-KĀ-shŭn) (p. 3) Any small molecule that changes any body function by working at the chemical and cell levels (same as a drug).

**metabolism** (mĕ-TĂB-ō-lĭz-ĭm) (p. 15) (drug metabolism) Chemical reaction in the body that changes the chemical shape and content of a drug, preparing the drug for inactivation and elimination.

**minimum effective concentration (MEC)** (MĬN-ĭ-mŭm ĕf-FĔK-tĭv kŏn-sĕn-TRĀ-shŭn) (p. 11) The smallest amount of drug necessary in the blood or target tissue to result in a measurable intended action.

**over-the-counter (OTC)** (Ō-vŭr THĒ KOWN-tŭr) (p. 4) Drugs that are approved for purchase without a prescription.

**parenteral route** (pă-RĔN-tĕr-ăl ROWT) (p. 12) Movement of a drug from the outside of the body to the inside of the body by injection (intra-arterial, intravenous, intramuscular, subcutaneous, intracavitary, intraosseous, intrathecal).

**peak** (PĒK) (p. 18) Maximum blood drug level.

**percutaneous route** (pĕr-kū-TĀN-ē-ŭs ROWT) (p. 12) Movement of a drug from the outside of the body to the inside through the skin or mucous membranes.

**personal responses** (PŬR-sŭn-ăl rē-SPŎN-sĕz) (p. 10) Unexpected adverse effects that are unique to the patient and not related to the mechanism of action of the drug. They are also called *idiosyncratic responses*.

**pharmacodynamics** (făr-mă-kō-dī-NĂM-ĭks) (p. 6) Ways in which drugs work to change body function.

**pharmacokinetics** (făr-mă-kō-kĭn-ĔT-ĭks) (p. 11) How the body changes drugs; drug metabolism.

**pharmacology** (făr-mă-KŎL-ō-jē) (p. 3) The science and study of drugs and their actions on living animals.

**physiologic effect** (fĭ-zē-ō-LŎ-jĭk ĕf-FĔKT) (p. 8) The change in body function as an outcome of the mechanism of action of a drug.

**potency** (PŌ-tĕn-sē) (p. 11) The strength of the intended action produced at a given drug dose.

**prescription** (prē-SKRĬP-shŭn) (p. 5) An order written or dictated by a state-approved prescriber for a specific drug therapy for a specific patient.

**prescription drugs** (prē-SKRĬP-shŭn DRŬGZ) (p. 5) The legal status of any drug that is considered unsafe for self-medication or has a potential for addiction and is only available by prescription written by a state-approved health care professional.

**receptors** (rē-SĔP-tŭrz) (p. 6) Physical place on or in a cell where a drug can bind and interact.

**sequestration** (sē-kwĕs-TRĀ-shŭn) (p. 15) The "trapping" of drugs within certain body tissues, delaying their elimination and extending their duration of action.

**side effects** (SĪD ē-FĔKTS) (p. 3) Any minor effect of a drug on body cells or tissues that is not the intended action of a drug.

**steady state** (STĔD-ē STĀT) (p. 11) Point at which drug elimination is balanced with drug entry, resulting in a constant effective blood level of the drug.

**target tissue** (TĂR-gĕt TĬ-shū) (p. 6) The actual cells or tissues affected by the mechanism of action or intended actions of a specific drug.

**transdermal** (trănz-DŬR-mŭl) (p. 12) Type of percutaneous drug delivery in which the drug is applied to the skin, passes through the skin, and enters the bloodstream.

**trough** (TRŎF) (p. 18) The lowest or minimal blood drug level.

**vaporized** (VĂ-pŭr-īzd) (p. 17) Changing of a drug from a liquid form to a gas that can be absorbed into the body by inhalation.

---

⊖-Learning Activity 1-1 ►

# DRUG THERAPY

## OVERVIEW

Nurses work with physicians and other health care professionals to assist a patient who is injured, ill, or at risk of becoming ill to achieve the best possible level of health. Sometimes the health problem is minor or temporary. Other times the health problem is complicated, serious, or chronic and requires long-term treatment and monitoring. Drugs are often used to diagnose or treat health problems. A **drug** is any small molecule that changes a body function by working at the chemical and cell levels. By this definition many everyday substances are drugs, including caffeine, alcohol, and nicotine. Some drugs are manufactured from chemicals, others are taken from plants, and still others are taken from a person or animal to be used by another person. For example, insulin can be made in a laboratory, or it can be taken from the pancreas of a cow or pig and given to humans. (There are no plant sources of insulin.)

Some people use the term medication to describe substances that are used to treat health problems and the term *drug* to describe substances that are harmful or can be abused. However, in health care these terms mean the same thing, and any drug or medication can be misused or abused.

When a plan to prevent or improve a health problem includes the use of drugs, it is called **drug therapy.** Drug therapy includes these factors:

- Identifying the specific health problem
- Determining what drug or drugs would be the best treatment for the problem
- Deciding the best delivery method and schedule
- Ensuring that the proper amount of the drug is given
- Helping the patient become an active participant in his or her drug therapy

The prescriber's role in drug therapy is to select and order specific drugs. State-approved prescribers may include physicians, dentists, podiatrists, advanced practice nurses, and physician's assistants. The pharmacist's role is to mix (compound) and dispense prescribed drugs. The nurse's role is to administer prescribed drugs directly to the patient. Because nurses are the last checkpoint for safe drug therapy, they must know the purposes, actions, side effects, problems, delivery methods, and necessary follow-up care for different drugs. Along with prescribers and pharmacists, nurses teach patients about the drugs they have been prescribed.

It is important to understand the interactions and mechanisms by which various types of drugs influence body activity. Drugs are prescribed or used to improve some body condition or function. But the body actually makes some of its own drugs in the form of hormones, enzymes, growth factors, and other substances that change the activity of cells. The chemicals the body makes are called **intrinsic drugs**—the insulin made by the pancreas is one example of an intrinsic drug. Other drugs are made outside of the body and must be taken into the body to change cell, organ, or body action. These drugs are known as **extrinsic drugs** because the body does not make them. For the most part the study of drugs and how they work (**pharmacology**) is concerned with extrinsic drugs. However, many of the most effective extrinsic drugs are nearly identical to the drugs created by the body. For example, the body makes endorphin, which is very similar to the extrinsic drug morphine. Morphine is a very effective pain reliever because it has the same action as endorphin at the cell level.

Any drug affects some tissue or organ in the body. The reason a drug is prescribed is that it has at least one desired effect that improves body function; this is called the **intended action** or the *therapeutic response*. Think about a drug that widens (dilates) blood vessels and thereby lowers blood pressure. The therapeutic response of such a drug is to lower blood pressure; thus it is classified as an antihypertensive drug. In addition to its intended action or therapeutic response, there may be many minor changes in body function that occur when the drug is taken. These minor effects of a drug on body cells or tissues that are not the intended actions are known as **side effects.** Side effects can be helpful or may cause problems. For example, a drug to treat high blood pressure (hypertension) that widens blood vessels also may cause dizziness and ankle swelling. All drugs have at least one intended action and at least one side effect. The safety of any drug is determined by balancing the seriousness of the side effects against the benefit of the therapeutic effect.

## DRUG NAMES

Most official drugs have more than one name, which can be confusing. There are three types of drug names: the chemical name, the generic name, and the brand

**Memory Jogger**

Any drug (medication) can be misused or abused and harm a person.

**Memory Jogger**

Your body actually makes drugs. Drugs made by the body are called *intrinsic drugs*.

**Memory Jogger**

All drugs have at least one intended action and at least one side effect.

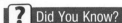

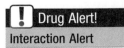

name. The *chemical name* of a drug describes the exact chemical composition of atoms and molecules for the main ingredient of the drug. Often the result is a very long name that is hard to pronounce or remember such as the chemical name for Lipitor: [R-(R*,R*)]-2-(4-fluorophenyl)-β,δ-dihydroxy-5-(1-methylethyl)-3-phenyl-4-[(phenyl amino)carbonyl]-lH-pyrrole-1-heptanoic acid, calcium salt (2 : 1) trihydrate. This name is used only by the chemists who develop the drug and oversee its manufacture.

The **generic name** of a drug is a shorter, simpler name that is commonly used by pharmacists, physicians, other prescribers, nurses, and other health care professionals. The generic name for Lipitor is atorvastatin. A special council (United States Adopted Names [USAN]) creates the generic names used for all drugs made in the United States. The rules used to name drugs help to ensure that the generic name is relatively short and easy to pronounce, gives some clue as to its use or chemical composition, and does not sound too much like any other known drug name. Often some part of all generic names for drugs of one class will be the same (suffix). For example, all the generic names for lipid-lowering drugs that are HMG-CoA reductase inhibitors end in "-statin," (such as atorvastatin, lovastatin, and simvastatin). Most beta-blockers end in "-olol" (such as atenolol, metoprolol, and propranolol). Once the generic name is approved, it is public and not owned by any one drug company. When a generic drug name is written, the first letter is not capitalized.

**Brand names** are created by each drug company that makes and sells a specific drug. Other terms for "brand name" are *proprietary name* and *trade name*. Each company owns its brand names. For example, aspirin is made by many drug companies, and each one has its own recognized brand name for it. St. Joseph Aspirin is the aspirin made by the McNeil Company; Bufferin is the aspirin made by Bristol-Myers Squibb. The first letter of a brand name is always capitalized, and the name will often be followed by either the symbol ® (for registered trademark) or ™ (for trademark).

## DRUG CATEGORIES

Any drug has the potential to harm a person if it is taken improperly or in large quantities. Some drugs have more powerful and dangerous effects than others. The United States government has classified drugs into two categories based on their potential for harm. These categories are over-the-counter drugs and prescription drugs.

### Over-the-Counter Drugs

Drugs that are weaker and have less potential for harmful side effects are available for purchase without a prescription. These drugs are called **over-the-counter (OTC)** drugs. OTC drugs are considered safe for self-medication when the package directions for dosage and schedule are followed. Examples of OTC drug types include aspirin, antacids, vitamin supplements, and antihistamines. These drugs may be sold at a drug store (pharmacy), grocery store, convenience store, department store, and at almost any other site.

Some drugs that were available only by prescription for many years have been reclassified as OTC. Most of these drugs are used for very common conditions, and extensive use has not shown the drugs to have dangerous side effects at low doses. Examples of drugs that were once available only by prescription and are now available OTC include diphenhydramine (Benadryl), ranitidine (Zantac), omeprazole (Prilosec), and cortisone creams.

OTC drugs are convenient and allow you to control your own health care to some extent. However, some problems do exist with OTC drugs. Many patients do not consider them to be even slightly dangerous. All drugs, even vitamins, can be abused and cause harmful side effects when taken too often or in high doses. In addition, some people do not consider OTC drugs to really be drugs and may not mention them when they are asked what drugs they take on a daily basis. An OTC drug can cause health problems and may interact with prescription drugs. Always specifically ask whether a patient takes any OTC drugs daily.

## Prescription Drugs

Drugs that have a greater potential for harm, strong sedating effects, or a potential for addiction are considered too dangerous for self-medication. These drugs are classified as **prescription drugs** and are available only from a pharmacy with a drug order from a state-authorized prescriber. A **prescription** is an order written or dictated by a state-approved prescriber for a specific drug therapy for a specific patient. Each state determines who has the authority to write drug orders (such as physicians, advanced practice nurses, dentists, podiatrists, physician's assistants, and veterinarians) and sets any limits on a prescriber's authority.

**Memory Jogger**

Professionals who may prescribe drugs vary by state and may include physicians, advanced practice nurses, dentists, podiatrists, physician's assistants, and veterinarians.

## High-Alert Drugs

Some prescription drugs have the designation of high-alert drugs. A **high-alert drug** has an increased risk of causing a patient harm if it is used in error. The error may be a dose that is too high, a dose that is too low, a dose given to a patient for whom it was *not* prescribed, and a dose *not* given to a patient for whom it was prescribed. Some of these high-alert drugs are used in special areas, such as anesthetics, imaging procedures, total parenteral nutrition solutions, and intensive care units. Other high-alert drugs are prescribed more commonly and are used on standard care units. One way to remember the more commonly prescribed high-alert drugs is with the term "PINCH." In this term, *P* is for potassium, *I* is for insulin, *N* is for narcotics (more commonly called opioids), *C* is for cancer chemotherapy agents, and *H* is for heparin or any other drug that strongly affects blood clotting. Although calculating drug dosages and administering drugs always requires care and concentration, extra care is needed when calculating and administering high-alert drugs. When possible, always check the order for a high-alert drug with another nurse or pharmacist. Specific high-alert drugs are highlighted throughout the clinical chapters of this textbook.

**Memory Jogger**

One way to remember the more commonly prescribed high-alert drugs is with the term PINCH: *P*otassium, *I*nsulin, *N*arcotics (more commonly called opioids), *C*ancer chemotherapy agents, and *H*eparin or any other drug that strongly affects blood clotting.

## Herbal Products

**Herbals** are natural products made from plants that cause a response in the body similar to that of a drug. Many herbal products, also called *botanicals*, have been used as drug therapy for centuries. This area of drug therapy is the least defined, least understood, and least controlled. Such products are available for sale almost everywhere; and individuals may even grow, collect, or make their own. Use of these products with or without the supervision of a prescriber is often termed *herbal therapy*, *homeopathic therapy*, *natural therapy*, or *alternative therapy*.

An even bigger problem is that most people who use herbal preparations consider them to be "natural" and therefore safe. In reality many of these products do have cellular effects that can be harmful or can interact with other drugs. For example, both white willow bark products and gingko biloba reduce blood clotting. If either of these is taken by a person who is also taking the prescription drug warfarin (Coumadin), the risk for a brain hemorrhage is high. When asked what drugs he or she is taking, a patient may not even mention herbal preparations that are taken on a daily basis, increasing the risk for an interaction with a prescribed drug.

In addition, because many people consider herbal products to be safe, they may take large quantities of the products, believing that if one dose is good, five doses must be even better. For example, juice of the stinging nettle is used by many people as a natural diuretic. It does increase urine output, but excessive doses cause dehydration and very low blood potassium levels *(hypokalemia)*, which can then make a normal dose of the prescribed drug digoxin toxic.

Your responsibility with herbal therapy is to obtain correct information about what specific herbal products a patient is using and make sure that the prescriber is aware of this information. You also can help a patient understand the proper uses for and potential problems of specific herbal therapies.

**Memory Jogger**

Herbal preparations are not regulated for effectiveness, purity, or drug strength.

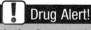
**Drug Alert!**
**Action/Intervention Alert**

When taking a history, always be sure to ask what specific herbal products the patient uses on a daily basis, including the brand names and the amounts.

## DRUG REGULATION

The United States Pharmacopeia (USP) is a national group responsible for developing standards for drug manufacturing, including purity, strength, packaging, and

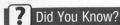 Did You Know?

Any change in drug standards, labeling, safety, or testing really does require "an act of Congress."

ⓔ-Learning Activity 1-2 ▶

labeling. The Food and Drug Administration (FDA) is an agency of the U.S. government that is responsible for enforcing the standards set by the USP. Both the FDA and the USP work together with the U.S. Congress and the U.S. Supreme Court to ensure continuing public protection and drug safety. Any changes in drug standards, labeling, safety, or testing must be approved by the U.S. Congress before they can be enacted.

## WAYS IN WHICH DRUGS AFFECT THE BODY (PHARMACODYNAMICS)

### MECHANISMS OF ACTION

An important aspect of drug therapy is **pharmacodynamics,** or how the drug works to change body function. Think of this as what the drug does to the body. Drugs change body function by changing the activity levels of individual cells. Remember that each body cell has at least one job that it must perform to make the whole body function correctly. The job that any cell performs can be slowed, stopped, or speeded up when that cell is exposed to a specific drug. Exactly how a drug changes the activity of a cell is the **mechanism of action** of the drug. Most cells have receptors that control their activity. The actual cells or tissues affected by the mechanism of action or intended actions of a drug are known as the **target tissues.**

### Receptors

**Receptors** are places on or in a cell to which a drug can bind (attach itself) and control cell activity. In this way the receptor acts as an ignition site for the cell motor. When the right key (drug) is placed in the ignition (receptor) and turned, the cell motor starts, and the cell performs its special job better or faster. The right key for the ignition can be either an intrinsic drug such as the adrenalin made by the adrenal glands or an extrinsic drug such as epinephrine. (Chemically epinephrine is almost identical to human adrenalin.) When the adrenal glands make and release adrenalin, it binds to adrenalin receptor sites on the heart muscle cells and makes those cells contract more strongly and rapidly. This action causes increased heart rate and higher blood pressure. When epinephrine is injected into a person, it binds to those same adrenalin receptor sites on the heart muscle cells and causes the same effects that adrenalin does. Figure 1-1 shows how cell receptors are used to control cell activity.

A cell can have more than one type of receptor; thus different drugs can affect the same cell in different ways. Figure 1-2 shows why a cell can respond to more than one drug. A cell can only respond to a drug by changing its activity when the proper drug fits into its receptor. If the wrong drug attempts to bind to a receptor,

💡 Memory Jogger

Receptors are physical places on or in cells that can bind with and respond to naturally occurring body chemicals. Their purpose is to control cell activity to meet the body's needs.

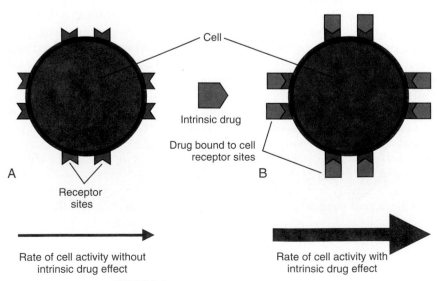

FIGURE 1-1 Receptors controlling cell activity.

it will not activate that receptor—just as using the wrong key in a car ignition will not start the motor.

Many different types of drugs work through cell receptors. These receptors can be on the surface of a cell or actually inside the cell. A cell with a receptor for a specific drug is known as the *target* for that drug. For example, the target of morphine is most brain cells (neurons) that perceive pain. Drug types that work by affecting cell receptors include opioid pain drugs, drugs for high blood pressure, diuretics, insulin, antihistamines, anti-inflammatory drugs, and antidiabetic drugs, to name only a few. For example, cells that are targets for antihistamines are those that have histamine receptors on their surfaces such as mucous membrane cells, blood vessel cells, cells that line the airways, and stomach lining cells.

*Receptor Agonists.*   When an extrinsic drug binds to the receptor of a cell and causes the same response that an intrinsic drug does, the extrinsic drug is called a receptor **agonist** because it is the right key to turn on that cell's ignition. Extrinsic drugs that are agonists have the same effects as the body's own hormones or natural substances (intrinsic drugs) that activate or turn on a specific receptor type in or on a cell (Figure 1-3).

Agonist drugs must interact with the correct receptor for the drug to change the activity of the cell. Some agonist drugs change this activity to the same degree that intrinsic drugs do (see Figure 1-3, *B*). Other agonist drugs work but not quite as well as the intrinsic drug. Still other agonist drugs work more powerfully than intrinsic drugs (see Figure 1-3, *C*). Agonist drug strength is determined by how tightly it binds to the receptor and how long it stays bound. Usually the more tightly bound a drug is to its receptor and the longer it stays attached to the receptor, the stronger the effect of the drug on the activity of the cell. For example, hydromorphone (Dilaudid) is an opioid agonist that binds to the opioid receptor better than morphine does. As a result, hydromorphone provides longer pain relief at lower doses than morphine.

*Receptor Antagonists.*   Sometimes the goal of drug therapy is to *slow* the activity of a cell. One way drugs can do this is by blocking the receptors of the cell so the intrinsic drug cannot bind with and activate the receptor. An extrinsic drug that works by blocking the receptor sites is called a receptor **antagonist**. An antagonist drug must be similar enough in shape to the intrinsic drug so it will bind with the receptor but not tightly enough or correctly enough to activate it. Antagonist action is like taking the key from one Chevrolet Impala and trying to start the motor of a different Chevrolet Impala. The key may fit into the ignition slot, but it will not turn on the motor. Instead, as long as the wrong key is in the ignition slot, the correct key cannot be placed in the slot, and the car does not run. The antagonist competes with

**Memory Jogger**

A cell can only respond to a drug by increasing its activity when the drug fits into the receptor of the cell.

**Memory Jogger**

The effectiveness of an agonist drug depends on how tightly and how long it binds to its receptor.

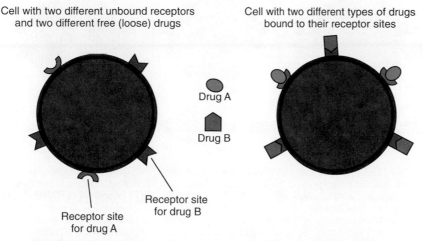

Cell with two different unbound receptors and two different free (loose) drugs

Cell with two different types of drugs bound to their receptor sites

Drug A

Drug B

Receptor site for drug B

Receptor site for drug A

**FIGURE 1-2** Cell with two different types of receptors, unbound and bound.

the intrinsic drug for the receptor site, blocking the receptor and slowing or stopping the activity of the cell. Antagonists have effects that are opposite of agonists. Figure 1-4 shows how antagonist drugs exert their effects on cells.

Receptors are the sites of direct action for most drugs. The final cell action when a drug binds to its receptor depends on both the nature of the drug (agonist or antagonist) and the nature of the receptor. Some drugs can act as agonists for certain cells and as antagonists for other cells. For example, epinephrine acts like an agonist when it binds to its receptors on heart muscle cells, making them contract more strongly and quickly. However, when epinephrine binds to muscle cells in the airways, it acts like an antagonist, causing these cells to relax rather than contract. Thus sometimes the same drug speeds up the activity of some cells and at the same time slows the activity of other cells. This is why you need to know the mechanism of action for each drug to understand both its intended actions and side effects. For example, when a person uses an epinephrine inhaler to widen the lung airways and breathe more easily, this is the intended action of the drug. The side effects are a more rapid heart rate and higher blood pressure.

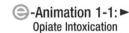-Animation 1-1: ►
Opiate Intoxication

### Nonreceptor Actions

Although most drugs work by affecting cell receptors, some drugs exert their effects differently. Examples of drug types that do not use cell receptors to exert their effects include antibacterial drugs, cancer chemotherapy drugs, and most drugs that reduce blood clotting. The exact mechanism of action varies for each drug type that does not use receptors. For example, the targets of antibacterial drugs are bacteria. These drugs are either deadly (cytotoxic) to these organisms or prevent them from reproducing. Cancer chemotherapy drugs have cancer cells as their main targets. The intended action of chemotherapy drugs is to kill cancer cells.

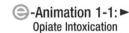-Learning Activity 1-3 ►

### PHYSIOLOGIC EFFECTS

The outcome of the mechanism of action of a drug is its physiologic effect. Usually this effect can be felt by the patient or measured or observed by another person. For example, a drug that binds to airway receptors and dilates the airways has the physiologic effect of improving airflow in the airways. The improved airflow leads to better gas exchange. The patient notices easier breathing; you, as the nurse, observe improved oxygen saturation ($SpO_2$).

Both expected and unexpected patient responses are part of physiologic effects. These include intended actions, side effects, and adverse effects. Two

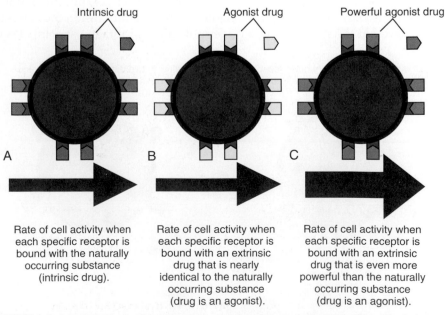

| Intrinsic drug | Agonist drug | Powerful agonist drug |

A — Rate of cell activity when each specific receptor is bound with the naturally occurring substance (intrinsic drug).

B — Rate of cell activity when each specific receptor is bound with an extrinsic drug that is nearly identical to the naturally occurring substance (drug is an agonist).

C — Rate of cell activity when each specific receptor is bound with an extrinsic drug that is even more powerful than the naturally occurring substance (drug is an agonist).

**FIGURE 1-3** Comparison of cell activity when receptor sites are bound with different substances.

specific types of adverse effects are allergic responses and personal (idiosyncratic) responses.

### Intended Actions

The intended actions or therapeutic responses of a drug are the desired effect that improves body function and are the reason a drug is prescribed. All approved drugs have at least one expected intended action, and many have more than one.

### Side Effects

Drug side effects are one or more effects on body cells or tissues that are not the intended action of drug therapy. All drugs have side effects. Generally side effects are the most common *mild* changes that occur in at least 10% of patients receiving a drug. *These effects are expected but do not occur in all patients.* Many are related to the mechanism of action of the drug and are temporary, resolving when the drug is discontinued. Although some side effects may be uncomfortable and may cause the patient to avoid a specific drug, they usually are not harmful and do not cause extensive tissue or organ damage. Examples of common side effects include:

- Constipation with the use of opioid analgesics.
- Sexual disinterest or impotency with the use of certain antidepressants.
- Diarrhea with the use of penicillin and other antibacterial drugs.
- Drowsiness with the use of certain antihistamines.
- Decreased blood clotting with the use of aspirin.

Some drug side effects may even become a therapeutic effect. For example, aspirin has several therapeutic effects involved with pain relief, fever reduction, and reduction of inflammation. One of its side effects—decreased blood clotting, is now an intended action for prevention of heart attack *(myocardial infarction)*.

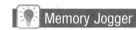
**Memory Jogger**

Drug side effects are expected, are mild, and do not occur in all patients.

### Adverse Effects

A drug **adverse effect** or an **adverse drug reaction (ADR)** is a harmful side effect that is more severe than expected and has the potential to damage tissue or cause serious health problems. It may also be called a *toxic effect* or a *toxicity*. Often these effects occur with higher drug doses and are rare when the patient is taking normal doses of a specific drug. For example, many patients have the side effect of diarrhea when taking an antibacterial drug for 10 to 14 days. A few may have such

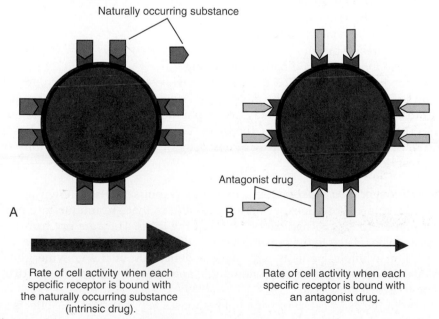

Rate of cell activity when each specific receptor is bound with the naturally occurring substance (intrinsic drug).

Rate of cell activity when each specific receptor is bound with an antagonist drug.

**FIGURE 1-4** Comparison of cell activity when receptor sites are bound with the naturally occurring substance (intrinsic drug) **(A)** and with an extrinsic drug that is an antagonist **(B)** (blocks the receptor site, preventing the naturally occurring substance from binding).

severe diarrhea that they become dehydrated. At higher doses a very few patients may develop the adverse effect of *pseudomembranous colitis*, which is profound bloody diarrhea and infection that can lead to complications such as perforation of the colon.

Although adverse effects are not common, it is important to know what types of ADRs and their signs and symptoms may occur with a specific drug so any problems are identified and managed early. Examples of ADRs include:

- Muscle breakdown with the use of "statin-type" cholesterol-lowering drugs.
- Lung fibrosis with the use of amiodarone (a drug to correct abnormal heart rhythms).
- Pseudomembranous colitis with the use of antibacterial drugs such as amoxicillin and vancomycin
- Seizures and life-threatening heart rhythm problems (dysrhythmias) with the use of theophylline (a bronchodilator)

Usually, when a patient has an adverse effect to a drug, he or she is taken off the drug. However, at times the intended action is needed so much that the drug is not discontinued, but other precautions are taken to limit tissue and organ damage.

Some adverse effects occur so commonly with a specific drug that the drug is removed from the market. Other drugs may continue to be prescribed but carry a black box warning. A **black box warning** means that a drug may produce serious or even life-threatening effects in some people in addition to its beneficial effects. This warning is printed on the package insert sheet and is bordered in black. Prescribers are instructed to make certain that such drugs are prescribed only for patients who meet strict criteria and who understand the serious nature of the possible adverse effects.

*Allergic Responses.*   An **allergic response** is a type of adverse effect in which the presence of the drug stimulates the release of histamine and other substances that cause inflammatory reactions. It may be as mild as a skin rash or as severe and life threatening as anaphylaxis. Anaphylaxis is a severe inflammatory response with these symptoms:

- Tightness in the chest
- Difficulty breathing
- Low blood pressure
- Hives on the skin
- Swelling of the face, mouth, and throat
- Weak, thready pulse
- A sense that something bad is happening

If not recognized and treated quickly, anaphylaxis can lead to vascular collapse, shock, and death. The patient who develops a skin rash, hives, or mild throat swelling within days of taking a drug may develop a more severe response and anaphylaxis the next time he or she takes the drug. Usually, when the person has a true allergic response to a drug, that drug or any drug from the same drug family should not be prescribed for him or her.

*Personal/Idiosyncratic Responses.*   **Personal responses**, also known as *idiosyncratic responses*, are those unexpected adverse effects that are unique to the patient and not related to the mechanism of action of the drug. They are not true allergies but appear to be related to the person's genetic differences in metabolism or immune function. For example, patients who have a deficiency of the enzyme glucose-6-phosphate dehydrogenase develop hemolytic anemia when they take the drug primaquine to prevent malaria.

Although the exact cause of personal responses is not known, the effects can be very severe and life threatening. For the purposes of prevention, they are documented in the patient's chart in the same way as severe drug allergies.

 **Memory Jogger**

An ADR is rare and serious and has the potential to damage organs (cause toxicities). Usually when a patient has an ADR, the drug is stopped.

 **Memory Jogger**

Drugs that carry a black box warning have more severe side effects and should only be used in patients for whom the potential benefits outweigh the possible drug risks.

 **Memory Jogger**

Anaphylaxis is the most severe type of allergic reaction to a drug and can lead to death if not treated quickly.

 **Drug Alert!**

**Administration Alert**

When a person has a true allergic response to a drug, do not administer that drug or any drug from the same drug family without additional precautions.

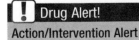 **Drug Alert!**

**Action/Intervention Alert**

Ask the patient about any adverse reactions, including allergic and personal reactions (idiosyncratic reactions), and record these in the patient's chart.

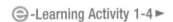-Learning Activity 1-4 ►

## HOW THE BODY USES AND CHANGES DRUGS (PHARMACOKINETICS)

Except for a few drugs that work just on the external skin surface, most drugs must enter the body to produce their intended actions (therapeutic responses). Once a drug enters a living human body, the body exerts its effects on the drug. This process is known as **pharmacokinetics.** After absorption, the drug is affecting the body at the same time the body is affecting the drug. Most of the time the body affects a drug by changing the structure of the drug so it can be inactivated and eliminated from the body. This "processing" of drugs by the body is why drugs must be taken repeatedly (for days and sometimes more than once each day) to continue to exert their intended actions. If drugs were never inactivated or eliminated, one dose would last for years and so would its intended actions and side effects.

A drug must enter the body and reach a high enough constant level in the blood or target tissue to produce the intended action. The lowest blood level needed to cause the intended action is known as the **minimum effective concentration (MEC)** (Figure 1-5). If the body eliminates the drug faster than it enters the body, the drug level at any given time will not be great enough to produce the intended action. If the body eliminates the drug more slowly than it enters the body, the drug level could become high enough to cause more side effects or adverse effects. For a drug to do its job and produce the intended action without causing harm to the patient, its level in the blood has to be maintained by balancing drug entry with drug elimination. This balance, known as a **steady-state** drug level, keeps the amount of drug in the body high enough to produce the intended action continuously (Figure 1-6). The body processes drugs through the stages of absorption, distribution, metabolism, and elimination.

How long a drug remains in the blood at the MEC is its **duration of action.** The duration of action is one way to describe the **potency** of a drug. Drug potency is the strength of the intended action produced at a given dose. Drugs that have higher potency need lower doses to produce an intended action. Drugs that are less potent require higher doses to produce the same intended action. The longer a drug dose stays active in the body at or above the MEC, the more potent it is. In general, less potent drugs have fewer expected side effects but may need to be taken more often. A more potent drug may need to be taken only once or twice daily to achieve the intended action.

 **Memory Jogger**

At the same time that a drug is having an effect on the body, the body is also having an effect on the drug.

 **Memory Jogger**

Drugs that have higher potency need lower doses to produce an intended action. Drugs that are less potent require higher doses to produce the same intended action.

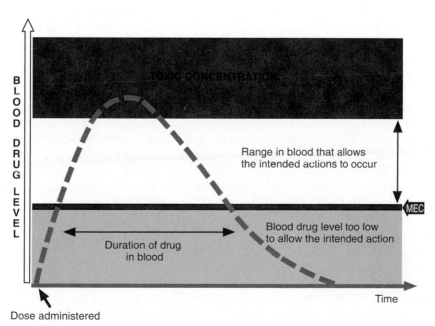

**FIGURE 1-5** Minimum effective concentration *(MEC)* and blood level needed to allow the intended action to occur.

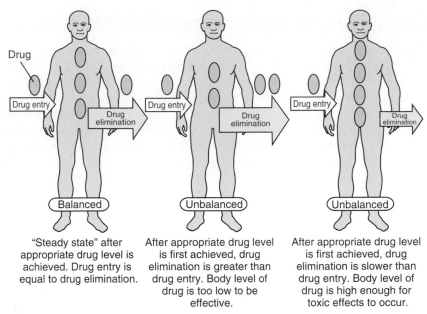

**FIGURE 1-6** Comparison of body levels of drug when drug entry and elimination are balanced and unbalanced.

## ABSORPTION

Drugs must come into contact with their target cells to cause a cell to change its activity. Extrinsic drugs must enter the body and get into the bloodstream to find their target cells. The movement of a drug from the outside of the body into the bloodstream is called **absorption.** The amount of a drug dose that actually reaches the blood is its **bioavailability.** If an entire drug dose reaches the bloodstream, its bioavailability is 100%. When only part of a drug dose gets into the blood, that drug is less than 100% bioavailable.

Drugs can enter the body in many ways:
- The **percutaneous route** means that the drug enters through the skin or mucous membranes.
- The **enteral route** refers to the gastrointestinal tract.
- The **parenteral route** means that the drug is injected into the body.

Table 1-1 lists the different routes of drug entry and their advantages and disadvantages. Chapter 2 describes how to administer drugs by these routes, along with any specific precautions needed.

Drugs are prepared differently by the manufacturer, depending on their intended routes. For example, drugs given by the parenteral route must be sterile, but those given by the enteral route only need to be clean, not sterile. A drug prepared to be given by the parenteral route is usually more expensive than the same drug prepared to be given orally. Some drugs prepared for the enteral route may have special coatings *(enteric coatings)* on them. These coatings either prevent the drugs from harming the stomach lining or prevent some of the enzymes and other substances in the digestive tract from destroying the drug before it can be absorbed. Most drugs processed for the enteral route are not absorbed through skin.

### Percutaneous Route

The percutaneous route of drug entry is the movement of the drug from the outside of the body to the inside through the skin or mucous membranes. Only lipid-soluble drugs—those that easily dissolve in lipids (fats) rather than water—can be absorbed percutaneously.

One method of the percutaneous route is **transdermal** delivery. In this method the drug is applied to the skin, passes through the skin, and enters the bloodstream. Some drugs can affect even deep body tissues when applied transdermally. For

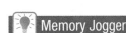
**Memory Jogger**

The three main drug entry routes are the percutaneous route, the enteral route, and the parenteral route.

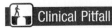
**Clinical Pitfall**

Do not give a drug that is prepared to be given by one route by any other route.

**Table 1-1** Advantages and Disadvantages of Drug Entry Routes

| ROUTE | ADVANTAGES | DISADVANTAGES |
|---|---|---|
| Percutaneous | Convenient | Absorption dependent on circulation |
| Transdermal | Bypasses gastrointestinal tract<br>Large selection of body areas | Absorption less predictable<br>Can lead to skin breakdown |
| Sublingual | Less invasive<br>Rapid absorption | Effect is reduced when patient eats or drinks |
| Buccal | Less invasive/obtrusive | Effect is reduced when patient eats or drinks |
| Rectal* | Usually painless | Embarrassing |
| Enteral | Convenient<br>High patient acceptance<br>Least expensive route<br>Large surface area for absorption | Can cause gastrointestinal disturbance<br>First pass loss<br>Can bind to other substances in the tract and not get absorbed<br>Absorption dependent on motility; has great individual variation |
| Parenteral | Speed<br>100% bioavailability<br>Decreased first pass loss | Speed<br>Invasive administration<br>Increased cost<br>Discomfort |

*Rectal drug delivery can be either percutaneous or enteral, depending on how far into the rectum the drug is placed. Drugs placed within the lowest 1.5 inches are considered to be delivered by the percutaneous route. Those placed higher in the rectum are considered to be delivered by the enteral route.

example, nitroglycerin paste applied to the skin dissolves through the skin, then enters the bloodstream, and finally exerts its effect on blood vessels in the heart. Other drugs that are often given by this route using skin patches include certain types of pain medications and continuous hormone treatments.

Some drugs can be given through the mucous membranes of the mouth, nose, lungs, rectum, or vagina and have effects on deeper tissues. Mucous membranes have many blood vessels close to the surface, making movement of the drug through the membranes and into the bloodstream rapid and easy. Drugs given this way can be placed as tablets under the tongue or between the gum and the cheek, sprayed in the nose or under the tongue, inhaled through the nose or mouth, or placed as a liquid or a suppository in the rectum or vagina (see Figures 2-5, 2-16, and 2-17). Examples of drugs that can be given this way include hormones (even insulin), pain medications, drugs for nausea and vomiting, and anesthetic agents.

### Enteral Route

The enteral route of drug delivery is the movement of drugs from the outside of the body to the inside using the gastrointestinal (GI) tract. It is the most commonly used route of drug administration. Usually enteral drugs are swallowed as liquids, tablets, or capsules. Most drugs that can be taken by mouth can also be placed directly into the stomach or intestines through a tube or into the rectum (when prescribed to do so). Once the drug is in the GI tract, it must dissolve and enter the bloodstream before it can exert its effects on target cells. Usually not all of a drug taken enterally enters the blood. Drugs given by the enteral route have *less* bioavailability than those given by the parenteral route and must be given in higher doses than the same drug given parenterally.

Absorption of oral drugs is affected by anything occurring in the stomach or intestines. Diarrhea can move drugs through the intestine so quickly that they are eliminated in the stool rather than absorbed. Food in the stomach or intestines slows or delays absorption. Substances such as calcium bind with drugs and prevent them from being absorbed. For these reasons some drugs such as the tetracycline antibiotics are not to be taken with food or milk. On the other hand, taking oral drugs when

 **Memory Jogger**

Mucous membranes have many blood vessels close to the surface, making movement of the drug through the membranes and into the bloodstream rapid and easy.

 **Memory Jogger**

Oral drugs have the least predictable absorption pattern.

 **Memory Jogger**

Drugs given by mouth usually require higher doses than those given intravenously.

the stomach is empty can cause such rapid absorption that the effects can occur too quickly and harm the patient.

Rectal drug delivery can be either percutaneous or enteral, depending on how far into the rectum the drug is placed. Drugs placed within the lowest 1.5 inches are considered to be delivered by the percutaneous route. Those placed higher in the rectum are considered to be delivered by the enteral route. The reason for this difference is the way venous blood leaves these areas. Venous blood from the last half of the mouth, the esophagus, the stomach, the intestines, and the higher part of the rectum drains into the liver system before it returns to the heart as part of systemic circulation. This means that the liver has a chance to metabolize drugs from the gastrointestinal tract *before* they get to their target tissues. Blood from the lowest part of the rectum does *not* enter the gastrointestinal circulation, and drugs absorbed there do not get metabolized before they reach their target tissues.

### Parenteral Route

The parenteral route involves giving drugs by injection, which bypasses the intestinal tract and other organs of digestion such as the liver, placing drugs more directly into the blood or target cells. Drugs can be injected into many different structures:

- An artery, called an *intra-arterial injection* (administered by the prescriber)
- A vein, known as *intravenous injection*
- The skin, known as *intradermal injection*
- The fatty tissue below the skin, called a *subcutaneous injection*
- A muscle, or *intramuscular injection*
- A body cavity, known as *intracavitary injection* (administered by the prescriber)
- A joint, known as *intra-articular injection* (administered by the prescriber)
- A bone, or *intra-osseous injection* (administered by the prescriber)
- The fluid of the brain or spinal cord, known as *intrathecal* (administered by the prescriber)
- Directly into specific tissues or organs

The parenteral route gets the drug into the bloodstream more quickly and more completely than other routes. For example, the dose of a drug given intravenously is entirely in the blood immediately after injection and then is 100% bioavailable. Not only do drugs work more quickly when given this way, but any problems the drugs may cause also occur more quickly. Drugs made to be given parenterally are more expensive than oral drugs because they require more processing and must be sterile. The parenteral route is more invasive and more dangerous to the patient than other routes. Only give drugs parenterally that are made to be given by the parenteral route.

### DISTRIBUTION

Once drugs are in the blood, they must be distributed to their target tissues, where the intended action is supposed to occur. Most drugs do not exert their mechanisms of action while in the blood. The bloodstream is just the "roadway" used by the body to get the drug to its target cells. Drugs can be distributed or spread to different body areas. Distribution of a drug is the extent that a drug spreads into three specific compartments. The *bloodstream* or *blood volume* (sometimes called the plasma volume) is the first drug compartment. This area is made up of the spaces in all the arteries, veins, and capillaries. The second drug compartment includes both the blood volume and the watery spaces between all body cells, also known as the *interstitial space*. The third drug compartment is the largest, including the blood volume, the watery spaces between the cells, and the space inside the cells (*intracellular space*).

Some drugs are limited in how far they get distributed, and others can be distributed easily throughout the body. Most drugs can only be distributed to watery compartments of the body. How well a drug is distributed is determined by the size and chemical nature of the drug.

---

**Memory Jogger**

The most rapid drug entry routes are intra-arterial and intravenous.

---

**Clinical Pitfall**

Drugs prepared for the enteral route should never be given by the parenteral route.

Drug size is based on its chemical composition and weight. Small drugs may have only a few molecules or parts. The smallest drug is lithium, which is made up of a molecule of the element lithium (Li) attached to a carbonate molecule ($Li_2CO_3$). Because of its small size, it can fit through cell pores and channels, entering any drug compartment. Large drugs may be composed of many molecules and have greater weight. These drugs do not fit easily through cell pores or channels and have a more limited distribution within the body.

Some large drugs bind to proteins in the blood. These drugs do not touch or enter other cells; they can only exert their effects on cells in the blood. An example of this type of drug is an antibiotic that stays in the blood and affects only the microorganisms that are also in the blood. Drugs that distribute only to the blood volume are eliminated more rapidly than those that are distributed more widely. Thus drugs that distribute only to the blood volume may have to be taken three or four times a day to keep the drug level high enough to be effective.

Smaller drugs that are water seeking are called *hydrophilic*. Hydrophilic drugs distribute to both the plasma volume and the watery spaces between cells. Because they may not enter cells, the effectiveness of these drugs is limited.

Very small drugs and those that easily dissolve in fats can cross cell membranes and enter cells. Drugs that dissolve easily in fats are known as *lipid-soluble* drugs. These drugs are distributed the most widely, staying in the body longer and affecting more tissues and organs.

Some places in the body are more difficult for drugs to enter (such as the brain, eye [actually inside the eye], sinuses, and prostate gland). In addition, some body conditions can reduce drug distribution (such as when the patient is *dehydrated* [when he or she has too little body water] or has low blood pressure [*hypotension*]). If a person is taking more than one drug, the drugs can interact (meaning that the presence of one drug can change the distribution of another drug). This issue is a type of drug interaction and must be considered whenever the patient is taking more than one drug.

Another issue related to drug distribution is the "trapping" of drugs in certain tissues. This is called **sequestration.** Drugs that are more easily dissolved in fat often enter body fat cells and are sequestered there, with the drug being slowly released over time. Completely eliminating these drugs may take a long time. So the effects of sequestered drugs may be present for weeks or longer after the person has stopped taking the drug.

## METABOLISM

Drugs that enter the body are considered "foreign." The normal response of the body to the presence of any drug is to inactivate and eliminate it. Before most drugs can be eliminated, they must first be metabolized. **Metabolism** is a chemical reaction in the body that changes the chemical shape and content of the drug. Usually the changing of a drug by the body inactivates the drug and makes it easier to eliminate. A few drugs are actually activated by body metabolism before they can exert their effects and then are remetabolized or reprocessed for elimination.

A comparison of the use of the opioid drugs morphine and codeine is a clinical example of how metabolism works for drug elimination and drug activation. When a patient receives morphine for pain management, it is distributed throughout the body, including the brain. In the brain it binds to receptor sites to reduce the patient's perception of pain. At the same time the liver inactivates the morphine through metabolism and readies it for elimination. This is why the effects of morphine wear off in a few hours and another dose of the drug then has to be given for the patient to remain comfortable. Codeine is another opioid drug given for pain. However, when codeine is first taken into the body, it is not active and does not bind to the receptor sites in the brain. It must be activated by metabolism and converted to morphine before it can relieve pain. Once this conversion takes place, codeine binds to receptor sites in the brain and reduces pain perception. When the metabolized codeine (now morphine) is remetabolized, it is ready to be eliminated from the body.

 **Memory Jogger**

Drug distribution and activity are reduced in a patient who is dehydrated or has a very low blood pressure.

**? Did You Know?**

Body fat is a "time-release" capsule for drugs that have a fat base, retaining them for weeks to months.

 **Memory Jogger**

Metabolism changes the chemical structure of drugs; it can activate drugs, inactivate them, and prepare them for elimination.

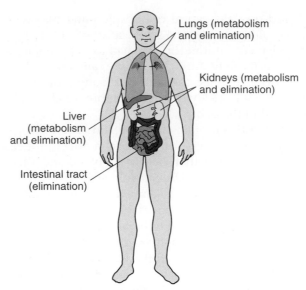

**FIGURE 1-7** Major sites of drug metabolism and elimination.

The fact that codeine first has to be activated by metabolism before it can work as a pain reliever explains why morphine relieves pain faster than codeine.

Drugs can be metabolized to different degrees by different body tissues. The organs and cells most involved in drug metabolism are the liver, kidneys, lungs, and white blood cells. All these tissues contain special enzymes that break down and change the chemicals in the drugs.

Some factors that determine how fast and how well drugs are metabolized include genetic differences between people, whether or not the person has been exposed to that specific drug or similar drugs before, and the health of the liver and kidneys. Some people have genetic differences that allow them to make more of the enzymes used in drug metabolism. These people may need higher-than-average doses of drugs for the drugs to work well and may also need to take the drugs more often to keep a steady-state level. Other people have genetic differences that reduce the amount of enzymes they make for drug metabolism. These people need lower doses for the same effect compared with the "average" person.

The liver and kidneys are the most important organs for drug metabolism (Figure 1-7). If a patient has a problem with either the liver or the kidneys, drugs may be metabolized slowly and remain active longer. In this situation high levels of a drug can build up in the patient very quickly, often leading to toxic side effects.

### ELIMINATION

Elimination is the inactivation or removal of drugs from the body accomplished by certain body systems. Just like metabolism, many body systems eliminate drugs to some degree; however, the most active routes for drug elimination are the intestinal tract, the kidneys, and the lungs (see Figure 1-7). Drugs leave the body in the feces, urine, exhaled air, sweat, tears, saliva, breast milk, and semen.

Drugs metabolized by the liver are sent to either the intestinal tract or the blood and then to the kidney for elimination. Even drugs given parenterally can be eliminated through the intestinal tract. When a drug is given orally, some of the drug is metabolized very quickly by the liver and rapidly eliminated from the body. This rapid inactivation and elimination of oral (enteral) drugs is called first-pass loss. This is the reason an enteral drug is less bioavailable and the dosage is higher compared with the same drug given intravenously.

Drugs that are dissolved in the blood may leave the body in the urine. The drugs may change the color or smell of the urine. (This is why urine tests can determine whether a person is using certain illegal drugs.)

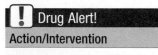

**Drug Alert!**

**Action/Intervention**

Anyone who has either liver or kidney problems must have the dosage and timing of drugs adjusted by the prescriber. Watch these patients carefully for signs of drug overdose.

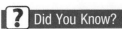

**Did You Know?**

Drugs administered intravenously can be eliminated through the intestinal tract.

**Table 1-2** Time Needed to Completely Eliminate a Drug with a Half-Life of 6 Hours

| TIME PASSED (HR) | AMOUNT OF DRUG REMAINING IN THE BODY | TIME PASSED (HR) | AMOUNT OF DRUG REMAINING IN THE BODY |
|---|---|---|---|
| 0 (time of drug administration) | 500 mg | 30 | 7.875 mg |
| | | 36 | 3.9375 mg |
| 6 | 250 mg | 42 | 1.969 mg |
| 12 | 125 mg | 48 | 0.984 mg |
| 18 | 62.5 mg | 54 | 0.492 mg |
| 24 | 15.75 mg | 60 | 0.264 mg |

A few types of drugs are metabolized and eliminated through the lungs and leave the body in the exhaled air. Drugs that are small and easily turned into gases (vaporized) are eliminated by the lungs. This is why a Breathalyzer test can measure blood alcohol levels.

Just as for metabolism, the liver and kidneys are the most important organs for drug elimination. The liver metabolizes the drug to make it ready for elimination, which often is performed by the kidney. If a patient has a problem with either the liver or the kidneys, drugs may take a longer time to be eliminated from the body and can build up to toxic levels quickly. Liver damage is called *hepatotoxicity*, and kidney damage is called *nephrotoxicity*. Drugs that can cause liver damage are called *liver toxic* or *hepatotoxic*. Drugs that can cause kidney damage are called *kidney toxic*, *renal toxic*, or *nephrotoxic*.

## Half-Life

The half-life of a drug is the time span needed for one half of the individual drug dose given to be eliminated. When multiple doses are given over time, the half-life for the total dosage also can be calculated. For example, suppose that an antibiotic has a half-life of 6 hours and the first dose of the drug was 500 mg. Six hours after the drug was given, 250 mg of the drug remains in the body. Half of the remaining 250 mg is eliminated in the next 6 hours so that, 12 hours after the first dose, 125 mg of the drug remains in the patient's body. Thus if you received only a single 500-mg dose of a drug that has a half-life of 6 hours, it would take more than 48 hours for you to completely eliminate the drug (Table 1-2). The drug is considered eliminated when less than 10% of the drug remains, which would be between 18 and 24 hours for this example. In general, at least five half-lives after the last dose are needed to eliminate a drug.

The half-life of a drug is related to how fast it is eliminated. Drugs that are eliminated rapidly have a short half-life; drugs eliminated slowly have a long half-life. The half-life of any drug is calculated based on research. The half-life is used to determine how much drug should be prescribed and how often it should be taken to get to and stay at a steady-state level (that is, a point at which drug elimination is balanced with drug entry). This steady-state level must be maintained at or above the minimum effective concentration (MEC). However, calculation of the MEC is based on the "average" response of the drug when it was given to a large number of test subjects. The same drug may have a different half-life in some patients because of differences in the patients' age, size, gender, race/ethnicity, metabolism, genetic heritage, and health and the presence of other drugs. Drugs with a short half-life are often prescribed to be taken more than once per day to get to and keep a steady-state level long enough to make the drug effective (produce its therapeutic effect). Drugs with a long half-life may be prescribed so the first dose is larger than the rest of the prescribed doses. This larger first dose is known as a loading dose. It is used to get the blood level up to the MEC as fast as possible. Once the MEC is achieved, all other doses can be smaller and still maintain the MEC because the drug has a long

 **Memory Jogger**

A drug with a half-life of 4 hours is *not* eliminated in 8 hours. Each portion *remaining* after a half-life time has passed is eliminated one half at a time.

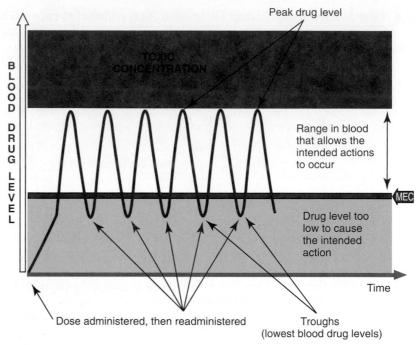

FIGURE 1-8 Peaks and troughs of blood drug levels. *MEC*, Minimum effective concentration.

half-life and is eliminated slowly. One example of a drug that is usually pre-scribed with a higher loading dose than a maintenance dose is theophylline, a drug used for asthma.

### Peaks and Troughs

Peaks and troughs describe the relationship between the actual dose of drug given and the blood drug level over time (Figure 1-8). The **peak** is the maximum blood drug level (like the very top of a mountain), and the **trough** is the lowest or minimal blood drug level (like the bottom of a water trough for animals). When patients have no severe health problems or unusual reactions to a drug and its metabolism, the peaks and troughs of a specific drug are already known (they have been worked out for the average person).

@-Learning Activity 1-5 ▶

## LIFE SPAN CONSIDERATIONS

### SIZE

*Pediatric Considerations.*   Children are smaller than most adults. Most drugs are given in smaller doses in proportion to the child's size, especially weight. Some drugs are prescribed in milligrams (mg) per kilogram (kg). Some prescribed drug doses are based on *body surface area (BSA)*—that is, they are calculated in milligrams per kilogram of body weight or milligrams per square meter ($m^2$). Either calculation must be made carefully and accurately because a math error of even one decimal place results in tremendous overdosing or underdosing. If you wish to review math facts and drug calculations before working with these calculations, see Chapter 5. Weights and measures are reviewed in Chapter 4.

The calculation of drug dose based on kilogram of body weight is made by first converting the child's weight in pounds (lbs) to kilograms. One kilogram is equal to 2.2 lbs. For example, if a child weighs 32 lbs, the kilogram calculation is made by dividing 32 by 2.2 (32 ÷ 2.2). This child's weight in kilograms is 14.6 kg. So for a drug dose of 3 mg/kg, multiply the weight in kilograms by 3 (14.6 kg × 3 mg); the correct dose is 43.8 mg, rounded up to 44 mg.

The calculation of drug dosage by BSA is a little more involved. This calcula-tion first requires converting the patient's height in inches to centimeters (cm) and converting his or her weight in pounds to kilograms. These numbers are then plugged into an equation for square meters. This calculation is usually performed by the prescriber. Just remember that the square meters for an average-size adult is not much over 1.2, and the square meters for a child or infant is considerably less than 1.

Correctly calculating drug dosages for children is critical for preventing drug overdose. Follow these rules for pediatric drug administration:

- Always compare the drug dose prescribed for an infant or child with the recommended dose for the child's size.
- Question any drug prescription for a child in which the prescribed dose is greater or lesser than the recommended dose.
- Double-check your drug dose calculation for an infant or child with a colleague or a pharmacist.

Drugs that have a specific type of effect or response on adults may have the opposite effect on children (these actions are called *paradoxical*). For example, the drug methylphenidate (Ritalin) stimulates the central nervous system of an adult and causes an overall increase in excitability and activity. This same drug reduces excitability and activity in children. Some drugs that cause drowsiness in adults may cause hyperactive behavior in children.

Other drug side effects that occur in children but not in adults can be related to the growth and maturity of specific tissues. For example, when teeth are developing, the antibiotic tetracycline changes the density of the tooth enamel and can result in tooth darkening. After teeth are mature, they are no longer at risk for this side effect. As a result the drug tetracycline is rarely used for pregnant women (when the first teeth are forming) or in children under the age of 12 years (when the permanent teeth are forming). Another example of a drug affecting development is the quinolone type of antibiotics. These drugs damage bone growth in children and are not prescribed for them unless an infection is life threatening and the organism only responds to a quinolone.

## ORGAN HEALTH

The health of the organs most involved in drug distribution, metabolism, and elimination affect drug actions. These organs include the liver, kidney, heart, lungs, and white blood cells. Along with physical immaturity and age-related changes in organ function, diseases can have an impact on organ function.

### Liver Health

A healthy liver is important for good drug metabolism and elimination. The liver health status of any person should be known before drug therapy is started. Table 1-3 lists the normal values for tests of liver function.

***Pediatric Considerations.***   Drug metabolism in children varies, depending on age and organ maturity. A premature infant or newborn may have a slower rate of metabolism than an adult because the enzyme systems of the liver may not yet be fully active. Toddlers, preschool children, school-age children, and adolescents usually have *higher* rates of metabolism than do adults. A child may receive a much lower dose of a drug than an adult, but the dose may need to be given more often because it is metabolized and eliminated more rapidly.

***Considerations for Older Adults.***   Many older adults have serious damage to the liver, making drug metabolism and elimination slower. Even older adults in good health have reduced liver function as a result of the aging process. Thus all older adults metabolize and eliminate drugs more slowly than younger adults, although this problem is greater in adults who have actual organ damage. Slow metabolism and elimination increase the half-life of a drug and make it easier to develop toxic drug levels in older adults. Table 1-4 lists examples of drugs that have longer half-lives on older adults.

 **Memory Jogger**

One inch is equal to 2.4 cm. So a person's height in centimeters is always a larger number than his or her height in inches.

 **Memory Jogger**

Children may have completely different responses to a drug than an adult would have to the same drug.

**Table 1-3** Laboratory Values for Liver Function

| TEST | NORMAL VALUES | SIGNIFICANCE OF ABNORMAL VALUES |
|---|---|---|
| Albumin | 3.5-5.0 g/dL | Decreased values indicate possible liver disease. |
| Alanine aminotransferase (ALT) | 3-35 international units/L or 8-20 units/L (SI units) | Increased values indicate possible liver disease. |
| Aspartate aminotransferase (AST) | 5-40 units/L | Increased values indicate possible liver disease. |
| Lactate dehydrogenase (LDH) | 115-225 international units/L | Increased values indicate possible liver disease. |
| Alkaline phosphatase | 30-85 international units/L or 42-128 units/L (SI units) | Increased values indicate possible liver disease. |
| Bilirubin total serum | 0.1-1.0 mg/dL | Increased values indicate possible liver disease. |
| Ammonia | 15-110 mg/dL | Increased values indicate possible liver disease. |

**Table 1-4** Examples of Drugs with Longer Half-Lives in Older Adults

| HALF-LIFE | DRUGS |
|---|---|
| Half-life increased by less than 3 hours | acetaminophen (Datril, Panadol, Tylenol) ampicillin (Ampicin, Omnipen, Principen) lidocaine (LidoPen, Xylocaine) |
| Half-life increased by 3 to 10 hours | gentamicin (Garamycin) kanamycin (Kantrex) metoprolol (Lopressor, Toprol) propranolol (Inderal) |
| Half-life increased by 10 to 25 hours | amitriptyline (Elavil) cyclophosphamide (Cytoxan) imipramine (Tofranil) thioridazine (Mellaril) |
| Half-life increased by 25 or more hours | amobarbitol (Amytal) chlorthalidone (Hygroton, Thalitone) diazepam (Diastat, Valium) digoxin (Lanoxin, Lanoxicaps) spironolactone (Aldactone) |

**Table 1-5** Laboratory Tests Assessing Kidney Function

| SUBSTANCE | NORMAL VALUES |
|---|---|
| Blood urea nitrogen (BUN) | 10-20 mg/dL |
| Creatinine | Males: 0.6-1.3 mg/dL Females: 0.5-1 mg/dL |
| Sodium | 135-145 mEq/L |
| Potassium | 3.5-5 mEq/L |

## Kidney Health

Some drugs are metabolized and eliminated by the kidney. Others are metabolized elsewhere and just eliminated by the kidney. Thus a healthy kidney is important for drug elimination and prevention of toxic drug levels. The kidney (renal) health status of any person should be known before drug therapy is started. Table 1-5 lists the normal values for tests of kidney function.

***Pediatric Considerations.***   An infant's kidneys do not concentrate fluids well. In addition, infants have a greater proportion of total body water than older children or adults. This means that drugs easily dissolved in water spread through proportionally more water and drugs are lost by the kidney route more rapidly. Thus an infant may need a higher dose in terms of milligrams per kilogram than would a toddler or an older child. Water-soluble drugs are eliminated more rapidly in infants and young children than they are in adults.

***Considerations for Older Adults.***   About two thirds of all adults over age 60 have reduced kidney size and kidney function. Because the kidney is important in eliminating drugs from the body, reduced kidney function in the older adult causes an increase in drug half-life. This means that one dose of a drug lasts much longer in the blood of an older adult than in a younger adult. As long as the drug is present in the blood, it continues to have intended actions and side effects. Refer to Table 1-4 for examples of drugs that have longer half-lives in older adults.

## Cardiopulmonary Health

The cardiovascular system ensures that drugs reach their target sites of action and sites for metabolism and elimination. The lungs and pulmonary system help metabolize and eliminate some drugs. Red blood cells (RBCs) carry oxygen, and white blood cells (WBCs) are sites of drug metabolism. Together the heart, blood, and lungs promote the health of all organs by ensuring adequate oxygenation. Thus a healthy heart, adequate blood pressure, and good oxygenation are needed for optimum drug therapy. Table 1-6 lists normal values for tests of cardiac, blood, and lung function.

***Considerations for Older Adults.***   Many adults over age 70 years have some degree of heart failure and poor blood flow to the liver and other body areas. This reduced blood flow both decreases drug effectiveness and limits how well drugs are distributed, metabolized, and eliminated.

The respiratory changes that occur with aging reduce lung volume and function to some degree in all older patients. These effects are made worse by a lifetime of exposure to inhaled irritants such as cigarette smoke, bacteria, air pollutants, and industrial fumes. These changes reduce lung metabolism and elimination of some drugs. Lung problems may reduce the effectiveness of drugs taken by inhalation.

Older adults often have fewer RBCs and WBCs than younger adults. These changes reduce oxygenation of all organs and limit drug metabolism.

## PREGNANCY AND BREASTFEEDING

### Pregnancy

Pregnancy is the time for development of a new human being. Nearly every organ forms in the 9 months before birth. During pregnancy the mother's bloodstream is separated from the unborn baby's bloodstream by the placenta. However, the placenta is not a perfect barrier. Some drugs can cross the placenta and may affect the unborn baby, although not all drugs taken during pregnancy have harmful effects on the fetus. Regardless of the presumed safety of a drug, no prescribed or OTC drug should be taken during pregnancy unless it is clearly needed and its benefits outweigh any risks to the fetus.

Drugs that can cause birth defects are *teratogenic* or *teratogens*. Some drugs are more teratogenic than others, and even one dose can cause a severe birth defect. Other drugs are less teratogenic and require either many doses or very high doses to cause even a minor birth defect. Not all pregnant women who take a teratogenic drug during pregnancy have a child with birth defects, but the *risk* for birth defects is higher.

The FDA has developed specific drug *pregnancy categories* based on the risk for causing birth defects (Table 1-7). Although drugs should be avoided during pregnancy, certain health problems may need to be managed with drug therapy. For a list of highly and moderately teratogenic drugs that should be avoided during

 **Memory Jogger**

Older adults may need a lower drug dosage than younger adults because of reduced kidney or liver function, and they are at a higher risk for dosage-related side effects.

 **Memory Jogger**

No prescribed or OTC drug is considered to be *completely* safe to take during pregnancy.

| Table 1-6 | Laboratory Tests Assessing Cardiovascular Function and Oxygenation |
|---|---|
| **TEST** | **RANGE** |
| **BLOOD CELLS** | |
| Red blood cells | |
| Women | 4.2 to 5.4 million per cubic millimeter ($mm^3$) of blood |
| Men | 4.7 to 6.1 million/$mm^3$ of blood |
| Platelets | 150,000 to 400,000/$mm^3$ of blood |
| White blood cells, total | 5,000 to 10,000/$mm^3$ of blood |
| Neutrophils | 5,000 to 7,000/$mm^3$ of blood |
| Eosinophils | 75 to 150/$mm^3$ of blood |
| Basophils | 25 to 50/$mm^3$ of blood |
| Monocytes | 150 to 500/$mm^3$ of blood |
| Lymphocytes | 1,400 to 2,800/$mm^3$ of blood |
| | |
| **OXYGENATION** | |
| Hematocrit | |
| Women | 37% to 47% |
| Men | 42% to 45% |
| Newborn to 6 months | 44% to 64% |
| Over 6 months | 30% to 44% |
| Hemoglobin | |
| Women | 12-16 g/dL |
| Men | 14-18 g/dL |
| Newborn to 6 months | 10-17 g/dL |
| Over 6 months | 10-15.5 g/dL |
| Oxygen saturation ($SpO_2$) | 95% to 100% |
| Arterial oxygen ($PaO_2$) | 80-100 mm Hg |
| Arterial carbon dioxide ($PaCO_2$) | 35-45 mm Hg |
| | |
| **CARDIAC FUNCTION** | |
| Brain natriuretic peptide (BNP) | Less than 100 pg/mL |
| Creatine kinase (CK) | |
| Women | 30-135 units/L |
| Men | 55-170 units/L |
| Newborns | 68-580 units/L |
| Children | Same as adults |
| Creatine kinase-MM | 100% |
| Creatine kinase-MB | 0% |
| Creatine kinase-BB | 0% |

pregnancy and breastfeeding, go to the Evolve website at http://evolve.elsevier.com/Workman/pharmacology/.

An unborn baby goes through different stages of development. The risk for any drug to cause harm to the unborn baby when taken during pregnancy depends on the nature and dosage of the drug and the developmental stage of the fetus. The third to the eighth week of pregnancy (days 15 though 60) is the *embryonic stage* and the time when most of the important organs are beginning to form. This is the most sensitive time, and drugs taken during this period can interrupt organ development. Unfortunately it is also the time that a woman may not even be aware that she is pregnant.

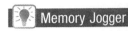 **Memory Jogger**

The risk for drugs to cause birth defects is highest from the third week to the eighth week of pregnancy.

## Table 1-7   Drug Pregnancy Categories

| PREGNANCY CATEGORY | DESCRIPTION AND RECOMMENDATION |
| --- | --- |
| A | Adequate well-controlled research studies that have included pregnant women have not shown the drug to have an increased risk for birth defects or problems in the fetus. |
| B | A drug is placed in this category if either of the following statements is true:<br>There have been no adequate or well-controlled studies in pregnant women, but animal studies have been done and do not show the drug to have an increased risk for birth defects or other problems in the fetus.<br>or<br>Animal studies do show an increased risk for birth defects or other problems in the fetus; but adequate, well-controlled studies that have included pregnant women have not shown the drug to have an increased risk for birth defects or other problems in the fetus. |
| C | A drug is placed in this category if either of the following statements is true:<br>There have been no adequate or well-controlled studies in pregnant women, but animal studies have been done and show the drug to have an increased risk for birth defects or other problems in the fetus.<br>or<br>No animal studies have been done, and there are no adequate or well-controlled studies testing this drug that have included pregnant women. |
| D | Adequate well-controlled or observational studies of this drug have been done in pregnant women and show it to have an increased risk for birth defects or other problems in the fetus.<br>Although the risk for fetal problems is increased with the use of drugs in this category, the benefits of treatment may outweigh the risk in a life-threatening situation or when the mother has a serious disease for which safer drugs are not available or are ineffective. |
| X | Adequate well-controlled or observational studies of this drug have been done in pregnant women or in animals and show this drug to have a greatly increased risk for fetal abnormalities.<br>Drugs in this category are not to be given to women who are pregnant or who may become pregnant. |

Modified from Meadows, M. (2001). Pregnancy and the drug dilemma. *FDA Consumer Magazine*, *35*(3). http://www.fda.gov/fdac/301_toc.html.

From the ninth week of pregnancy until birth, known as the *fetal stage*, most organ structure is complete, and the organs just grow larger. The fetus is less likely to be damaged at this time, but it is still possible; therefore unnecessary drugs should be avoided. Drugs have the same effects on the fetus as on the mother but can cause more problems. For example, when a pregnant woman takes the anticoagulant warfarin, the unborn baby's blood is also less able to clot, and the fetus can bleed to death. Drugs that lower blood pressure can lower the fetus's blood pressure so much that the brain does not receive enough oxygen and brain damage results.

### Breastfeeding
Some drugs taken by a breastfeeding woman cross into the milk and are ingested by the infant. The effects of the drugs on the baby are the same as on the mother. For example, lipid-lowering drugs taken by a breastfeeding woman will lower her infant's blood lipid levels. Although the mother may need to lower her blood lipid levels, the infant does not. Low lipid levels in an infant may cause poor brain development and mental retardation.

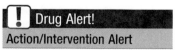

### Drug Alert!
**Action/Intervention Alert**

Before administering any newly prescribed drug, ask any female patient between the ages of 10 to 60 years if she is pregnant, likely to become pregnant, or breastfeeding.

| Box 1-1 | Recommended Methods of Reducing Infant Exposure to Drugs During Breastfeeding |

- For drugs that should not be given to infants:
  - Switch the infant to formula feeding temporarily or to breast milk obtained when you were not taking the drug.
  - Maintain your milk supply by pumping your breasts on a regular schedule and discard the pumped milk.
  - When you are no longer taking the drug and it has been eliminated, resume breastfeeding.
- For drugs that do not have to be avoided but should have levels reduced:
  - Nurse your baby right before taking the next dose of the drug.
  - Drink plenty of liquids to dilute the amount of drug in the breast milk.
  - Take the drug just before the baby's longest sleep period.

When a breastfeeding woman has an infection, usually the infant does not; however, the antibiotic the mother takes can enter the breast milk and affect the infant. Some antibiotics such as penicillin may not cause a problem. Other antibiotics such as the quinolones, even taken for a short time, can disrupt bone development. The "sulfa" class of antibiotics causes *jaundice* (yellowing of the skin) in the infant because the infant's liver is too immature to metabolize and eliminate the drug. The jaundice can become severe enough to cause brain damage.

Before a drug is selected and prescribed for a breastfeeding woman, the effects on the infant must be considered. The mother's prescriber, the infant's health care provider, and the mother must discuss the issues together. For a list of drugs to avoid while breastfeeding, go to the Evolve website at http://evolve.elsevier.com/Workman/pharmacology/.

Although breastfeeding is ideal nutrition for an infant, other means are also safe. Breastfeeding is not recommended for mothers with chronic disorders (such as seizures, hypertension, and hypercholesterol) that require daily drug therapy. For short-term health problems (such as infection) that require less than 2 weeks of drug therapy, the breastfeeding woman can make adjustments to reduce the infant's exposure to the drug (Box 1-1).

**![] Drug Alert!**

**Action/Intervention Alert**

If a woman is breastfeeding, urge her to discuss any drugs that she may be taking with her pediatrician.

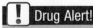-Learning Activity 1-6 ▶

**![] Drug Alert!**

**Teaching Alert**

Warn patients taking prescribed drugs to check with the prescriber before starting any OTC drugs, vitamins, or herbal supplements.

## DRUG INTERACTIONS

Drugs taken into the body can interact with other extrinsic drugs, intrinsic drugs, food, vitamins, and herbal compounds. These interactions can change the way a drug works or the timing of its action. Some interactions actually increase the activity of the drug, whereas others decrease it. Some drugs and herbal compounds are not compatible with each other and can lead to adverse effects. Always ask patients who are being prescribed a new drug what other drugs (prescribed or OTC), vitamins, and herbal supplements they are taking currently. Because the number of possible problem interactions is huge, always check with the pharmacy or a drug handbook for potential drug interactions.

Examples of interactions between drugs and between drugs and other common agents follow:

- Cimetidine (Tagamet) enhances the action of quinidine (Quinadure, Quinidex), increasing the risk for adverse effects.
- Ciprofloxacin (Cipro) increases the blood concentration of warfarin (Coumadin), increasing the risk for bleeding.
- Ibuprofen (Advil) and naproxen (Aleve) reduce the effectiveness of angiotensin-converting enzyme inhibitor antihypertensives such as captopril (Capoten) and lisinopril (Zestril), increasing the risk for heart failure and strokes.
- Grapefruit juice greatly increases the activity of many drugs, including felodipine (Plendil), midazolam (Versed), and lovastatin (Mevacor), increasing the risks for overdose and adverse effects.

- St. John's wort, an herbal preparation, reduces the effectiveness of many drugs, including digoxin (Lanoxin), warfarin (Coumadin), and oral contraceptives (birth control pills). Reducing the effectiveness of digoxin may worsen heart failure; reducing the effectiveness of warfarin increases the risk for clot formation, strokes, and pulmonary embolism; reducing the effectiveness of oral contraceptives may lead to unplanned pregnancies.

## Get Ready for Practice!

### Key Points

- The prescriber's role in drug therapy is to select and order specific drugs. Prescribers may include physicians, dentists, podiatrists, advanced practice nurses, and physician's assistants.
- The pharmacist's role is to mix (compound) and dispense prescribed drugs.
- The nurse's role is to administer prescribed drugs directly to the patient.
- The health care professionals responsible for teaching patients about their drugs include the prescriber, the pharmacist, and the nurse.
- Generic drug names are spelled with all lowercase letters; brand names have the first letter capitalized.
- When possible, always check the order and dosage calculation of a high-alert drug with another nurse or with a pharmacist.
- Herbal products can cause problems if taken too often or with prescribed drug therapy.
- Drugs often work in the same way that body hormones, enzymes, and other proteins do.
- For a drug to work on body cells, it must enter the body.
- Most drugs exert their effects by binding to a cell receptor.
- Although some drug side effects may be uncomfortable and may cause the patient to avoid a specific drug, they usually are not harmful and do not cause extensive tissue or organ damage.
- True allergic drug reactions result when the presence of the drug stimulates the release of histamine and other body chemicals that cause inflammatory reactions. They may be as mild as a skin rash or as severe as anaphylaxis.
- Anaphylaxis is the most severe type of allergic reaction to a drug and can lead to death if not treated quickly.
- At the same time that a drug is changing body activity, the body is processing the drug for elimination.
- Drugs have to reach a high enough level in the blood to exert their effects.
- The three main drug entry routes are percutaneous, enteral, and parenteral.
- A drug prepared to be given by one route often may not be given by any other route.
- Any problem with the gastrointestinal tract can interfere with how fast a drug is absorbed.
- Never give by injection any drug made to be given by the enteral route.
- The side effects of a drug given intravenously can occur very rapidly.
- Drugs may take a longer time to work when a patient is dehydrated or has very low blood pressure.
- Taking more than one drug at the same time can change the effectiveness of both drugs.
- Drug metabolism reduces its bioavailability.
- The most important organs for drug metabolism and elimination are the liver and kidneys.
- Drugs that have a long half-life stay in the body longer and are more likely to build up to toxic levels more quickly.
- Although the expected actions and patient responses are known for all approved drugs, some patients may react differently than expected. Whenever a patient receives the first dose of a drug, be alert to the possibility of unique responses.
- Although the peak and trough times for most drugs are known, these times can vary for any one patient, depending on his or her unique characteristics and the presence of other drugs.
- An infant may need a higher drug dose (in terms of milligrams per kilogram) than toddlers or older children because infants have a greater proportion of total body water.
- Unless a serious health problem exists in the pregnant woman, all types of drugs should be avoided (except for prenatal vitamins and iron supplements).
- When a female patient is prescribed to take a drug that is known to cause birth defects, be sure that she understands the risks, that her pregnancy test is negative, and that she is using a reliable method of birth control (or completely abstains from sex) during treatment.
- Urge breastfeeding women to consult with their infant's health care provider before taking any prescribed or OTC drug.
- Always ask patients who are being prescribed a new drug what other drugs (prescribed or OTC), vitamins, and herbal supplements they are taking currently.
- Check with the pharmacy or a drug handbook for potential drug interactions.
- Warn patients taking prescribed drugs to check with the prescriber before starting any OTC drugs, vitamins, or herbal supplements.

### Additional Learning Resources

evolve Go to your Evolve website (http://evolve.elsevier.com/Workman/pharmacology/) for the following FREE learning resources:
- eLearning Activities
- Animations
- Video Clips

- Interactive Review Questions
- Audio Key Points
- Audio Glossary
- Audio Glossary—Spanish-English
- Drug Dosage Calculators
- Patient Teaching Handouts

**SG** Go to your Study Guide for additional learning activities to help you master this chapter content.

## Review Questions

1. Which is the broadest and most accepted definition of the term *drug?*
   A. Any chemical substance that is either harmful or can be abused
   B. An agent available by prescription that is used to treat a specific health problem
   C. A substance that, when it enters the body, changes the action of any body system
   D. Any natural or synthetic chemical substance with potential for abuse or addition

2. Which action is primarily the role of the nurse in drug therapy?
   A. Administering a prescribed drug directly to the patient
   B. Teaching a patient the possible side effects of a prescribed drug
   C. Changing the dose of a prescribed drug based on a patient's response
   D. Dispensing a drug according to the instructions written in the prescription

3. Which patient response is a side effect rather than an intended action or adverse effect of a drug used to treat hypertension?
   A. Lower blood pressure
   B. Flushing of the skin
   C. Slower heart rate
   D. Dizziness

4. Which substance is always an extrinsic drug?
   A. Aspirin
   B. Insulin
   C. Endorphin
   D. Histamine

5. What is the expected response of the heart rate when a patient is taking a drug that is an adrenalin antagonist?
   A. It is unchanged.
   B. It increases.
   C. It decreases.
   D. It is louder.

6. Which patient response is a personal (idiosyncratic) adverse response to a drug rather than a true allergic reaction or general side effect?
   A. Prolonged hiccoughing while taking a drug to reduce nausea and vomiting
   B. A change in urine color to reddish orange while taking a bladder anesthetic for 3 days
   C. Development of a vaginal yeast infection while taking a tetracycline antibiotic for the past 10 days
   D. Swelling of the lips, tongue, and lower face while taking an angiotensin-converting enzyme inhibitor type of antihypertensive for 2 weeks

7. What action or condition is a major disadvantage of the percutaneous drug delivery route?
   A. First pass loss of drug is extensive.
   B. Drug must be sterile rather than clean.
   C. Only lipid-soluble drugs can be absorbed.
   D. Adverse effects occur more rapidly than with other routes.

8. Which two organs are the most important in drug metabolism and elimination?
   A. Skin and lungs
   B. Liver and kidneys
   C. Heart and pancreas
   D. Stomach and intestines

9. What is meant by the term *drug half-life?*
   A. The amount of time it takes for half of the drug dose to be absorbed
   B. The amount of time it takes for half of the drug dose to be eliminated
   C. The amount of time required for the body to be completely free of the drug
   D. The amount of time the drug remains in the "steady-state" range

10. Which principle of pharmacology do you always need to use or consider when administering drugs to infants or children?
   A. Drugs for newborns and young children must be given by the parenteral route.
   B. Children eliminate drugs through the skin rather than through the liver or kidneys.
   C. Drugs are distributed and eliminated more rapidly in newborns and young children.
   D. Newborns and young children have less total body water, so more water must be given with drugs.

11. How does reduced liver function affect drug therapy in the older adult?
    - **A.** Drugs are absorbed more slowly.
    - **B.** Drug doses must be reduced to prevent reaching toxic levels.
    - **C.** Drugs are distributed only to the first and second drug compartments.
    - **D.** Drugs must be given by the parenteral route rather than by the enteral route.

12. A patient who is breastfeeding her 6-week-old infant is prescribed to take montelukast sodium (Singulair) 10 mg orally daily (at 9:00 AM) for control of asthma. Which action should you teach her to reduce the infant's exposure to this drug?
    - **A.** Breastfeed the infant no sooner than 1 hour after taking the drug
    - **B.** Avoid drinking fluids for 6 hours after taking the drug
    - **C.** Breastfeed the infant right before taking the drug
    - **D.** Take the drug on an empty stomach

13. What potential problem can occur when ciprofloxacin (Cipro) is prescribed for 2 weeks to a patient who takes warfarin (Coumadin) daily?
    - **A.** Ciprofloxacin levels can become too high and lead to an increased risk for adverse reactions.
    - **B.** Ciprofloxacin levels can become too low, and the infection is not adequately treated.
    - **C.** Warfarin levels are too low, and the risk for stroke or embolism increases.
    - **D.** Warfarin levels are too high, and the patient is at risk for hemorrhage.

14. A drug is prescribed at 250 mg every 4 hours. How many total milligrams are given in a 24-hour period?
    - **A.** 500
    - **B.** 1000
    - **C.** 1500
    - **D.** 2000

15. A patient receives 100 mg of a drug at noon, 6 PM, and midnight. The drug has a half-life of 6 hours. How much of the drug remains in the patient at 6 AM the next day?
    - **A.** 50 mg
    - **B.** 75 mg
    - **C.** 87.5 mg
    - **D.** 95.5 mg

16. What is the weight in kilograms for a child who weighs 56 lb? _____ kg

## Critical Thinking Activities

The patient is a 2-day-old baby girl born 2 months premature. Her liver is not yet functioning at the normal level for a newborn. She is prescribed an antibiotic and a cardiac drug.

1. What type of dosage adjustment would you expect for this patient?

2. What problems could occur if the drug dosages are not adjusted?

3. What route would you expect to be used for administration of these drugs and why?

# Safely Preparing and Giving Drugs

## Objectives

*After studying this chapter you should be able to:*

1. List the six "rights" of giving drugs.
2. Identify four types of drug orders.
3. Describe ways to prevent drug errors.
4. List important principles related to preparing and giving drugs.
5. Describe responsibilities related to giving enteral drugs.
6. Describe responsibilities related to giving parenteral drugs.
7. Describe responsibilities related to giving drugs through the skin and mucous membranes.
8. Describe responsibilities related to giving drugs through the ears and eyes.
9. List responsibilities before and after a drug has been given.

## Key Terms

**buccal route** (BŬK-ŭl ROWT) (p. 42) Application of a drug within the cheek or the cavity of the mouth.

**drug error** (DRŬG ĂR-ŭr) (p. 31) Any preventable event that may cause inappropriate drug use or patient harm while the drug is in the control of the health care professional, patient, or consumer. A drug error may cause a patient to receive the wrong drug, the right drug in the wrong dose, the wrong route, or at the wrong time.

**enteral route** (ĔN-tŭr-ŭl ROWT) (p. 33) Delivery of drugs from the outside of the body to the inside of the body through the GI tract.

**intradermal route** (ĭn-tră-DŬR-mŭl ROWT) (p. 37) Injection of drugs within or between the layers of the skin.

**intramuscular (IM) route** (ĭn-tră-MŬS-kyū-lŭr ROWT) (p. 38) Injection of drugs into a muscle.

**intravenous (IV) route** (ĭn-tră-VĒ-nŭs ROWT) (p. 40) Injection of drugs directly into a vein.

**nasogastric (NG) tube** (nă-zō-GĂS-trĭk) (p. 35) A tube inserted through the nostril into the stomach to deliver drugs.

**onset of action** (ŎN-sĕt ŭv ĂK-shŭn) (p. 33) The length of time it takes for a drug to start to work.

**oral route** (ŌR-ŭl) (p. 33) Administration of drugs by way of the mouth.

**parenteral route** (pŭr-ĔN-tŭr-ŭl ROWT) (p. 36) Movement of a drug from the outside of the body to the inside of the body by injection (intra-arterial, intravenous, intramuscular, subcutaneous, intracavitary, or intra-osseous).

**percutaneous route** (pŭr-kū-TĂN-ē-ŭs ROWT) (p. 41) Movement of a drug from the outside of the body to the inside of the body through the skin or mucous membranes.

**percutaneous endoscopic gastrostomy (PEG) tube** (pŭr-kū-TĂN-ē-ŭs ĕn-dō-SKŌP-ĭk găs-TRŎS-tō-mē) (p. 35) A surgically implanted tube placed through the abdomen into the stomach.

**per os (PO)** (PŬR ŎS) (p. 33) Giving drugs by way of the mouth.

**PRN order** (p. 31) An order written to administer a drug to a patient as needed.

**rectal route** (RĔK-tŭl ROWT) (p. 36) Movement of a drug from outside of the body to the inside of the body through the rectum.

**single-dose order** (SĬN-gŭl DŌS ŌR-dŭr) (p. 31) An order written to administer a drug one time only.

**standing order** (STĂN-dĭng) (p. 30) An order written when a patient is to receive a drug on a regular basis.

**STAT order** (STĂT) (p. 31) An order written to administer a drug once and as soon as possible.

**subcutaneous route** (sŭb-kū-TĂN-ē-ŭs ROWT) (p. 37) Injection of drugs into the tissues between the skin and muscle.

**sublingual (SL) route** (sŭb-LĬN-gwŭl ROWT) (p. 42) Administration of drugs by placing them underneath the tongue.

**suppository** (sŭ-PŎZ-ĭ-tōr-ē) (p. 36) A small medication plug designed to melt at body temperature within a body cavity other than the mouth.

**topical route** (TŎP-ĭ-kŭl ROWT) (p. 41) Application of drugs directly to the skin.

**transdermal route** (trănz-DŬR-mŭl ROWT) (p. 41) A type of percutaneous drug delivery in which the drug is applied to the skin, passes through the skin, and enters the bloodstream.

**unit-dose drugs** (YŪ-nĭt DŌS) (p. 31) Drugs that are dispensed to fill each patient's drug orders for a 24-hour time period.

⊖-Learning Activity 2-1 ▶

## OVERVIEW

Nurses work with physicians and other health care professionals to assist a patient who is injured, ill, or at risk of becoming ill to achieve the best possible level of health. The drug therapy role of prescribers, including physicians and other health care providers, is to select and prescribe specific drugs. The role of the pharmacist is to mix (compound) and dispense the prescribed drugs. The role of the nurse is to give or "administer" the prescribed drugs directly to the patient. Thus, although other health care professionals also have major roles in the drug therapy process, you, as the nurse, are responsible for providing competent and safe patient care.

Nurses, along with prescribers and pharmacists, must teach patients about the drug or drugs that have been prescribed.

Administering drugs is one of the nurse's most important responsibilities. But his or her responsibilities are more than just "giving" the drug to the patient. Every nurse should be familiar with the nurse practice act for the state in which he or she works.

To give drugs safely, you must understand the basic principles of drug administration. Check the expiration date to be sure that the drug is not outdated. Look carefully at intravenous (IV) drugs for any sediment or discoloration that may indicate that the drug is unstable and should not be used. Be sure to wash your hands and follow the six "rights" of drug administration.

After giving a drug, you must check the patient for the expected results and for any side effects or adverse effects. You also have a duty to teach patients and their families about drugs, including the desired action and side effects and when to call the prescriber.

## THE SIX RIGHTS OF SAFE DRUG ADMINISTRATION

When preparing and giving drugs to patients safely, follow the six "rights" for drug administration:

1. Right patient
2. Right drug
3. Right dose
4. Right route
5. Right time
6. Right documentation

Some sources cite two additional rights to follow when giving drugs: the right diagnosis to match the drug's purpose, and the patient's right to refuse a drug.

### THE RIGHT PATIENT

To make sure that the right patient is receiving any drug that has been prescribed, The Joint Commission (TJC) recommends checking two unique patient identifiers (name and birth date) before medication administration. An alert and oriented patient can be asked directly. If the patient is confused, hard of hearing, unconscious, or otherwise unable to reply, wash your hands first and then check the name, birth date, and identification number on his or her wristband. Some long-term care facilities such as nursing homes use pictures of patients to ensure that the correct patient receives the correct drugs. If a patient does not have an identification wristband, have one made and place it on his or her wrist. As an added safety measure, be sure to check the medication administration record (MAR) and the label on the patient's medication box with the wristband.

### THE RIGHT DRUG

Each drug that is prescribed has a particular intended action. You must be sure that the drug being given is correct. Carefully compare the drug you are about to administer with the drug order. Thousands of drugs are available today, and many of their names are so similar that they can be confusing. Be aware of these easily confused

 **Memory Jogger**

Safe drug administration requires that the person administering the drug be knowledgeable about these drug features:
- Purpose(s)
- Actions
- Side effects
- Abnormal reactions
- Delivery methods
- Necessary follow-up care

 **Memory Jogger**

Be sure to review the nurse practice act for your state on the state board of nursing website.

 **Memory Jogger**

Remember to use the six "rights" every time you prepare and administer drugs.

◄ ⊖-**Video 2-1:** Ensuring the Six Rights of Medication Administration

drug names. For more information about them, see "Confusing Drug Name Lists" later in this chapter.

## THE RIGHT DOSE, ROUTE, AND TIME

A prescriber's drug order should be in written form and include all the minimum information required by the U.S. government. Verbal orders should be accepted only in emergency situations. As soon as the emergency has been resolved, verbal orders must be written and signed. Contact the prescriber whenever a drug order seems unclear or if a drug dosage is higher or lower than expected. For safety, when you contact the prescriber by telephone or follow a verbal order, be sure to write the order, read it back, and ask for confirmation that what you wrote is correct before administering any drug. Be sure to document that you read back the order to the prescriber.

## THE RIGHT DOCUMENTATION

When you give a drug, record it immediately. This is essential for all drugs, but it is especially important for drugs given on an as-needed (PRN) basis. Many pain-relieving drugs are prescribed to be given as needed. These drugs often require 20 to 30 minutes to take effect. If you fail to document giving one of these drugs, a patient may request and receive a second dose from another health care worker. When a patient is receiving a narcotic pain drug, a second dose can cause complications such as a decreased respiratory rate. Documenting that a drug has been given may prevent another nurse or health care worker from mistakenly repeating the dose.

## THE RIGHT DIAGNOSIS

Before giving a drug, you must be familiar with the patient's medical diagnosis. The diagnosis should match the purpose of the drug. If the diagnosis does not match its purpose, question the prescription.

You should also check any related laboratory tests before giving a drug. For example, if a patient's diagnosis is digitalis toxicity, be sure to check the digitalis level before giving this drug. If the drug you are giving may cause adverse effects on a major body organ, be sure to check laboratory values related to that organ. For example, before giving an aminoglycoside drug such as gentamicin, you should be sure to check kidney function test results such as creatinine and blood urea nitrogen (BUN).

Many drugs affect blood pressure, heart rate, or respiratory rate. Be sure to check a patient's vital signs before giving these drugs. If the patient's vital signs are outside of the normal limits, you should hold the drug and notify the prescriber. Be sure to check the patient's vital signs again after giving the drug.

## THE RIGHT TO REFUSE

A patient has the right to refuse any drug. Be sure that he or she understands why the drug has been prescribed and the consequences of refusing to take it. When a patient refuses to take a drug, document the refusal, including the fact that the patient understands what may happen if the drug is not taken.

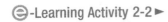
-Learning Activity 2-2 ▶

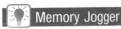

## TYPES OF DRUG ORDERS

Remember, a drug order from a qualified prescriber is needed before any drug may be administered to a patient. Drug orders may be written by different types of health care providers, including physicians, dentists, and some advanced practice nurses. Common types of drug orders include standing orders, PRN orders, single-dose orders, and immediate (STAT) orders.

A **standing order** is written when a patient is receiving a drug on a regular basis. These drugs are prescribed for a specific number of days or until discontinued by the prescriber. Certain drugs such as narcotics can only be prescribed as standing orders for a certain number of days. If the patient is to continue taking the drug after that number of days, the prescription must be renewed.

A **single-dose order** is an order to give a drug once only. A **PRN order** is given to the patient as needed. Prescribers usually designate a time interval between doses of these drugs. **STAT orders** are given one time as soon as possible.

## DRUG ERRORS

A **drug error** is a preventable event that leads to inappropriate drug use or patient harm. A drug error can occur while the drug is in the control of the health care professional, the patient, or the consumer.

*Drug errors are a leading cause of death and injury.* Each year as many as 98,000 deaths result from drug errors in hospitals in the United States. Errors can occur when the prescriber writes the drug order, when the pharmacist dispenses the drug, or when the nurse or health care worker administers the drug. *Because nurses give most drugs to patients, they are the final defense for detecting and preventing drug errors.*

### PREVENTING DRUG ERRORS

When administering drugs, always follow the six "rights." Many drug errors occur because one or more of the "rights" was not followed. If a drug prescription does not make sense, contact the prescriber to ensure that the order is correct. Always check drug dosage calculations with a coworker. Listen to the patient's questions about a drug or a drug dose. Administer drugs only after the patient's questions have been researched and answered appropriately. While giving drugs, concentrate on the task at hand. Often drug errors result from distractions or interruptions.

### Bar-Code Systems

Hospitals that use bar-code systems add a bar code to each patient's identification wristband on admission. **Unit-dose drugs** (drugs dispensed to fill a patient's drug orders for a 24-hour period) and IV fluids are all bar coded. A bar-code scanner is used to ensure that each patient receives the right drug doses at the right time. Take the scanner to each patient's bedside to scan the identification band and the drugs that are given (Figure 2-1). Scanning automatically documents the drugs that have been given. Standing order, one-time, PRN, and STAT drugs are scanned. Research shows that bar-code systems dramatically decrease the number of drug errors.

◀ⓔ-Learning Activity 2-3

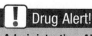
**Memory Jogger**

Eight categories of drug errors include:
- Omission
- Wrong patient
- Wrong dose
- Wrong route
- Wrong rate
- Wrong dosage form
- Wrong time
- Error in preparation of dose

---

**⚠ Drug Alert!**
**Administration Alert**

Most drug errors are made while giving drugs. Common errors include giving the wrong drug or giving the wrong dose. Follow the six "rights" to prevent drug errors.

◀ⓔ-Learning Activity 2-4

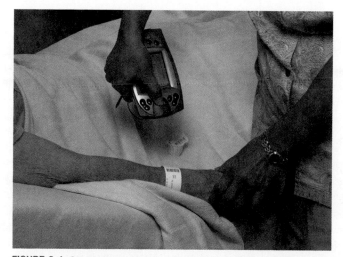

**FIGURE 2-1** Checking a patient's wristband with a bar-code scanner.

## Box 2-1   Examples of Easily Confused Drug Names

**ACCUPRIL** (quinapril) for hypertension
**ACIPHEX** (rabeprazole) for heartburn and ulcers

**AMBIEN** (zolpidem) for insomnia
**AMEN** (medroxyprogesterone) to control menstrual cycles

**CELEBREX** (celecoxib) for arthritis
**CELEXA** (citalopram) for depression

**CLOZARIL** (clozapine) for schizophrenia
**COLAZAL** (balsalazide) for ulcerative colitis

Deltasone, Orasone, others (**PREDNISONE**) for
      inflammation
Mysoline (**PRIMIDONE**) for seizures

Flumadine (**RIMANTADINE**) for influenza
Zantac (**RANITIDINE**) for heartburn and ulcers

**FOSAMAX** (alendronate) for osteoporosis
**FLOMAX** (tamsulosin) for enlarged prostate

**LAMICTAL** (lamotrigine) for epilepsy
**LAMISIL** (terbinafine) for fingernail fungus

**OXYCONTIN** (oxycodone) for pain
Ditropan (**OXYBUTYNIN**) for urinary incontinence

**PAXIL** (paroxetine) for depression
**PLAVIX** (clopidogrel) to prevent heart attack and stroke

**PRAVACHOL** (pravastatin) for high cholesterol
Inderal (**PROPRANOLOL**) for hypertension

**SINGULAIR** (montelukast) for asthma
**SINEQUAN** (doxepin) for depression and anxiety

Thorazine (**CHLORPROMAZINE**) for severe psychotic
      behavior
Diabinese (**CHLORPROPAMIDE**) for diabetes

Valium (**DIAZEPAM**) for anxiety, muscle spasms
Ativan (**LORAZEPAM**) for anxiety

**XANAX** (alprazolam) for anxiety
**ZANTAC** (ranitidine) for heartburn and ulcers

**ZYPREXA** (olanzapine) for bipolar mania, and schizophrenia
**ZYRTEC** (cetirizine) for allergies

---

**? Did You Know?**

You can find lists of confused drug names on the Internet at the website for the Institute for Safe Medication Practices (ISMP) (www.ismp.org).

**! Drug Alert!**

**Action/Intervention Alert**

Always report drug errors *immediately* so appropriate actions can be taken to counteract possible adverse reactions to the drug.

### Confusing Drug Name Lists

Lists of drug names that have been confused and involved in drug errors are published by organizations such as the Institute for Safe Medication Practices (ISMP). A partial list is provided in Box 2-1. As you read through this text, be sure to check the "Do Not Confuse" boxes for additional hints on how to avoid confusing drug names.

### REPORTING DRUG ERRORS

When a drug error is made, report it immediately. Carefully watch the patient for any signs of an adverse reaction. Drug errors may result in life-threatening complications such as coma or death. Most patient care facilities have a form and standard procedure that are used to report a drug error. The patient's prescriber must also be notified.

### PRINCIPLES OF ADMINISTERING DRUGS

You must know the drug that you are administering, including its uses, actions, and common adverse reactions and any special precautions. You will probably become familiar with the drugs given most often in your institution. However, many drugs are not given on a daily basis, and new drugs are constantly being developed. Before giving a drug with which you are not familiar, seek out information from dependable sources such as pharmacists, drug inserts, and manufacturers' websites. In addition, *know the patient's drug history, allergies, previous adverse reactions, and pertinent laboratory values and any important changes in his or her condition* before administering a drug.

Often prescribers put limitations on when a drug should be given. For example, the prescriber may order that the drug be given only if the patient's blood pressure is above or below a particular value. Similar limitations may be based on heart rate, respiratory rate, or pain level. Be aware of the prescribed limitations and check them before giving the drug. If the patient's condition or vital signs are outside of the set limits, you must hold the drug and document the reason for your action.

When giving drugs, listen to your patient. Patient comments give clues to adverse reactions such as nausea, dizziness, unsteady walking, and ringing in the ears. These comments indicate that the patient may be having an adverse reaction, and you should hold the drug while you notify the prescriber.

## GETTING READY TO GIVE DRUGS

There are several important guidelines to follow before preparing to give drugs.
- Always check the written order.
- Limit interruptions and distractions.
- Wash your hands.
- Keep drugs in their containers or wrappers until at the patient's bedside.
- Avoid touching pills or capsules.
- Never give drugs prepared by someone else.
- Follow sterile technique when handling syringes and needles.
- Remain alert to drug names that sound or look alike. Giving the wrong drug can have serious adverse effects.

Some pills and capsules are prepared for slow absorption. These drugs are often labeled enteric-coated, time-release, or slow-release. If crushed or opened, these drugs may be absorbed too rapidly. This can irritate the gastrointestinal (GI) system or cause symptoms of overdose. If a patient cannot take pills or capsules, a liquid form of the drug may be a better option. A prescriber's order is needed to change the drug form.

Giving drugs to children can be challenging and difficult. Tips that may help you give drugs to children are listed in Box 2-2.

## GIVING ENTERAL DRUGS

A drug given by the **enteral route** is delivered from the outside of the body to the inside of the body using the GI tract. Enteral drugs enter the body in one of three ways: through the mouth (oral), by feeding tube (nasogastric or percutaneous endoscopic gastrostomy), or through the rectum.

### ORAL DRUGS

Drugs are most commonly given by mouth or the **oral route.** Orders for oral drugs are written as "PO," which means **per os** or "by mouth." Most drugs are available in one or more oral forms: tablets, capsules, and liquids. They are relatively inexpensive when compared to other drug forms. Oral drugs are easy to give as long as the patient can swallow. A major advantage of PO drugs is that, if a patient receives too much, the drug can be removed by pumping the stomach or causing the patient to vomit. Oral drugs do not work well for patients suffering from nausea and vomiting. Onset of action for these drugs is slow because they must be absorbed through the GI tract.

### What To Do *Before* Giving Oral Drugs

Be sure that the patient can swallow. Check the drug order. Wash your hands. Check the patient's wristband and ask the patient's name and date of birth for identification. Follow the six "rights" for giving drugs. Sit the patient upright and have a full glass of water ready. Tell the patient what drugs you will be giving and answer any questions asked. Tell the patient if there are any special instructions related to the drugs (e.g., getting up slowly from bed after new antihypertensive drugs are given). Ask the patient to place the tablets or capsules in the back of the mouth, take a few sips of water, and swallow the drugs. Have the patient drink the entire glass of water because oral drugs dissolve better and cause less GI discomfort when they are given with enough water. Stay at the patient's bedside until the drugs are swallowed. Do not leave drugs at the patient's bedside to be taken later. An exception may be made

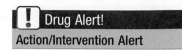

**Drug Alert!**
**Action/Intervention Alert**

Always listen to patients when giving drugs because their actions and comments can be clues to adverse or side effects of drugs.

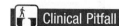

**Clinical Pitfall**

Never crush tablets or open capsules without first checking with the drug guide.

◄ⓔ-Learning Activity 2-5

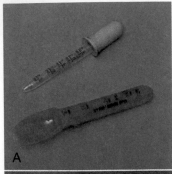

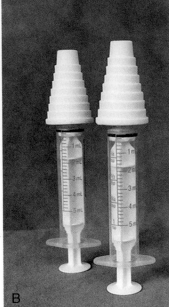

FIGURE 2-2 Calibrated devices for delivery of liquid oral drugs. **A,** Calibrated dropper and calibrated spoon. **B,** Calibrated oral syringe.

## Box 2-2   Tips for Administering Drugs to Children

### DO'S

- Keep drugs in their original containers and never in dishes, cups, bottles, or other household containers.
- When dosage calculations are needed, have another nurse, prescriber, or pharmacist also perform the calculation to ensure accuracy.
- Check with a drug guide for information on dosage by milligrams per kilogram and ensure that the calculated dosage is within the guidelines.
- Question any order in which the prescribed dosage does not match the recommended dosage for body weight or size.
- Use appropriate measuring devices (see Figure 2-2) to ensure accurate doses of liquid drugs.
- Work with the pharmacist to ensure that a liquid oral drug or a crushed oral tablet is mixed with a small amount of pleasant, delicious-tasting liquid.
- Keep all drugs out of reach of children.
- Before crushing a tablet, check with the pharmacist or drug resource book to determine whether it should be crushed.
- Apply transdermal patch drugs to a child's back between the shoulder blades.
- Use two identifiers, including the child's name band, to identify him or her before administering any drug (this can include asking a parent the child's full name and date of birth).
- Position children in a sitting or semisitting position when administering an oral drug (to avoid aspiration or choking).
- Help a child rinse his or her mouth after taking an oral liquid drug.
- Watch an infant or child closely (at least every 15 minutes) for the first 2 hours after giving the first dose of a newly prescribed drug for expected and unexpected or unusual responses to the drug.
- Offer creative choices for the child who is old enough to understand such as:
  - Which drug to take first if more than one drug will be administered at the same time.
  - Which type of drink the child would like as a follow-up after a drug is administered.
  - Which leg or arm (when appropriate) the child would prefer be used for an injection.
  - What toy to hold during an injection.
- When an infant or child is prescribed to take a drug at home, demonstrate to the parents exactly how to measure and give the drug. Have the parents demonstrate these acts.
- Obtain the assistance of another adult when administering a parenteral drug, drops or ointment to the eye, or drops to the ear of an infant or child.
- Select the smallest gauge and shortest needle that will safely deliver the injection.
- If possible, change needles after injecting the drug into the syringe (prevents any irritating drug residue from contacting the child's tissues).
- Follow agency policy for site selection of injectable drugs for a child.
- Use diversion during an injection.
- Try to avoid having the child see the needle or the actual injection.

### DON'TS

- Don't refer to drugs as "candy."
- Don't place liquid drugs in a large bottle of formula (unless the child drinks the entire amount, he or she will not receive the correct dose).
- Don't place crushed drugs into the child's *favorite* food or snack (he or she may never eat that food again).
- Don't threaten a child with an injection in place of an oral drug.
- Don't lie to a child.

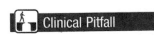 Clinical Pitfall

Never leave drugs at the bedside for the patient to take at a later time or ask someone else to administer drugs that you have prepared.

for antacids or nitroglycerin tablets *if* there is an order permitting this. You are responsible for documenting that drugs have been taken and must witness that this has occurred.

When giving oral liquid drugs, be sure to use a calibrated device to measure the correct dose (Figure 2-2) because household devices such as spoons or cups vary widely in size and their use can result in giving inaccurate doses. Always hold a calibrated medicine cup at eye level to measure the dose (Figure 2-3).

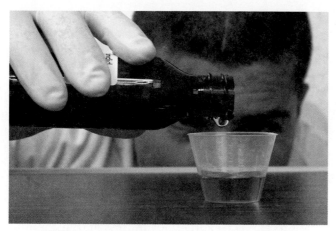

FIGURE 2-3 Checking the drug dose in a medicine cup.

### What To Do *After* Giving Oral Drugs

Document that the drug was given. If a drug was refused or not given, document the reason. Be sure to check the patient later for side effects, adverse effects, and the desired effect. For example, check the patient taking hypertensive drugs for decreased blood pressure. Document your findings.

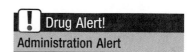
◀ ⊜-**Video 2-2:** Administering Oral Medications

### ORAL DRUGS GIVEN BY FEEDING TUBE

Oral drugs may be given by feeding tubes. Patients who are unable to swallow or who have nausea may be given oral drugs by a nasogastric tube. A nasogastric (NG) tube delivers drugs by a tube inserted through the nostrils to the stomach. A percutaneous endoscopic gastrostomy (PEG) tube is surgically implanted through the abdomen into the stomach.

### What To Do *Before* Giving Drugs by NG or PEG Tube

As with all oral drugs, check the drug orders that may be written as PO or by feeding tube. Check your drug book or with the pharmacist before crushing tablets or opening capsules. Wash your hands and place the patient upright. Check to make sure that the tube is located in the stomach by withdrawing (*aspirating*) stomach contents with a syringe, or you can attach an end-tidal carbon dioxide ($CO_2$) detector to the feeding tube. The presence of carbon dioxide indicates that the tube is in the trachea rather than the stomach.

    If the patient is receiving a tube feeding, check the amount of tube feeding remaining in the stomach (*residual*). Some drugs are not well absorbed when food is in the stomach (e.g., phenytoin [Dilantin]), and the tube feeding must be stopped for a period before and after administration. Liquid drugs should be diluted and flushed through the tube. Crushed tablets and the contents of opened capsules are first dissolved in water before being given through the tube. To give the drugs, attach a large syringe to the tube, pour the liquid or dissolved drug into the syringe, and let it run in by gravity.

**[⫩] Clinical Pitfall**

Do *not* give a drug by NG tube if $CO_2$ is present when the tube is tested with an end-tidal $CO_2$ detector.

◀ ⊜-**Learning Activity 2-6**

**[!] Drug Alert!**
**Administration Alert**

Always check for correct placement of a feeding tube before giving drugs by this route to ensure that the drugs do not go into the lungs.

### What To Do *After* Giving Drugs by NG or PEG Tube

After giving drugs by this route, flush the tube well to make sure that it is clear. Use at least 50 mL of water to prevent the tube from becoming clogged. If the patient's NG tube is connected to suction, the tube should be clamped for at least 30 minutes after administering drugs before reattaching it to suction. This allows time for the drugs to be absorbed from the GI system. As with oral drugs, document what has been given and watch the patient for side effects, adverse effects, and the desired effects. Document your findings.

## GIVING RECTAL DRUGS

Patients who are unable to swallow or have severe nausea and vomiting may need to have drugs given by the rectal route. These drugs may come as suppositories or in the form of an enema. A suppository is a small drug plug designed to melt at body temperature when placed within the rectum or vagina. With drugs given by this route, absorption is not as dependable or predictable as when drugs are given orally. The patient with diarrhea cannot hold them long enough for absorption to take place. The rate of absorption is also affected by the amount of stool present.

### What To Do *Before* Giving Rectal Drugs

Always check the drug order. Ask whether the patient has any health problems such as diarrhea that may make using this route undesirable. Other reasons for not giving a rectal drug include recent rectal surgery or trauma and history of vasovagal reactions (slowed heart rate and dilation of blood vessels, which can lead to fainting, sometimes called *syncope*).

Wash your hands. Check the patient's wristband for identification and follow the six "rights" as you would when giving any drug. Bring the drug, some lubricant, and a pair of disposable gloves to the bedside. Assist the patient to turn to the side with one leg bent over the other (Sims' position) (Figure 2-4). The left Sims' position is best for giving rectal suppositories.

Protect the patient's privacy by closing doors or drapes and keeping as much of the patient covered as possible. Explain what you will be doing and be sure to include any special instructions such as how long the drug must be held inside the rectum. Put on your gloves. Take the wrapper off the suppository and coat the pointed end with a small amount of water-soluble lubricant. Also apply a small amount of lubricant to the finger that you will be using to insert the drug. Hold the suppository next to the anal sphincter and explain that you are ready to insert the drug. Ask the patient to take a deep breath and bear down a little. With the pointed end first, push the suppository into the rectum about one inch (Figure 2-5).

### What To Do *After* Giving Rectal Drugs

Remind the patient to remain on his or her side for about 20 minutes. Clean the patient's anal area with tissue. Remove gloves and wash your hands. Immediately document that the drug was given. Check the patient for any expected or unexpected responses and chart these. For example, if the patient was given a suppository to relieve constipation, be sure to note whether or not the patient had a bowel movement.

## GIVING PARENTERAL DRUGS

Drugs given by the parenteral route are injected through the skin. They may be injected intradermally, subcutaneously, intramuscularly, or intravenously. There are four primary reasons for giving drugs parenterally. The patient may:

- Be unable to take oral drugs.
- Need a drug that acts rapidly.
- Need a constant blood level of a drug.
- Need drugs such as insulin, which are not made in an oral form.

Standard precautions from the Centers for Disease Control and Prevention (CDC) recommend wearing gloves whenever you are exposed to blood or other body fluids, mucous membranes, or any area of broken skin.

Giving parenteral drugs requires that you use needles and syringes safely. Do not recap needles and always dispose of needles and syringes in labeled containers. "Sharps" containers are located in every patient room. Many hospitals use needles with plastic guards that slip over the needle to protect against needlesticks.

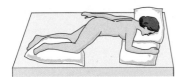

**Memory Jogger**

Vasovagal reactions are a common cause of fainting from a decrease in heart rate and blood pressure.

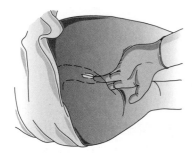

**FIGURE 2-4** Sims' left position. For this position, the patient lies on one side with the knee and thigh drawn upward toward the chest.

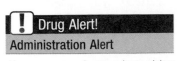

**FIGURE 2-5** To administer a rectal suppository, push the suppository into the rectum about 1 inch.

⊖-Video 2-3: Inserting a ▶ Rectal Suppository

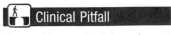

**Drug Alert!**

**Administration Alert**

Always wear gloves when giving parenteral drugs to avoid exposure to blood and other body fluids.

**Clinical Pitfall**

To avoid needlesticks, do not recap needles.

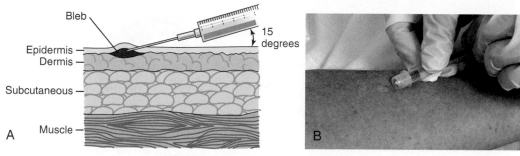

FIGURE 2-6 **A** and **B,** Intradermal injection.

In 2001 the Occupational Safety and Health Administration (OSHA) developed guidelines to help prevent needlesticks. OSHA advises that prevention of needlesticks is best and recommends that health care employers select safer needle devices. Needlestick injuries should be tracked using a Sharps Injury Log. The purpose of this log is to identify problem areas. In addition, OSHA recommends that employers have a written Exposure Care Plan that is updated on an annual basis.

## GIVING INTRADERMAL DRUGS

A drug administered by the intradermal route is administered by an injection between the layers of the skin. The most common site for intradermal injections is the inner part of the forearm. The primary uses of intradermal injections are for:
* Allergy testing.
* Local anesthetics.
* Testing for tuberculosis (TB).

The TB test is done with purified protein derivative. A very small amount of drug is injected into the space between the epidermis and the dermis layers of the skin (Figure 2-6). This results in a bump *(bleb)* that looks like an insect bite. The volume of drug injected is very small (0.01 to 0.1 mL), and the needle used is short and small (⅜ inch, 25 gauge).

### What To Do *Before* Giving Intradermal Drugs

Check the drug order and the patient's wristband. Follow the six "rights." Put on gloves. Cleanse the injection site in a round motion, beginning from the center and moving outward. Insert the needle at a 15-degree angle with the bevel facing up (Figure 2-7). Do not pull back (aspirate) on the plunger of the syringe. Inject the drug so a little bump forms and remove the needle. *Do not massage the area.* If the little bump does not form, the drug has probably been injected too deeply into the subcutaneous tissue, and test results will not be accurate. When this happens, discard the used equipment and use a different site with a new sterile needle and syringe for the intradermal injection.

### What To Do *After* Giving Intradermal Drugs

Document the drug administration immediately. Check the patient for allergic or sensitivity reactions to the injection. These reactions may take several hours to days. Making a circle around the injection site with a pen may help to accurately check the site. Document any reactions and notify the prescriber. TB tests must be checked and read three days (72 hours) after the injection.

## GIVING SUBCUTANEOUS DRUGS

A drug given by the subcutaneous route is injected into tissues between the skin and muscle (Figure 2-8). Two drugs that are commonly given subcutaneously are insulin and heparin. Subcutaneous drugs are absorbed more slowly than

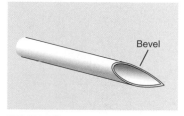

FIGURE 2-7 Close up of a needle with the bevel up.

**Drug Alert!**

**Administration Alert**

Use a small needle and a 15-degree angle for intradermal drugs. Do not aspirate before injecting the drug or massage afterward.

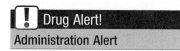

◄ ⊜-**Video 2-4:** Administering an Intradermal Injection

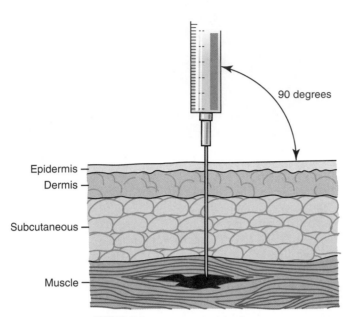

FIGURE 2-9 Intramuscular injection.

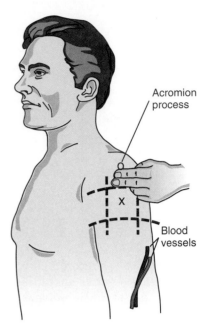

FIGURE 2-10 Deltoid (arm) intramuscular injection site landmarks.

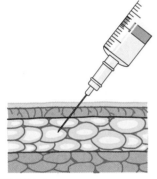

FIGURE 2-8 Subcutaneous injection.

### Clinical Pitfall

Do not aspirate when giving subcutaneous heparin. Aspirating causes a vacuum and can lead to tissue damage and bruising when the heparin is injected.

ⓔ-Video 2-5: Administering a ▶ Subcutaneous Injection

### Drug Alert!
**Administration Alert**

IM injections of more than 3 mL are rare. To ensure that the drug dose is correct, carefully calculate and check it with another nurse.

intramuscular drugs. Typically these injections are from 0.5 to 1 mL. When a larger volume of drug is ordered, give the injection in two different sites with different syringes and needles. Small, short needles are used (⅜ to ⅝ inch, 25 to 27 gauge). Sites for subcutaneous injections include the upper arms, the abdomen, and the upper back. Rotate the sites for the injections to avoid damage to the patient's tissues.

### What To Do *Before* Giving Subcutaneous Drugs

Check the order and the patient's wristband for identification. Follow the six "rights." Insert the needle at a 45-degree angle for most patients. If the patient is obese, you may need to use a 90-degree angle. If the patient is thin, you may need an angle that is less than 45 degrees. Before giving some subcutaneous injections, aspirate (pull back on the plunger of the syringe) to make sure that the needle is not in a vein. Do not aspirate the syringe before giving an injection of heparin or insulin. Inject the drug and remove the needle.

### What To Do *After* Giving Subcutaneous Drugs

Apply pressure to prevent bleeding. If a patient has a bleeding disorder or is receiving anticoagulation therapy, you may have to apply pressure longer until bleeding is stopped. Document giving the drug immediately, including the site used for injection. Check the patient for side effects, adverse effects, and expected effects. Document your findings.

### GIVING INTRAMUSCULAR DRUGS

A drug given by the intramuscular (IM) route is given by injection deep into a muscle (Figure 2-9). Because of the rich blood supply in the muscles, IM drugs are absorbed much faster than subcutaneous drugs. IM injections can also be much larger than subcutaneous injections (1 to 3 mL). Infants and children usually do not receive more than 1 mL. If an injection order is for more than 3 mL, divide the dose and give two injections. Injections of more than 3 mL are not as well absorbed.

Needles for these injections are longer (1 to 1.5 inches) and larger (20 to 22 gauge). Sites for IM injections include the upper arm deltoid muscle, the thigh vastus lateralis muscles, and the dorsogluteal muscles in the buttocks (Figures 2-10

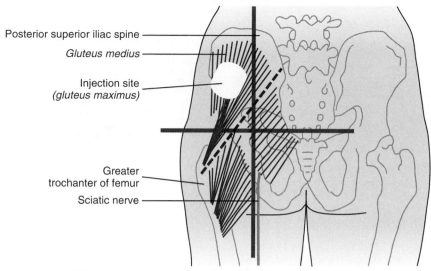

FIGURE 2-11 Dorsogluteal intramuscular injection site landmarks.

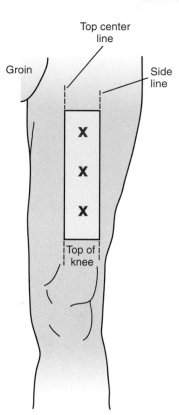

FIGURE 2-12 Vastus lateralis (thigh) intramuscular injection site landmarks.

### Table 2-1 Intramuscular Injection Site Advantages and Disadvantages

| INJECTION SITE | ADVANTAGES | DISADVANTAGES |
|---|---|---|
| Deltoid (upper arm) | Easily accessible<br>Useful for vaccinations in adolescents and adults | Poorly developed in young children<br>Only small amounts (0.5 to 1 mL) can be injected |
| Vastus lateralis (thigh) | Preferred site for infant injections<br>Relatively free of large blood vessels and nerves<br>Easily accessible | |
| Dorsogluteal (buttocks) | | Presence of large blood vessels and sciatic nerve<br>Should not be used in children under 3 years of age |

through 2-12). Be sure to rotate injection sites when multiple IM injections are prescribed. Table 2-1 describes the advantages and disadvantages of IM injection sites.

### What To Do *Before* Giving Intramuscular Drugs

Check the order and the patient's identification wristband. Follow the six "rights." Help the patient into a comfortable position that is appropriate for the site you plan to use. Select the injection site by identifying the correct anatomic landmarks. Be sure to wear gloves. Cleanse the injection site. Using a 90-degree angle, insert the needle firmly into the muscle. Aspirate the syringe (pull back on the plunger) to make sure that the needle is not in a vein. If the needle is in a vein, blood will appear in the syringe. Remove the needle and discard the drug if this happens. Get a new dose of the drug and a sterile needle and syringe and give the injection in another site. Once you have determined that the needle is not in a blood vessel, inject the drug and remove the needle.

Use the Z-track method of IM injection for drugs that are irritating to subcutaneous tissue or that may permanently stain the tissues (Figure 2-13). After drawing the drug into the syringe, draw in 0.1 to 0.2 mL of air. The air follows the drug into the muscle and stops it from oozing through the path of the needle. After you select and cleanse the site, pull the tissue laterally and hold it. Insert the needle into the muscle;

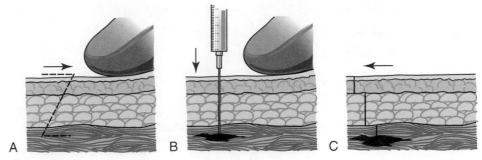

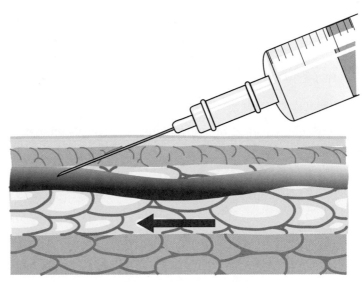

**FIGURE 2-13** Z-track intramuscular injection. **A,** Displace the tissue downward, away from the injection site. **B,** Inject while holding the tissue away. **C,** Allow the displaced tissue to move back into place.

**FIGURE 2-14** Intravenous injection.

inject the drug and release the tissue as you remove the needle. Releasing the tissue allows the skin to slide over the injection and seal the drug in the muscle.

### What To Do *After* Giving Intramuscular Drugs

Apply pressure after removing the needle to prevent bleeding. When charting the drug administration, be sure to include the injection site. Check the patient for adverse effects, side effects, and expected effects of the drug. Document your findings.

### GIVING INTRAVENOUS DRUGS

A drug given by the intravenous (IV) route is injected directly into a vein (Figure 2-14). This route is selected when a drug needs to enter the bloodstream rapidly or when large doses of a drug must be given. The rates of absorption and action are very rapid with this route. Emergency drugs may be given by a needle and syringe directly into a vein; however, most IV drugs are given slowly through a needle or catheter that has been inserted into a vein. The needle or catheter is attached to IV tubing with an injection port. IV drugs may be pushed slowly over 1 or more minutes, pushed rapidly over a few seconds, or given slowly by IV piggyback. They may be given through an IV line or a saline lock.

### What To Do *Before* Giving Intravenous Drugs

Check the drug order and the patient's identification wristband. Follow the six "rights." Wash your hands. Put on gloves. Check the IV site to make sure that it is patent. Document the condition of the IV site. If the drug has been added to IV fluid, be sure to remove all air from the tubing. (This is called *"priming"* the IV tubing.) If

⊖-**Video 2-6:** Administering an ▶
Intramuscular Injection

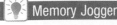 Memory Jogger

IV drugs may be given continuously or intermittently.

⊖-**Video 2-7:** Administering ▶
Medications by IV Piggyback

⊖-**Video 2-8:** Administering ▶
Medications by IV Bolus

the drug is to be administered in a continuous IV infusion or an IV piggyback, it should be placed on an infusion pump to control the rate.

In most cases registered nurses (RNs) will give IV push and IV piggyback drugs. Be sure to check the scope of practice laws of your state. In some states licensed practical nurses or licensed vocational nurses may administer IV drugs with additional training.

### What To Do *After* Giving Intravenous Drugs

Document that the drug has been given, including the site and flow rate. Continue to check the IV site for signs of these conditions:
- Infection
- Escape of fluid from the vein into tissue (*extravasation*)
- Collection of fluid in the tissues (*infiltration*)

If fluid escapes or collects in the tissues, the IV catheter must be discontinued and replaced in a different vein. As with administration of any drug, check the patient for side effects, adverse effects, or expected effects of the drug. Document these effects. To learn more about IV fluids, see Chapter 6.

## GIVING PERCUTANEOUS DRUGS

A drug given by the **percutaneous route** is applied to and absorbed through the skin and mucous membranes. Absorption of these drugs is affected by several factors:
- Size of area covered by the drug
- Concentration or strength of the drug
- Time the drug remains in contact with the skin or mucous membranes
- Condition of the skin (breakdown, thickness, hydration, nutrition, and skin tone)

### GIVING TOPICAL OR TRANSDERMAL DRUGS

A drug given by the **topical route** is applied directly to the skin for local effects. Topical drugs include creams, lotions, and ointments. They soften or lubricate the skin. Some are used to treat superficial infections of the skin. Topical drugs are applied in a thin, even layer over the affected area of skin.

A drug given by the **transdermal route** is applied to the skin, but it is absorbed and enters the bloodstream. The transdermal route allows the patient to maintain a steady blood level of the drug. For this reason toxicity and adverse effects can usually be avoided. Examples of transdermal drugs are:
- Nitroglycerin to treat cardiac problems.
- Scopolamine to treat dizziness and nausea.
- Birth control.
- Nicotine patches for smoking cessation.
- Long-term pain drugs.

They are applied as patches or ointments. Drug patches have a semipermeable membrane and an adhesive that attaches to the skin (Figure 2-15). Common sites of application include the chest, flank, back, and upper arms.

### What To Do *Before* Giving Topical or Transdermal Drugs

Check the drug order and the patient's identification wristband. Follow the six "rights." Wash your hands. Put on gloves. Clean the area of skin where the drug will be applied. Apply topical drugs in a smooth, thin layer, and cover the area. When administering transdermal drugs, remove old patches or doses of the drug. Be sure to remove all traces of the drug from the previous dosage site, and rotate sites to avoid skin irritation or breakdown.

### What To Do *After* Giving Topical or Transdermal Drugs

Document that the drug has been given, including the site where it was applied. Be sure to write the date, time, and your initials on the new patch. Check the patient

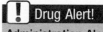
**Drug Alert!**
**Administration Alert**

Always check the IV site before administering IV drugs. If an IV line is not patent, the drug will go into the tissue instead of the vein and may cause tissue damage.

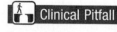
**Clinical Pitfall**

Do not shave skin before applying topical or transdermal drugs. Shaving may cause skin irritation and change the absorption of the drug.

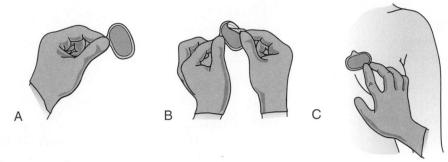

**FIGURE 2-15** Applying a transdermal patch. **A,** Nitroglycerin patch. **B,** Remove plastic backing carefully, taking care not to touch the medication. **C,** Place the medication side of the patch on the patient's skin and press the adhesive to stay in place.

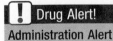

⊖-Video 2-9: Administering ▶ Topical Medications

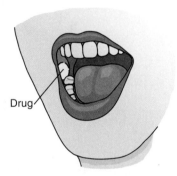

Drug

**FIGURE 2-16** Giving buccal drugs.

⊖-Learning Activity 2-7 ▶

**❗ Drug Alert!**

**Teaching Alert**

Teach the patient to avoid swallowing any buccal or sublingual drugs.

**❗ Drug Alert!**

**Administration Alert**

Before giving ear drops to children younger than 3 years, pull the ear lobe down and back to straighten the ear canal. Before giving ear drops to older children and adults, pull the ear lobe up and out to straighten the ear canal.

for adverse effects or expected effects and document these. For example, headache and dizziness related to decreased blood pressure are common side effects of nitroglycerin ointment.

### GIVING DRUGS THROUGH THE MUCOUS MEMBRANES

Drugs may be absorbed through the mucous membranes. The following are examples of drug forms used for the different mucous membranes found in the body:

- Buccal or sublingual drugs are used in the mouth.
- Drops and ointments are applied to the eyes, nose, or ears.
- Inhalation drugs are drawn into the lungs.
- Suppositories and creams are used in the vagina.

Drugs are usually well absorbed through these areas; however, the blood supply to mucous membranes varies. When you administer a drug through mucous membranes, be sure to use a sterile or clean procedure.

#### What To Do *Before* Giving Drugs Through the Mucous Membranes

Always check the order and the patient's identity. Wash your hands and wear gloves. Follow the six "rights."

*Buccal and Sublingual Drugs.*    Drugs given by the buccal route, such as lozenges, are placed between the cheek and molar teeth of the upper jaw (Figure 2-16). A drug given by the sublingual route, such as nitroglycerin, is placed under the tongue (Figure 2-17). The blood supply is very good in the mouth; therefore these drugs dissolve and are absorbed quickly. The patient should not eat or drink until the drug is completely dissolved. Teach the patient not to swallow or chew while the drug is in the mouth because these drugs are not effective if absorbed through the GI tract.

*Ear Drops.*    Ear drops are drugs given to treat local infection or inflammation and should be kept at room temperature. Help the patient to lie on one side with the affected ear up. For children younger than 3 years, pull the ear lobe (*pinna*) down and back. For older children and adults, pull the ear lobe up and out (Figure 2-18). This straightens the ear canal. Do not let the ear dropper touch the ear. Have the patient stay in the same position for at least 5 minutes so the drug can coat the inner ear canal. Sometimes a cotton ball is ordered to be placed in the ear canal. Repeat this procedure for the other ear when both ears are affected.

*Eye Drops and Ointments.*    Administration of eye drops and ointments is discussed in detail in Chapter 26.

*Nose Drops.*    Nose drops or sprays are given to treat congestion or infection. To give nose drops, draw the drops into a dropper. Ask the patient to gently blow his or her nose and then lie down with the head hanging over the edge of the bed. Hold

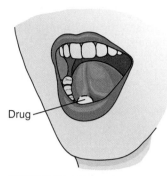

Drug

**FIGURE 2-17** Giving sublingual drugs.

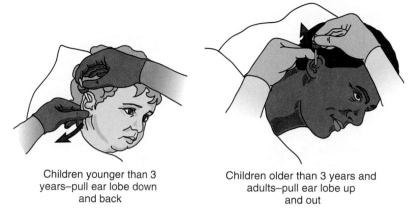

Children younger than 3 years—pull ear lobe down and back

Children older than 3 years and adults—pull ear lobe up and out

**FIGURE 2-18** Giving ear drops.

the dropper over a nostril and give the ordered number of nose drops. Do not let the dropper touch the nose. Repeat for the second nostril if needed.

To give nasal spray, position the patient sitting up with one nostril blocked by a finger. Place the tip of the spray in the other nostril. Ask the patient to take a deep breath. During the deep breath, squeeze a puff of spray into the nostril. Wipe the spray bottle tip if it is to be used with both nostrils. Nasal sprays are absorbed quickly from the nasal mucosa. Do not use the same spray container for any other patient.

*Inhalers.* Drugs may be inhaled through the respiratory tract. Different types of devices are used for delivery of inhaled drugs. Specific techniques for administering inhaled drugs are presented in Chapter 18.

*Vaginal Drugs.* Vaginal drugs are given to treat irritation or infection. Types of vaginal drugs include creams, jellies, tablets, foams, or suppositories. These drugs should be kept at room temperature. Ask the patient to empty her bladder then lie down. Be sure to put on gloves after washing your hands. Suppositories are lubricated and given in the same way as rectal suppositories. Creams, jellies, tablets, and foams are given with a special applicator that is placed in the vagina as far as possible. The plunger of the applicator is pushed to give the drug. Be sure to have the patient lie down for 10 to 15 minutes after receiving these drugs.

**What To Do *After* Giving Drugs Through the Mucous Membranes**

Always document that the drugs have been given, including the route. Check the patient for any expected or unexpected actions of the drug that you have given. Document these effects.

## Get Ready for Practice!

### Key Points

- Always follow the procedures of the six "rights" when giving drugs (right patient, right drug, right dose, right route, right time, right documentation).
- The four types of drug orders are standing, single dose, PRN, and STAT.
- Most drug errors occur while giving drugs. Following the procedure of the six "rights" helps prevent drug errors.
- Nurses give most drugs to patients, and they are the final defense for detecting and preventing drug errors.

- Bar-code systems for giving drugs have led to decreases in drug errors.
- Always report a drug error immediately so actions can be taken to counteract any possible adverse drug reactions.
- Always listen to patients for clues to adverse effects when giving drugs.
- Always check the written order and pertinent laboratory values and vital signs before giving a drug.
- Always check the patient for expected effects, side effects, and adverse effects after giving a drug.

- Never crush tablets or open capsules without checking with the pharmacist first.
- Check the patient's ability to swallow before giving oral drugs.
- Always wear gloves and use standard precautions to protect yourself from the risk of exposure to body fluids when giving drugs.
- To avoid needlesticks, do not recap needles.

## Additional Learning Resources

**evolve** Go to your Evolve website (http://evolve.elsevier.com/Workman/pharmacology/) for the following FREE learning resources:
- eLearning Activities
- Animations
- Video Clips
- Interactive Review Questions
- Audio Key Points
- Audio Glossary
- Audio Glossary—Spanish-English
- Drug Dosage Calculators
- Patient Teaching Handouts

**SG** Go to your Study Guide for additional learning activities to help you master this chapter content.

## Review Questions

1. Which is the best action to take to determine if you are giving a drug to the right patient?
   A. Ask the patient's name
   B. Look at the patient's bedside chart
   C. Check the patient's wristband
   D. Check the drug order

2. A patient needs a dose of oral potassium for a low serum potassium level (3.4 mEq/dL). Which type of order does the prescriber use?
   A. Standing order
   B. Single order
   C. PRN order
   D. STAT order

3. Which is the best way to prevent drug errors?
   A. Double check the written drug order
   B. Follow the procedure of the six "rights"
   C. Recheck drug dosage calculations
   D. Check the patient's wristband for identification

4. Before giving a drug, what should you do? (Select all that apply.)
   A. Check the order
   B. Wash your hands
   C. Instruct the patient that he or she must take the drug
   D. Find out the patient's diagnosis
   E. Check the patient's identification band

5. The patient with an NG tube has orders for several enteral drugs (i.e., capsules, tablets, and liquids). What should you do before giving these drugs? (Select all that apply.)
   A. Check with the pharmacist about crushing the tablets
   B. Follow the procedures of the "six" rights
   C. Aspirate to check for stomach contents
   D. Open the extended-release capsules
   E. Inject 50 mL of water to check tube patency

6. Which statement accurately describes the correct technique for giving subcutaneous drugs?
   A. Use a ⅜-inch, 25-gauge needle and a 15-degree angle for injection.
   B. Use a ⅜-inch, 25-gauge needle and a 45-degree angle for injection.
   C. Use a 1-inch, 22-gauge needle and a 90-degree angle for injection.
   D. Use a ½ inch, 25-gauge needle and a 45-degree angle for injection.

7. You are teaching a patient about a prescribed sublingual drug. What will you be sure to tell the patient? (Select all that apply.)
   A. "Don't swallow this drug."
   B. "Do not drink anything until the drug is completely dissolved."
   C. "Place this drug between your jaw and your molar teeth."
   D. "Notify your physician if you experience side effects."
   E. "Place the drug beside or above the tongue."

8. You are to give ear drops to a 2-year-old child. Which technique will you use?
   A. Pull the ear lobe up and out
   B. Pull the ear lobe down and back
   C. Pull the ear lobe out and back
   D. Pull the ear lobe up and back

9. What should you do immediately after giving a PRN pain drug?
   A. Ask if the patient's pain has been relieved
   B. Check the patient's vital signs
   C. Notify the prescriber
   D. Document the action

# Teaching Patients About Drug Therapy

## Objectives

*After studying this chapter you should be able to:*

1. Define the key terms important to teaching and learning.
2. Explain the role of communication in teaching and learning.
3. Use culturally sensitive body language and spoken language during the communication process.
4. Identify which type of learning activities belong to each domain of learning.
5. Explain the seven principles of adult education.
6. Identify when a patient is and is not actively participating in the teaching-learning process.
7. Describe any changes you would make to improve learning when teaching older adults.

## Key Terms

**active listening** (ĂK-tĭv LĬS-ĕn-ĭng) (p. 46) The type of listening in which your full attention is given to the speaker; you restate back to the person what he or she said and ask if your interpretation of what is said is what was actually meant.

**affective domain** (ĂF-fĕk-tĭv dō-MĂN) (p. 49) The learning area concerned with attitudes, values, interests, and adjustment.

**andragogy** (ĂN-drĕ-gō-jē) (p. 50) The study and principles of how adults learn.

**cognitive domain** (KŎG-nĭ-tĭv dō-MĂN) (p. 48) The learning area of intellectual ability.

**cultural sensitivity** (KŬL-chŭr-ŭl sĕn-sĭ-TĬV-ĭ-tē) (p. 46) Responding in an appropriate, accepting, and nonjudgmental way to cultural differences.

**learning** (LŬR-nĭng) (p. 45) The acquiring of new knowledge that results in a persistent change of behavior.

**pedagogy** (PĔD-ĕ-gō-jē) (p. 50) The study and principles of how children learn.

**psychomotor domain** (sī-kō-MŌ-tŭr dō-MĂN) (p. 48) The learning area concerned with motor skills.

**teaching** (TĒ-chĭng) (p. 45) The art and science of helping a person learn.

## OVERVIEW

◄ *e*-Learning Activity 3-1

As a nurse you will help patients understand information about their health, illness, or drug therapy on a daily basis. This process is called teaching, the art and science of helping a person learn. The people you teach include patients, patients' families or friends, the people with whom you work, your family, and your friends or neighbors. Usually you will teach adults rather than children. If the patient is a child, the parents, who are responsible for the child's care at home, may be the focus of your teaching efforts. However, whenever possible, the child also should be included in the teaching session. When teaching children, ensure that your method of teaching and use of terminology are appropriate for the child's age and developmental stage. Consult a pediatric textbook or a growth and development text for specific information on this topic.

Your patient may have more education than you do. He or she may have medical training. Try not to be intimidated by this issue. Even very educated people may have little or no knowledge about their own health care and drug therapy. For example, a critical care nurse may not be familiar with the thyroid replacement therapy drugs needed after his or her thyroid surgery.

### COMMUNICATION FOR TEACHING AND LEARNING

Learning means to acquire new knowledge that results in a persistent change of behavior. Teaching—helping a person to learn this new knowledge—requires good communication skills. The better your communication skills are, the more effective you will be as a teacher. During the teaching process you will send messages to and receive messages from your patient. In sending messages you provide the information to be learned. In receiving messages you get cues to help you know whether the patient is actually learning what you are teaching or if you need to change your teaching method. By using good communication to give and receive messages, you make the patient the center of your teaching efforts and tailor your teaching to meet individual learning needs. After all, you may think that you're teaching; but if you don't communicate well, no one may be learning.

Teaching and learning communication occur best when your patient knows and trusts you. This can be hard to accomplish in today's health care environment in which office visits and hospital stays are short. Trust occurs when a patient believes that you are professional and competent and that you genuinely care. Part of developing trust includes being courteous, kind, truthful, and sensitive to cultural differences and doing what you say you will do. (If the patient has previously had a bad health care experience, you may be helping him or her regain trust in the entire health care system.)

Remember that listening is the key to knowing whether what you are teaching actually is being learned. You must use active listening, in which you give your full attention to what the patient is saying. When actively listening, you restate what the patient says and ask whether you understand correctly what he or she is telling you. You must also let the patient take time to answer questions. Don't jump ahead and answer for the patient.

Effective communication is difficult in a noisy and busy hospital or when the patient doesn't feel well. It is also more difficult if you are not organized. To make patient teaching as effective as possible, carefully plan the time and place. Choose a time of day when the patient is not too busy with visitors, tired, sick, having a treatment, or experiencing side effects of drug therapy. Ensure that the room is quiet with few distractions. Turn off the television or radio, close the door or privacy curtain, and turn up the lights. Help the patient to a position of comfort. Sit or stand where you can best be seen and heard. Have all the necessary equipment, pamphlets, and other teaching devices with you and ready to use.

## CULTURAL SENSITIVITY AND COMMUNICATION

Cultural sensitivity means responding in an appropriate, accepting, and nonjudgmental way to cultural differences. It also includes avoiding words or actions that are offensive to other people. We usually think of race and ethnicity as the major parts of a person's culture; but culture includes many other aspects, including communication.

*Language* plays a role in culture. A patient's primary language may not be English, the dominant language of the United States. This can affect that patient's level of trust and safety. Trust is easier to earn when the health care worker speaks the patient's primary language, but this may not always be possible. In addition, language differences can pose a risk in health care settings if the patient and health care worker cannot understand one another. Speaking slowly and clearly can help a person with limited English understand the conversation better; however, speaking louder doesn't help.

It is important to recognize when a patient does not understand enough English to communicate needs or be able to participate in his or her own care. Many large hospitals have a variety of appropriate interpreters, including certified medical translators. Other communication aids include asking bilingual family members for assistance (with the patient's permission to share information with a family member) and using the language service offered by AT&T. This service, called *Language Line Services,* can be reached at (800)752-6096. For a fee Language Line Services translates more than 150 different languages. Using English–foreign language dictionaries or

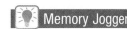

**Memory Jogger**

Always use active listening skills during patient teaching sessions.

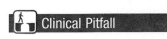

**Clinical Pitfall**

Language differences are *not* a reason to break a patient's confidentiality. The patient must give permission for a non–health care professional or family member to be involved in discussions of the patient's health status and personal information.

picture boards can also be helpful. Whatever method is used, be sure to maintain patient confidentiality.

Even when a patient's language is the primary language of the country, he or she may not be familiar with medical terminology. For example, most nonhealth care people are not familiar with the use of the word *void* for urination or the word *prophylactic* for prevention of health problems. For them, these words may have completely different meanings. In addition, when a disorder is more common within a specific culture, it may be referred to by a culturally specific word. Some examples include the term *sugar* for diabetes mellitus, *high blood* for high blood pressure, *free bleeder* for a blood-clotting problem, *catarrh* for cold, *consumption* for tuberculosis, and *dropsy* for generalized edema from heart failure. Use words that the patient understands and with which he or she is comfortable. When using any medical terminology, explain it in common, everyday words. Avoid medical jargon and abbreviations.

Language and communication also include body language and gestures. It may be tempting to use hand gestures and facial expressions to communicate with a patient who does not speak your language. Use this method cautiously to avoid appearing threatening. Do not get too close to the patient's face when gesturing and avoid touching his or her head. In addition, remember that some gestures that have harmless meanings in one country may have altogether different and insulting meanings in the society or culture of another country. A few examples of gestures or body language that can be misunderstood are as follows:

- In the United States direct eye contact indicates interest and respect. However, in many other cultures direct eye contact is considered disrespectful, intimidating, or rude (such as Asian, Hispanic, Islamic), especially when done by a woman.
- Head nodding may mean that a person is paying attention but does not indicate that he or she understands or agrees with what is being said.
- In the United States people often indicate the sign for "okay" by making a circle touching the thumb and forefinger together while extending the remaining fingers. In many other cultures this is seen as a rude or even obscene gesture.
- Pointing at a person with the index finger is considered impolite or threatening in most African cultures. Pointing with the chin or head is acceptable.
- The United States is a high-touch or "huggie" country, fond of handshakes, shoulder grips, back slaps, actual hugs, and many other forms of touching to convey understanding and comfort. Many other countries and cultures consider touching by strangers or anyone but family members to be disrespectful or threatening. In addition, other cultures may consider adult touching to be sexually provocative.
- Most Americans do not consider the hand that is used to communicate to be of special significance (that is, the right and left hands are considered equal). In some cultures, however, only the right hand is considered "clean." In these cultures the left hand is used to clean oneself after using the toilet, and this hand is always considered "dirty." People from these cultures would be insulted if anyone touched them, their food, their medications, or their belongings with the left hand.
- Modesty is a form of communication and varies in degree and in the definition of acceptable behavior, particularly for women, from culture to culture.

The use of silence also varies with culture. In the United States silence is often associated with negative issues such as disagreement or misunderstanding. Other cultures (such as American Indians) may use silence as a sign of agreement with or respect for the speaker. Silence may also indicate that the person is taking the time to give a statement thoughtful consideration. A person whose native language is not English may need time to translate your question or statement and formulate a response. Allow time for silence before assuming that the person did not hear or understand what was said.

 **Memory Jogger**

Avoid medical jargon and abbreviations when talking with patients and explain any medical terms or words carefully.

 **Memory Jogger**

When caring for a person from a culture that is unfamiliar to you, keep hand gestures, touching, and skin exposure to a minimum.

 **Clinical Pitfall**

Do not assume that silence indicates disagreement or misunderstanding and do not interrupt the patient's silent periods.

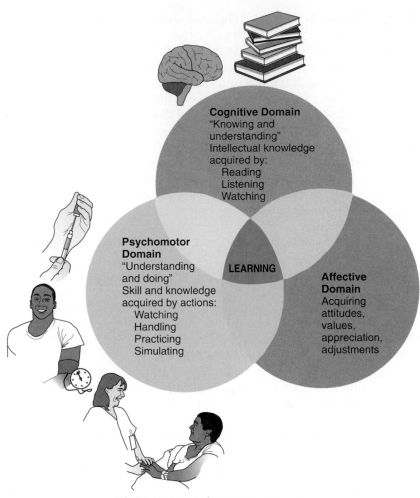

**FIGURE 3-1** The three domains of learning.

## DOMAINS OF LEARNING

Learning is divided into three areas or domains: cognitive, psychomotor, and affective (Figure 3-1). These three domains correspond to areas of the brain where each type of learning occurs or is stored. A person usually has one domain that is most comfortable as a type of learning but also is able to use the other domains. When teaching patients you will be most involved in the cognitive and psychomotor domains, but you must be aware of the affective domain. The most effective learning makes use of all three domains, although not necessarily to the same degree. Box 3-1 lists examples of actions or behaviors that demonstrate learning within the three domains.

The **cognitive domain** is the intellectual learning area. Basic knowledge is learned and understood in this domain. The types of activities used to teach topics or content in the cognitive domain are well defined. Examples of patient teaching that belong in the cognitive domain include:

- How drugs work.
- Why a patient is taking a specific drug.
- Instructions for taking a drug properly.

The **psychomotor domain** is concerned with motor skills or activities. This domain is just as important for health care as the cognitive domain and often involves *applying* knowledge from the cognitive domain. Manual dexterity works with intellectual understanding of a physical task to create a skill. Examples of the types of patient teaching that belong in the psychomotor domain include:

Box 3-1    Examples of Learning in the Different Domains

The cognitive domain is focused on intellectual knowledge and includes:
- Knowing how drugs work.
- Explaining why a specific drug is needed.
- Listing drug side effects
- Describing when to call the prescriber.
- Knowing when to adjust insulin dosage based on blood glucose levels.

The psychomotor domain is focused on skill activities and includes:
- Taking a pulse.
- Drawing up drugs into a syringe.
- Self-injecting parenteral drugs.
- Applying transdermal patches.
- Mixing two different types of insulin in the same syringe.
- Applying eye drops

The affective domain helps the patient value learning about health care and drug therapy and includes:
- Testing blood glucose levels daily on awakening, before meals, and at bedtime.
- Keeping a diary of daily blood pressure measurements and daily weights.
- Teaching another person a specific skill.
- Walking for 30 minutes daily to maintain body weight and muscle tone.

- Taking a pulse.
- Drawing up drugs into a syringe.
- Self-injecting parenteral drugs.

The **affective domain** is concerned with attitudes, values, interests, appreciation, and adjustment. The major use of this domain in patient teaching is to help the patient value information on health care and drug therapy. Therefore motivation is part of the affective domain. The affective domain is more personal than the other domains, and affective learning is a little harder to determine, but this type may be the longest-lasting form of learning. Examples that demonstrate learning in the affective domain include consistent behaviors on the part of the learner, showing that what was learned is valued. (Remember, just because a patient knows how and when to take a drug or perform a skill does not mean that he or she will actually do it!) Some examples are:
- Testing blood glucose levels daily on awakening, before meals, and at bedtime.
- Keeping a diary of daily blood pressure measurements and daily weights.
- Teaching another person a specific skill.

## TEACHING AND LEARNING

Some of your teaching will be unplanned and very informal. Unexpected "teachable moments" often occur while you are performing another task. For example, while you are changing a dressing or giving a bath, the patient may ask a question about his or her drug therapy or health promotion strategy. Be sure to take advantage of these moments because patient interest usually means that the patient is motivated and ready to learn. At other times you will teach more formally with a written plan and outcome goals. The whole point of any type of teaching is for someone to learn something new.

One way to know if a person has learned what was taught is to observe the person using the new knowledge. For example, suppose that you taught a nursing assistant that the best way to prevent the spread of infection from person to person is good hand washing. How can you check whether learning occurred? One way is to ask, "What is the best way to prevent spread of infection from one person to another?" The nursing assistant should answer "good hand washing" (an example of learning in the cognitive domain). A better way is to see the nursing assistant washing his or her hands before touching a patient or the patient's belongings (an example of learning in the psychomotor domain). When the nursing assistant consistently uses good hand washing before touching any patient or the patient's belongings, he or she is demonstrating learning that also is part of the affective domain, indicating that the nursing assistant values this behavior.

Patient teaching can be done in a hospital or an outpatient setting, clinic, or provider's office. In most cases the nurse conducts patient teaching. However, sometimes you will work with other health care professionals such as physicians, nutritionists, pharmacists and social workers to provide the best information to your patient. Whether you teach alone or in a group, you must know and use the principles of adult learning discussed in the following paragraphs.

**⊖-Learning Activity 3-2 ▶**

## PRINCIPLES OF ADULT LEARNING: PATIENT TEACHING

Adults and children learn differently and have different expectations when learning. Box 3-2 lists some of the characteristics and expectations of adult learners. **Andragogy** is the study of how adults learn and the application of the principles of adult learning. This concept differs from **pedagogy,** which is the study of how children learn. Whether you are teaching adults or teaching children, learning is more likely to occur if you focus on the learner.

The principles of learning (and teaching) come from research done within childhood education. These principles have been modified for use with adults. Some principles sound like common sense, and you may already use them. Others may be less obvious but are helpful tips when used correctly.

Seven major principles of learning form the basis of successful teaching of adults (Box 3-3). These principles were first identified by Malcolm Knowles who examined

---

**Box 3-2** Adult Learner Characteristics and Expectations

**CHARACTERISTICS**
The adult:
- Understands why learning is necessary in a specific situation.
- Wants or chooses to learn the information being taught.
- Takes an active part in the learning experience.
- Takes responsibility for learning.
- Wants to know how and if he or she is progressing in his learning.
- Feels a sense of accomplishment when learning has taken place.

**EXPECTATIONS**
The adult expects that:
- Teaching will occur in a setting that promotes learning.
- The information being taught applies directly to his or her situation and needs.
- The teacher knows the content being taught.
- The teacher enjoys the content and enjoys teaching.
- The teacher will use the right method to teach the content.

---

**Box 3-3** Principles for Adult Learning

Learning occurs best when:
- The adult feels a need to know the information.
- Teaching starts with what the learner already knows and progresses to what he or she does not know.
- Simple concepts are presented before complex concepts.
- The adult actively participates in the teaching-learning process.
- A new skill is practiced.
- The information, skill, or behavior is reinforced.
- Feedback is fast, and mistakes or misconceptions are corrected early.

Adapted from Knowles, M. (1980). *The modern practice of adult education.* New York: Cambridge.

the methods used by people and corporations who taught adults new knowledge and skills. The same principles apply whether you teach one patient or a group.

## BELIEVE IN THE NEED TO KNOW

Learning occurs best when the adult believes that information being taught is necessary or useful. This principle means that the patient must want to learn the information that you are teaching. Part of teaching is to motivate the person to want to learn the information. For example, motivation to learn is very high in parachute packing class—everyone pays attention. This is because the person taking sky-diving lessons is required to pack his or her own parachute and use it when jumping out of an airplane. Clearly the learner believes that knowing the right way to pack a parachute is very important.

Motivating a patient to want to learn can be more difficult and requires trust. During motivation focus on the positive aspects of the new knowledge or skill. Scaring a patient with possible negative outcomes is not true motivation. Helping patients see the benefits of sticking to drug therapy is more helpful than scaring them with the costs of not sticking to it. For example, a scare tactic is telling a patient that, if she doesn't take her antidiabetic drug, a foot or leg may have to be amputated. Scaring people does not always make them want to learn. In fact, it can have the opposite effect, and may make them want to forget about health problems.

One way to motivate is to ask the patient for any questions before you begin teaching. Giving information relevant to the first question can increase the patient's interest in the topic, trust in you, and motivation to learn.

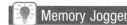

**Memory Jogger**

To motivate a patient to want to learn about drug therapy, stress the positive aspects of the therapy.

## START WITH THE KNOWN BEFORE MOVING TO THE UNKNOWN

Learning occurs best when the teacher starts with what the learner already knows and progresses to what the learner does not yet know. Starting with what is more familiar to a person makes it easier to relate to the new information and promotes the learner's confidence. In addition, you do not waste time reteaching something the patient already knows. Instead you can use that time to teach more new information.

Before beginning any lesson, determine what the patient already knows about the health problem and drug therapy. Also ask what concerns the patient most about his or her specific health problem and the prescribed drugs.

Because the adult learner is most interested in information that applies directly to his or her situation, ask what the patient wants to learn. For example, if you have a male patient beginning antihypertensive drug therapy, ask him what he knows about high blood pressure. If he tells you that his father had high blood pressure and died of a stroke, he may already understand that high blood pressure should be treated. Ask him how blood pressure becomes high. He may already know; if he doesn't, you can tell him that having the blood vessels constrict and get narrow is the most common cause of high blood pressure. Then, when you explain that the prescribed drug will help his blood vessels relax and dilate, he is more likely to understand how that will lower his blood pressure.

Determining what the patient already knows and doesn't know is important, regardless of his or her education level. Another nurse who works in a different specialty might not know about a newly prescribed drug used often in your area; the nurse may be able to use the medical terminology correctly but may need as much information about the drug as any other patient.

**Memory Jogger**

When starting a patient teaching session, ask what the patient already knows about the health problem and its treatment.

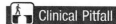

**Clinical Pitfall**

Never assume that a highly educated patient does not need to be taught about the prescribed drug therapy.

## LEARNING GOES FROM THE SIMPLE TO THE COMPLEX

Learning occurs best when simple concepts are presented before complex concepts. This principle is related to starting with what is known before trying to teach what the patient doesn't know.

To go from simple to complex, keep your language simple. Most patients are not used to medical terms for disease, treatments, body functions, or body parts. Even a person who has a great deal of education (for example, a lawyer or an

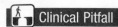

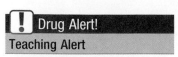

engineer) may not know the word *hypercortisolism* or the health problem *Cushing's disease*. You also must decide what the patient does not need to know. For example, a hypertensive patient may not know the term *hypertension*. Does the patient need to know that term? Or is it enough to know that his or her blood pressure is too high?

Before you begin to teach, you may have to "interpret" what the prescriber has said. Patients often look to the nurse for this type of help. Many feel most free to ask questions of the nurse; and they expect honest, understandable answers.

Be very clear in your directions for drug use. There are many sad and funny stories about mistakes made by patients who were not told clearly about their drug therapy. For example, patients have been known to swallow rectal suppositories because they were merely told to "take" the drug. At the very least the drug was not effective. At worst it may have caused harm when taken incorrectly.

Important information about drug therapy that must be given clearly includes:
- The drug name.
- The purpose of the drug (what is the health problem being treated).
- How the drug works.
- Exactly how to take the drug (what route, what dose, how many, how often).
- Any special instructions (for example, take on an empty stomach, do not take with milk).
- What the expected response(s) (intended action) is.
- What side effects may occur.
- What adverse effects may occur.
- When to call the prescriber.

## ACTIVE PARTICIPATION IS NEEDED

Learning occurs best when the learner actively participates in the teaching-learning process. Sometimes a patient may not want to be an active participant and may just want you to "pour in" the information or give it to someone else. Such a patient may say, "Tell my daughter about this because she is the one who will be giving me the drug," or "My wife always takes care of those things." Whoever is the learner, whether it is the patient or someone else, needs to be active in learning.

You can pick up clues about how active the person is in the learning process from his or her face, the questions asked (or not asked), the body language used, and the response to your questions. The learner who is engaged in the teaching-learning process will:
- Watch your face and mouth (if this is culturally acceptable for him or her).
- Ask questions.
- Repeat what you say.
- Sit forward.
- Stay focused on you.
- Write things down.
- Answer questions with phrases or complete sentences.

The learner who is not taking an active role will:
- Look away from you.
- Check the door or clock often.
- Watch television.
- Push the chair away from you or lower the head of the bed.
- Not respond to questions.

## PRACTICE MAKES PERFECT

Learning occurs best when a new skill is practiced. This point is especially true when an activity or skill is involved. Break any skill down into its basic parts. Demonstrate each part separately. Have the patient (or other learner) demonstrate each part back to you (known as a *return demonstration*). Have him or her work with one skill part until it is mastered before moving on to the next part.

## REINFORCE LEARNING

Learning occurs best when the information, skill, or behavior is reinforced. Part of this principle involves practice. It also means providing more than one reminder of what was learned. The more senses that are stimulated during teaching and learning, the more the learner will remember the information. For example, a female patient needs to take the drug cyclosporine for the rest of her life. You know that mixing this oral drug correctly is important for its effectiveness. You may first show the patient a video about how to mix and take the drug. Second, correctly demonstrate these tasks and have her demonstrate them back to you. Give her a colored pamphlet or video (if available) to take home. The pamphlet uses words and pictures to show the exact steps for this task. Videos show the actual skill. Some patients may even want an audio recording of your voice as you are teaching. Encourage this behavior. Using these techniques stimulates several of the patient's senses and provides multiple reinforcement opportunities.

Each patient learns in an individual way. One patient may learn best by hearing information, and another may learn best by seeing or reading the information. Because patients may not know their learning styles, combining several teaching methods is more likely to be successful. Learning is enhanced when actual equipment is handled, success is rewarded, and errors are corrected quickly.

 **Memory Jogger**

The more senses that are stimulated during teaching and learning, the more likely it is that the information will be remembered.

## PROVIDE EARLY FEEDBACK AND CORRECTIONS

Learning occurs best when feedback is fast and mistakes or misconceptions are corrected early. Remember that it is hard to "unlearn" something that was thoroughly learned but was incorrect. Learners like to feel a sense of accomplishment when they have learned a new skill or concept. Immediately after teaching a section, ask the patient to repeat what you have just said. Then ask him or her to put the information into his or her own words. This is also a good time to ask what the patient may have heard about the topic from friends, television, or the Internet. You can use this time to separate facts from "wives' tales."

When teaching a patient, do not be afraid to correct misconceptions or mistakes in performing a skill, but do so kindly and gently. Try to say something positive at the same time such as, "You did a really good job wiping the vial with alcohol; now let's work on being a little more careful not to touch the needle."

 **Memory Jogger**

Give feedback early and often to correct mistakes. Provide positive reinforcement.

 ◄ ⓔ-Learning Activity 3-3

## LIFE SPAN CONSIDERATIONS

Communicating with and teaching older adults may require special considerations. In addition to physiologic differences (discussed in Chapter 1), behavior and views also change as a person ages. Older people have had more life experiences that have contributed to their views and values (good and bad). It is important to remember not to prejudge a person by age. Not all older people have hearing or vision problems, although many do. Some are frugal and try to save money by not taking prescribed drugs as often as they should, but not all of them think this way. Remember that an older person is an individual. The only way to know a person's beliefs and views on drug therapy is to ask.

Many older adults are resentful when strangers call them by their first name rather than by their last name and title. Until invited to call any patient by his or her first name, always address the person by the last name and title (for example, Miss Purple, Mr. Brown, Mrs. Green, Dr. Blue, Rev. Yellow). If you are aware of the patient's nationality and are familiar with the correct terminology, use the accepted form of address to show respect (such as Señor, Señora, Monsieur, Madame). Avoid referring to a patient of any age as "sweetie" or "honey."

Many older adults are prescribed multiple drugs, a practice termed *polypharmacy*. They may not have been taught when and how to take each drug, what effects to

**Clinical Pitfall**

Do not prejudge any individual because of age. Not every older person has hearing or vision problems.

 **Memory Jogger**

Until invited to call any patient by his or her first name, always address the person by the last name and title (for example, Miss Purple, Mr. Brown, Mrs. Green, Dr. Blue, Rev. Yellow).

Box 3-4    Tips for Teaching Older Adults

- Sit in an area with good lighting.
- Try to find a place where it is quiet and there are few distractions.
- Sit facing the patient so he or she can see your face and mouth.
- If needed, make sure that the patient wears glasses, contacts, or a hearing device during the teaching time.
- If the patient sees better with one eye or hears better with one ear, sit on the side that has the better vision or hearing.
- Get the patient's attention before you start teaching.
- Use a normal tone of voice for the patient who has a vision problem but has normal hearing.
- Use language and terminology with which the patient is comfortable.
- Use a certified interpreter if language is a barrier.
- Speak slowly and clearly.
- Take your time; do not hurry the patient.
- Give the patient several opportunities to ask questions.
- Have the patient repeat your statements (using his or her own words) rather than just nodding yes.
- Rephrase sentences and repeat information to aid in understanding.
- If there is a skill to learn, show the patient how to perform it and then have the patient demonstrate the skill back to you.
- When possible, have the patient's spouse or other family member be a part of the teaching session.
- When possible, repeat the teaching daily. At the beginning of each session, have the patient tell you what he or she learned previously before you repeat the information.
- Teach an older adult with vision problems who is taking more than one drug ways to identify different drugs such as placing a rubber band around one drug bottle; marking another bottle with a large, brightly colored symbol; or keeping different drugs in different drawers or on different shelves.
- Have an older adult patient tell you in his or her own words about each drug prescribed (how much and when to take it, side effects, and when to call the prescriber).
- Tell an older patient to take a forgotten drug dose as soon as it is remembered and to take the next scheduled dose as usual (unless the missed dose is remembered within 4 hours of the next scheduled dose). If he or she remembers the forgotten dose within 4 hours of the next scheduled dose, the forgotten dose should be skipped and the next dose taken on schedule.
- Teach an older patient who is discontinuing an old drug and starting a new one to discard the old drug as instructed or give it to the pharmacist to discard so there less chance of accidentally taking the discontinued drug.
- If an older adult living at home has prescriptions for more than one drug, make a chart in large print for him or her that outlines when to take each drug, the exact dose of each drug (including number of tablets or capsules), special instructions (such as "take with food," or "drink a full glass of water"), possible side effects, what to do if a dose is missed, and when to call the prescriber.
- Determine whether the use of a weekly pill dispenser or organizer may help an individual older adult manage his or her daily drugs safely.

expect, and when to notify the prescriber. Older adults can learn, but you may need to take more time and care when teaching about the drugs, especially if the patient is hard of hearing or does not see well. Often older adults may not ask questions of a prescriber or nurse because questioning the health care professional is not part of their upbringing. They may become confused about their drugs and be ashamed to ask questions. Box 3-4 lists many tips to use to enhance learning for an older adult.

## Get Ready for Practice!

### Key Points

- Teaching is more effective, and learning is more likely to occur if the teacher focuses on the learner.
- Adjust the environment and timing of teaching sessions to make them as quiet, private, and free of distractions as possible.
- Ask the patient what concerns him or her most about his or her specific health problem and about the prescribed drugs.
- Never assume that a highly educated patient, including a health care professional, does not need to be taught about his or her drug therapy.
- Do not assume that silence indicates disagreement or misunderstanding and do not answer for patients or interrupt them.
- Break down tasks or information to be learned into simple steps and teach one step at a time.
- Be very clear in your directions for how and when to take a drug.
- Watch your patient's eye contact, body language, the questions asked, and the responses to your questions during teaching to determine whether he or she is actively participating.
- Have the patient work with one skill part at a time and practice until it is mastered; then move on to the next skill part.
- Learning is enhanced when actual equipment is handled, success is rewarded, and errors are corrected quickly.
- Do not be afraid to correct a patient's misconceptions or skill mistakes, but do so kindly and gently, always including praise for something that is correct.

### Additional Learning Resources

**evolve** Go to your Evolve website (http://evolve.elsevier.com/Workman/pharmacology/) for the following FREE learning resources:
- eLearning Activities
- Animations
- Video Clips
- Interactive Review Questions
- Audio Key Points
- Audio Glossary
- Audio Glossary—Spanish-English
- Drug Dosage Calculators
- Patient Teaching Handouts

**SG** Go to your Study Guide for additional learning activities to help you master this chapter content.

### Review Questions

1. How does andragogy differ from pedagogy?
   A. Andragogy is the study of men, and pedagogy is the study of women.
   B. Andragogy is the science of learning, and pedagogy is the science of teaching.
   C. Pedagogy is the science of learning, and andragogy is the science of teaching.
   D. Pedagogy is the teaching of children, and andragogy is the teaching of adults.

2. Which cue best indicates to you that the patient is actively trying to learn what is being taught?
   A. The patient is awake.
   B. The spouse is answering for the patient.
   C. The patient restates what you said in his or her own words.
   D. You sit in a chair to be physically at the same level with the patient.

3. You speak only English and work in a facility that does not have access to a translator. What is your best method of communication with a non-English speaking woman who is having an abortion in this facility?
   A. Do nothing; no communication is needed.
   B. Ask her bilingual teenage daughter to translate for her.
   C. Use the AT&T Language Line Services with an anonymous interpreter.
   D. Attempt to use hand gestures and facial expressions to tell her what is happening.

4. Which patient actions indicate learning in the affective domain? (Select all that apply.)
   A. Believing that taking an antibiotic will cure an infection
   B. Understanding the need to take the entire antibiotic prescribed for a bladder infection even though the symptoms are gone after just two doses
   C. Drinking a full glass of water when taking a diuretic
   D. Inserting a vaginal suppository as far back as possible into the vagina
   E. Accepting that he or she has high blood pressure
   F. Correctly using a spacer with an aerosol inhaler

5. Which principle of adult learning are you using when giving the patient, who is severely allergic to bee stings, an empty Epi-Pen (for self-injection of adrenalin) to assemble after the patient has been shown a video about it?
   A. Reinforcing learning
   B. Motivating the patient to learn
   C. Correcting misinformation or mistakes
   D. Starting with the known before moving to the unknown

6. Which actions during a patient teaching session indicate to you that the patient is actively participating in the teaching-learning process? (Select all that apply.)
   A. Smiling at you
   B. Asking to touch the insulin syringe
   C. Telling you that his wife takes charge of all the health care problems at home
   D. Watching a soap opera during the session
   E. Asking you to slow down so he can write the important points in a notebook
   F. Telling you that he is afraid he will lose his sight from diabetes just like his mother did

7. An 88-year-old patient is to be discharged from the hospital with a variety of drugs. How can you help the patient take the drugs safely at home?
   A. Include the patient's children in discussions regarding proper drug administration.
   B. Have the patient practice opening and closing the drug containers over and over again.
   C. Give the patient a pamphlet outlining the actions, side effects, and doses of all prescribed drugs.
   D. Make a chart for the patient, showing exactly which drugs are to be taken at different times during the day.

## Critical Thinking Activities

You are teaching a 16-year-old girl how to self-administer insulin. This is the second teaching session, and she can draw up the correct amount and maintain sterility. She has not been able to actually inject the needle into her skin, saying, "It doesn't hurt, but I just can't stand to push that needle in." She has not had any difficulty when her mother or the nurse has injected the insulin.

1. What should your immediate response be?

2. What modifications in your teaching technique can you make?

3. Is it critical that the patient learn to inject herself at this session?

4. Is there any type of adaptation that can help with this problem?

# Medical Systems of Weights and Measures

evolve

## Objectives

*After studying this chapter you should be able to:*

1. Define common units of measure for liquids and solids.
2. Convert from the household system of measurement to the metric system of measurement.
3. Solve dosage problems using the household system.
4. Identify the three basic units of measure in the metric system.
5. Using a prefix and a root word, identify the unit of measure.
6. Convert milliliters to liters; convert liters to milliliters.
7. Convert ounces and pounds to grams and kilograms.
8. Solve dosage problems using the metric system.
9. Solve drug calculation problems using units.

## Key Terms

**centigrade or Celsius** (SĚN-tĭ-grād, SĚL-sē-ŭs) (p. 58) Metric or hospital scale of temperature measurement based on 100. Zero (0) degrees is the freezing point of water, and 100° is the boiling point of water. Normal human body temperature ranges between 36.1° and 37.8°.

**equivalent** (ē-KWĬV-ĕ-lĕnt) (p. 57) To be equal in amount or to have equal value.

**Fahrenheit** (FĂR-ĕn-hīt) (p. 58) System of temperature measurement used in the United States in which the freezing point of water is 32° above zero and the boiling point of water is 212°. Normal human body temperature ranges between 97° and 100°.

**gram (g)** (GRĂM) (p. 60) The basic metric unit for measurement of weight.

**liter (L)** (LĒ-tŭr) (p. 60) The basic metric unit for measurement of liquids.

**meter (m)** (MĒ-tŭr) (p. 60) The basic metric unit for measurement of length or distance.

◀ⓔ-Learning Activity 4-1

## OVERVIEW

Systems of weights and measures were invented so there could be standard ways of comparing two or more objects for size, strength, function, and condition. The first measuring system discussed in this chapter is the one used to check a patient's temperature. All systems that follow are used in prescribing drugs. For solving the conversion problems in this chapter, you will need to apply the math principles presented in Chapter 5, including using proportions.

For the most part, drugs are measured by weight (for example, an extra-strength Tylenol tablet contains 500 mg of drug) or liquid volume (5 mL or 1 tsp of Benadryl). For each measuring system, this chapter identifies which units are used for *dry weights* and which are used for *liquids*. After each system is presented, there will be practice problems to work so you can see exactly how each system is used.

To convert from one system to another, values that are equal to each other, known as **equivalents,** are used. You need to understand and either memorize the equivalents in each system or carry a conversion card with you so you can convert from one system to another quickly and easily. It is a good idea to make up your own conversion card with equivalents listed so you can take it with you to the clinical area. If you are still not sure of the conversions, look them up in a drug reference guide or ask for help. As the United States moves closer to accepting the metric system for all weights and measures, there will be less need to learn the other systems or memorize the conversions. For now, understanding each system and being able to make conversions are still necessary.

## MEASURING SYSTEMS

### TEMPERATURE: FAHRENHEIT AND CELSIUS

When measuring temperature, the symbol ° is used in place of the word "degree." Many hospitals use the metric system for measuring temperature (Celsius [C]), and other health care settings use the Fahrenheit [F] system. Health care workers must be familiar with both systems of measurement. You are probably familiar with the Fahrenheit system since it is used most often for temperature measurement in American culture. In the Fahrenheit system the freezing point of water is 32° above zero, and the boiling point of water is 212°. The normal human body temperature ranges between 97° and 100°. The Centigrade or Celsius is based on the number 100. Zero (0) ° is set as the freezing point of water, and 100° is used for the boiling point of water. Normal human body temperature ranges between 36.1° and 37.8°.

Digital thermometers are often used to check body temperature and can be set for either system. For learning purposes, though, it is helpful to picture the old mercury thermometers such as the one shown in Figure 4-1. As you can see in the figure, there is a big difference in ranges between Centigrade (Celsius) and Fahrenheit temperatures. To change from one system to another, use the following two equations or a conversion chart (available in most hospital units). It is often necessary to convert because patients usually report their temperatures from home using a thermometer with a Fahrenheit scale.

### Equation 1: Fahrenheit to Centigrade

$$(\text{Fahrenheit temperature} - 32) \times \frac{5}{9} = \text{Degrees Centigrade}$$

First, subtract 32° from 102° (102° − 32°) for an answer of 70 and plug that number into the formula:

$$70 \times \frac{5}{9}$$

Multiply 70 by 5, which equals 350. Divide 350 by 9, which equals 38.88°.

If the answer has more than one decimal place, round to the nearest tenth of a degree (for example, 38.9°, not 38.88°).

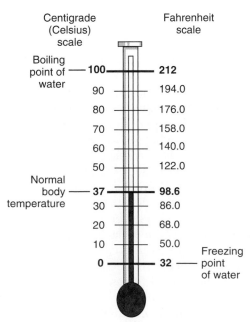

**FIGURE 4-1** Comparing Centigrade to Fahrenheit values with a mercury thermometer.

### Equation 2: Centigrade to Fahrenheit

$$(\text{Centigrade temperature}) \times \frac{9}{5} + 32 = \text{Degrees Fahrenheit}$$

Place the centigrade temperature of 41° C into the formula:

$$41 \times \frac{9}{5} + 32$$

Multiply 41 by 9, which equals 369. Divide 369 by 5, which equals 73.8. Add 32, which makes the answer 105.8.

If the answer has more than one decimal place, round to the nearest tenth of a degree (for example, 100.6°, not 100.59°).

## HOUSEHOLD SYSTEM FOR LIQUID AND DRY MEASUREMENTS

You have probably cooked at one time or another and have had to measure ingredients for a recipe. This same household system is the one most used by patients when they are taking *liquid* drugs at home.

The household system uses drops (gtts), teaspoons (tsp), tablespoons (Tbs), ounces (oz), and cups (c) to measure liquids. Note that a liquid ounce is *not* equal to a dry ounce such as flour. In cooking, liquid ounces are measured in a one-piece measuring cup (often made of glass), and dry ounces are measured in nested cups. In health care liquid drugs have their own special measuring tools. Table 4-1 lists household abbreviations and equivalents.

 **Try This!**

**TT-1**  Convert the Fahrenheit temperature to Centigrade and the Centigrade temperature to Fahrenheit.

a.  101.4° F = _____ ° C

b.  97° F = _____ ° C

c.  103.8° F = _____ ° C

d.  40° C = _____ ° F

e.  35° C = _____ ° F

f.  39.2° C = _____ ° F

Answers are at the end of this chapter.

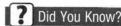 **Did You Know?**

Tableware teaspoons and tablespoons used for eating are only names that indicate that the two spoon types are different in size. They do not reflect the actual liquid amount that either one can hold, and they do not hold the same volume from one brand of tableware to another.

**Table 4-1   Abbreviations and Equivalents for the Household System of Measure**

| ABBREVIATION | MEANING | EQUIVALENT |
|---|---|---|
| **DRY MEASURE (SMALLEST TO LARGEST)** | | |
| oz | Ounce | 16 oz = 1 lb |
| lb | Pound | 1 lb = 16 oz |
| **LIQUID MEASURE (SMALLEST TO LARGEST)** | | |
| gtts | Drops | 60 gtts = 1 tsp |
| tsp | Teaspoon | 3 tsp = 1 Tbs |
| tbs | Tablespoon | 2 Tbs = 1 oz |
| fl oz | Fluid ounces | 8 oz = 1 c |
| | | 16 oz = 1 pt |
| | | 32 oz = 1 qt |
| | | 64 oz = ½ gal |
| | | 128 oz = 1 gal |
| c | Cup | 2 c = 1 p |
| | | 4 c = 1 qt |
| | | 8 c = ½ gal |
| | | 16 c = 1 gal |
| pt | Pint | 2 pts = 1 qt |
| | | 4 pts = ½ gal |
| | | 8 pts = 1 gal |
| qt | Quart | 4 qts = 1 gal |
| gal | Gallon | 1 gal = 4 qts |
| **LENGTH (SMALLEST TO LARGEST)** | | |
| in | Inch | 12 in = 1 ft |
| ft | Foot | 3 ft = 1 yd |
| | | 5280 ft = 1 mile |
| yd | Yard | 1 yd = 3 ft |
| | | 1760 yds = 1 mile |

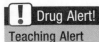

**Drug Alert!**

**Teaching Alert**

Teach patients who are taking liquid drugs to buy and use only measuring tools that are designed and calibrated for liquid drugs. Remind them *never* to use tableware spoons to measure liquid drugs.

**Drug Alert!**

**Administration Alert**

Be sure that the patient has a good swallow reflex before administering a liquid drug using an oral syringe, dropper, small medicine cup, or hollow-handle spoon.

**Drug Alert!**

**Administration Alert**

When using a dropper to administer liquid drugs, place it into the side of the patient's mouth rather than in the middle, where it can move down the throat too quickly and cause choking.

**Drug Alert!**

**Administration Alert**

Always double check the amount of drug in any measuring device against the amount ordered to prevent giving an overdose.

**Try This!**

**TT-2** Calculate the response in teaspoons or drops. (NOTE: "How to" math steps for conversion of *want* versus *have* problems are in Chapter 5.)

a. *Want* ampicillin 500 mg; *Have* ampicillin 250 mg/tsp

b. *Want* guaifenesin 50 mg; *Have* guaifenesin 100 mg/60 gtts

c. *Want* milk of magnesia 1 Tbs; *Have* milk of magnesia 1 tsp

Answers are at the end of this chapter.

The only *dry* measures used in the household system for health care purposes are ounces and pounds. Patients usually report their weight in pounds (lb). The reported weight often must be converted to kilograms (kg) in the hospital or other health care setting.

Larger liquid household measures include the pint, quart, and gallon. These larger measures will be discussed later in the chapter under the metric system.

Patients often use the teaspoons and tablespoons from tableware to measure liquid drugs. However, these spoons are *not* accurate, and patients should be instructed *not* to use them to measure drugs. Measuring-spoon sets are more accurate than tableware, but it is best to use measuring tools that are designed and *calibrated* (marked in accurate units) for liquid drugs. These include the dropper, oral syringe, hollow-handle spoon, and small medicine cup and (see Figure 2-2 in Chapter 2). All of these can be purchased in any pharmacy or drug store and even in many grocery stores.

We will talk about each of these in turn. Becoming familiar with them will help you teach patients how to take and give oral liquid drugs safely. Many of these items can deliver liquid drugs quickly into the mouth, which may be a choking hazard. Be sure that the person who is swallowing the liquid drug has a good swallow reflex before using these items.

*Droppers* are marked in both teaspoons and milliliters (mL) (metric). Check the drug order carefully to determine which measurement is correct. Place the dropper into the side of the patient's mouth so the liquid can slide with more control down the throat to prevent choking or *aspiration* (inhaling something into the lungs).

The most common device for measuring oral drugs in the hospital is the *oral syringe* (similar to a dropper). Oral syringes are marked in both teaspoons and milliliters. The rubber stopper is small enough to be aspirated (inhaled) into the lungs, so be sure to remove the stopper before you attempt to use the syringe.

*Hollow-handle spoons* are useful for giving small doses between 1 and 2 tsp (5 to 10 mL). Mark the desired dose with your finger and hold the spoon at eye level to ensure that the dose you pour is accurate. When administering the drug to the patient, allow enough time to ensure that all the drug in the handle is in the patient's mouth before disposing of the spoon.

*Medicine cups* are useful to measure and give liquid doses from 1 tsp to 1 oz. The cup is marked around its sides in teaspoons, tablespoons, and ounces. Note that the ounce is marked "FL OZ" to indicate that this cup is for liquids only. The other marks indicate the liquid unit of the metric system: the milliliter (mL).

To use the cup accurately, fill while holding it at eye level. Either place the cup on a table and bend to look straight at the mark or hold it up to your eyes as you fill it (see Figure 2-3 in Chapter 2). Looking down at the mark or from an angle will result in an inaccurate dose.

All of the devices described previously are small. They are meant to administer small doses of drugs. When using a larger device for small doses, it is easy to measure out too much drug and give an overdose.

## METRIC SYSTEM

Most of the world uses the metric system for all types of measuring. It is the most used system worldwide for drug prescriptions because it is accurate even in small doses. The metric system is based on the number 10 and uses the decimal system (multiples of ten). (See Chapter 5 for a review of decimals.) In giving drugs, only a few of the possible metric measurements are used. For a more complete discussion of the metric system, consult a mathematics text. This system is not difficult, and you *can* learn it!

### Metric Basics

The three basic units of the metric system are the **meter** (length), the **liter** (liquid), and the **gram** (weight). Each of these three words forms the *root* (that part or

| Box **4-1** | Metric Equivalents | | |
|---|---|---|---|

**DRY**

1 kg = 1000 g

1 g = 1000 mg

    = $\frac{1}{1000}$ kg

1 mg = $\frac{1}{1000}$ g

**LIQUID**

1 L = 1000 mL

1 mL = $\frac{1}{1000}$ L

**LENGTH**

1 m (meter) = 100 cm

    = 1000 mm

1 cm = 10 mm

    = $\frac{1}{100}$ meter

1 mm = $\frac{1}{10}$ cm

    = $\frac{1}{1000}$ meter

parts of a multiple-part word that indicates the basic meaning) of every metric measuring unit. Always look for these root words in each metric measurement. They indicate whether you are measuring a length, a liquid volume, or a weight. For example:

- Your height can be measured in either inches or centi*meters.*
- Your weight can be measured in pounds or kilo*grams.*
- Penicillin is prescribed in 250-milli*gram tablets.*
- A household quart is slightly less than a *liter.*

Box 4-1 lists basic metric equivalents.

Just as in decimals, there are measurements for *less than* and *more than* the basic unit. These descriptive words are called *prefixes* because they come before the root of a word. Which prefix is attached to the root explains how much larger or smaller each unit is in relation to the basic unit. For example, weight can be written in *kilo*grams, in which a kilogram is 1000 times heavier or *larger* than a gram. Drugs are often prescribed using the *milli*gram, which is 1000 times *smaller* than a gram. See Table 4-2 for a list of the prefixes most commonly used in health care, listed from large to small.

### Metric Abbreviations

The basic metric unit abbreviations are meter (m), liter (L), and gram (g). Note that the "L" for liter is capitalized to avoid confusion with other abbreviations.

Every health care workplace has a list of accepted abbreviations for drugs. Be sure to use only these abbreviations and to write them clearly. Mistakes can result in serious drug errors. Table 4-2 lists the abbreviations most often used.

The metric units for liquids are used for liquid oral drugs and intravenous (IV) fluids. The metric units for weight are used for drug doses and to weigh objects, including the human body. Two prefixes for weights are very small, the microgram (mcg) and the nanogram (ng). A few drugs currently are administered in microgram doses. At this time no drugs used for normal administration are measured in nanogram amounts. Both micrograms and nanograms are the exceptions to the "three decimal place" rule discussed in Chapter 5.

### SWITCHING BETWEEN HOUSEHOLD AND METRIC SYSTEMS

Working in health care means that you live in at least two worlds of measuring systems: metric and household. For the most part your patients live only in one, the household measure. Because you are often the medical interpreter for your patients, you must be able to quickly switch or convert between metric and household measurements. Unfortunately only practice will make you comfortable with

 **Memory Jogger**

Remember from the drug dosage calculations that **L** stood for liquid dose. This will help you to remember that liters (L) are a way of measuring liquids.

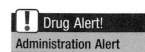 **Drug Alert!**

**Administration Alert**

The milligram is 1000 times *stronger* than the microgram. Confusion could lead to a BIG overdose. If any drug dose order is written using an abbreviation, always clarify with the prescriber which unit is meant before giving the drug.

## Table 4-2   Metric Prefixes and Abbreviations

| PREFIX | ABBREVIATION | MEANING |
|---|---|---|
| **WEIGHT (GRAM) (g)** | | |
| "kilo" | kg | 1000 g |
| "milli" | mg | 0.001 or $\frac{1}{1000}$ of a gram |
| "micro" | mcg | 0.000001 or $\frac{1}{1,000,000}$ of a gram |
| | | $\frac{1}{1000}$ of a milligram |
| "nano" | ng | 0.000000001 or $\frac{1}{1,000,000,000}$ of a gram |
| **LIQUIDS (LITER)** | | |
| "deci" | dL | 100 mL |
| | | 0.1 or $\frac{1}{10}$ of a liter |
| "milli" | mL | 0.001 or $\frac{1}{1000}$ of a liter |
| **LENGTH (METER)** | | |
| "kilo" | km | 1000 meters |
| "centi" | cm | 0.01 or $\frac{1}{100}$ of a meter |
| "milli" | mm | 0.001 or $\frac{1}{1000}$ of a meter |

## Box 4-2   Household-to-Metric Equivalents

| DRY WEIGHT | | LIQUID | |
|---|---|---|---|
| 1 oz | = 30 g (30,000 mg) | 15 gtts | = 1 mL |
| 16 oz | = 1 lb | 1 tsp | = 5 mL |
| | = 454 g | 1 Tbs | = 15 mL |
| 2.2 lb | = 1 kg | 2 Tbs | = 30 mL |
| | | 1 fl oz | = 30 mL |
| **LENGTH** | | 8 fl oz | = 1 c |
| 1 in | = 2.54 cm | | = 240 mL |
| 1 ft | = 30.48 cm | 1 pt | = 500 mL (slightly less) |
| | | | = 0.5 L (slightly less) |
| | | 1 qt | = 1000 mL (slightly less) |
| | | | = 1 L |

### Memory Jogger

A person's weight in kilograms is less than half his or her weight in pounds.

### Try This!

**TT-3** Convert the following weights in pounds to kilograms and the weights in kilograms to pounds.

| a. | 98 lb | f. | 68 kg |
|---|---|---|---|
| b. | 52 lb | g. | 12 kg |
| c. | 315 lb | h. | 122 kg |
| d. | 2.9 lb | i. | 52 kg |
| e. | 147 lb | j. | 80 kg |

Answers are at the end of this chapter.

### Drug Alert!

**Administration Alert**

Switching from one measuring system to another is only approximately right. Always apply the DIMS test ("does it make sense") when converting between systems. If an answer does not make sense to you (for example, give 50 tsp), redo the math and ask for help.

the conversion (switching) process. Begin with the smaller equivalents and move to the larger ones. Build an equivalents table that makes sense to you. Box 4-2 shows household-to-metric equivalents.

One of the most common switching situations is changing a patient's weights between pounds and kilograms. One kilogram is equal to 2.2 lb. So a person's weight in kilograms is *always* less than half of his or her weight in pounds. To obtain the kilogram weight, first weigh the patient on a standard pound scale and then *divide* this number by 2.2. For example, a patient who weighs 232 lb weighs 105.45 kg (round to 105.5 kg). A patient who weighs 120 lb weighs 54.5 kg. To change weight in kilograms to pounds, *multiply* the kilogram number by 2.2. For example, the patient who weighs 90 kg weighs 198 lb. The infant who weighs 1.6 kg weighs 3.5 lb.

A problem with switching between household and metric measurements is that the metric measurements are precise and the household measurements are only approximate. If you bought different brands of household measuring spoons and compared the exact volume of each spoon in milliliters, there would be considerable differences among them. For example, some teaspoons would measure just about 5 mL, others 4 mL, and others somewhere in between. When using household measuring containers or instruments for drugs, the dose may be close to the one ordered in milliliters but may not be exact.

## THE MILLIEQUIVALENT SYSTEM

Milliequivalents (mEq) are used to measure electrolytes. *Electrolytes* are minerals and chemicals in the body that have a positive or negative charge. The electrolytes most often calculated in milliequivalents are potassium chloride (KCl), potassium phosphate ($KPO_4$), and different types of IV calcium ($Ca^{++}$). The electrolyte most often prescribed is KCl, which can be given orally or mixed with IV fluid. Whichever way it is given, it is irritating to the body.

Potassium can be given as a tablet, an extended-release tablet, an effervescent (fizzy) tablet, in a liquid, as a powder, or dissolved in IV fluids. The different types are *NOT interchangeable*. Do not substitute a different potassium type for the one prescribed.

Although drugs measured and prescribed in milliequivalents sound different than those measured and prescribed in milligrams, the dosage calculations are performed exactly the same way. Once again, you are determining the amount of tablets or milliliters to administer based on what you *want* versus what you *have* on hand. (If necessary, review drug dosage calculations in Chapter 5.) For example, the order reads "potassium chloride (Slow-K) 40 mEq orally," and you have Slow-K tablets that contain 20 mEq/tablet. Divide the number you want by the number you have.

$$\frac{Want}{Have} = \text{Number of tablets to give! } Want \text{ 40 mEq; } Have \text{ 20 mEq.}$$

$$\text{So, } \frac{40 \text{ mEq}}{20 \text{ mEq/1 tablet}} = (\text{chop off the end zeroes}) \frac{4}{2} = 2 \text{ tablets!}$$

## THE UNIT SYSTEM

Drugs measured in units come in either plain or international units. The most common drugs measured in units are insulin and heparin (a drug to reduce blood clotting, sometimes called a *blood thinner* by patients, even though it does not really thin the blood). Others include injectable penicillin and some vitamins. Curious? Check your vitamins at home to see how they are measured.

### Insulin

Insulin is a drug used by some patients with diabetes to replace the insulin their bodies no longer make. (Chapter 25 has more information about diabetes and insulin.) The drug insulin is very concentrated and requires special syringes. The most common insulin syringe holds 50 units in one small 0.5-mL syringe. Each unit on the syringe is marked up to 50. However, there are many different types of insulin syringes. Some are measured up to 100 units, and others are measured up to 500 units. These syringes *cannot* be interchanged with one another or with noninsulin syringes. Carefully check the concentration of insulin in the bottle with the type of syringe chosen to make sure that you have the correct syringe. Do not go by the color of the syringe to determine whether the syringe is a 50-unit insulin syringe. *There is no common color for insulin syringe types.* Different equipment companies use different colors for their syringes. Check the specific markings on the syringe rather than going by the color of the cap, needle hub, or box label. If the incorrect dose of insulin is given, severe hypoglycemia and death can result. Chapter 25 discusses safe insulin administration in detail.

◄ ⊖ -Learning Activity 4-2

⊚ **Try This!**

**TT-4** Convert these household measures into metric equivalents, rounding to the nearest tenth when necessary.

a. 250 lb         d. 4 Tbs

b. 12 oz (liquid)   e. 2 tsp

c. 17 in

Answers are at the end of this chapter.

⊚ **Try This!**

**TT-5** Convert these metric measures into household equivalents.

a. 45 g          d. 100 kg

b. 90 mL         e. 780 g

c. 1500 mL

Answers are at the end of this chapter.

⊚ **Try This!**

**TT-6** Calculate how much drug you should administer.

a. *Want* potassium 16 mEq in extended-release tablet; *Have* potassium 8 mEq in extended-release tablet

b. *Want* potassium 10 mEq effervescent tablet; *Have* potassium 20 mEq scored effervescent tablet

c. *Want* potassium 10 mEq in an oral solution; *Have* potassium 20 mEq dissolved in 8 oz of water

Answers are at the end of this chapter.

❗ **Drug Alert!**

**Administration Alert**

To prevent insulin dose errors, check the specific markings on the syringe rather than relying on the color of the cap, needle hub, or box label.

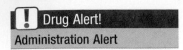

## Drug Alert!

**Administration Alert**

Always write out the word *unit* or the words *international units*.

## Try This!

**TT-7** Calculate how many milliliters you should give.

a. *Want* heparin 7500 units subcutaneously; *Have* heparin 10,000 units/mL

b. *Want* heparin 1000 units; *Have* heparin 5000 units/mL

c. *Want* heparin 300 units/kg body weight; *Have* heparin 20,000 units/mL. The patient weighs 250 lb.

Answers are at the end of this chapter.

## Try This!

**TT-8** Calculate how many milli-grams in how many teaspoons that you should give to a baby who weighs 7 lb.

*Want* amoxicillin 50 mg/kg; *Have* amoxicillin 50 mg/mL (Remember to round up or down.)

Answers are at the end of this chapter.

@-Learning Activity 4-3 ►

Always write out the word *unit* or the words *international units*. Errors are made when the written "U" is mistaken for a zero. For example, 5U could be read as 50 units! The abbreviation "IU" could be mistaken for the Roman numeral IV (4).

### Heparin

Heparin is a fast-acting anticoagulant (drug to slow or prevent blood clotting) that leaves the body quickly. The major use of heparin is to prevent clots from forming during heart surgery and to prevent extension of a clot that has already formed in the deep veins. A more complete discussion of heparin and heparin-like drugs can be found in Chapter 17.

Heparin is only given by subcutaneous injection or into an IV site. It comes in single- and multiple-dose vials. In addition, weaker solutions of heparin are available already loaded in single-use syringes. Strengths of heparin vary from 10 units/mL to 40,000 units/mL.

Although drugs measured and prescribed in units sound different from those measured and prescribed in milligrams, the dosage calculations are performed exactly the same way. Once again, you are determining the milliliters to administer based on what you *want* versus what you *have* on hand. (If necessary, review drug dosage calculations in Chapter 5.) For example, the order reads "heparin 2000 units subcutaneously," and you have heparin 5000 units/mL. Divide the number you want by the number you have.

$$\frac{Want}{Have} = \text{Number of milliliters!}$$

*Want* 2000 units, *Have* 5000 units

$$\frac{2000}{5000/mL} \text{ (chop the zeroes)} = \frac{2}{5} = 0.4 \text{ mL}$$

Because heparin is such a fast-acting drug, the rate of infusion for IV therapy must be watched closely even if it is on a pump or controller. See Chapter 17 for more details about IV heparin calculations and administration.

## TWO-STEP DRUG DOSAGE CALCULATIONS

When you have two measurements that are in different systems, dosage calculation becomes a two-step problem similar to the proportion calculations presented in Chapter 5. First find how the two measurements are related to one another.

The equivalent tables shown earlier will help convert one measurement into another. For example, dextromethorphan comes in solutions of 3.5 mg per 5 mL (or written as a ratio of $\frac{3.5 \text{ mg}}{5 \text{ mL}}$. You want to give 7 mg, but you need the final dose expressed in teaspoons. How do you determine how many teaspoons to give?

The Household-to-Metric Equivalents table (see Box 4-2) tells us that 1 tsp = 5 mL.

Step 1: Convert the system you *have* into the system you *want* using proportion calculations.

$$1 \text{ tsp} = 5 \text{ mL, then } 3.5 \text{ mg} = 5 \text{ mL} = 1 \text{ tsp}$$

Step 2: Plug the numbers into the formula for liquids.

$$\frac{Want}{Have} \times \textbf{\textit{Liquid}} = \frac{7 \text{ mg}}{3.5 \text{ mg}} \times 1 \text{ tsp} = 2 \text{ tsp}$$

## Get Ready for Practice!

### Key Points

- A liquid ounce is not equal to a dry ounce.
- Always double check the amount of drug in a measuring device with the amount ordered to prevent giving an overdose.
- Before using a measuring device (oral syringe, dropper, medicine cup) to administer a liquid drug, check the patient's swallow reflex.
- The household measurement system is not as precise as the metric system.
- Do not substitute one type of potassium for another.
- When calculating doses for drugs that are manufactured in milliequivalents or units, determine the amount of tablets or milliliters to administer based on what you *want* versus what you *have* on hand, in the same way as for drugs manufactured in milligrams.
- To prevent insulin dose errors, check the specific markings on the syringe rather than going by the color of the cap, needle hub, or box label.
- Always write out the word *unit* or the words *international units* rather than using abbreviations.

### Additional Learning Resources

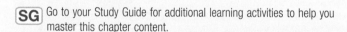 Go to your Evolve website (http://evolve.elsevier.com/Workman/pharmacology/) for the following FREE learning resources:
- eLearning Activities
- Animations
- Video Clips
- Interactive Review Questions
- Audio Key Points
- Audio Glossary
- Audio Glossary—Spanish-English
- Drug Dosage Calculators
- Patient Teaching Handouts

**SG** Go to your Study Guide for additional learning activities to help you master this chapter content.

### Review Questions

1. If there are 60 gtts in a tsp, how many gtts are there in a Tbs?
   - A. 600
   - B. 300
   - C. 180
   - D. 120

2. You prepare to mix dry amoxicillin into a solution by adding 150 mL of water to the bottle containing the dry amoxicillin. How many ounces of water will you add to the bottle?
   - A. 5
   - B. 10
   - C. 30
   - D. 50

3. The patient is to take 30 mg of a drug that comes as 5 mg/tsp. How many Tbs is this? _____ Tbs

4. Which unit is the basic measure of liquid in the metric system?
   - A. Dram
   - B. Gram
   - C. Liter
   - D. Meter

5. Which weight is the smallest?
   - A. 1 kg
   - B. 10 mg
   - C. 100 mcg
   - D. 1000 g

6. Convert 0.7 L into milliliters. _____ mL

7. The patient weighs 115 lb. Convert this weight to kilograms. _____ kg

8. The drug and dose prescribed is cortisol 40 mg by injection. The dose available is 50 mg/mL. How many milliliters will you draw up into the syringe? _____ mL

9. The patient is to receive 15,000 units of heparin intravenously. The vial contains heparin 20,000 units/mL. How many milliliters will you draw up into the syringe? _____ mL

### Answers To *Try This!* Problems

**TT-1** Convert the Fahrenheit temperature to Centigrade and the Centigrade to Fahrenheit.

101.4° F = 38.6° C
97° F = 36.1° C
103.8° F = 39.9° C
40° C = 104° F
35° C = 95° F
39.2° C = 102.6° F

**TT-2** Calculate the response in teaspoons or drops.

a. *Want* ampicillin 500 mg; *Have* ampicillin 250 mg/tsp

2 tsps = 500 mg

b. *Want* guaifenesin 50 mg; *Have* guaifenesin 100 mg per 60 gtts

50 mg in 30 gtts or in 0.5 tsp

c. *Want* milk of magnesia 1 Tbs; *Have* milk of magnesia 1 tsp

3 tsp of milk of magnesia = 1 Tbs

**TT-3** Convert the following weights in pounds to kilograms and the weights in kilograms to pounds.

a. 98 lb = 44.5 kg
b. 52 lb = 23.6 kg
c. 315 lb = 143.2 kg
d. 2.9 lb = 1.3 kg
e. 147 lb = 66.8 kg
f. 68 kg = 149.6 lb
g. 12 kg = 26.4 kg
h. 122 kg = 268.4 kg
i. 52 kg = 114.4 lb
j. 80 kg = 176 lb

**TT-4** Convert these household measures in metric equivalents, rounding to the nearest tenth when necessary.

a. 250 lb = 113.6 kg
b. 12 oz (liquid) = 360 mL
c. 17 in = 43.2 cm
d. 4 Tbs = 60 mL
e. 2 tsp = 10 mL

**TT-5** Convert these metric measures into household equivalents.

a. 45 g = 1.5 oz (dry weight)
b. 90 mL = 3 oz
c. 1500 mL = 1 qt and 1 pt, or 6 c
d. 100 kg = 220 lb
e. 780 g = 1.7 lb

**TT-6** Calculate how much drug you should administer.

a. *Want* potassium 16 mEq in extended-release tablet; *Have* potassium 8 mEq in an extended-release tablet

   Give two extended-release tablets

b. *Want* potassium 10 mEq effervescent tablet; *Have* potassium 20 mEq scored effervescent tablet

   Give one half ( ½ ) of the effervescent tablet

c. *Want* potassium 10 mEq in an oral solution; *Have* potassium 20 mEq dissolved in 8 oz of water as an oral solution

   Give 4 oz of the oral solution (you could add more water to the solution *after* you have measured out the 4 oz to give the patient a more dilute dose).

**TT-7** Calculate how many milliliters you should give.

a. *Want* heparin 7500 units subcutaneous; *Have* heparin 10,000 units/mL

$$\frac{7500}{10,000/mL} = \frac{75}{100} = 0.75 \text{ mL}$$

b. *Want* heparin 1000 units; *Have* heparin 5000 units/mL

$$\frac{1500}{5000/mL} = \frac{1}{5} = 0.2 \text{ mL}$$

c. *Want* heparin 300 units/kg body weight; *Have* heparin 20,000 units/mL. The patient weighs 250 lb

250 lb = 250 divided by 2.2 = 113.6 kg, round to 114 kg

114 kg × 300 units = need 34,200 units

34,200 divided by 20,000 = 1.71 mL, round to 1.7 mL

**TT-8** Calculate how many milligrams in how many teaspoons you should give to a baby who weighs 7 lb.

*Want* amoxicillin 50 mg/kg; *Have* amoxicillin 50 mg/mL (Remember to round up or down.)

7 lb = 3.18 kg, round to 3.2 kg
50 mg × 3.2 kg = 160 mg; want 160 mg
5 mL = 1 tsp; 50 mg/mL = 250 mg/5 mL (1 tsp)

$$\frac{160}{250} \times 1 \text{ tsp} = 0.64 \text{ tsp}; \text{ not easy to measure, better to use a medicine dropper (in mL)}$$

$$\frac{Want}{Have} \times 1 \text{ mL} = \frac{160 \text{ mg}}{50 \text{ mg}} \times 1 \text{ mL} = 3.2 \text{ mL}$$

# Mathematics Review and Introduction to Dosage Calculation

## Objectives

*After studying this chapter you should be able to:*

1. Identify the numerator and denominator of a fraction.
2. Identify a proper and an improper fraction.
3. Change a whole number into a fraction.
4. Change a mixed number into a fraction.
5. Reduce a fraction to its lowest terms.
6. Calculate the lowest common denominator of a series of fractions.
7. Add two or more fractions and subtract two or more fractions.
8. Multiply two fractions and divide two fractions.
9. Identify the divisor and the dividend of a decimal problem.
10. Multiply two decimals and divide two decimals.
11. Change a fraction into a decimal and a decimal into a fraction.
12. Calculate a given percentage of a number.
13. Compare the dose on hand (what you have) with the dose that has been prescribed (what you want).
14. Calculate the number of tablets or amount of liquid drug needed to make the prescribed dose.
15. Convert a set of fractions into a proportion.
16. Solve for "*X*" (the unknown) in a math problem.

## Key Terms

**decimal** (DĔS-ĭ-mŭl) (p. 72) The part of a whole number based on a system of units of ten (for example, 0.5 is 5 tenths of 1).

**decimal point** (DĔS-ĭ-mŭl PŌYNT) (p. 72) The dividing point between whole numbers and parts of numbers in a system based on units of ten.

**denominator** (dē-NŎM-ĭn-ā-tŭr) (p. 69) The bottom number in a fraction, the dividing number (for example, in $\frac{3}{4}$ the denominator is 4); same as divisor.

**dividend** (DĬ-vĭ-dĕnd) (p. 74) The number to be divided in a division problem (for example, in $\frac{3}{4}$ the dividend is 3); same as numerator.

**divisor** (dĭ-VĪ-zŭr) (p. 74) The number the dividend is divided by (or that is divided into the dividend) (for example, in $\frac{3}{4}$ the divisor is 4); same as denominator.

**fraction** (FRĂK-shŭn) (p. 68) A part of a whole number obtained by dividing one number by a larger number.

**improper fraction** (ĭm-PRŎ-pŭr FRĂK-shŭn) (p. 69) A fraction that has a top number (numerator) that is larger than the bottom number (denominator). The final answer to an improper fraction is always greater than the number 1.

**intradermal (ID)** (ĭn-trĕ-DŬR-mŭl) (p. 77) Drug delivery into the body by injection just under the top part of the skin.

**intramuscular (IM)** (ĭn-trĕ-MŬS-kyū-lŭr) (p. 77) Drug delivery into the body by injection into the muscle.

**mixed-number fractions** (MĬKST NŬM-bŭr FRĂK-shŭnz) (p. 69) Whole numbers with a fraction attached.

**numerator** (NŪ-mŭr-ā-tŭr) (p. 69) The top number in a fraction that is divided by the bottom number (denominator) (for example, in $\frac{3}{4}$ the numerator is 3; same as dividend.

**parenteral** (păr-ĔN-tŭr-ŭl) (p. 77) Drug delivery to the body that does not use the gastrointestinal tract.

**percent** (pŭr-SĔNT) (p. 75) The expression of how a number is related to 100; literally "for each hundred."

**proper fraction** (PRŎ-pŭr FRĂK-shŭn) (p. 69) A fraction in which the top number is smaller than the bottom number. The final answer to a proper fraction is always less than the number 1.

**proportion** (prō-PŌR-shŭn) (p. 77) An equal mathematic relationship between two sets of numbers.

**quotient** (KWŌ-shĕnt) (p. 74) The answer to a division problem.

**reduced fractions** (rē-DŪST FRĂK-shŭnz) (p. 69) Fractions that have been changed to their lowest common denominator (that is, both the numerator and the denominator of a fraction have been divided by the same number evenly).

**scored tablet** (SKŌRD TĂB-lĕt) (p. 76) A tablet that has a line etched into it marking the exact midpoint. Cutting (or breaking) a tablet along this line gives you two halves with known dosages.

**subcutaneous** (sŭb-kyū-TĂN-ē-ŭs) (p. 77) Drug delivery into the body by injection just below the skin into the fat.

◄ ⊖-Learning Activity 5-1

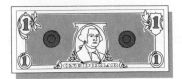

A one-dollar bill representing the whole number one

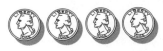

Four quarters, each representing 1/4 or 25% (0.25) of the whole one-dollar bill

**FIGURE 5-1** Comparison of part of a number to a whole number.

## WHY DO NURSES NEED MATHEMATICS?

You have probably taken drugs at some time in your life, either over-the-counter or prescription drugs. As a nurse you will be responsible for giving drugs to others safely and accurately.

All drugs work better if they are given at the right dose. This is one of the eight rules for drug administration that have traditionally been known in nursing as the *six rights*. Understanding math helps to ensure that a drug is given at the right dose.

Drugs do not usually come from the pharmacy prepared in exactly the right dose to give to a patient. You will have to calculate *how much to give* from what you *have on hand* (available). Dosage calculations are performed in the same way whether the drug is a tablet, oral liquid, injectable liquid, or suppository.

This chapter and Chapter 6 contain all the basic skills and equivalencies needed to solve any drug dosage problem. Traditional math terms will be used only when they help you to understand the dosage calculation concept. Basic math is logical, and you *can* understand it.

Of course you can use a calculator to work all of these problems, but beware! For a calculator to arrive at the correct answer, you must be sure to set the problem up correctly. This involves entering the numbers into the calculator in the right order. Entering the numbers into the calculator in the correct order is known as the *order of operation*. If you understand the math principle, you will be more likely to enter the numbers correctly. The location of the keys on a calculator can differ from one brand to another. So be sure to practice with your calculator before you use it at work to calculate drug dosages. *Practice makes perfect!*

Remember that math problems are punched into a calculator just like they are written or just like you would say them aloud. For example, 24 × 12 is punched in as 2, 4, ×, 1, 2 = *answer*. If you punch in any of the numbers backwards (for example, 4, 2, ×, 1, 2 or 2, 4, ×, 2, 1), the answer will be wrong.

Always use common sense whether you are using a calculator or a paper and pencil. Always ask yourself, *DOES IT MAKE SENSE?* Some people refer to this thinking as the "DIMS test." If the answer doesn't look right (for example, give 15 tablets), it probably isn't right! Think about it again and rework the problem.

Some types of drugs are *high-alert drugs* and are very dangerous if the dosage is miscalculated. These include *p*otassium, *i*nsulin, *n*arcotics, *c*hemotherapy and *c*ardiac drugs, and *h*eparin or other anticlotting drugs. Remember these dangerous drugs with the term *PINCH*. After you calculate one of these drug doses, always have another health care professional independently double check your calculation.

## TALKING ABOUT NUMBERS: A WHOLE NUMBER VERSUS A PART OF A NUMBER

If you are comfortable with the difference between whole numbers and a part of a number, just skip to the next section. Let's review whole numbers versus fractions. A **fraction** is a part of a whole number obtained by dividing one number by a larger number. The simplest way to do this is to think about money. A $1 bill represents the whole number one (1). A $1.25 amount is both a whole dollar (1) and a part of another dollar. The 25 cents is a fraction of the second $1. If you wrote it out, it would be 25 out of 100 cents, or $\frac{25}{100}$. The same amount written as a decimal would be $0.25. Both express the exact same amount of money. So the dollar is a *whole number*, and the 25 cents is a *part or fraction* of another whole number. Figure 5-1 shows the relationship of a fraction (part of a whole number) to a whole number.

### FRACTIONS

A fraction is a part of a whole number obtained by dividing one number by a larger number. Any fraction (for example, $\frac{25}{100}$) is actually a division problem. The fraction

$\frac{25}{100}$ is the same as $100\overline{)25}$ or $25 \div 100$. So any number *over* another number is a fraction. The top number in a fraction, in this example 25, is called the **numerator**. Remember the numerator as being "numero uno," No. 1, the best! The number on the bottom in a fraction is the **denominator**. In the example $\frac{25}{100}$, the denominator is 100.

Any number can be expressed as a fraction, even a whole number. To make a whole number a fraction, simply make the denominator of the fraction 1. Thus the whole number 2 has the same value when written as the fraction $\frac{2}{1}$. When any whole number is written as a fraction, the whole number is always on top (numerator), and the denominator (1) is always on the bottom. Remembering this concept will help you solve drug dosage problems using fractions.

### Different Types of Fractions

There are several types of fractions, including proper fractions, improper fractions, mixed-number fractions, and reduced fractions. The differences are simple, and you can do it!

***Proper Fractions.***   A **proper fraction** is one in which the top number is smaller than the bottom number. So $\frac{25}{100}$ is a proper fraction. A proper fraction is the most common type of fraction. The value of a proper fraction is always less than the number 1. For example, the answer to $\frac{25}{100}$ (which is really $100\overline{)25}$ or $25 \div 100$) is **0.25**, a number less than 1.

***Improper Fractions.***   Improper fractions didn't do anything wrong. They are just different from proper fractions, which represent only part of a whole number. A fraction can also have a top number (numerator) that is *bigger* than the bottom number (denominator) (for example, $\frac{125}{100}$). This number is still a fraction, but it represents *more* than the number 1. So an **improper fraction** is a fraction that has a top number (numerator) that is larger than the bottom number (denominator), meaning that the value is greater than 1. For example, $\frac{125}{100}$ is really $100\overline{)125}$ or $125 \div 100$, and the answer is **1.25.**

***Mixed-Number Fractions.***   **Mixed-number fractions** are whole numbers with a fraction attached. For example $1\frac{2}{4}$ is a mixed-number fraction; 1 is a whole number, and $\frac{2}{4}$ is a fraction. A mixed-number fraction can be changed into an improper fraction by multiplying the denominator (4) times ($\times$) the whole number (1) and adding the numerator (2). $4 \times 1 = 4 + 2 = 6$. Now make 6 the new numerator (top number) with the same denominator (4) and you get $\frac{6}{4}$, an improper fraction. Being able to convert mixed-number fractions into improper fractions is useful when you have to multiply proper and improper fractions together.

***Reduced Fractions.***   Reducing fractions is a way to make fractions "simpler" and easier to use. **Reduced fractions** have been changed to their lowest common denominator. This means that both the top number (numerator) and the bottom number (denominator) of a fraction have been divided by the same number evenly. For example, the part of a dollar ($\frac{25}{100}$, or 25 cents out of 100 cents in a dollar) is also equal to $\frac{1}{4}$ of a dollar. To change $\frac{25}{100}$ into $\frac{1}{4}$, *divide both* the numerator and the denominator by the largest number possible that will go evenly into both numbers. In this example both 25 and 100 can be divided evenly by 25. You have just *reduced* this fraction to its lowest common denominator! When you are working with a drug dosage problem, wouldn't it be easier to work with $\frac{1}{4}$ rather than with $\frac{25}{100}$? The final dosage answer is the same either way.

If you find it hard to think of a large number that can be divided evenly into both the numerator and the denominator, start with several small numbers. For example, in $\frac{25}{100}$ each number can be divided evenly by 5. This answer, $\frac{5}{20}$, can then be divided by 5 again to get to $\frac{1}{4}$. Does this make sense? Do whatever is easier for you. The final answer is the same.

 **Memory Jogger**

Remember the word *NUDE*. The top number in a fraction is the **numerator** (NU), and the bottom number is the **denominator** (DE): NU/DE

 **Memory Jogger**

Whenever a whole number is written as a fraction, the whole number is on top, and the denominator is always 1.

 **Memory Jogger**

The value of a proper fraction is always less than 1; for example, $\frac{1}{5}$.

 **Memory Jogger**

The value of an improper fraction is always greater than 1; for example, $100\overline{)125}$, or 1.25.

 **Try This!**

**TT-1** Change these mixed-number fractions into improper fractions.

a. $1\frac{3}{4}$      d. $6\frac{7}{8}$

b. $2\frac{5}{8}$      e. $7\frac{1}{3}$

c. $4\frac{1}{5}$

Answers are at the end of this chapter.

 **Try This!**

**TT-2** Reduce each of these fractions to their lowest common denominators.

a. $\frac{10}{24}$      d. $\frac{9}{15}$

b. $\frac{50}{100}$      e. $\frac{115}{130}$

c. $\frac{36}{84}$

Answers are at the end of this chapter.

### Memory Jogger

When dividing a fraction with both the top and bottom numbers ending in zero, you can chop the same number of zeros off of both numbers.

---

### Try This!

**TT-3** How many zeros can you chop and drop?

a. $\frac{230}{3500}$     d. $\frac{500}{100}$

b. $\frac{1400}{10}$     e. $\frac{50,000}{100,000}$

c. $\frac{20}{500}$

Answers are at the end of this chapter.

---

### Memory Jogger

When the numerator of a fraction is 1, the bigger the denominator, the smaller the fraction.

---

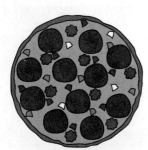

Whole pizza
(1/1)

1/2 pizza
slice

1/4 pizza          1/8 pizza
slice              slice

**FIGURE 5-2** Fraction sizes.

*Reducing Special Fractions.* How do you manage fractions with larger numbers such as $\frac{240}{120}$? You could reduce it the way it is (dividing 240 by 120), and the answer is 2. There is a way to make it a little easier. Because *both* the top number (numerator) and the bottom number (denominator) end in *zero*, you can "chop off" both zeros and be left with $\frac{24}{12}$. By chopping off the zeros, you are actually dividing both the numerator (240) and the denominator (120) by 10, resulting in a new numerator of 24 and a new denominator of 12. The answer is still 2 because you divided both the numerator and the denominator by 10. *However, be very careful because this shortcut only applies to zeros.* You can use it with any number of zeros as long as there are an *equal* number of them on both the top and bottom of a fraction. For example, $\frac{3500}{4600}$ can be chopped off to $\frac{35}{46}$. The answer to reducing both fractions is the same! When reducing a fraction by 10, chop one zero off both the numerator and the denominator. For example, this reduces $\frac{30}{50}$ to $\frac{3}{5}$. When reducing a fraction by 100, chop two zeros off both the numerator and the denominator. For example, this reduces $\frac{300}{500}$ to $\frac{3}{5}$. When reducing a fraction by 1000, chop three zeros off both the numerator and the denominator (for example, $\frac{3000}{5000}$ is reduced to $\frac{3}{5}$).

### Comparing Fractions

There may be times when you must compare several drugs and determine which dose is the strongest (or weakest). What if the dose comes in $\frac{1}{4}$, $\frac{1}{2}$, and $\frac{1}{8}$ strengths? How are you going to decide which is the strongest dose?

If the numerators (top numbers) are all 1, you can just think of slices of a pizza. Would you get a bigger slice if you had $\frac{1}{8}$ or $\frac{1}{4}$ of the pizza? Figure 5-2 shows the comparison of sizes by fractions. Don't be fooled into thinking that the biggest denominator gives the biggest slice. It is actually the other way around! As you can see in Figure 5-2, if the numerators are all the same (in this case they are all equal to 1), the *smallest* denominator gives the biggest slice (or the strongest dose).

But what if the denominators AND the numerators are different? Consider the fractions $\frac{2}{3}$ and $\frac{3}{4}$. How can these fractions be compared? Because they are different, you cannot compare them until you first rewrite the fractions to find the lowest common denominator. As you recall from the section on reducing fractions, this means that, to be able to compare the two strengths, you first have to convert both of them to the same denominator. Once you convert them to the same denominator, you can figure out exactly how they are related by comparing their numerators.

The best way to make them have a common denominator is to determine the *lowest* bottom number that both can be divided into evenly. For 3 and 4, that number is 12. To determine the lowest common denominator, start writing all the multiples of both denominators. Multiples of 3 are 3, 6, 9, 12, 15, 18, and so on because $1 \times 3 = 3$, $2 \times 3 = 6$, $3 \times 3 = 9$, $4 \times 3 = \mathbf{12}$, $5 \times 3 = 15$, and $6 \times 3 = 18$. Multiples of 4 are 4, 8, 12, 16, 20, 24, and so on because $1 \times 4 = 4$, $2 \times 4 = 8$, $3 \times 4 = \mathbf{12}$, $4 \times 4 = 16$, $5 \times 4 = 20$, and $6 \times 4 = 24$. When you compare the multiples of 3 with the multiples of 4, the first number that appears on both lists is **12**. For denominators of 3 and 4, then, the lowest common denominator is 12. This means that you will now use 12 as the *new* denominator for both fractions. Now, take each original denominator (3 and 4) and divide it into 12. Take each answer and multiply it by its numerator. That number becomes the *new* numerator for each fraction. For example, for the first fraction $\frac{2}{3}$, when you divide the new denominator 12 by the old denominator (3), you get 4. Now multiply the old numerator (2) by 4 and you get 8. So, when the common denominator is 12, $\frac{2}{3}$ is equal to $\frac{8}{12}$. Those of you who love math may have noticed that the cross products are equal ($2 \times 12$ is equal to $3 \times 8$)! That will tell you that your answer is correct.

Next try the fraction $\frac{3}{4}$. Did you get $\frac{9}{12}$? Now that both the original fractions have the same denominator ($\frac{8}{12}$ and $\frac{9}{12}$), you can easily see which one is the strongest or biggest ($\frac{9}{12}$)! Do you see that $\frac{9}{12}$ (or $\frac{3}{4}$) has more parts of the whole ($\frac{12}{12}$) than $\frac{8}{12}$ (or $\frac{2}{3}$) and so it is the strongest dose?

## Adding Fractions

Adding fractions that have the same denominator is as simple as adding whole numbers. The math symbol for addition is a plus sign (+). When adding fractions that have the same denominator, you only add the numerators (top numbers). For example, when adding $\frac{2}{4}+\frac{1}{4}$, just add the numerators (2 + 1 = 3) and place that answer (the sum) on top of the original denominator. (The denominator does not change.) The result is $\frac{2}{4}+\frac{1}{4}=\frac{3}{4}$. You can add any amount of fractions with the same denominators in this way. For example, the answer to the addition problem $\frac{2}{6}+\frac{2}{6}+\frac{4}{6}+\frac{5}{6}$ is $\frac{13}{6}$. When the sum of fractions is an improper fraction, convert it to a mixed fraction. In this case the answer ($\frac{13}{6}$) can be converted to the mixed-number fraction of $2\frac{1}{6}$.

Adding fractions that have different denominators requires that they all first be converted to the same lowest common denominator, just as is necessary when comparing fractions. Then the numerators can be added in the same way as for fractions that started out with the same denominators. How would you add $\frac{1}{2}+\frac{4}{5}+\frac{3}{4}$? First, calculate the multiples of each denominator. For the denominator of 2 the multiples are 2, 4, 6, 8, 10, 12, 14, 16, 18, **20**, 22, 24, and so on. For the denominator of 5 the multiples are 5, 10, 15, **20**, 25, 30, 35, and so on. The numbers 10 and 20 are common to both 2 and 5. However, the multiples of 4 are 4, 8, 12, 16, **20**, 24, 28, and so on. The number 10 is not a multiple of 4, but **20** is a multiple of all three denominators. So **20** is now our common denominator. To make the fraction $\frac{1}{2}$ have a common denominator of 20, multiply both its numerator (1) and its denominator (2) by 10 to get $\frac{10}{20}$. To make the fraction $\frac{4}{5}$ have a common denominator of 20, multiply both its numerator (4) and its denominator (5) by 4 to get $\frac{16}{20}$. To make the fraction $\frac{3}{4}$ have a common denominator of 20, multiply both its numerator (3) and its denominator (4) by 5 to get $\frac{15}{20}$. Next add $\frac{10}{20}+\frac{16}{20}+\frac{15}{20}$, which equals $\frac{41}{20}$. Then change this improper fraction to the mixed-number fraction of $2\frac{1}{20}$.

## Subtracting Fractions

The need to subtract fractions is rare for drug calculations or drug preparation, so this review of subtracting fractions is brief. Not only is subtracting fractions rare in drug calculation, negative numbers are not used. This means that you would not need to subtract the larger numerator from the smaller numerator.

The math symbol for subtraction is a minus sign (−). When subtracting two fractions that have the same denominator (bottom number), subtract the smaller numerator (top number) from the larger one. For example, when subtracting $\frac{2}{4}-\frac{1}{4}$, simply subtract 1 from 2 (2 − 1) and place that answer on the original denominator. The result is $\frac{2}{4}-\frac{1}{4}=\frac{1}{4}$.

Subtracting fractions that have different denominators first requires their conversion to the same lowest common denominator, just as you did when adding fractions with different denominators. After they have been converted to the lowest common denominator, the numerators can be subtracted in the same way as for fractions that began with the same denominators. For example, to subtract $\frac{4}{7}-\frac{2}{5}$, first find the lowest common denominator (as described under "Comparing Fractions" on p. 70), which is 35. Then multiply the numerators by the amount needed to make their denominators become 35. (That would be 5 for the first fraction and 7 for the second fraction). Multiply the numerator (4) in $\frac{4}{7}$ by 5 and place that number on the new denominator to get $\frac{20}{35}$. Then multiply the numerator (2) in $\frac{2}{5}$ by 7 and place that number on the new denominator to get $\frac{14}{35}$. Subtract $\frac{14}{35}$ from $\frac{20}{35}$ ($\frac{20}{35}-\frac{14}{35}=\frac{6}{35}$).

## Multiplying Fractions

Multiplying fractions is fairly straightforward. The math symbol for multiplication is "×." Look at all the fractions in an equation that you need to multiply. For example, multiply $\frac{3}{9}\times1\frac{5}{6}$. First make sure that all the fractions are reduced to their lowest possible terms (but you do not have to find the lowest *common* denominator). So reduce $\frac{3}{9}$ to $\frac{1}{3}$. Then see if there are any mixed-number fractions and change them to improper fractions. For this example, change the mixed-number

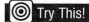

## Try This!

**TT-8** Subtract these fractions. If a fraction is a mixed-number fraction, first convert it to an improper fraction. Reduce answers to their lowest common denominators.

a. $\frac{3}{4} - \frac{2}{3}$          d. $2\frac{1}{2} - \frac{3}{4}$

b. $2\frac{2}{3} - 1\frac{1}{2}$          e. $6\frac{1}{3} - 2\frac{1}{2}$

c. $\frac{4}{5} - \frac{1}{3}$

Answers are at the end of this chapter.

## Try This!

**TT-9** Multiply these fractions.

a. $1\frac{3}{4} \times 5\frac{6}{7}$          d. $\frac{1}{2} \times 10\frac{1}{3}$

b. $2\frac{2}{4} \times 6\frac{7}{8}$          e. $4\frac{5}{8} \times \frac{2}{3}$

c. $\frac{3}{4} \times 9\frac{11}{16}$

Answers are at the end of this chapter.

## Try This!

**TT-10** Divide these fractions.

a. $3 \div \frac{1}{2}$          d. $10 \div \frac{2}{3}$

b. $\frac{3}{4} \div \frac{1}{2}$          e. $6\frac{3}{4} \div 2\frac{1}{3}$ (More difficult, but try it!)

c. $5\frac{1}{4} \div \frac{6}{8}$

Answers are at the end of this chapter.

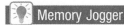
**Memory Jogger**

Decimal places are always written in (and represent) multiples of 10.

fraction $1\frac{5}{6}$ into an improper fraction ($6 \times 1 + 5 = \frac{11}{6}$). Now you have $\frac{1}{3} \times \frac{11}{6}$. To get the answer, just multiply all the numerators (top numbers) straight across the top ($1 \times 11 = 11$). Doing this makes a *new* numerator. Now do the same thing with the denominators ($3 \times 6 = 18$). Doing this makes a *new* denominator. The new total is now $\frac{11}{18}$. That's it!

## Dividing Fractions

Fractions that need to be divided are usually written out with the math symbol for division (÷), (for example, $\frac{5}{8}$ divided by $\frac{2}{3}$, or $\frac{5}{8} \div \frac{2}{3}$). To divide these fractions, flip (invert) the second fraction so the problem now reads $\frac{5}{8} \times \frac{3}{2}$. Multiply across the numerators and denominators as you did when multiplying two fractions. The answer is $\frac{15}{16}$. If possible, reduce the fraction answer to its lowest terms. In this case $\frac{15}{16}$ cannot be reduced further.

If your division involves a whole number to be divided by a fraction (for example, $2 \div \frac{3}{4}$), change the whole number 2 into a fraction by putting it over 1. The whole number 2 is the fraction $\frac{2}{1}$. (Remember that all whole numbers can be expressed as fractions by putting the whole number over 1.) Therefore the problem is now $\frac{2}{1} \div \frac{3}{4}$. After you invert (flip) the second fraction, the problem is $\frac{2}{1} \times \frac{4}{3} = \frac{8}{3}$. Reduce this fraction to $2\frac{2}{3}$. That's it!

Dividing a fraction by a whole number works the same way. For the problem $\frac{1}{3} \div 4$, first convert it to $\frac{1}{3} \div \frac{4}{1}$ and flip (invert) the second fraction, converting the problem to $\frac{1}{3} \times \frac{1}{4}$. The answer is $\frac{1}{12}$!

## DECIMALS

A **decimal,** like a fraction, describes parts of a whole. Decimals and fractions are related because decimals can be written as fractions and fractions can be written as decimals. To understand how to change from one to the other, you must first understand that the place value of decimals is based on multiples of 10. We will talk about the relationship between fractions and decimals a little later.

The key to understanding decimals is to understand the way they are written. A **decimal point** is the dividing point between whole numbers and parts of numbers in a system based on units of 10 (Table 5-1). It is located between the whole number and the part of the whole number.

Any number to the *left* of a decimal point is a *whole* number. So the whole number 125 is written from left to right as 1 one hundred, 2 tens, and 5 ones (or right to left as 5 ones, 2 tens, and 1 one hundred). By now you do this instinctively because you started doing it in first grade!

Any number to the *right* of the decimal point is a *part* of the whole number. So the decimal 0.25 is 25 parts of 100 because the place value of the 5 is hundredths, and 0.025 is 25 parts of a thousand because the third place after the decimal point (in this case the 5) has a place value of thousandths. The place to the right or left of the decimal determines the value of a number.

When working with drug dosages, *always* put a *zero before* the decimal point of any number less than 1 to indicate that there are no whole parts (for example, write .5 mg as 0.5 mg. When you are tired, reading a fax order, or reading an order written on no-carbon-required (NCR) paper, the numbers may not be clear; a decimal point could easily be missed, leading to a serious drug dosage error.

*Never* put any extra zeros (which are useless) at the end of a decimal when writing a drug dose. For example, although 0.25 is equal to 0.250, 0.250 could be easily misread as 250 instead of 25 parts when measuring drugs. Always chop off those end zeros to the right of the decimal point (but only the *end* zeros).

### Adding and Subtracting Decimals

Adding and subtracting decimals is exactly the same as adding and subtracting whole numbers. The key to ensuring that you obtain the correct answer when adding or subtracting decimals is to keep the decimal points in all the numbers that you are

## Table 5-1   Decimal Table and Conversions

| WORD DESCRIPTION | NUMBER | FRACTION | WORD DESCRIPTION | NUMBER | FRACTION |
|---|---|---|---|---|---|
| Hundred thousands | 100,000 | $\frac{100,000}{1}$ | Tenths | 0.1 | $\frac{1}{10}$ |
| Ten thousands | 10,000 | $\frac{10,000}{1}$ | Hundredths | 0.01 | $\frac{1}{100}$ |
| Thousands | 1,000 | $\frac{1000}{1}$ | Thousandths | 0.001 | $\frac{1}{1000}$ |
| Hundreds | 100 | $\frac{100}{1}$ | Ten thousandths | 0.0001 | $\frac{1}{10,000}$ |
| Tens | 10 | $\frac{10}{1}$ | Hundred thousandths | 0.00001 | $\frac{1}{100,000}$ |
| Ones/Units | 1 | $\frac{1}{1}$ | Millionths | 0.000001 | $\frac{1}{1,000,000}$ |
| Decimal point | . | | | | |

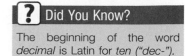

**Did You Know?**

The beginning of the word *decimal* is Latin for *ten* ("dec-").

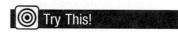

**Clinical Pitfall**

The places to the right or left of the decimal point determine the value of a number. So always put a zero before the decimal point of any proper fraction written as a decimal. If you don't, 0.25 g of a drug written as .25 could be misread as 25 g of a drug: a *BIG* overdose. For example, an adult morphine dose of 5 mg is normal, but a pediatric morphine dose might be .5 mg and should be written as 0.5 mg. If this dose is read as 5 mg, it is ten times the normal dose, which could be lethal.

adding in the same position. For example, when adding 7.25, 9.3, and 11.71, position the decimal points as shown in the following problem.

$$\begin{array}{r} 7.25 \\ +9.3 \\ +11.71 \\ \hline 28.26 \end{array}$$

Follow the same procedure when subtracting decimals (for example, 42.22 from 98.61).

$$\begin{array}{r} 98.61 \\ -42.22 \\ \hline 56.39 \end{array}$$

## Multiplying Decimals

Multiplying decimals is almost as easy as multiplying whole numbers. The only difference is that your answer has to contain the right number of decimal places for it to make sense. The key is to count the total number of decimal places (the number of digits after the decimal point) in the whole problem and then make sure that the same amount of decimal places are in the answer. So you do not need to keep track of the decimals until you have an answer!

To multiply 2.4 × 4, treat the numbers as 24 × 4 and multiply, which equals 96. Now add the number of decimal places in both numbers. There is only one decimal place for this problem (it is in 2.4). Starting from the far right of 96, count one space to the left and place the decimal point; 9.6 is the correct answer. Try multiplying a decimal by another decimal. For example, when multiplying 2.4 × 3.6, treat it as 24 × 36; 964 is the correct answer. Add the number of decimal places in both numbers that were multiplied. There is one decimal place in 2.4 and one decimal place in 3.6, for a total of two decimal places. Starting from the far right of 964, count two spaces to the left and place the decimal point; 9.64 is the correct answer. Now multiply 4.3 × .21 by treating it as 43 × 21, with 903 being the answer. There are three decimal places in the number being multiplied (one in 4.3 and two in .21). So, starting from the far right of 903, count spaces to the left and place the decimal point for 0.903 as the correct answer. Remember, just as when you multiply whole numbers, it is important to line up your numbers properly when you are doing the problem without a calculator.

**Try This!**

**TT-11** Decimals as parts of a whole:

a. 0.3 = How many parts of a whole?

b. 0.75 = How many parts of a whole?

c. 5.1 = How many whole numbers and how many parts of a whole?

d. 2.2 = How many whole numbers and how many parts of a whole?

e. 2.48 = How many whole numbers and how many parts of a whole?

Answers are at the end of this chapter.

**Try This!**

**TT-12** Multiply these decimals.

a. 100 × 0.25     d. 40.5 × 2.4

b. 51.2 × 2.1     e. 1.2 × 1.2

c. 15.5 × 10

Answers are at the end of this chapter.

## Dividing Decimals

Let's start by dividing a decimal by a whole number: $\frac{36.48}{2}$ , or, to put it another way, $2\overline{)36.48}$ or 36.48 ÷ 2. The number being divided (or divided into) is 36.48 and is known as the **dividend**. The number doing the dividing (in this case 2) is the **divisor**. The answer to a division problem is the **quotient**.

The problem works like any other division problem except that *you must be sure that the decimal point in the answer is placed exactly above the one in the dividend*. So first put the decimal point for the answer *exactly above* the one in the dividend (36.48):

$2\overline{)36.48}$ . Then complete the division: $2\overline{)36.48}^{\,18.24}$ . Does this make sense?

To check division, multiply the divisor (2) and the quotient (18.24). Your answer should equal the dividend (36.48). If you don't get the dividend, your division was wrong, and you must redo it.

Dividing a decimal by a decimal is a little harder, but the principle is the same. Keep in mind that you always have to *divide by a whole number*. If your divisor is a decimal, you have to move the decimal point all the way to the right to make it a whole number. Whatever you do to the divisor you also must do to the dividend. So move the decimal point in the dividend the *same number* of decimal spaces. For example, in the problem $\frac{32.4}{1.6}$ or $1.6\overline{)32.4}$ , moving the decimal point in the divisor all the way to the right involves moving it one place: changing 1.6 to the whole number 16. Now move the decimal point in the dividend (32.4) one place to the right (an equal number of places) so 32.4 becomes 324, giving you $16\overline{)324}$ . Divide as usual and you should get $16\overline{)324.00}^{\,20.25}$ . Check your answer in the same way as mentioned previously: multiply the divisor (16) and the answer (quotient, 20.25). The result should equal the dividend (324).

Dividing a whole number by a decimal also requires moving the decimal points to make things even. In a whole number the decimal point is located at the *end* of the number. For example, the whole number 4 actually equals 4. Using $\frac{4}{2.5}$ , which is the same as $2.5\overline{)4}$ or 4 ÷ 2.5, move the decimal point one place to the right in the divisor. *Add* a decimal place after 4 and move it one place to the right, making it 40. The resulting problem is $25\overline{)40.0}$ . Now work the problem the way you would any division problem. Did you get $25\overline{)40.0}^{\,1.6}$ ? To divide a whole number by a decimal, add as many extra zeros to the whole number after the decimal as you need until the division ends or repeats. For drug calculations you will not need to work a decimal problem through more than the thousandth (third) place.

## Changing Fractions into Decimals

Decimals and fractions are related because they are both parts of a whole. For example, decimals change the fraction $\frac{25}{100}$ into 0.25 (see Table 5-1). Because both decimals and fractions are a part of the whole, you can change fractions into decimals and decimals into fractions. You do this every time you turn $\frac{25}{100}$ into 0.25. To do this, just divide the numerator (in this case 25) by the denominator (in this case 100). This step is written as $100\overline{)25}$ or 25 ÷ 100. To divide, place a decimal point after the 25 and add zeros until the division ends. The answer is .25, but when writing drug dosages, remember to write it as 0.25 to avoid any confusion.

## Changing Decimals into Fractions

To change a decimal to a fraction, drop the decimal point and make this number the numerator (top number) of the fraction. The denominator (bottom number) of the fraction is the place value of the last digit (number) of the decimal. Determine the place value of the last number (digit) after the decimal point. For example, the decimal 0.25 is 25 parts of 100 because the place value of the 5 is hundredths. Then reduce the fraction to its lowest terms. For example, to change 0.25 to a fraction, drop

---

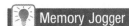

**Memory Jogger**

Divisor × Quotient (answer) = Dividend (if you divided correctly).

---

**Memory Jogger**

Add as many extra zeros (decimal places) to the right of the dividend (whole number) as you need to make the answer accurate.

---

**Try This!**

**TT-13** Divide these decimals.

a. 630 ÷ 0.3         d. 10 ÷ 0.25
b. 0.125 ÷ 0.5       e. 1.4 ÷ 1.4
c. 2.5 ÷ 0.75

Answers are at the end of this chapter.

---

**Memory Jogger**

To turn a fraction into a decimal, always divide the numerator (top number) by the bottom number (denominator).

the decimal point and make 25 the numerator. The denominator becomes 100 because the place value of the 5 in 0.25 is hundredths and 0.25 is 25 out of 100 (see Table 5-1). Therefore the fraction is written as $\frac{25}{100}$ and is reduced to $\frac{1}{4}$. Another example is the conversion of the decimal 5.017 into a fraction. It becomes $5\frac{17}{1000}$ because the place value of the 7 in .017 is thousandths.

## ROUNDING PARTS OF NUMBERS

When giving drugs it may be necessary to decide how many milliliters to give if your calculated dose is uneven. For example, if you get an answer such as 2.17 mL, you must decide whether to give 2 mL or more than 2 mL, since the .17 is part of the next whole number. How do you decide which number to give? Usually liquid dosages are rounded to the tenth place rather than to a whole number.

The key concept in rounding decimals is to remember the number **5**! Any answer that ends in a number *below* .05 is *rounded down* to the next lower tenth. Any answer that ends in the number .05 or higher is *rounded up* to the next higher tenth. So, if your answer is 2.82 mL, you give 2.8 mL *(rounded down)*. If your answer is 2.17 mL, you give 2.2 mL *(rounded up)*. In clinical practice with drugs that come in tablet form, there is an exception. Some tablets can be cut in half.

## PERCENTS

You are probably familiar with percents from using them to decide how much money to tip a waiter in your favorite restaurant (10%, 15%, or 20%). Percent expresses a number as part of a hundred. The word *percent* literally means "for each hundred." In health care percents are used to calculate drug doses and the strength of solutions (for example, the percent [%] of salt in a salt-and-water solution).

Percents express the same idea as a fraction or decimal. They can be written as a whole number (20%), a mixed-number fraction ($12\frac{1}{2}$%), a decimal (0.9%) or a proper fraction ($\frac{1}{2}$%).

### Converting a Percent to a Decimal

Let's say we have a 9% salt solution. To change 9% to a decimal, drop the percent sign and multiply the number in the percent by 0.01. The 9% can then be written as 0.09, or 9 parts salt per 100 parts of water. A 0.9% salt solution (commonly called "normal saline" in the health care setting) when multiplied by 0.01 results in 0.009 or 0.9 parts of salt per 100 parts of water (also 9 parts of salt per 1000 parts of water). You can also change the 9% to a decimal just by moving the decimal point that is behind the 9 two places to the *left*. Thus 9% = 0.09 (see Table 5-1).

To change a decimal to a percent, reverse the process by moving the decimal point two places to the *right* (for example, 0.09 = 9%).

Be very careful to move the decimal point in the correct direction. Moving it in the wrong direction can result in a serious error. Work it out or *call the pharmacist if you are not sure*.

### Converting a Percent to a Fraction

The process of converting a percent to a fraction is the same whether you have a whole number, a mixed number, or a fraction of a percent.

To convert a whole number percent to a fraction, drop the percent sign and divide the percent whole number by 100. For example, to convert 20% to a fraction, drop the percent sign and divide 20 by 100 ($\frac{20}{100}$). Reduce this number to its lowest common denominator, $\frac{1}{5}$. So 20% of a pizza is the same as $\frac{1}{5}$ of a pizza (remember that 5% of a pizza is the same as $\frac{1}{20}$ of a pizza).

To convert a mixed number to a fraction, first drop the percent sign and change the mixed number to an improper fraction. Then divide that fraction by 100. So, to convert $12\frac{1}{2}$% to a fraction, convert it to an improper fraction ($\frac{25}{2}$) and divide that fraction by 100: $\frac{25}{2} \div \frac{100}{1} = \frac{25}{2} \times \frac{1}{100} = \frac{25}{200}$, which can then be reduced to $\frac{1}{8}$. So 12.5% or $12\frac{1}{2}$% of a pizza is $\frac{1}{8}$ of a pizza!

**Try This!**

**TT-14** Change the following fractions to decimals and the decimals to fractions.

a. $\frac{3}{4}$     d. 1.25
b. 0.55     e. $\frac{7}{8}$
c. 0.075     f. $\frac{300}{650}$

Answers are at the end of this chapter.

**Clinical Pitfall**

The *exception* to the rounding principle is when you get an answer of exactly half (0.5 or $\frac{1}{2}$) of a tablet. If the tablet can be cut, give $\frac{1}{2}$ tablet (see guidelines under Dosage and Calculation problems).

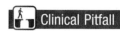

**Try This!**

**TT-15** Work to three places and then round to two places.

a. $\frac{58.4}{33}$     d. $\frac{25.4}{5}$
b. $\frac{6}{3.4}$     e. $\frac{26.8}{13.4}$
c. $\frac{27.5}{3.4}$

Answers are at the end of this chapter.

**Did You Know?**

*Percent* comes from Latin and means "for each hundred."

**Clinical Pitfall**

Moving the decimal point in the *wrong* direction is hazardous to your patient. If it is moved in error to the right, the dose will be too large and may cause serious or even lethal side effects. If it is moved in error to the left, the dose will be too small to be effective.

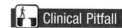

**Try This!**

**TT-16** Convert the following percents into fractions.

a. $\frac{1}{2}$%     d. 2.5%
b. 3%     e. 7%
c. $5\frac{3}{4}$%

Answers are at the end of this chapter.

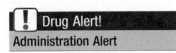 
You can use the same process to make a fraction of a percent. For example, to express $\frac{1}{4}$% as a fraction, divide it by 100 (which means multiplying it by $\frac{1}{100}$). $\frac{1}{4} \times \frac{1}{100} = \frac{1}{400}$, a mere crumb of a pizza!

### Finding the Percentage of a Number

Let's begin with what you already know: 50% of a number is $\frac{1}{2}$ of that number, right? In other words, 50% of 84 is 42. How did you get that answer? You either multiplied 84 by 0.50 or you divided 84 by 2.

What is 30% of 150? This "word" problem is the same as the one you just did in your head. You already know that 30% is equal to 0.3. So to find 30% of 150, just multiply $150 \times 0.3$. The answer is 45! Remember to count the total number of decimal places and put the decimal in the correct place in your answer.

## SOLVING DOSAGE AND CALCULATION PROBLEMS

### INTRODUCTION

In some health care settings most drugs come from the pharmacy in the correct dose, ready to give to the patients. However, remember that you are the *last check* in the system and are responsible for making sure that the patient not only gets the right drug but also gets the right dose. Always read each drug order carefully, watching for decimal points and zeros.

Sometimes a drug dose that you have on hand does not equal what you want to administer to the patient. You will need to calculate the correct drug dose from what you have on hand. The first thing you must do is write down all the information that you have and then *label* each number (that is, categorize each number as either *have* or *want*). For example, if you *have* Catapres (clonidine) 0.1 mg and you *want* to give 0.2 mg, first label all the information. Then you may proceed to plug the numbers into the following formulas and do the math. *Finally, do the DIMS (does it make sense) test to see if the answer makes sense!* You can use these formulas only when the drug dose that you have on hand is in the same measurement unit (for example, milligrams and milligrams) as the drug dose that you want to give.

### Oral Drugs

***Formula 1.*** This formula works for drug calculations involving dry pills (tablets, capsules, caplets). If the drug order is for 440 mg of naproxen and you have tablets that each contain 220 mg of naproxen, how many tablets should you give? Here is the easy way to know: divide the number you want by the number you have.

$$\frac{Want}{Have} = \text{Number of tablets to give!}$$

So, $\frac{440 \text{ mg}}{220 \text{ mg}} = (\text{chop off the end zeros}) \frac{44}{22} = 2$ tablets!

What happens if the dose of diazepam (Valium) you want is 15 mg and you have Valium 10-mg tablets? Use the formula:

$$\frac{15 \text{ mg}}{10 \text{ mg}} = 1\frac{1}{2} \text{ tablets}$$

You can cut a tablet in half and give a half tablet only if the tablet is scored. A **scored tablet** is one that has a line etched into it marking the exact center. Cutting (or breaking) a tablet along this line gives you two halves of equal known dosages. If you cut or break a tablet that is not scored, the dose will not be correct, and you will have uneven halves. If tablets are not scored, call the pharmacy to see if the drug comes either in a smaller strength or as a liquid.

Other types of drugs that should not be cut or broken include capsules, long-acting or sustained-release capsules or tablets, and enteric-coated tablets. Cutting a capsule allows the powder or tiny beads inside to spill. Long-acting or sustained-

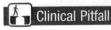

release drugs are made so small amounts of drug are released continuously through-out the day. Cutting this type of drug allows all of the drug to go into the patient's system rapidly and may cause an overdose. Enteric-coated drugs are meant to dissolve and be absorbed in the intestine rather than in the stomach. Cutting or crushing these drugs not only may cause stomach irritation, but the acid in the stomach may inactivate the drugs so they won't work. Always look up any new drug or one you are not familiar with to see if there is any reason that it should not be cut.

***Formula 2.*** This formula works for drug calculations involving oral liquids. These drugs may be called a *suspension* or an *elixir* (an old word for an alcohol-based liquid).

$$\frac{Want}{Have} \times \text{Liquid} = \text{Amount of liquid to give}$$

If an order reads, "Give Benadryl (diphenhydramine) 50 mg," and the diphenhydramine liquid comes in 25 mg/5 mL, 5 mL is the amount of liquid in one dose that you have on hand. In this example:

$$\frac{50 \text{ mg}}{25 \text{ mg}} \times 5 \text{ mL} = 2 \times 5 \text{ mL} = \text{Give } 10 \text{ mL}$$

Be sure to label both the numerator and the denominator of the formula to double check that the two dosage measurements you are working with are the same.

### Drugs Given by Injection

There are three major types of injectable drugs. These include **intramuscular (IM)**, which is injected into a muscle; **subcutaneous**, which is injected into the fat below the skin; and **intradermal (ID)**, which is injected just under the top part of the skin. All three types are **parenteral** forms of drug delivery that do not go through the gastrointestinal tract. These drugs may come in either single-dose containers (syringes, vials, or ampules) or multiple-dose bottles (vials).

All injectable drugs are liquids, so they follow the same formula as formula 2 for liquid drugs. For example, the unit-dose syringe that you *have* contains meperidine (Demerol) 100 mg/mL, and you are ordered *(want)* to give 50 mg IM. How should you set up the problem? You would set it up the same way as for other liquid drugs.

$$\frac{Want}{Have} \times \text{Liquid} = \text{Amount to pull up into a syringe}$$

$$\frac{50 \text{ mg}}{100 \text{ mg}} \times 1 \text{ mL} = \frac{1}{2} = 0.5 \text{ mL IM}$$

### USING PROPORTIONS TO SOLVE FOR *X*

A fraction uses a division line (called a *bar*) or slash to describe a mathematic relationship between two numbers (for example, $\frac{1}{2}$ or ½. A **proportion** describes an *equal* mathematic relationship between two *sets* of numbers (for example, $\frac{1}{2} = \frac{2}{4}$ ). If you look closely, you will see that, when you multiply *diagonally* across the equal sign, $1 \times 4$ *equals* $2 \times 2$! Another way of thinking of the proportion is that 1 is related to 2 in the same way as 2 is related to 4.

You can use proportions to solve for **X**, the unknown, as an alternate approach to drug calculations, especially if you don't want to memorize a formula. When you write a proportion as a set of fractions, be careful to label each piece of the equation. For example:

$$\frac{1 \text{ case}}{12 \text{ bottles}} = \frac{3 \text{ cases}}{36 \text{ bottles}}$$

**Try This!**

**TT-18** How many tablets should you give?

a. *Want* digoxin (Lanoxin) 0.25 mg; *Have* digoxin 0.125 mg

b. *Want* alendronate sodium (Fosamax) 5 mg; *Have* alendronate 10 mg

c. *Want* alprazolam (Xanax) 1.5 mg; *Have* alprazolam 0.5 mg

d. *Want* diphenhydramine (Benadryl) 75 mg; *Have* diphenhydramine 25 mg

e. *Want* estrogen 0.0625 mg; *Have* estrogen 0.125 mg

Answers are at the end of this chapter.

**Try This!**

**TT-19** How many milliliters should you give?

a. *Want* dextromethorphan (Robitussin) 7 mg; *Have* dextromethorphan 3.5 mg/5 mL

b. *Want* acetaminophen (Tylenol) 240 mg; *Have* acetaminophen 80 mg/2.5 mL

c. *Want* ibuprofen (Advil) 100 mg; *Have* ibuprofen 50 mg/1.25 mL

d. *Want* doxylamine (Aldex) 25 mg; *Have* doxylamine 6.25 mg/mL

e. *Want* chloral hydrate syrup 100 mg; *Have* chloral hydrate syrup 500 mg/5 mL

Answers are at the end of this chapter.

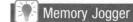

**Memory Jogger**

When dividing a fraction with both the top number (numerator) and the bottom number (denominator) ending in zero, the same number of zeros can be chopped off of both numbers.

**TT-20** How many milliliters should you give by injection?

a. *Want* hydromorphone (Dilaudid) 1 mg; *Have* a unit-dose syringe with 4 mg/mL

b. *Want* heparin 5000 units; *Have* a unit-dose syringe with 10,000 units/mL

c. *Want* trimethobenzamide 200 mg; *Have* a 20-mL vial with 100 mg/mL

d. *Want* morphine 15 mg; *Have* 50 mL vial with 10 mg/mL

e. *Want* prochlorperazine (Compazine) 10 mg; *Have* prochlorperazine 5 mg/mL

Answers are at the end of this chapter.

---

 **Try This!**

**TT-21** Express the following problems as a fractional proportion.

a. If 3 boats have 6 sails, then 9 boats have 18 sails.

b. If 1 case of IV fluids holds 12 bags, then 3 cases hold 36 bags.

c. If 5 mL have 325 mg of acetaminophen, then 2 mL have 130 mg.

d. If 1 mL has 2 mg of hydromorphone (Dilaudid), then 5 mL have 10 mg of hydromorphone.

Answers are at the end of this chapter.

---

 **Memory Jogger**

Remember to *label* your problem correctly or you might not know what the answer you get actually means!

---

Notice that in the fractions, *both* numerators identify the number of "cases," and *both* denominators identify the number of bottles. All fractional proportions must be set up this way for you to obtain the correct answer.

What if a piece of the proportion is missing? This is what happens when the prescriber orders a drug strength that is different from the one that you have on hand. To figure out how many of the drug tablets that you have on hand will be equal to the strength that is ordered, set up a proportion to solve for the missing piece.

For example, an order reads, "Give 500 mg of Primidone by mouth (orally)," and you have on hand primidone 250 mg per 1 caplet. How many caplets will you have to give the patient to equal 500 mg? Set the problem up as:

$$\frac{250 \text{ mg}}{1 \text{ caplet}} = \frac{500 \text{ mg}}{X \text{ caplets}}$$

The $X$ is what you need to give. By figuring out the "$X$" correctly, both sides of the proportion will be equal. You can cross out ("cancel") the word "mg" in the proportion equation because they are both known numbers. That leaves you with the word "caplets" as the missing part of the proportion. Therefore your answer must be the number of *caplets* needed.

Maybe you can do this in your head, but you need to understand how you get the 2 caplets. First, cross multiply to set up the equation $250 X = 500$. An easy way to work the problem is to remember that any time you bring the number in front of the $X$ (250 in this case) across the equals sign (or bring the 250 to the other side of the equals sign), it means *divide*.

$$\text{So, } X = \frac{500}{250} = 2 \text{ caplets}$$

Solving liquid drug problems by proportion involves two steps, but they are relatively easy. First label what you *have* and what you *want*, as usual. Then, set up the proportion. For example, you *want* to give diphenhydramine (Benadryl) 100 mg, and you *have* diphenhydramine 50 mg per mL. How would the proportion be set up?

Step 1: (cancel the mg):

$$\frac{50 \text{ mg}}{1 \text{ mL}} = \frac{100 \text{ mg}}{X \text{ mL}} \text{ (cancel the mg)}$$

$$50 X = 100 \text{ or } \frac{100}{50} \text{ (chop the zeros); } 5 X = 10 \text{ or } \frac{10}{5}; 10 \div 5 = 2$$

Step 2: Take the answer from step 1 and multiply that times the liquid dose that you have:

$$(\text{Liquid} = 1 \text{ mL}) : 2 \times 1 \text{ mL} = 2 \text{ mL}$$

---

 **Try This!**

**TT-22** How many milliliters should you give?

a. *Want* dextromethorphan (Robitussin) 7 mg; *Have* dextromethorphan 3.5 mg/5 mL

b. *Want* ibuprofen (Advil) 100 mg; *Have* ibuprofen 50 mg/1.25 mL

c. *Want* digoxin (Lanoxin) 0.03 mg; *Have* digoxin 0.05 mg/1 mL

d. *Want* hydromorphone (Dilaudid) 1 mg; *Have* hydromorphone 2 mg/1 mL

e. *Want* acetaminophen (Tylenol) 100 mg; *Have* acetaminophen 160 mg/5 mL

Answers are at the end of this chapter.

## Get Ready for Practice!

### Key Points

- The top number of a fraction is the numerator.
- The bottom number of a fraction is the denominator.
- If the numerator of a fraction is 1, then the larger the denominator, the smaller a part of the whole it is.
- A whole number is turned into a fraction by making the whole number the numerator and making "1" the denominator.
- Reducing fractions to their lowest terms (1 is the only number that can be evenly divided into the numerator and the denominator) helps simplify working with fractions.
- Adding fractions that have the same denominator involves only adding the numerators; the denominator remains the same.
- Adding fractions that have different denominators requires calculating the lowest common denominator, changing the numerators to proportionately match their new denominators, and adding the numerators.
- Subtracting fractions that have the same denominator involves only subtracting the smaller numerator from the larger numerator; the denominator remains the same.
- Subtracting fractions that have different denominators requires calculating the lowest common denominator, changing the numerators to proportionately match their new denominators, and subtracting the smaller numerator from the larger numerator.
- Multiplying fractions involves multiplying the numerators with one another and then multiplying the denominators with one another.
- When dividing fractions, the second fraction is inverted and multiplied by the first fraction.
- When dividing a fraction with both the top number and the bottom number ending in one or more zeros, the same number of zeros can be "chopped off" *both* numbers.
- Decimal places are always written in multiples of 10.
- The places to the right or left of the decimal determine the value of a number.
- Place a zero before the decimal point of any proper fraction written as a decimal.
- Never put a meaningless zero at the end of a decimal.
- To change a fraction into a decimal, always divide the bottom number into the top number.
- To check division of a decimal, multiply the divisor by your answer. If the division was performed correctly, you will get the dividend.
- Moving the decimal point in error to the right will make a drug dose too high and may cause serious or even lethal side effects.
- Moving a decimal point in error to the left will make a drug dose too small to be effective.
- If your drug calculation for tablets results in a decimal number below 0.5, round down to the next lowest whole number. If the calculation results in a decimal number above 0.5, round up to the next highest whole number.

- Do not attempt to cut a tablet that is not scored, a capsule, a gelcap, a drug that is enteric coated, or one that is long acting.
- Urge a patient to drink a full glass of water whenever he or she takes a tablet or capsule unless fluids must be restricted because of another medical problem.
- When reading a drug order, check and double check carefully for decimal points and zeros.
- Remember to label proportion problems so you know the correct units for your final answer.

### Additional Learning Resources

### Review Questions

1. In the formula $X = \frac{100}{25}$ , which element of the formula represents the denominator?

   A. X
   B. =
   C. The top number
   D. The bottom number

2. Why is $\frac{165}{33}$ an "improper" fraction?

   A. The answer is an odd number.
   B. Neither number can be divided evenly by 2.
   C. The numerator is greater than the denominator.
   D. The denominator is greater than the numerator.

3. Which fraction represents the whole number 16?

   A. $\frac{16}{1}$
   B. $\frac{16}{16}$
   C. $\frac{1}{16}$
   D. $\frac{16}{2}$

4. What fraction accurately represents $4\frac{1}{2}$ ?

   A. $\frac{9}{2}$
   B. $\frac{5}{16}$
   C. $\frac{16}{5}$
   D. $\frac{8}{1}$

**5.** Which fraction is reduced to its lowest terms?

   **A.** $\frac{5}{25}$

   **B.** $\frac{17}{29}$

   **C.** $\frac{2}{8}$

   **D.** $\frac{12}{16}$

**6.** What is the lowest common denominator for this series of fractions: $\frac{3}{4}$, $\frac{1}{4}$, $\frac{3}{5}$?

   **A.** 12

   **B.** 15

   **C.** 20

   **D.** 30

**7.** What is the sum of the fractions $\frac{3}{4}$, $\frac{1}{4}$, $\frac{3}{5}$?

   **A.** $\frac{32}{20}$ or $1\frac{3}{5}$

   **B.** $\frac{35}{20}$ or $1\frac{3}{4}$

   **C.** $\frac{64}{40}$ or $1\frac{3}{5}$

   **D.** $\frac{70}{40}$ or $1\frac{3}{4}$

**8.** What is the quotient of $\frac{1}{3} \div \frac{1}{2}$?

   **A.** $\frac{1}{6}$

   **B.** $\frac{1}{3}$

   **C.** $\frac{2}{3}$

   **D.** $\frac{6}{1}$

**9.** In the equation $75.5 \div 125.5 = 0.6016$, which element is the divisor?

   **A.** 0.6016

   **B.** 75.5

   **C.** 125.5

   **D.** $\div$

**10.** What is the quotient of $26.4 \div 16.22$ rounded to the tenth place?

   **A.** 0.163

   **B.** 1.628

   **C.** 16.280

   **D.** 162.800

**11.** Which number expresses the fraction $\frac{5}{8}$ as a decimal?

   **A.** 0.625

   **B.** 40.05

   **C.** 1.6

   **D.** 0.2

**12.** How much is 18% of 52?

   **A.** 2.889

   **B.** 9.36

   **C.** 288.89

   **D.** 936

**13.** The drug and dose prescribed are prednisone 20 mg. The dose of the drug on hand is prednisone 5-mg tablets. What is the relationship between the dose prescribed and the dose on hand?

   **A.** There is no relationship.

   **B.** Dose on hand is greater than dose prescribed.

   **C.** Dose prescribed is greater than dose on hand.

   **D.** Dose on hand is proportional to dose prescribed.

**14.** A patient is ordered 1000 mg of penicillin orally. Available are 250-mg tablets. How many tablets should you give to the patient?

   **A.** $\frac{1}{4}$ of a tablet

   **B.** $\frac{1}{2}$ of a tablet

   **C.** 2 tablets

   **D.** 4 tablets

**15.** Which response expresses the relationship "50 mL of morphine contains 500 mg of morphine" as a proportion?

   **A.** 1 mL of morphine contains 5 mg of morphine.

   **B.** 5 mL of morphine contains 100 mg of morphine.

   **C.** 10 mL of morphine contains 50 mg of morphine.

   **D.** 15 mL of morphine contains 150 mg of morphine.

**16.** You are ordered to give a patient with an allergic reaction 60 mg of diphenhydramine (Benadryl) by IM injection. The vial contains 10 mL of diphenhydramine solution with a concentration of 25 mg/mL. Exactly how many milliliters of diphenhydramine should you give to this patient?_____ mL

## Answers to *Try This!* Problems

**TT-1** Change these mixed-number fractions into improper fractions.

   a. $1\frac{3}{4} = \frac{7}{4}$

   b. $2\frac{5}{8} = \frac{21}{8}$

   c. $4\frac{1}{5} = \frac{21}{5}$

   d. $6\frac{7}{8} = \frac{55}{8}$

   e. $7\frac{1}{3} = \frac{22}{3}$

**TT-2** Reduce each of these fractions to their lowest common denominators.

   a. $\frac{10}{24} = \frac{5}{12}$

   b. $\frac{50}{100} = \frac{1}{2}$

   c. $\frac{36}{84} = \frac{3}{7}$

   d. $\frac{9}{15} = \frac{3}{5}$

   e. $\frac{115}{130} = \frac{23}{26}$

**TT-3** How many zeros can you chop and drop?

   a. $\frac{230}{3500}$ Chop one zero off the top and bottom to make $\frac{23}{350}$.

   b. $\frac{1400}{10}$ Chop one zero off the top and bottom to make $\frac{140}{1}$.

   c. $\frac{20}{500}$ Chop one zero off the top and bottom to make $\frac{2}{50}$.

   d. $\frac{500}{100}$ Chop two zeros off the top and bottom to make $\frac{5}{1}$ (or 5).

   e. $\frac{50,000}{100,000}$ Chop four zeros off the top and bottom to make $\frac{5}{10}$ (reduced to $\frac{1}{2}$).

**TT-4** Which fraction represents the largest part of the whole?

   a. $\frac{1}{2}$, $\frac{3}{4}$, or $\frac{7}{8}$? $\frac{7}{8}$ is the largest part of the whole. The lowest common denominator for these fractions is 8.

   b. $\frac{1}{5}$, $\frac{5}{15}$ or $\frac{6}{45}$? $\frac{5}{15}$ is the largest part of the whole. The lowest common denominator for these fractions is 15. (Hint: $\frac{6}{45}$ is not in lowest terms.)

   c. $\frac{2}{4}$, $\frac{6}{8}$, or $\frac{3}{24}$? $\frac{6}{8}$ is the largest part of the whole. The lowest common denominator for these fractions is 8.

Which fraction represents the smallest part of the whole?

d. $\frac{1}{3}$, $\frac{1}{5}$, or $\frac{1}{6}$? $\frac{1}{6}$ is the smallest part of the whole. The lowest common denominator for these fractions is 30.

e. $\frac{1}{2}$, $\frac{3}{8}$, or $\frac{3}{4}$? $\frac{3}{8}$ is the smallest part of the whole. The lowest common denominator for these fractions is 8.

f. $\frac{8}{9}$, $\frac{1}{3}$, or $\frac{3}{27}$? $\frac{3}{27}$ is the smallest part of the whole. The lowest common denominator for these fractions is 3.

**TT-5** Add these fractions. If a sum is an improper fraction, convert it to a mixed-number fraction.

a. $\frac{1}{7} + \frac{5}{7} = \frac{6}{7}$

b. $\frac{1}{5} + \frac{2}{5} + \frac{1}{5} = \frac{4}{5}$

c. $\frac{6}{8} + \frac{1}{8} + \frac{3}{8} + \frac{5}{8} = \frac{15}{8} = 1\frac{7}{8}$

d. $\frac{1}{4} + \frac{2}{4} + \frac{3}{4} = \frac{6}{4} = 1\frac{2}{4} \left(1\frac{1}{2}\right)$

e. $\frac{9}{9} + \frac{5}{9} + \frac{7}{9} + \frac{4}{9} = \frac{25}{9} = 2\frac{7}{9}$

**TT-6** Add these fractions. If the sum is an improper fraction, convert it to either a whole number or a mixed-number fraction.

a. $\frac{4}{7} + \frac{2}{5} = \frac{20}{35} + \frac{14}{35} = \frac{34}{35}$ (cannot be reduced further)

b. $\frac{3}{4} + \frac{1}{3} + \frac{5}{6} = \frac{9}{12} + \frac{4}{12} + \frac{10}{12} = \frac{23}{12}$; convert to $1\frac{11}{12}$

c. $\frac{1}{2} + \frac{1}{6} + \frac{1}{5} = \frac{15}{30} + \frac{5}{30} + \frac{6}{30} = \frac{26}{30}$; reduce to $\frac{13}{15}$

d. $\frac{2}{9} + \frac{1}{3} + \frac{3}{5} = \frac{10}{45} + \frac{15}{45} + \frac{27}{45} = \frac{52}{45}$; reduce to $1\frac{7}{45}$

e. $\frac{1}{9} + \frac{3}{4} + \frac{2}{3} = \frac{4}{36} + \frac{27}{36} + \frac{24}{36} = \frac{55}{36}$; reduce to $1\frac{19}{36}$

**TT-7** Subtract these fractions. If a fraction is a mixed-number fraction, first convert it to an improper fraction. Reduce answers to their lowest common denominators.

a. $\frac{4}{5} - \frac{1}{5} = \frac{3}{5}$

b. $1\frac{1}{3} - \frac{2}{3} = \frac{4}{3} - \frac{2}{3} = \frac{2}{3}$

c. $\frac{3}{4} - \frac{1}{4} = \frac{2}{4}$; reduce to $\frac{1}{2}$

d. $2\frac{1}{2} - 1\frac{1}{2} = \frac{5}{2} - \frac{3}{2} = \frac{2}{2} = 1$

e. $2\frac{5}{6} - 1\frac{3}{6} = \frac{17}{6} - \frac{9}{6} = \frac{8}{6} = 1\frac{2}{6} = 1\frac{1}{3}$

**TT-8** Subtract these fractions. If a fraction is a mixed-number fraction, first convert it to an improper fraction. Reduce answers to their lowest common denominators.

a. $\frac{3}{4} - \frac{2}{3} = \frac{9}{12} - \frac{8}{12} = \frac{1}{12}$ (cannot be reduced further)

b. $2\frac{2}{3} - 1\frac{1}{2} = \frac{8}{3} - \frac{3}{2} = \frac{16}{6} - \frac{9}{6} = 1\frac{1}{6}$

c. $\frac{4}{5} - \frac{1}{3} = \frac{12}{15} - \frac{5}{15} = \frac{7}{15}$ (cannot be reduced further)

d. $2\frac{1}{2} - \frac{3}{4} = \frac{5}{2} - \frac{3}{4} = \frac{10}{4} - \frac{3}{4} = \frac{7}{4} = 1\frac{3}{4}$

e. $6\frac{1}{3} - 2\frac{1}{2} = \frac{19}{3} - \frac{5}{2} = \frac{38}{6} - \frac{15}{6} = \frac{23}{6} = 3\frac{5}{6}$

**TT-9** Multiply these fractions.

a. $1\frac{3}{4} \times 5\frac{6}{7} = \frac{7}{4} \times \frac{41}{7} = \frac{287}{28}$; reduce to $10\frac{1}{4}$

b. $2\frac{2}{4} \times 6\frac{7}{8} = \frac{10}{4} \times \frac{55}{8} = \frac{550}{32}$, or $\frac{275}{16}$; reduce to $17\frac{3}{16}$

c. $\frac{3}{4} \times 9\frac{11}{16} = \frac{3}{4} \times \frac{155}{16} = \frac{465}{64}$; reduce to $7\frac{17}{64}$

d. $\frac{1}{2} \times 10\frac{1}{3} = \frac{1}{2} \times \frac{31}{3} = \frac{31}{6}$; reduce to $5\frac{1}{6}$

e. $4\frac{5}{8} \times \frac{2}{3} = \frac{37}{8} \times \frac{2}{3} = \frac{74}{24} = 3\frac{2}{24}$; reduce to $3\frac{1}{12}$

**TT-10** Divide these fractions.

a. $3 \div \frac{1}{2} = \frac{3}{1} \div \frac{1}{2} = \frac{3}{1} \times \frac{2}{1} = \frac{6}{1}$ or 6

b. $\frac{3}{4} \div \frac{1}{2} = \frac{3}{4} \times \frac{2}{1} = \frac{6}{4} = 1\frac{2}{4}$ or $1\frac{1}{2}$

c. $5\frac{1}{4} \div \frac{6}{8} = \frac{21}{4} \div \frac{6}{8} = \frac{21}{4} \times \frac{8}{6} = \frac{168}{24}$ or 7

d. $10 \div \frac{2}{3} = \frac{10}{1} \div \frac{2}{3} = \frac{10}{1} \times \frac{3}{2} = \frac{30}{2}$ or 15

e. $6\frac{3}{4} \div 2\frac{1}{3} = \frac{27}{4} \div \frac{7}{3} = \frac{27}{4} \times \frac{3}{7} = \frac{81}{28}$ or $2\frac{25}{28}$

**TT-11** Decimals as parts of a whole.

a. 0.3 = 3 parts of 10

b. 0.75 = 75 parts of 100

c. 5.1 = 5 whole numbers and 1 part of 10

d. 2.2 = 2 whole numbers and 2 parts of 10

e. 2.48 = 2 whole numbers and 48 parts of 100

**TT-12** Multiply these decimals.

a. $100 \times 0.25 = 100 \times 25 = 2500$, two decimal places, final answer is 25

b. $51.2 \times 2.1 = 512 \times 21 = 10752$, two decimal places, final answer is 107.52

c. $15.5 \times 10 = 155 \times 10 = 1550$, one decimal place, final answer is 155

d. $40.5 \times 2.4 = 405 \times 24 = 9720$, two decimal places, final answer is 97.20

e. $1.2 \times 1.2 = 12 \times 12 = 144$, two decimal places, final answer is 1.44

**TT-13** Divide these decimals.

a. $630 \div 0.3 = 3\overline{)6300}$, then divide $3\overline{)6300}^{\,2100}$

b. $0.125 \div 0.5 = 5\overline{)1.25}$, then divide $5\overline{)1.25}^{\,0.25}$

c. $2.5 \div 0.75 = 75\overline{)250}$, then divide $75\overline{)250}^{\,3.33}$

d. $10 \div 0.25 = 25\overline{)1000}$, then divide $25\overline{)1000}^{\,40}$

e. $1.4 \div 1.4 = 14\overline{)14}$, then divide $14\overline{)14}^{\,1}$

**TT-14** Change the following fractions to decimals and the decimals to fractions.

a. $\frac{3}{4} = 4\overline{)3} = 0.75$

b. $0.55 = \frac{55}{100}$; reduced to $\frac{11}{20}$

c. $0.075 = \frac{75}{1000}$; reduced to $\frac{3}{40}$

d. $1.25 = 1\frac{25}{100}$ or $1\frac{1}{4}$

e. $\frac{7}{8} = 8\overline{)7} = 0.875$

f. $\frac{300}{650} = 650\overline{)300}$ (or $65\overline{)30}$) $= 0.4615$

**TT-15** Work to three places and then round to two places.

a. $\frac{58.4}{33} = 33\overline{)58.4} = 330\overline{)584.000} = 1.769 = 1.77$

b. $\frac{6}{3.4} = 3.4\overline{)6} = 34\overline{)60.000} = 1.764 = 1.76$

c. $\frac{27.5}{3.4} = 3.4\overline{)27.5} = 34\overline{)275.000} = 8.088 = 8.09$

d. $\frac{25.4}{5} = 5\overline{)25.4} = 5\overline{)25.4} = 5.08$

e. $\frac{26.8}{13.4} = 13.4\overline{)26.8} = 134\overline{)268} = 2$

**TT-16** Convert the following percents into fractions.

a. $\frac{1}{2}\% = \frac{1}{2} \div \frac{100}{1} = \frac{1}{2} \times \frac{1}{100} = \frac{1}{200}$

b. $3\% = 3 \div 100 = \frac{3}{100}$ (cannot be reduced further)

c. $5\frac{3}{4}\% = \frac{23}{4} \div \frac{100}{1} = \frac{23}{4} \times \frac{1}{100} = \frac{23}{400}$ (cannot be reduced further)

d. $2.5\% = 2.5 \div 100 = \frac{2.5}{100}$ (can be reduced further to $\frac{1}{40}$)

e. $7\% = 7 \div 100 = \frac{7}{100}$ (cannot be reduced further)

**TT-17** Find the percentages of the whole numbers.

a. 25% of 300 = 0.25 × 300 = 75

b. 10% of $5.00 = 0.1 × $5.00 = $.50

c. 0.2% of 10 = 0.002 × 10 = 0.02

d. 300% of 5 = 3 × 5 = 15

e. 20% of 120 = 0.2 × 120 = 24

**TT-18** How many tablets should you give?

a. *Want* digoxin (Lanoxin) 0.25 mg; *Have* digoxin 0.125 mg tablet: $\frac{0.25\,mg}{0.125\,mg}$ = 2 tablets

b. *Want* alendronate sodium (Fosamax) 5 mg; *Have* alendronate 10 mg tablet: $\frac{5\,mg}{10\,mg} = \frac{1}{2}$ tablet

c. *Want* alprazolam (Xanax) 1.5 mg; *Have* alprazolam 0.5 mg tablet: $\frac{1.5\,mg}{0.5\,mg}$ = 3 tablets

d. *Want* diphenhydramine (Benadryl) 75 mg; *Have* diphenhydramine 25 mg capsule: $\frac{75\,mg}{25\,mg}$ = 3 capsules

e. *Want* estrogen 0.0625 mg; *Have* estrogen 0.125 mg tablet: $\frac{0.0625\,mg}{0.125\,mg} = \frac{1}{2}$ tablet

**TT-19** How many milliliters should you give?

a. *Want* dextromethorphan (Robitussin) 7 mg; *Have* dextromethorphan 3.5 mg/5 mL: $\frac{7\,mg}{3.5\,mg}$ × 5 mL = 2 × 5 mL = give 10 mL

b. *Want* acetaminophen (Tylenol) 240 mg; *Have* acetaminophen 80 mg/2.5 mL: $\frac{240\,mg}{80\,mg}$ × 2.5 mL = 3 × 2.5 mL = give 7.5 mL

c. *Want* ibuprofen (Advil) 100 mg; *Have* ibuprofen 50 mg/1.25 mL: $\frac{100\,mg}{50\,mg}$ × 1.25 mL = 2 × 1.25 mL = give 2.5 mL

d. *Want* doxylamine (Aldex) 25 mg; *Have* doxylamine 6.25 mg/mL: $\frac{25\,mg}{6.25\,mg}$ × 1 mL = 4 × 1 mL = give 4 mL

e. *Want* chloral hydrate syrup 100 mg; *Have* chloral hydrate syrup 500 mg/5 mL: $\frac{100\,mg}{500\,mg}$ × 5 mL = $\frac{1}{5}$ × 5 mL = give 1 mL

**TT-20** How many milliliters should you give by injection?

a. *Want* hydromorphone (Dilaudid) 1 mg; *Have* a unit dose syringe with 4 mg per mL: $\frac{1\,mg}{4\,mg}$ × 1 mL = 0.25 × 1 mL = inject 0.25 mL

b. *Want* heparin 5000 units; *Have* a unit dose syringe with 10,000 units/mL: $\frac{5000\,units}{10,000\,units}$ × 1 mL = 0.5 × 1 mL = inject 0.5 mL

c. *Want* trimethobenzamide 200 mg; *Have* 20 mL vial with 100 mg/mL: $\frac{200\,mg}{100\,mg}$ × 1 mL = 2 × 1 mL = inject 2 mL

d. *Want* morphine 15 mg; *Have* 50 mL-vial with 10 mg/mL: $\frac{15\,mg}{10\,mg}$ × 1 mL = 1.5 × 1 mL = inject 1.5 mL

e. *Want* prochlorperazine (Compazine) 10 mg; *Have* prochlorperazine 5 mg/mL: $\frac{10\,mg}{5\,mg}$ × 1 mL = 2 × 1 mL = inject 2 mL

**TT-21** Express the following problems as a fractional proportion.

a. If 3 boats have 6 sails, then 9 boats have 18 sails. $\frac{3}{6} = \frac{9}{18}$

b. If 1 case of IV fluids holds 12 bags, then 3 cases hold 36 bags. $\frac{1}{12} = \frac{3}{36}$

c. If 5 mL have 325 mg of acetaminophen, then 2 mL have 130 mg. $\frac{5\,mL}{325\,mg} = \frac{1\,mL}{65\,mg} = \frac{2\,mL}{130\,mg}$

d. If 1 mL has 2 mg of hydromorphone (Dilaudid), then 5 mL have 10 mg of hydromorphone. $\frac{1\,mL}{2\,mg} = \frac{5\,mL}{10\,mg}$

**TT-22** How many milliliters should you give?

a. *Want* dextromethorphan (Robitussin) 7 mg; *Have* dextromethorphan 3.5 mg/5 mL:

$\frac{3.5\,mg}{5\,mL} = \frac{7\,mg}{X\,mL}$ ; (cancel mg), 3.5 X = 35; $X = \frac{7}{3.5} = 2$; 2 × 5 mL = give 10 mL

b. *Want* ibuprofen (Advil) 100 mg; *Have* ibuprofen 50 mg/1.25 mL:

$\frac{50\,mg}{1.25\,mL} = \frac{100\,mg}{X\,mL}$; (cancel mg), 50 X = 125; $X = \frac{100}{50} = 2$; 2 × 1.25 mL = give 2.5 mL

c. *Want* digoxin (Lanoxin) 0.03 mg; *Have* digoxin 0.05 mg/1 mL:

$\frac{0.05\,mg}{1\,mL} = \frac{0.03\,mg}{X\,mL}$ ; (cancel mg), 0.05 X = 0.03; X = 0.6; 0.6 × 1 mL = give 0.6 mL

d. *Want* hydromorphone (Dilaudid) 1 mg; *Have* hydromorphone 2 mg/1 mL:

$\frac{2\,mg}{1\,mL} = \frac{1\,mg}{X\,mL}$ ; (cancel mg), 2 X = 1 mL; X = 0.5; 0.5 × 1 mL = give 0.5 mL

e. *Want* acetaminophen (Tylenol) 100 mg; *Have* acetaminophen 160 mg/5 mL:

$\frac{160\,mg}{5\,mL} = \frac{100\,mg}{X\,mL}$ ; (cancel mg), 160 X = 500 mL; $X = \frac{500}{160}$ ; X = 3.125; (round down), give 3 mL

# Dosage Calculation of Intravenous Solutions and Drugs

## Objectives

*After studying this chapter you should be able to:*

1. Identify three common problems of intravenous (IV) therapy.
2. Explain how the size of an IV fluid drop determines the flow rate for IV fluid infusion.
3. List the parts of an order for IV fluids that are necessary to determine the correct infusion rate.
4. Correctly calculate IV drug infusion problems when provided with the volume, hours to be infused, and drip factor.
5. Identify the signs and symptoms of fluid overload.
6. Use the "15-second" rule to determine an IV flow rate.
7. List the required parts of a valid IV therapy order.
8. Identify at least three drug categories that can cause chemical trauma to veins during IV therapy.
9. List three actions to prevent tissue damage with IV therapy.
10. Describe ways to check for a blood return at the IV site.
11. Explain how IV therapy should be modified for children and older adults.

## Key Terms

**administration set** (ăd-mĭn-ĭ-STRĀ-shŭn SĔT) (p. 84) The tubing and drip chamber used to administer an IV drip.

**drip chamber** (DRĬP CHĂM-bŭr) (p. 84) The clear cylinder of plastic attached to the IV tubing. It is filled no more than halfway so you can see the fluid dripping.

**drip rate** (DRĬP RĀT) (p. 85) The number of drops per minute needed to make an IV solution infuse in the prescribed amount of time.

**drop factor** (DRŎP FĂK-tŭr) (p. 84) The number of drops (gtts) needed to make 1 mL of IV fluid. The larger the drop, the fewer drops needed to make 1 mL.

**duration** (dŭr-Ā-shŭn) (p. 85) How long in minutes or hours an IV infusion is ordered to run.

**extravasation** (ĕks-tră-vă-SĀ-shŭn) (p. 86) Condition in which an IV needle or catheter pulls from the vein and causes tissue damage by leaking irritating IV fluids into the surrounding tissue.

**flow rate** (FLŌ RĀT) (p. 84) How fast an IV infusion is prescribed to run—the number of mL delivered in 1 hour.

**fluid overload** (FLŪ-ĭd Ō-vŭr-lōd) (p. 84) An accidental infusion of IV fluids at a much faster rate than was ordered, causing harm to the patient. Sometimes called a "runaway IV."

**infuse (infusion)** (ĭn-FYŪZ) (p. 83) To run IV fluids into the body.

**infiltration** (ĭn-fĭl-TRĀ-shŭn) (p. 86) Condition in which an IV needle or catheter pulls from the vein and begins to leak IV fluids into the surrounding tissue, resulting in tissue swelling.

**volume** (VŎL-yŭm) (p. 85) Amount of fluids ordered (for example, 1000 mL).

**VI** (p. 85) IV pump abbreviation for "volume infused."

**VTBI** (p. 85) IV pump abbreviation for "volume to be infused."

## OVERVIEW

◄ ⊝-Learning Activity 6-1

Administering intravenous (IV) fluids (IV therapy) is another parenteral drug delivery method. When delivered intravenously, the fluids, along with any drugs, go directly into a vein and thus *immediately* into the bloodstream. This process is called an **infusion**, which means to run **(infuse)** IV fluids into the body. IV fluids may be given alone to hydrate the patient, or they may be used to place drugs directly into the patient's system.

Fluids given intravenously (by IV) are also used for drugs that would not be absorbed if taken by mouth. However, because IV drugs act immediately, there is the potential for an immediate and severe problem if there is an adverse drug reaction. As discussed in Chapter 1, an *adverse drug reaction* is a severe, unusual, or life-threatening patient response to a drug that requires intervention. Another potential

 **Memory Jogger**

IV infusions are ideal for drugs or fluids that:
• Must get into the patient's system quickly.
• Need to be given at a steady rate.
• Are patient controlled (such as IV drugs for pain).

problem with IV fluid therapy is **fluid overload,** which is an accidental infusion of IV fluids at a much faster rate than was ordered, causing harm to the patient. Sometimes this problem is called a *runaway IV.*

How fast an IV infusion is prescribed to run depends on the reason for having it. For example, if a patient is dehydrated, the prescriber might want to run the fluids faster than if the IV is present just in case a problem might occur. So, not only must you know how fast an IV is prescribed to run, but you must know *why* IV therapy was prescribed. You are responsible not only for giving the correct fluids at the ordered rate, but for monitoring the patient's reaction to the IV infusion.

## IV MECHANICS

The IV **flow rate** is how fast the IV infusion is prescribed to run (that is, the number of milliliters delivered in 1 hour). The rate of an IV depends on the diameter of the tubing. Compare the tubing to a straw. A fat straw will suck up a larger amount of soda in 10 seconds compared with a thinner straw in the same 10 seconds. When you use your finger to make the soda drip out of the straw, the fatter the straw, the larger the drop. Ten fat drops have more fluid in them than ten thin drops. The same principle applies to IV fluids. Tubing with a larger diameter will let bigger drops into the vein and a larger amount of fluid into the body. The number of drops needed to make a milliliter of fluid is called the **drop factor.**

The diameter of the tubing varies according to the tubing manufacturer. Tubing sizes are divided into macrodrip and microdrip and have different types of drip chambers. A **drip chamber** is the clear cylinder of plastic attached to the IV tubing. It is filled not quite halfway so you can see the fluid dripping (Figure 6-1). The complete set of tubing and drip chamber used to administer an IV is the **administration set.** A *microdrip* tubing set delivers very small drops. It is most often used for children, older patients, and patients who cannot tolerate a fast infusion rate or a high volume of fluids. On the other hand, *macrodrip* sets deliver larger drops and are used when fast infusion rates or larger quantities of fluids or drugs are needed. Figure 6-1 shows the difference in drop size between a macrodrip chamber and a microdrip chamber.

Each company puts its drop factor (sometimes called *drip factor*) on every IV fluid administration set. Depending on the brand, macrodrip tubing delivers 10 drops/ mL, 15 drops/mL, or 20 drops/mL. Every microdrip tubing is 60 drops/mL, regardless of who makes it. *You must use the drop factor in every IV calculation.* Figure 6-2 shows different IV tubing administration sets. Administration sets for blood transfusions are larger to prevent damage to blood cells and also have some differences in the drip chamber. This chapter does not discuss administering blood or blood prod-

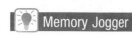
**Memory Jogger**

The larger the diameter of the IV tubing, the larger the drops.

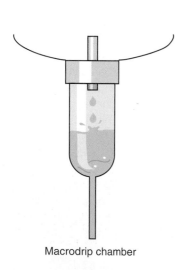
Macrodrip chamber

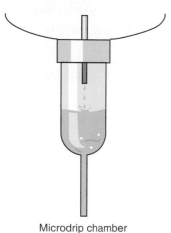
Microdrip chamber

**FIGURE 6-1** Drop size differences between a macrodrip chamber and a microdrip chamber on IV tubing.

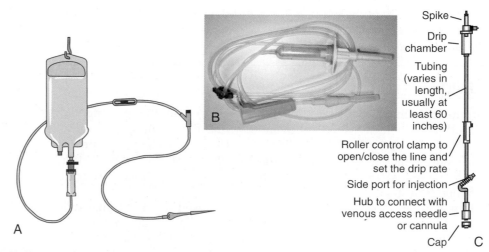

Spike

Drip chamber

Tubing (varies in length, usually at least 60 inches)

Roller control clamp to open/close the line and set the drip rate

Side port for injection

Hub to connect with venous access needle or cannula

Cap

B

A

C

**FIGURE 6-2** IV tubing administration sets. **A,** Administration set connected to an IV solution bag. **B,** Photo of an actual IV tubing administration set. **C,** Detail of IV tubing administration set.

ucts; however, flow rate calculations for any blood product are the same as for any other type of IV fluid.

## REGULATING IV FLUIDS

IV therapy involves calculating the **drip rate,** the number of drops per minute needed to make the IV infuse in the prescribed amount of time. Calculations for drip rates are very precise and must be made carefully. Although IV infusion rates can be controlled by adjusting the roller clamp, the vast majority of IV fluids today are regulated by either a pump or a controller. A *controller* is a simple device that uses gravity to control the flow of an IV. An *IV infusion pump* is a computer-based machine that pushes fluid into the vein by low pressure. The buttons used to program an IV pump are much like the ones you use to work the remote control to your television. Figure 6-3 shows examples of IV infusion pumps. All pumps have at least the following buttons:

- **ON/OFF** switch
- **Start/Enter**
- **STOP**
- **Delete or Clear**
- **Direction arrows: < > ∧**
- **Silence (MUTE)**
- **IV lock** (prevents patients and visitors from tampering with the IV pump)
- **Primary** (controller for the main IV bag—the bag hanging at the lowest point)
- **IVPB** (piggyback or secondary bag controller—the bag hanging at the highest point)

Because each brand of control device differs, always read and follow the manufacturer's directions. Even if you are not directly responsible for starting or maintaining the IV infusion, you may be responsible for checking that it is running smoothly and on time.

To understand the basics of IV fluid regulation, you need to understand these four important concepts:

- *What:* What type of fluid should be infused
- *Volume:* How much of the fluid should be infused
- *Duration:* For how long the fluid should be infused
- *Rate:* How fast the fluid should be infused

For example, a prescription reads "1000 mL of normal saline (NS) to be infused over 8 hours." The order already gives you the "What," "Volume," and "Duration." Using this information, you can determine the flow rate. As you prepare the IV infusion, check the clock to determine the start and stop time.

Once you know what kind of fluids to give, how much, and for how long, you can use this information to program the pump. Just remember that the accuracy of the pump depends on the information that you punch into it. Remember "GIGO!": "Garbage in, garbage out!" *If you make an error programming the pump, at least one factor will be incorrect, and a drug administration error will result.*

Be sure to understand all the abbreviations that are used and that may show up on the IV monitor screen. For example, a pump may use the abbreviations "VI" and "VTBI." The **VI** stands for "volume infused" and tells you how much has been infused up to that minute. **VTBI** means the "volume to be infused" or the amount that is left in the bag at any point. As the VI increases, the VTBI decreases. At any given time, if you add what has been infused (VI) to what is left in the bag (VTBI), you should have the total amount of fluid that was prescribed.

How will you know how much is really in the IV bag at any time during the infusion? Figure 6-4 shows a standard IV bag for NS (0.9% saline in water). In this illustration the black markings on the clear plastic bag are repeated in the box next to the bag so you can read them more easily. Note that there are numbers with horizontal lines going down the right side of the bag (and the label). These numbers indicate how much fluid has been infused from the bag. For example, if the fluid

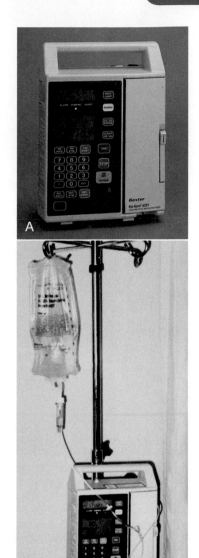

**FIGURE 6-3** Examples of IV infusion pumps. **A,** Pump alone, not in use. **B,** Pump with IV set attached.

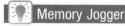 **Memory Jogger**

The four basic parts of IV fluid regulation are what type of fluid, how much (volume), for how long (duration), and how fast the fluids should be infused (rate).

**Memory Jogger**

Adding the VI and the VTBI should equal the total amount of fluid that was in the bag when it was first hung.

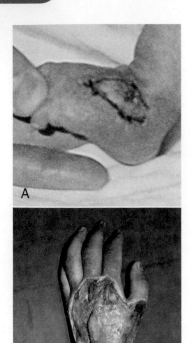

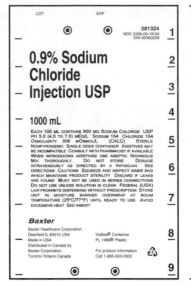

These numbers correspond to the volume (x 100) already infused. So, when the fluid level in the bag is even with the number 4, 400 mL of the solution has infused and 600 mL remains in the bag.

**FIGURE 6-4** An IV solution bag (1000 mL) with the label from the bag enlarged and illustrated on the right.

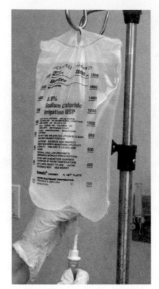

**FIGURE 6-5** Appearances of tissues after IV infiltration **(A)** and after extravasation **(B)**.

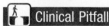 **Drug Alert!**

**Administration Alert**

Always calculate both the start and stop times and then mark the IV bag, even when the IV is on a controller or pump.

**Clinical Pitfall**

Never speed up an IV to make up for lost time when the infusion is behind schedule.

**Memory Jogger**

If an infiltration has occurred, a controller stops, but a pump can continue to push IV fluid into the surrounding tissue.

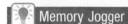-Video 6-1: Regulating an ▶
IV Infusion

line of solution in the bag is even with the line next to the number 4, 400 mL has been infused, and 600 mL (1000 mL – 400 mL) remains in the bag to be infused.

Mark the top line of the bag with the *start time* (the actual time when the IV infusion is started) and put a thick line with a pen or marker on the bag in 1-hour segments down the volume line, just like a ruler. Each hour marked should be right next to the volume to be infused for that hour. End with the *stop time*, the time when the IV bag is supposed to be empty (fluid is totally infused).

Always calculate both the start and stop times and mark the IV bag, even when it is on a controller or pump. Many things can happen to disturb the flow rate. For example, the tubing may kink, or the IV needle may get out of place and lead to infiltration. **Infiltration** is a condition that occurs when an IV needle or catheter pulls from the vein and begins to leak (infiltrate) IV fluids into the surrounding tissue. This condition prevents the patient from receiving the right dose of fluid or drug and causes swelling in the surrounding tissues. When the fluid or drug that infiltrates is irritating and leads to tissue damage or loss, the condition is called **extravasation.** Figure 6-5 shows the appearance of the tissue around an IV infusion that has infiltrated and the appearance of tissue where extravasation has occurred.

Never speed up an IV infusion to make up for lost time when the infusion is behind schedule. Playing "catch up" can cause fluids to enter the patient too fast. This can lead to fluid overload and other complications.

An IV infusion on a pump or controller can develop flow problems just as an IV without a pump can. A controller stops dripping if it encounters an obstruction. On the other hand, a pump actually uses pressure to push the drops in to get past the blockage. *This means that pumps can continue to push in drops even if the needle is no longer in the vein.* Thus, if an infiltration has occurred, a controller stops, but a pump continues to push IV fluid into the surrounding tissue. All pumps have a set limit to the pressure that can be used. This limit is displayed on the IV screen (for example, "Limit 600 mm Hg" [millimeters of mercury]). If the IV pump has to exert more pressure than the 600–mm Hg of pressure that was set to force the fluid into the vein, it will BEEP—loudly!

## IV CALCULATIONS

For you to correctly calculate the flow rate, every IV prescription must include (1) the total volume to be infused, and (2) the length of time the IV should run (in hours). You can then use the particular drop factor of the tubing that you are using to calculate how many *drops per minute* are needed to make the IV infuse in the ordered time. All IV rates that are controlled using the control roller or the control slide on the tubing are calculated by drops per minute. Some pump rates are calculated by drops per minute, and others are programmed by the pump computer in terms of milliliters per hour to be infused.

Now that you know the theory, let's work with the formula.

## Macrodrip Formula

The basic formula for determining how fast to run an IV infusion is $\dfrac{\text{Drop factor}}{\text{Minutes}}$.

Now let's break it down to make it easier!

*Step 1:* An IV infusion of 1000 mL is prescribed to run for 8 hours.

First find out how many milliliters should run in 1 hour *(flow rate)*. It is much easier to work with 1 hour than with 8 hours!

$$\text{Divide 1000 by 8:} \frac{1000}{8} = 125 \text{ mL/1 hr. Does it make sense (DIMS)?}$$

*Step 2:* Now calculate how many drops per minute are needed to make the IV infuse at 125 mL/hr (or 125 mL/60 minutes). This depends on the drop factor (drops/mL) of the IV tubing and drip chamber.

$$\frac{\text{Volume (milliliters)}}{\text{Time (minutes)}} \times \text{Drop factor (drops/milliliters)} = \text{Drops per minute}$$

You check the label information on the administration set and find that the drop factor is 15.

$$\frac{125}{60} \times 15 = 2.08 \times 15 = 31.2 \text{ drops/minute, round down to 31 drops/minute.}$$

## The Macrodrip Tubing Shortcut

Now that you know the macrodrip formula, here is a shorter way to calculate the drops per minute with macrodrip tubing. Because all of the diameters of tubing and drip chamber (10, 15, or 20) can be evenly divided into 60, you can use this relationship to calculate drip rates. Let's use these to calculate the original prescription of 1000 mL to infuse over 8 hours, which equals 125 mL/hr.

- Sets with 10 gtts/mL, divide milliliters per hour by 6 (because 6 × 10 = 60 minutes); 125 ÷ 6 = 12.5 drops/minute, round to 13 drops/minute
- Sets with 15 gtts/mL, divide milliliters per hour by 4 (because 4 × 15 = 60 minutes); 125 ÷ 4 = 31.2 drops/minute, round to 31 drops/minute
- Sets with 20 gtts/mL divide milliliters per hour by 3 (because 3 × 20 = 60 minutes); 125 ÷ 3 = 41.6 drops/minute, round to 42 drops/minute

Get the idea?

## Microdrip Formula

The microdrip formula is much easier. When using microdrip tubing, the drop factor of 60 drops/mL is the same as the number of minutes in 1 hour (60). Using the same formula as for macrodrip, you can see that the two 60s cancel each other out.

$$\frac{125}{60} \times \frac{60}{1} \text{ (drop factor)} = \frac{125}{1} = 125 \text{ microdrops/minute}$$

*This is why the flow rate for microdrip tubing always equals the drop rate!* Just calculate the milliliters needed per hour and you have the drops per minute!

## The 15-Second Rule

To see if the drip rate (for example, 42 gtts/min) is accurate, technically you should stand at the bedside and count the drops in the drip chamber for a full minute. When you are busy, a minute can seem like a very long time! Because a minute has 60 seconds, you can divide the drop rate by 4, round off the answer, and then count

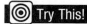

**TT-1** Calculate the milliliters to be infused in 1 hour given each of the following prescriptions.

a. 500 mL in 4 hours

b. 250 mL in 1 hour

c. 1000 mL in 6 hours

d. 1000 mL in 24 hours

Answers are at the end of this chapter.

**TT-2** Use the macrodrip tubing shortcut to calculate the drip rate for each of these prescriptions.

a. 1000 mL D₅W in 6 hours, drop factor 10

b. 500 mL lactated Ringer's in 5 hours, drop factor 15

c. 1000 mL NS in 24 hours, drop factor 20

Answers are at the end of this chapter.

**Try This!**

**TT-3** Calculate the drops per minute needed to get the right volume per hour for each of these prescriptions.

a. 500 mL D₅W in 24 hours with microdrip tubing

b. 1000 mL lactated Ringer's in 12 hours, drop factor = 15

c. 250 mL D₅W in 2 hours, drop factor = 20

Answers are at the end of this chapter.

**Try This!**

**TT-4** Calculate the 15-second drip rate for each of these problems.

a. 20 gtts/min

b. 56 gtts/min

c. 28 gtts/min

Answers are at the end of this chapter.

**Memory Jogger**

Remember that the 15-second drip rate check works only for *manually* controlled IV bags, not for those on a pump.

**Memory Jogger**

For an order to start IV therapy to be valid, it must contain the specific drug or IV solution to be infused, the dosage or volume, the duration, and the rate of infusion.

⊜-Video 6-2: Using an ▶
Infusion Pump

that number of drops for 15 seconds. Your answer will be very close to what it would have been if you had counted for the whole 60 seconds. For example, if the drop rate is the 31 gtts/min using the macrodrip tubing shortcut, divide 31 by 4: $\frac{31}{4} = 7.75$, and round that up to 8.

If you count 8 gtts when you count for 15 seconds, the IV infusion rate is correct! Be sure to check the IV rate every time that you are in the room. It only takes 15 seconds! Remember that this method only works for *manually* controlled IV bags, not those on a pump.

## MAINTAINING IV THERAPY

In some states an IV infusion can be started by a licensed practical nurse/licensed vocational nurse (LPN/LVN). In other states the person who starts the IV infusion must be a registered nurse. Before starting an IV infusion or giving drugs intravenously, check the nurse practice act in your state and the policy of your agency to determine your legal scope and expected practice for this issue.

IV drug therapy is an invasive procedure that requires a prescriber's order (prescription). Always double check the order before starting the procedure. Remember that the order must contain the specific drug or IV solution to be infused, the dosage or volume, the duration, and the rate of infusion.

### INFUSION CONTROL DEVICES

Many health care settings require a pump or controller to be used for all types of IV therapy. As described earlier, there are differences between a controller and a pump.

*Controllers* are gravity-run systems in which gravity makes the IV solution infuse into the arm. The nurse sets the rate on the device. (Controllers can be set at a maximum of about 400 mL/hr.) If resistance becomes too great to maintain the desired rate or if the fluid infuses at the wrong rate, an alarm will sound. This alarm is the primary benefit of a controller over a manually administered IV infusion.

*Pumps* push the fluid into the patient at a rate greater than gravity. They are better than a controller when the patient needs a precise amount of fluid or drug or when he or she receives hyperosmolar solutions (those that contain a higher concentration of particles dissolved in the solution than the patient's normal body fluid) such as fluids for total parenteral nutrition. A disadvantage of the pump is that an infiltration or extravasation may not be detected by the machine until it has become serious.

*Syringe pumps* (Figure 6-6) are used when the volume of drug to be given by IV push (IVP) is large (but too small for an IVPB bag) or when it should be given over more than 2 minutes. For example, a syringe pump would be helpful in a situation in which IV promethazine (Phenergan) must be diluted with NS to a volume of 10 mL and then given over a 5- to 10-minute period.

### IV THERAPY RESPONSIBILITIES

When a patient is receiving IV therapy, you must check the flow rate, equipment function, and site condition often. How often you perform these checks depends on the type of solution and equipment used, but it may be as often as every hour. During each check determine how much solution has been infused since the last check. Ensure that the flow rate and volume being delivered are maintained according to the prescriber's order.

Additional nursing responsibilities during IV therapy include assessing for and preventing complications. Common complications of IV therapy include infection, tissue damage, and imbalances of fluid and electrolytes.

#### Infection

Signs and symptoms of IV therapy–related infections may not be obvious until 24 hours after the infection begins. Check the insertion site at least every 4 hours for redness and heat and ask the patient about any discomfort at the site. Thick, purulent

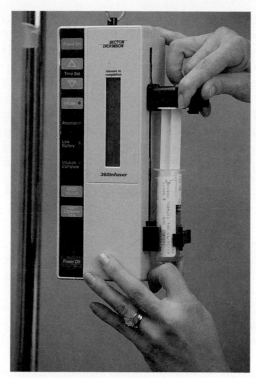

**FIGURE 6-6** Syringe pump used to control IV push drugs.

drainage (pus) may be present. If the infection becomes systemic, the patient may have chills and a low-grade fever. The most common organisms causing IV therapy–related infections are those that are normally present on the skin and often include the bacterium methicillin-resistant *Staphylococcus aureus*, also known as MRSA (see Chapter 9 for a discussion of this particular bacterial infection).

If you suspect that an IV infection is present, remove the needle immediately and document this action. A prescriber's order is not required for this action, but you must notify the prescriber about why the IV was discontinued. Apply ice or heat to the infected area, depending on how red and painful the area is. Apply a sterile dressing with antibiotic ointment to a draining IV site.

### Tissue Damage

The tissues most often damaged by IV therapy are the skin, blood vessels, and subcutaneous tissues. Tissue damage may be temporary or permanent. It always causes the patient to have discomfort. Most tissue damage can be avoided by proper technique and good observation.

*Skin* can be damaged by trauma when starting an IV. Bruising and clot formation at the IV site also can occur from improper needle removal. To prevent a bruise, remove the needle gently and apply direct pressure immediately with a sterile gauze for 1 to 2 minutes (or longer if the patient is receiving anticoagulants or platelet inhibitors). Also elevate the patient's arm while applying pressure to slow bleeding. After bleeding stops, apply a sterile gauze over the site.

*Vein* damage occurs as a result of chemical trauma related to the type and concentrations of IV solutions and to the infusion rate. Certain drugs are capable of causing irritation and phlebitis (vein inflammation) or thrombophlebitis (inflammation with clot formation). Common IV fluids or drugs capable of causing chemical trauma to veins are hypertonic solutions, potassium chloride, antibiotics, calcium, magnesium, alcohol, and chemotherapy drugs.

Chemical trauma can be reduced by diluting IV drugs and infusing them slowly into a large vein. Many known irritating solutions are given through a central venous catheter to avoid the risk of phlebitis.

 **Memory Jogger**

Signs and symptoms of IV site infection include redness, heat, and pain around the site. Wound drainage and a fever may also be present.

◄ⓔ-**Video 6-3:** Changing IV Tubing and Fluids

 **Memory Jogger**

IV fluids and drugs that can damage veins include hypertonic solutions, potassium chloride, antibiotics, calcium, magnesium, alcohol, vasoconstrictive drugs, and chemotherapy drugs.

Check for phlebitis by looking for one or more reddened and warm areas or hard streaks that follow the vein path. The patient usually reports burning or pain in the area. If phlebitis occurs, remove the IV needle immediately and notify the prescriber. Apply ice or heat, depending on the amount of inflammation present.

*Subcutaneous tissues* are most commonly damaged during IV therapy by infiltration or extravasation. Infiltration occurs when chemically irritating IV fluids or drugs, called *vesicants*, leak into the subcutaneous tissues, causing tissue damage. Some fluids can cause tissue death *(necrosis)* and sloughing wherever they contact healthy tissue (see Figure 6-5). This damage is painful and may require grafting for healing. When strong drugs or fluids enter deeper tissues such as muscles, nerves, and even bones, these tissues can be damaged permanently. Drugs that constrict blood vessels can lead to tissue necrosis when infiltration occurs. These drugs can constrict local blood vessels so severely that oxygen and other nutrients cannot reach the tissues and tissue death occurs.

Prevent infiltration or extravasation by checking the IV site at least every 2 hours to ensure that the needle is completely in the vein. (When a vesicant drug is infusing, check the site hourly.) Use any of the following methods for checking for blood return (backup):

- Lower the IV bag or bottle below the level of the IV site and look for blood return. When the IV needle is in a small vein or if the patient has low blood pressure, blood return may not be evident, even when the needle is in the vein.
- Stop the IV infusion, wrap a tourniquet around the arm above the IV site, and look for blood return.
- Use a syringe to aspirate blood back into the tubing.
- Always listen to a patient's report of pain associated with an IV site. Remember that infiltration and extravasation can be present even though a blood return is obtained.
- Do not depend solely on blood return for assurance that the needle is in the vein. If the needle is partly in the vein and partly in the tissues, a blood return may be present, but the fluid is still leaking into the tissues. Another way to check for proper placement is to apply pressure on the vein about 2 inches above the IV site. The IV rate should decrease when pressure is applied.

Check for signs and symptoms of infiltration, which include swelling, pain, or burning at the IV site, paleness of the skin, coolness or warmth around the site, lack of blood return, and leakage around the needle. The IV rate is not always affected by infiltration or extravasation when an IV pump is used. The alarm on a pump may not be sensitive to the problem until it is severe. If infiltration is present or if extravasation is suspected, stop the IV infusion immediately. Remove the needle if there is any doubt that it is in the vein. Apply compresses to the IV site area for 2 to 3 days. Whether the compresses are hot or cold depends on the specific solution infiltrated; check with the pharmacist.

Document carefully when infiltration or extravasation occurs. Describe the area thoroughly and accurately when the infiltration or extravasation is discovered and then every 8 hours until the patient is discharged. Depending on the policies of the institution, daily photographs of the site may be taken and become part of the patient's permanent record.

### Imbalances of Fluid and Electrolytes

Because IV therapy involves infusion of fluids directly into the bloodstream, the potential risk for rapid changes in blood volume and composition is great. The effects of these changes depend on how rapidly the change occurs and what specific electrolytes are out of balance.

*Fluid overload* is the most common imbalance among patients receiving IV therapy. Usually fluid overload occurs because fluid is infused too rapidly. These factors can lead to fluid overload:

- Position changes of the patient or the IV bag

- Infusing IV fluids without using a controller or a pump
- A change made in the infusion rate by patients or visitors

Fluid overload can cause circulatory overload when the patient (especially an older patient) has cardiac or kidney problems. Carefully monitor intake and output and observe for symptoms of fluid overload (rapid pulse, elevated blood pressure, bulging hand veins, bulging neck veins in the sitting or standing positions, shortness of breath, coughing, and pitting edema). Fluid overload can occur quickly. In a patient who has kidney or heart problems, it may be life threatening. *You must report fluid overload immediately.*

*Electrolyte imbalances* may result in blood electrolyte levels that are too low or too high. Too much IV fluid can dilute the blood electrolytes. When the infusing fluid contains a high concentration of an electrolyte, rapid infusion can increase the blood electrolyte concentration to life-threatening levels. For example, if a solution is 40 mEq of potassium chloride in 1000 mL of 0.9% saline, rapid infusion can greatly increase the blood potassium to dangerous levels that can cause cardiac rhythm problems and death. For this reason any IV fluid containing potassium should always be given with a controller or pump.

## LIFE SPAN CONSIDERATIONS

***Pediatric Considerations.***   IV sites are difficult to access in younger children and infants. Although infants and younger children tend to have healthier tissues and veins than adults, their veins are small and can be very difficult to access. Veins on the scalp are most commonly used for IV therapy in infants. For younger children the top of the foot is a common site.

Young children and infants usually must be restrained to some degree to prevent accidental dislodging of the needle. Elbow restraints can prevent an infant with a scalp IV from rubbing or touching the IV site. When a foot, leg, or arm is used, limb motion must be limited. Consult a pediatric textbook for the best methods of limb restraint in young children. When the fluid being infused is known to be irritating or is a vesicant, check the site for a blood return and possible infiltration hourly. If infiltration occurs, discontinue the IV immediately and notify the prescriber.

Infants and young children have a narrow range of normal fluid volume, and the risk for fluid overload is great, especially in an infant. Always use microdrip tubing and a volume-controlled IV administration set with an infant or small child. These sets hold no more than 100 to 150 mL of fluid, so the maximum amount that could accidentally be infused is limited. Teach parents not to regulate the IV and to immediately report any observed change in the flow rate.

***Considerations for Older Adults.***   IV therapy in older adults may be especially difficult to start and maintain without complications. The skin on the forearm and hand may be thin and fragile from sun exposure and age. In addition, as a person ages, veins lose elasticity and become fragile, making vein damage easier. Box 6-1 offers tips to make IV therapy safer for older patients.

The older patient may be less able to tolerate rapid changes in fluid volume, and fluid overload can occur more easily. Always use a controller or pump with an older

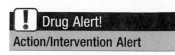

**Action/Intervention Alert**

Report signs and symptoms of fluid overload (rapid pulse, elevated blood pressure, bulging hand and neck veins, shortness of breath, coughing, and pitting edema) in a patient receiving IV therapy to the prescriber or charge nurse immediately.

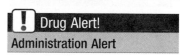

**Administration Alert**

Always use a controller or pump when infusing IV fluids that contain potassium.

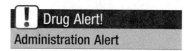

**Administration Alert**

Always use microdrip tubing and a volume-controlled IV administration set with an infant or small child.

---

**Box 6-1**   IV Therapy Safety for the Older Adult

- Check the older patient's mental status every 4 hours while on IV therapy.
- Use controllers, pumps, or small-volume containers to limit the possibility of fluid overload.
- Check the site and the patient hourly.
- Ask a coworker to stabilize the needle while you remove the tape or anchoring materials.
- Carefully remove the tape or anchoring materials from the sides inward toward the needle.
- Remove the needle gently while supporting the skin around it.
- Apply gentle but firm pressure over the insertion site for at least 2 to 5 minutes after removing the needle (longer if the patient is taking an anticoagulant).

patient to prevent accidental rapid infusion. Check the older patient receiving IV therapy every hour for signs and symptoms of fluid overload (rapid pulse, elevated blood pressure, bulging hand and neck veins, shortness of breath, coughing, and pitting edema). If these symptoms occur, slow the rate and notify the prescriber immediately.

## Get Ready for Practice!

### Key Points

- The rate of an IV infusion depends on the diameter of the tubing. The larger the diameter of IV tubing, the larger the drops.
- Report signs and symptoms of fluid overload (rapid pulse, elevated blood pressure, bulging hand and neck veins, shortness of breath, coughing, and pitting edema) in a patient receiving IV therapy to the prescriber or the charge nurse immediately.
- Because each brand of IV pump or control device differs, always read and follow the manufacturer's directions.
- Always calculate both the start and stop times and then time-tape the IV bag, even when it is on a controller or pump.
- Never speed up an IV to make up for lost time when the infusion is behind schedule.
- An IV controller works by gravity and only controls the rate that the fluid drips into the vein. A pump actually forces drops. Thus, if an infiltration has occurred, a controller stops, but a pump can continue to push IV fluid into the surrounding tissue.
- Always double check the order before starting an IV infusion.
- Signs and symptoms of phlebitis include burning and pain at the site, reddened and warm areas, or hard streaks that follow the vein path.
- Signs and symptoms of infiltration include pain or burning at the IV site, paleness of the skin, coolness or warmth around the site, lack of blood return, and leakage around the needle.
- A prescriber's order is not required to discontinue an IV that is infiltrated or infected at the insertion site.
- Always use a controller or pump with IV fluids that contain potassium.
- Use a controller or pump when giving IV fluids to an older adult.
- Use a volume-controlled IV administration set when giving IV fluids to infants and young children.

### Additional Learning Resources

e**volve** Go to your Evolve website (http://evolve.elsevier.com/Workman/pharmacology/) for the following FREE learning resources:
- eLearning Activities
- Animations
- Video Clips
- Interactive Review Questions
- Audio Key Points
- Audio Glossary
- Audio Glossary—Spanish-English
- Drug Dosage Calculators
- Patient Teaching Handouts

**SG** Go to your Study Guide for additional learning activities to help you master this chapter content.

### Review Questions

1. Which is a common health problem resulting from IV therapy?
   A. The patient is more likely to gain weight when receiving IV therapy.
   B. Adverse drug reactions happen more quickly with IV drugs.
   C. Patients are required to stay in bed during IV therapy.
   D. IV drugs cost more than oral drugs.

2. Why does a drop factor of 10 result in a faster infusion at the same number of drops per minute than a drop factor of 15?
   A. A drop factor of 10 is a bigger individual drop than a drop factor of 15.
   B. An infusion set with a drop factor of 10 has more drops per milliliter than an infusion set with a drop factor of 15.
   C. An infusion set with a drop factor of 10 has macrotubing, and an infusion set with a drop factor of 15 has microtubing.
   D. An infusion set with a drop factor of 15 has macrotubing, and an infusion set with a drop factor of 10 has microtubing.

3. Which parts of an order are needed to correctly calculate the flow rate?
   A. Drop factor, drop rate
   B. Specific fluid, number of hours
   C. Specific fluid, total volume to be infused.
   D. Total volume to be infused, number of hours

4. Calculate the flow rate for 1000 mL of dextrose 5% in NS to be infused over 6 hours. The tubing that is available has a drop factor of 20 gtts/mL. _____ gtts/min.

5. Which signs and symptoms are associated with fluid overload? (Select all that apply.)
   A. Hypotension
   B. Leg and ankle swelling
   C. Coughing
   D. Bulging neck veins in the sitting position
   E. Rapid pulse
   F. Shortness of breath

6. A patient's IV infusion is supposed to have a drip rate of 31 gtts/min. You count 6 gtts/15 seconds. What is your best action?

   A. Nothing; the IV flow rate is correct
   B. Increase the drip rate to 8 gtts/15 seconds
   C. Increase the drip rate to 10 gtts/15 seconds
   D. Decrease the drip rate to 4 gtts/15 seconds

7. Which parts of a written order for IV therapy are needed for it to be a valid order?

   A. Drop factor, flow rate, IV site
   B. Specific fluid, number of hours, drop rate
   C. Specific fluid, total volume to be infused, number of hours
   D. Total volume to be infused, number of hours, specific drop factor

8. With which IV drug type are you especially alert for chemical trauma if infiltration occurs?

   A. Anti-inflammatories
   B. Blood products
   C. Chemotherapy
   D. Antihypertensives

9. Which action do you implement to prevent tissue damage during IV therapy?

   A. Use a soft restraint to restrict the patient's arm movement
   B. Complete the infusion within the prescribed time frame
   C. Use a pump to ensure fluid infusion at the proper rate
   D. Check the IV site for a good blood return hourly

10. What action do you use to determine whether the blood return of an IV is adequate?

    A. Lowers the IV bag to a level below the insertion site and observes for blood rising in the tubing
    B. Closes the control roller and squeezes the patient's arm above the IV site until the side port fills with blood
    C. Disconnects the tubing from the needle hub and watches for at least 1 full mL of blood to drip out within 10 seconds
    D. Applies a tourniquet above the IV insertion site and asks the patient whether he or she is experiencing any pain or throbbing

11. What factor is most important for you to consider when maintaining IV therapy with a 5-month-old infant?

    A. Infants have small veins.
    B. Infants are at risk for fluid overload.
    C. Infants cannot verbally express their discomfort.
    D. Infants have healthier skin and veins than older patients.

## Critical Thinking Activities

The patient is a 250-pound, 22-year-old college student who was practicing football in 100° F heat. He comes to the health clinic and is diagnosed as being dehydrated. The order reads 1000 mL NS IV over 2 hours.

1. You have your choice of all administration sets (drop factors of 10, 15, and 20). Which one would be the most appropriate for this patient and this IV order? Provide a rationale for your answer.

2. Using the specific administration set with the drop factor that you selected, calculate the drops per minute needed to infuse the correct volume within the time ordered.

3. Is this patient at risk for fluid overload with the prescribed IV therapy? Why or why not?

## Answers To *Try This!* Problems

**TT-1** Calculate the milliliters to be infused in 1 hour given the following orders.

   a. 500 mL in 4 hours: $\frac{500}{4}$ = 125 mL in 1 hour
   b. 250 mL in 1 hour: $\frac{250}{1}$ = 250 mL in 1 hour
   c. 1000 mL in 6 hours: $\frac{1000}{6}$ = 166.66 mL, round to 167 mL in 1 hour
   d. 1000 mL in 24 hours: $\frac{1000}{24}$ = 41.66 mL, round to 42 mL in 1 hour

**TT-2** Calculate the drip rate using the macrodrip tubing shortcut.

   a. 1000 mL $D_5W$ in 6 hours, drop factor 10: $\frac{1000}{6}$ = 167 mL/hr ÷ 6 = 28 gtts/min
   b. 500 mL lactated Ringer's in 5 hours, drop factor 15: $\frac{500}{5}$ = 100 mL/hr ÷ 4 = 25 gtts/min
   c. 1000 mL NS in 24 hours, drop factor 20: $\frac{1000}{24}$ = 42 mL/hr ÷ 3 = 14 gtts/min

**TT-3** Calculate the drops per minute needed to get the right volume per hour.

   a. 500 mL $D_5W$ in 24 hours with microdrip tubing

   $\frac{500}{24}$ = 20.8 mL/hr, round up to 21 mL/hr and 21 gtts/min

   b. 1000 mL lactated Ringer's in 12 hours, drop factor = 15

   $\frac{1000}{12}$ = 83.33 mL/hr, round down to 83 mL per hour

   $\frac{\text{Volume (milliliters)}}{\text{Time (minutes)}}$ × Drop factor (drops per milliliter) = Drops per minute

   $\frac{83}{60}$ × 15 = 1.38 × 15 = 20.7 gtts/min, round up to 21 gtts/min

   c. 250 mL $D_5W$ in 2 hours, drop factor = 20

   $\frac{250}{2}$ = 125 mL/hr

   $\frac{\text{Volume (milliliters)}}{\text{Time (minutes)}}$ × Drop factor (drops per milliliter) = Drops per minute

   $\frac{125}{60}$ = 2.08 × 20 = 41.6 gtts/min, round up to 42 gtts/min

**TT-4** Calculate the 15-second drip rate for each of these problems.

   a. 20 gtts/min = 5 gtts/15 seconds
   b. 56 gtts/min = 14 gtts/15 seconds
   c. 28 gtts/min = 7 gtts/15 seconds

# Drugs for Pain and Sleep Problems

evolve

http://evolve.elsevier.com/Workman/pharmacology/

## Objectives

*After studying this chapter you should be able to:*

1. Identify personal factors that affect a patient's perception of pain.
2. Compare the features of acute pain with those of chronic pain.
3. Describe the different types of pain-control drugs.
4. Compare the features of drugs classified as controlled substances.
5. Explain what to do before and after giving an opioid drug for pain control.
6. List the names, actions, usual adult dosages, possible side effects, and adverse effects of commonly prescribed opioid drugs for pain control.
7. Explain what to teach patients about opioid drugs for pain control, including what to do, what not to do, and when to call the prescriber.
8. List the names, actions, usual adult dosages, possible side effects, and adverse effects of commonly prescribed nonopioid drugs for pain control.
9. Explain what to teach patients about nonopioid drugs for pain control, including what to do, what not to do, and when to call the prescriber.
10. Describe life span considerations for pain-control drugs.
11. List the names, actions, usual adult dosages, possible side effects, and adverse effects of drugs for sleep problems.
12. Explain what to do before and after giving a drug for sleep problems.
13. Explain what to teach patients about drugs for sleep problems.
14. Describe life span considerations related to drugs for sleep problems.

## Key Terms

**acute pain** (ă-KYŪT PĂN) (p. 99) Pain that has a sudden onset, an identifiable cause, and a limited duration; triggers physiologic changes; and improves with time even when it is not treated.

**addiction** (ă-DĬK-shŭn) (p. 105) The psychologic need or craving for the "high" feeling that results from using opioids when pain is not present.

**analgesics** (ăn-ăl-JĒ-zē-ŭ) (p. 101) Drugs that provide pain relief by either changing the perception of pain or reducing its source.

**antihistamines** (ăn-tĭ-HĬS-tă-mēnz) (p. 113) Drugs used to treat allergies and allergic reactions.

**benzodiazepine receptor agonists** (běn-zō-dī-ĂZ-ĕ-pēn rē-SĔP-tŭr Ă-gŏn-ĭsts) (p. 113) Drugs that depress the central nervous system and induce sleep by binding with gamma-aminobutyric acid (GABA) receptors.

**benzodiazepines** (běn-zō-dī-ĂZ-ĕ-pēnz) (p. 113) A class of psychotropic drugs with hypnotic and sedative effects, used mainly as tranquilizers to control symptoms of anxiety or stress and as sleeping aids for insomnia.

**chronic pain** (KRŎN-ĭk PĂN) (p. 100) Pain that has a long duration, may not have an identifiable cause, does not trigger physiologic changes, and persists or increases with time.

**controlled substance** (kŏn-TRŌLD SŬB-stěns) (p. 101) A drug containing ingredients known to be addictive that is regulated by the Federal Controlled Substances Act of 1970.

**dependence** (dē-PĔN-děns) (p. 105) Physical changes in autonomic nervous system function that can occur when opioids are used long term.

**insomnia** (ĭn-SŎM-nē-ŭ) (p. 112) Inability to go to sleep or to remain asleep throughout the night.

**narcolepsy** (NĂR-kō-lěp-sē) (p. 116) A sleep problem with sudden, uncontrollable urges to sleep, causing the person to fall asleep at inappropriate times.

**nociceptors** (nō-sĭ-SĔP-tŭr) (p. 98) Free sensory nerve endings that, when activated, trigger a message sent to the brain that allows the perception of pain.

**nonopioid analgesic** (NŎN-Ō-pē-ōyd ăn-ăl-JĒZ-ĭk) (p. 107) A drug that reduces a person's perception of pain; it is not similar to opium and has little potential for psychologic or physical dependence.

**opioid analgesic** (Ō-pē-ōyd ăn-ăl-JĒZ-ĭk) (p. 103) A drug containing any ingredient derived from the poppy plant (or a similar synthetic chemical) that changes a person's perception of pain and has a potential for psychologic or physical dependence.

**pain** (PĂN) (p. 95) An unpleasant sensory and emotional experience associated with acute or potential tissue damage; pain is whatever a patient says it is and exists whenever a patient says it does.

**pain threshold** (PĂN THRĔSH-hōld) (p. 99) The smallest amount of tissue damage that must be present before a person is even aware that he or she is having pain.

**pain tolerance** (PĂN TŎL-ŭr-ĕns) (p. 99) A person's ability to endure or "stand" pain intensity.

**sedatives** (SĔD-ĕ-tĭvz) (p. 113) Drugs that promote sleep by targeting signals in the brain to produce calm and ease agitation.

**sleep** (SLĒP) (p. 112) A natural and necessary periodic state of rest for the mind and body, in which consciousness is partly or completely lost, eyes close, metabolism slows,

body movements decrease, and responsiveness to external stimuli declines.

**sleep deprivation** (SLĒP dĕp-rĭ-VĀ-shŭn) (p. 112) A shortage of quality, undisturbed sleep with detrimental effects on physical and mental well-being; also known as sleep debt.

**tolerance** (TŎL-ŭr-ĕns) (p. 105) The adjustment of the body to long-term opioid use that increases the rate that a drug is eliminated and reduces the main effects (pain relief) and side effects of the drug. More drug is needed to achieve the same degree of pain relief.

**withdrawal** (wĭth-DRŌ-ĕl) (p. 105) Autonomic nervous system symptoms occurring when long-term opioid therapy is stopped suddenly after physical dependence is present. Symptoms include nausea, vomiting, abdominal cramping, sweating, delirium, and seizures.

◀ⓔ-Learning Activity 7-1

## PAIN

Pain, like life, is personal and subjective with no objective measures. It is common, and everyone experiences it in a different way. Therefore pain is what the patient says it is. The best way to describe and monitor pain is through the patient's own report.

Pain is an unpleasant sensory and emotional experience associated with tissue damage. We perceive pain with all our senses. How we feel and react to pain depends on our emotional makeup along with our previous experiences with pain. Issues such as culture, age, gender, and our interactions with society also affect our responses to pain.

Pain is called the *fifth vital sign* because unrelieved or undertreated pain is a common but avoidable health problem. In addition, the presence of some types of pain changes the other four vital signs (pulse, respiratory rate, temperature, blood pressure). Checking for pain as often as we check other vital signs increases our awareness of its presence and of the patient's actual responses to drugs and other interventions.

Pain is divided into *acute* and *chronic*, with chronic pain having additional divisions. Acute pain is the most common reason that patients seek medical help. The five most common sources of acute pain are muscle, gastrointestinal, chest pain, headache, and injuries (especially when bones are broken or tissues are swollen).

Chronic pain changes a person's life and affects not only those with pain but their families. *Chronic* means that a person lives with pain all day, just about every day, and has done so for at least 6 months. One type of chronic pain is the pain caused by cancer.

Pain is often both underreported and undertreated, leading to poor pain control. Box 7-1 lists factors that contribute to the poor reporting and treatment of pain. One factor in good pain control is recognizing the severity of the patient's pain, even when he or she cannot describe it.

How much pain the patient feels is called *pain intensity*. There are several ways to work with the patient to determine pain intensity. Figure 7-1 shows examples of common pain scales that are useful for an alert patient to rate his or her pain. When the patient cannot speak or when you are working with young children, a nonverbal scale called FACES may be used (Figure 7-2). The patient picks the face on the scale that best represents how he or she is feeling. Another scale, the FLACC scale, is often

**Memory Jogger**

Pain is whatever the patient says it is and exists whenever he or she says it does.

**Memory Jogger**

Assess the patient for pain whenever you check his or her vital signs.

Box **7-1**    Barriers to Good Pain Management

- Patient's and health care worker's fear of addiction
- Patient's fear of meaning of pain, for example:
  - Worsening of condition
  - Threats to independence
  - Impending death
- Patient's and health care worker's belief that pain is an expected part of aging
- Patient's fear of testing
- Health care worker's fear of "drugging the older adult"
- Health care provider's fear of overdosing a patient

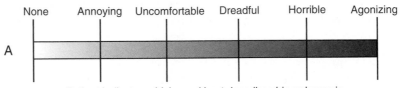

None    Annoying    Uncomfortable    Dreadful    Horrible    Agonizing

**A**

Patient indicates which word best describes his or her pain

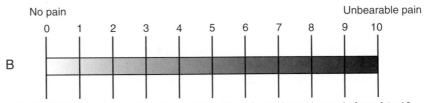

No pain                                          Unbearable pain

0    1    2    3    4    5    6    7    8    9    10

**B**

Patient indicates the number that matches his or her pain on the scale from 0 to 10

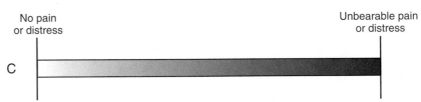

No pain                                          Unbearable pain
or distress                                        or distress

**C**

Patient marks a place on the line that matches his or her level of pain

**FIGURE 7-1** Examples of patient pain-rating scales. **A,** Simple descriptive pain scale. **B,** Numeric pain distress scale. **C,** Visual analog scale.

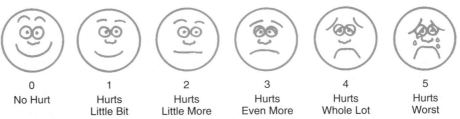

| 0 | 1 | 2 | 3 | 4 | 5 |
| No Hurt | Hurts Little Bit | Hurts Little More | Hurts Even More | Hurts Whole Lot | Hurts Worst |

**FIGURE 7-2** The Wong-Baker FACES Pain Rating Scale for children and nonverbal adults.

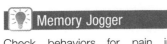

**Memory Jogger**

Check behaviors for pain in patients who cannot point or express pain in words.

used for infants, very young children, and any patient who cannot express pain in words or point to a face (Figure 7-3). This scale uses observations and scoring of behaviors to establish a pain intensity level.

Follow the guidelines set by your workplace for the treatment of pain. Reassure the patient that you know that the pain is real and you will do whatever you can to relieve it.

| Category | Score | | |
|---|---|---|---|
| | **0** | **1** | **2** |
| Face | No particular expression or smile | Occasional grimace or frown, withdrawn, disinterested | Frequent-to-constant quivering chin, clenched jaw |
| Legs | Normal position or relaxed | Uneasy, restless, tense | Kicking, or legs drawn up |
| Activity | Lying quietly, normal position, moves easily | Squirming, shifting back and forth, tense | Arched, rigid, or jerking |
| Cry | No cry (awake or asleep) | Moans or whimpers, occasional complaint | Crying steadily, screams or sobs, or frequent complaints |
| Consolability | Content, relaxed | Reassured by occasional touching, hugging, or being talked to, distractible | Difficult to console or comfort |

Each of the five categories–(F) Face, (L) Legs, (A) Activity, (C) Cry, (C) Consolability–
is scored from 0-2, which results in a total score between 0 and 10.

**FIGURE 7-3** The FLACC pain rating scale for infants and patients who are not alert.

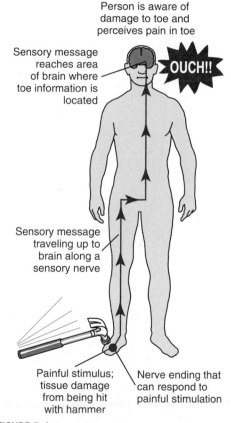

**FIGURE 7-4** A sensory pathway for pain perception.

# REVIEW OF RELATED PHYSIOLOGY AND PATHOPHYSIOLOGY

## PAIN ORIGIN AND TRANSMISSION

Acute pain, although uncomfortable, can be a helpful response because it tells us that something is wrong and often where it is wrong. The brain is the place where pain is actually "felt" (Figure 7-4). If you stub your toe, the damage stimulates nerve endings that send messages along a sensory nerve to the place in your brain where that particular nerve stops. The message triggers your brain to know that your toe hurts. So, even though the damage causing the pain occurs in the toe, it is your brain

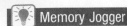
that *perceives* the pain. If the sensory nerve between your toe and your brain were severed, you would not feel pain in your toe no matter how badly you injured it. Also, if the area of your brain that is connected to the sensory nerve of the toe were damaged or destroyed, you would not feel pain as a result of hurting your toe.

**Nociceptors** are sensory nerve endings that, when activated, trigger the message sent to the brain that allows the perception of pain (Figure 7-5). Nociceptors can be activated when body chemicals called *mediators* bind to them. The mediators for pain include substance P ("P" is for "pain") and many of the same mediators that cause the symptoms of inflammation, especially bradykinin (see Chapter 8). When mediators are released from damaged tissue (such as when you stub your toe), they bind to the nociceptors and activate them (see Figure 7-5). Once activated, the receptor starts electrical changes that send the message along the nerve to the brain.

Other ways that the receptors can be triggered include changing their shapes (by stretching or applying pressure), exposing them to extreme heat or cold, and reducing the oxygen level in the tissue surrounding them. For example, when you have a large amount of intestinal gas, the wall of the intestine and the nociceptors in the

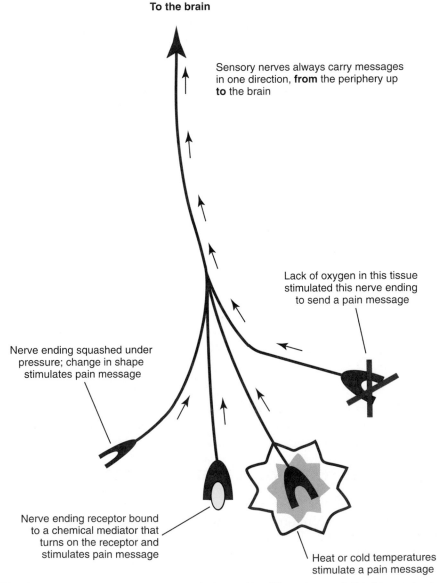

**To the brain**

Sensory nerves always carry messages in one direction, **from** the periphery up **to** the brain

Lack of oxygen in this tissue stimulated this nerve ending to send a pain message

Nerve ending squashed under pressure; change in shape stimulates pain message

Nerve ending receptor bound to a chemical mediator that turns on the receptor and stimulates pain message

Heat or cold temperatures stimulate a pain message

**FIGURE 7-5** Sensory nerve endings (nociceptors) triggered by different types of stimuli to send pain messages to the brain.

intestinal walls are stretched. This stretching activates the nociceptors, which makes you feel abdominal pain.

Different types of nerve fibers transmit pain messages to the brain. These fibers differ in how fast they transmit the message, where they are located, and what type of pain sensation is transmitted. This is one reason why not all pain drugs work in the same way and why some drugs are very effective in relieving one type of pain and not effective at all for another.

## PAIN PERCEPTION

Different nerve fibers end in different areas of the brain. This means that the brain perceives pain on different levels. At lower brain levels the person may not know exactly what is wrong but will try to move away from a pain source. This type of response can occur even when the person is asleep or not fully conscious. At the highest brain levels the person can pinpoint the location of pain and describe it.

Some fibers pass through areas of the brain where emotions and memories are stored, allowing emotions, memories, and behavior to affect pain perception. In addition, because nerve fibers pass through many body areas on the way to the brain and interact with other nerves, the perception of pain location is not always direct. Pain may be *localized*, which means that the patient feels pain that is confined to the site where the tissue damage is located. For example, when you stub your toe, you know which foot and which toe are affected. Other times the patient feels the pain all along the path of the nerve from the point of the damaged tissue to the spinal cord. For example, an injury to the little finger in the left hand may cause a person to have pain all along the underside of the left forearm. This type of pain is called *projected pain*. Sometimes a person feels the pain all around and extending out from the problem causing the pain. For example, the pain of a heart attack is often felt as chest pain that extends up the jaw and down the left arm. This type of pain is called *radiating pain*. A person may sense pain in an area that is not close to the tissue causing the pain (*referred pain*). For example, pain from gallstones is often felt under the right shoulder blade instead of directly at the location of the gallbladder.

Each person's pain perception is different. The smallest amount of tissue damage that makes a person aware of having pain is known as the **pain threshold**. It is the point that a person first feels any pain. The pain threshold is different for every person and varies from one body site to another. Factors such as age and the presence of other diseases also affect pain threshold. Most drugs used for pain control change (raise) the patient's pain threshold.

Related to pain threshold is **pain tolerance**, which is a person's ability to endure or "stand" the pain intensity. Behavioral and emotional factors rather than physical factors are more likely to affect a person's pain tolerance. These factors are modifiable and include what the person thinks the pain means, how family and friends expect the patient to behave while in pain, and previous experience with pain. This makes pain tolerance unique to each person. Fear, anxiety, and lack of sleep are a few factors that reduce a person's pain tolerance. Relaxation and distraction increase pain tolerance.

Pain tolerance is so personal that you cannot determine a person's level of pain on the basis of behavior. You must always ask patients about their pain. Just because a person tolerates pain does not mean that he or she isn't suffering!

## TYPES OF PAIN

Pain also is divided into types on the basis of its cause, how long it lasts, and whether it is present continuously or comes and goes (*intermittent*). The three main types of pain are acute, chronic, and cancer. Table 7-1 lists the features of acute and chronic pain.

### Acute Pain

**Acute pain** has a sudden onset, an identifiable cause, and a limited duration; triggers physiologic changes; and improves with time even when it is not treated. It is the

 **Memory Jogger**

Different types of nerve fibers are responsible for the type of pain felt and which type of pain drug is most effective at relieving the pain.

 **Memory Jogger**

Nonmodifiable factors affecting pain perception are age and the presence of disease. These factors cannot be changed.

 **Clinical Pitfall**

Do not assume that a patient who is tolerating pain well is comfortable.

Table **7-1** Comparison of Acute and Chronic Pain Features

| ACUTE PAIN | CHRONIC PAIN |
| --- | --- |
| Sudden onset | Intermittent or persistent |
| Often has an identifiable cause | Exact cause may or may not be known |
| Limited duration | Unlimited duration |
| Triggers physiologic responses:<br>  Increased heart rate and breathing<br>  Increased blood pressure<br>  Sweating | Physiologic responses disappear with time |
| Improves with time | Does not improve and may even worsen |
| Variable intensity | Intensity may increase over time |
| Relatively superficial | Deeper pain |
| Described as sharp, stabbing, pricking, or electric | Described as burning, aching, throbbing |

 **Memory Jogger**

Common physiologic changes with acute pain include elevated heart rate, blood pressure, and respiratory rate; cool, clammy skin; dry mouth; restlessness; and inability to concentrate.

 **Memory Jogger**

The four most common sources of chronic pain are:
• Neck and back pain.
• Arthritis pain.
• Migraine headaches.
• Nerve pain.

**Clinical Pitfall**

Do not rely on changes in vital signs to indicate the intensity of chronic pain.

most common pain type; typical causes include trauma, surgery, heart attack, inflammation, and burns. Even though acute pain is temporary and decreases as the damaged tissue heals, it can be severe and should be treated.

One of the main features of acute pain is the physical response of the body to it. Pain is a stressor, and acute pain triggers the stress response (sometimes called the *fight or flight* response). This response occurs whenever the sympathetic part of the autonomic nervous system is activated. The stress response includes elevated heart rate, respiratory rate, and blood pressure. Skin becomes cool and clammy with increased sweating of the hands and feet. The mouth becomes dry, and usually the pupils of the eyes dilate. A person's behavioral responses when the stress response is triggered by acute pain include restlessness, inability to concentrate, general distress, and a sense that something bad is happening (sometimes called a sense of *impending doom*).

### Chronic Pain

A traditional definition for separating acute pain from chronic pain is that **chronic pain** is present daily for 6 months. It persists or increases with time, may not have an identifiable cause, and does not trigger the stress response. Chronic pain may hurt less on some days than others but is usually always present. Causes may be difficult to find. This problem has often led to family members and health care workers not believing the patient's reports of pain and its intensity.

One of the most important differences between acute and chronic pain is that chronic pain is present so long that the stress response of the body is no longer triggered. This means that a person with chronic pain can have severe pain intensity without changes from the normal ranges for heart rate, breathing rate, or blood pressure.

### Cancer Pain

Cancer pain, sometimes called *malignant pain*, has both unique features and features in common with acute and chronic pain. Not every person with cancer has pain. Box 7-2 lists the main features of cancer pain.

Cancer pain has many causes and is complex. This means that more than one pain strategy and often more than one type of drug for pain control are needed. In addition, the diagnosis of cancer may increase this patient's anxiety and fear, making the pain worse.

Often the patient with cancer receives traditional pain-control drugs but at much higher doses than those prescribed for other types of pain. The drug therapy plan may include every type of pain-control drug given in combination to ensure ade-

---

Box **7-2**   Main Features of Cancer Pain

- The most distressing and most feared complication of cancer
- Complex, with many emotional and physical issues
- More than one cause
- Shares features with acute pain and chronic pain
- Can be present in more than one body area at the same time
- Usually occurs later in cancer progression
- Can be managed but usually requires more than one drug type for adequate control
- Type of pain in which nonopioid miscellaneous drugs play a major role

---

quate pain relief. Drug therapy for cancer pain must be tailored to each patient for the most effective pain control.

◄ -Learning Activity 7-2

## GENERAL ISSUES RELATED TO ANALGESIC DRUG THERAPY

Pain is the number one health problem that drives people to seek medical help. It interferes with every aspect of a person's life and usually decreases the quality of life. Pain control involves many different approaches. Drug therapy is one approach. *Usually the nondrug therapies for pain control are used along with drug therapy, not in place of it.* The use of other therapies such as relaxation, massage, distraction, guided imagery, and application of electrical stimulation to the skin over a painful area can reduce the amount of drugs or change the type of drugs needed to help control pain.

Analgesics are drugs that control pain, by changing either the perception or the source of pain. Different types of drugs are used for pain control based on their composition and how they work. The three main types of pain control drugs include opioids, nonsteroidal anti-inflammatory drugs, and nonopioid miscellaneous drugs. Different types of pain respond differently to each drug type.

All analgesic drugs provide some degree of pain relief; but some drugs are stronger than others, and it may take a greater amount of a weaker drug to provide the same amount of pain relief that a stronger drug provides.

Drugs prescribed for pain control have traditionally been ordered on a PRN or "as needed" basis, usually with a range of doses permitted (for example, "Give morphine sulfate 2 to 6 mg IV every 4 to 6 hours PRN"). Such drug orders, known as *range orders*, are not always effective for controlling acute pain because there is too much variation in the timing and dose of the drug. Patients often try to go as long as possible before accepting another dose, or health care workers may stick to the lowest doses and the longest durations.

Better pain-control plans involve two techniques: doses are given on a schedule around the clock to prevent complete elimination of the drug before the next dose, or the patient is given a machine to "punch in" a small intravenous (IV) dose whenever the need arises. This is called *patient-controlled analgesia (PCA)*. Sometimes these two techniques are used at the same time for personalized and effective pain control.

Many drugs used for pain control have ingredients that may be addictive. In the United States any drug that contains ingredients known to be addictive is classified by the federal government as a controlled substance and is regulated by the Federal Controlled Substances Act of 1970. This act classifies controlled substances into five different schedules based on how likely they are to result in addiction. The drugs most likely to lead to addiction are in schedule I. Those with the least potential for addiction are in schedule V. Table 7-2 describes and lists examples of drugs in each category.

The agency with the responsibility for enforcing the distribution of controlled substances in the United States is the Drug Enforcement Administration (DEA). The DEA reviews the actions of individual prescribers and investigates when the amount or type of drugs prescribed for a patient or a group of patients suggests controlled-substance abuse.

 **Clinical Pitfall**

Do not rely on nondrug therapies alone for pain control.

 **Memory Jogger**

Analgesics include:
- Opioids.
- Nonsteroidal anti-inflammatory drugs (NSAIDs).
- Nonopioid miscellaneous drugs.

**Clinical Pitfall**

Pain drugs have varying strengths and dosages to achieve the same level of pain relief.

 **Memory Jogger**

In the United States drugs and drug products with the highest potential for addiction or abuse are classified as schedule I; those with the lowest potential for addiction or abuse are classified as schedule V.

Table **7-2**    **Classification of Controlled Substances (United States)**

| SCHEDULE | DESCRIPTION | EXAMPLES |
|---|---|---|
| I | High potential for abuse<br>No accepted medical use in treatment in United States<br>Lack of accepted safety for use of the drug or other substance under medical supervision | More than 80 drugs or substances of which the following are the most well known:<br>Alpha-acetylmethadol; gamma-hydroxybutyric acid (GBH); heroin; lysergic acid diethylamide (LSD); marijuana; mescaline; peyote; "quaaludes" |
| II | High potential for abuse<br>Currently accepted use for treatment in United States<br>Abuse may lead to severe psychologic dependence or physical dependence | More than 30 drugs or substances of which the following are the most well known:<br>Amphetamines; cocaine; codeine; fentanyl; hydromorphone (Dilaudid); meperidine (Demerol); methadone; methylphenidate (Ritalin); morphine; oxycodone (Percodan); pentobarbital; secobarbital |
| III | Potential for abuse is less than the drugs or substances in schedules I and II<br>Currently accepted medical use for treatment in the United States<br>Abuse may lead to moderate or low physical dependence or high psychologic dependence | Most drugs are compounds containing some small amounts of the drugs from schedule II along with acetaminophen or aspirin such as Tylenol No. 3 or No. 4, Fiorinal<br>Other drugs include anabolic steroids such as testosterone preparations and sodium oxybate [Xyrem], a drug containing GHB for use with the sleep disorder narcolepsy |
| IV | Low potential for abuse relative to the drugs or substances in schedule III<br>Currently accepted medical use for treatment in the United States<br>Abuse may lead to limited physical dependence or psychologic dependence relative to the drugs or substances in schedule III | Include diet drugs with propionic acid<br>Other well-known drugs include benzodiazepines (lorazepam [Ativan], flurazepam [Dalmane], diazepam [Valium], midazolam [Versed], alprazolam [Xanax]); chloral hydrate; paraldehyde; pentazocine (Talwin); phenobarbital |
| V | Low potential for abuse relative to the drugs or substances in schedule IV<br>Currently accepted medical use in the United States<br>Abuse may lead to limited physical dependence or psychologic dependence relative to the drugs or substances in schedule IV | Include cough preparations with small amounts of codeine and drugs for diarrhea that also contain small amounts of opioids such as diphenoxylate with atropine (Lomotil) |

Source: United States Drug Enforcement Administration (DEA), Title 21, Section 812.

Many different drug types can be used as analgesia for pain control. Each type has both different and common actions and effects. The *intended response* of all pain-control drugs is to reduce pain. General nursing responsibilities for safe administration of drugs for pain control are listed in the following paragraphs. Specific nursing responsibilities are listed with each individual drug class.

*Responsibilities before administering pain-control drugs* include checking the patient's pain intensity using the pain scale preferred by your workplace (see Figures 7-1 through 7-3). Checking the pain level before you give a drug helps to determine how effective the drug is in relieving the patient's pain.

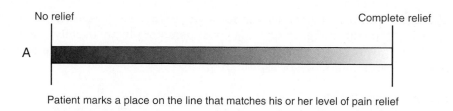

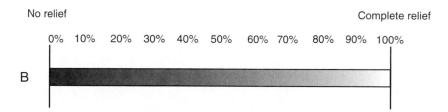

Patient indicates the number that matches his or her relief from pain in percentages

**FIGURE 7-6** Examples of patient pain-relief rating scales. **A,** Pain-relief visual analog scale. **B,** Percent pain-relief scale.

Check to see when the patient last received the drug for pain control. Giving doses too close together can lead to more side effects or toxic levels. Giving doses too far apart can lead to pain and suffering for the patient. If the patient is to receive a drug on a regular schedule rather than PRN, try to keep on schedule even if the patient is sleeping or is not reporting pain. *A sleeping patient is not necessarily comfortable or pain free.*

*Responsibilities after administering a pain-control drug* include asking how much pain relief the patient has received as a result of the drug. This helps to determine if the drug is right for the patient's pain, if the dose needs to be changed, or if the pain control strategy must be adjusted. Figure 7-6 shows two scales to determine how well a drug may relieve a patient's pain. Check pain relief after 30 minutes and then hourly until the next dose is scheduled.

*Teach the patient taking a pain-control drug* that the best pain relief occurs when drugs are taken on a regular schedule rather than PRN. If the patient thinks that the pain is improving and less drug is needed, tell him or her to first reduce the dose but maintain the schedule. If the pain continues to improve, the time between doses may be increased. Remind the patient that addiction will not occur if the drugs are taken to relieve pain.

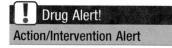

**Drug Alert!**

**Action/Intervention Alert**

Check the patient's pain level 30 minutes *after* giving a pain-control drug and then hourly.

## OPIOIDS (NARCOTICS)

Opioid analgesics, also called *narcotics*, are drugs that contain any ingredient derived from the poppy plant (or a similar synthetic chemical) that change a person's perception of pain and have the potential for psychologic or physical dependence. All opioids work in the same way and have similar side effects. The main difference among various types of opioids is the strength of the drug.

Opioids can be addictive and are classified by the U.S. federal government as schedule II drugs. They also have a high potential for abuse that can lead to psychologic or physical dependence. The fear of addiction to opioids is one cause of poorly treated pain. In addition, opioids are *high-alert drugs* that have an increased risk of causing patient harm if used in error. The error may be giving too high a dose, giving too low a dose, giving a dose to a patient for whom it was not prescribed, and not giving it to a patient for whom it was prescribed.

The following table describes opioids most commonly used for pain control. Be sure to consult a drug reference for more information about any specific opioid. The dosages listed are those recommended for acute pain. The dosages used for other pain types may be much higher. Opioids given parenterally are usually single-agent drugs. When given orally, opioid tablets, capsules, or liquids may contain other drugs such as acetaminophen or aspirin.

### Dosages for Common Opioids

| Drug | Dosage |
|---|---|
| morphine ❶ (Morphine Sulfate, Duramorph, Epimorph🍁, Morphitec🍁, Roxanol, MS Contin) | *Adults:* 10-30 mg orally every 4 hr (Children's oral dose calculated individually based on the child's age, size, and pain severity) *Adults:* 5-20 mg IM or 4-10 mg IV every 4 hr *Children:* 100-200 mcg/kg IM or 50-100 mcg/kg IV every 4 hr |
| hydromorphone ❶ (Dilaudid, Hydrostat) | *Adults:* 2-7.5 mg orally every 3-6 hr; 1-4 mg IM every 4-6 hr; 500 mcg-1 mg IV every 3 hr as needed Safety and efficacy in children not established |
| meperidine ❶ (Demerol) | *Adults:* 50-150 mg orally, IM, or IV every 3-4 hr *Children:* 1.1-1.7 mg/kg orally or IM every 3-4 hr |
| codeine ❶ (Paveral🍁) | *Adults:* 15-60 mg orally or IM every 3-6 hr *Children:* 0.5 mg/kg orally or IM every 3-6 hr |
| fentanyl ❶ (Fentanyl, Actiq, Oralet) | Oral lozenges and lollipops vary in strength; check carefully |
| fentanyl transdermal ❶ (Duragesic) | *Adults:* 0.05-0.1 mg IM every 1-2 hr, or 2.5-10 mg patch every 72 hr |
| oxycodone **TOP 100** ❶ (OxyContin, OxyFast, Supeudol🍁) | *Adults:* 10-160 mg orally every 12 hr |
| oxycodone with acetaminophen ❶ (Endocet🍁, Percocet, Tylox) | *Adults:* 1.5-10 mg orally every 4-6 hr |
| oxycodone with aspirin ❶ (Endodan🍁, Oxycodan, Percodan) | *Adults:* 1.5-10 mg orally every 4-6 hr |
| oxymorphone ❶ (Opana, Numorphan) | *Adults:* 10-20 mg orally every 4-6 hr |
| hydrocodone **TOP 100** ❶ (Lortab, Vicodin) | *Adults:* 5-10 mg orally every 4-6 hr *Children:* 2-5 mg orally every 4-6 hr |
| hydrocodone with acetaminophen ❶ (Dolacet, Polygesic, Vicodin) | *Adults:* 5-7 mg orally every 4-6 hr *Children:* 2.5 mg orally in solution every 4-6 hr |
| tramadol **TOP 100** ❶ (Ultram) | *Adults:* 50-70 mg orally every 6 hr |

❶ High-alert drug; **TOP 100** Top 100 drugs prescribed.

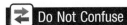

### Do Not Confuse

**OxyContin** *with* **MS Contin**

An order for OxyContin can be confused with MS Contin. Although both drugs are opioids, the large differences in dosages make underdosing or overdosing possible.

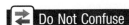

### Do Not Confuse

**hydromorphone** *with* **morphine**

An order for hydromorphone can be confused with morphine. Although both drugs are opioids, hydromorphone is five times stronger than morphine. Giving hydromorphone in place of morphine could result in a serious overdose.

### Do Not Confuse

**tramadol** *with* **Toradol**

An order for tramadol can be confused with Toradol. Tramadol is an oral opioid analgesic. Toradol is a nonsteroidal anti-inflammatory drug (NSAID) that can be given orally or parenterally.

### ? Did You Know?

You make your own opioids when you have pain and during extreme physical labor.

### How Opioids Work

The classic opioid is morphine. Morphine and all other opioids work by binding to opioid receptor sites in the brain and other areas. When specific opioid receptor sites are bound by morphine, they are activated and alter a person's perception of pain. *Opioids only alter the perception of pain; they do nothing at the site of damaged tissue to reduce the cause of pain.*

We have opioid receptor sites because the body makes its own opioid-like chemicals called *endorphin* and *enkephalin*. When these two substances bind to opioid receptors, they activate these receptors, decreasing pain and increasing the feeling of well-being. This means that opioids are receptor agonists because they work in the same way as endorphins and enkephalins to activate opioid receptors.

***Side Effects***.   The most common side effect of opioids is constipation. Some patients may have nausea and vomiting if intestinal motility is affected. At higher dosages drowsiness is common.

***Adverse Effects.***   *Respiratory depression* is possible when opioids are used, especially at higher doses and when the drugs are given intravenously. Most patients only have mild respiratory depression, with respirations dropping to 7 to 12 breaths/minute. If severe (less than 8 breaths/minute), action must be taken to prevent hypoxia (low tissue oxygen levels).

*Addiction, dependence, tolerance,* and *withdrawal* can occur with opioid use. **Dependence** is the physical changes in autonomic nervous system function that can occur when opioids are used long term (more than a few weeks, especially after pain is reduced or no longer present). **Addiction** is the psychologic need or craving for the "high" feeling resulting from the use of opioids when pain is not present. When opioids are needed for pain, their use seldom causes either dependence or addiction.

Two other adverse effects or problems of opioid use are tolerance and withdrawal. **Tolerance** is the adjustment of the body to long-term opioid use that increases the rate that the drug is eliminated and reduces the main effect (pain relief) and side effects of the drug. It occurs with anyone who is taking opioids for a long period of time, whether or not he or she has pain. More drug is needed to achieve the same degree of pain relief.

**Withdrawal** is the occurrence of autonomic nervous system symptoms when long-term opioid therapy is stopped suddenly after physical dependence is present. Symptoms include nausea, vomiting, abdominal cramping, sweating, delirium, and seizures. This reaction seldom occurs in a patient who is taking opioids for pain. It is common among people who are not in pain but who take opioids for the psychologic "high" that they can produce.

## What To Do *Before* Giving Opioids

Be sure to review the general nursing responsibilities related to analgesic therapy for pain (p. 102) in addition to these specific responsibilities for opioid drugs.

Check the patient's respiratory rate and oxygen saturation. Opioids can cause some degree of respiratory depression.

Check the dose and the specific drug name carefully. *Opioids are not interchangeable because the strength of the drugs varies. Only the prescriber can change the drug order.* Drug doses must be recalculated by the prescriber when one opioid is switched to another.

## What To Do *After* Giving Opioids

Be sure to review the general nursing responsibilities related to analgesic therapy for pain (p. 103) in addition to these specific responsibilities for opioids.

Monitor the patient's respiratory rate and oxygen saturation at least hourly. If the respiratory rate is 8 or less and the patient is sleeping, try to wake him or her. First call the patient's name. If there is no response, gently shake his or her arm. Shake more firmly if needed. If the patient does not respond to these actions, use a slightly stronger trigger (without using enough force to cause harm) such as:

- Squeezing the trapezius muscle (located at the angle of the shoulder and neck muscle).
- Applying pressure to the nail bed.

If the patient cannot be aroused, immediately call for help. If the patient's oxygen saturation is below 95% or is five percentage points lower than his or her normal saturation, arouse the patient and check the saturation when fully awake. If the saturation does not improve when fully awake, apply supplemental oxygen and notify the charge nurse or prescriber.

When respiratory depression is severe, the opioid effects may need to be reversed by giving an opioid blocker (antagonist) such as naloxone (Narcan). When an IV

---

**Common Side Effects**

**Opioids**

Constipation, Nausea/   Drowsiness
Vomiting

 **Memory Jogger**

Drug dependence is a physical problem; drug addiction is a psychologic problem.

 **Clinical Pitfall**

Never substitute one opioid for another without an order from the prescriber that includes a recalculation of the dose. Strengths vary.

⊖-Animation 7-1: Opiate ►
Intoxication

opioid blocker is given, it displaces opioids on the opioid receptors. When the opioid is off the receptors, all the effects of the opioids are reversed within 1 minute, including respiratory depression. Unfortunately the pain control effects are also reversed. Watch the patient who has received an opioid receptor blocker for respiratory depression very closely for several hours in case respiratory depression recurs.

A patient receiving an opioid may become very drowsy and is at risk for falling. Be sure to raise the side rails. Place the call light button within easy reach for the patient. Remind him or her to call for help to get out of bed for any reason.

When a patient is receiving opioids for several days, ask about constipation daily. Most patients taking opioids for 2 days or longer have constipation. Urge the patient to drink plenty of fluids and be sure to give any prescribed stool softeners or laxatives.

Opioids can cause a sudden lowering of blood pressure, especially when the patient changes position *(orthostatic hypotension)*. Help the patient change position slowly. When getting out of bed, he or she should sit for a few minutes on the side of the bed before attempting to get up. Help him or her during walking to help prevent falling.

### What To *Teach* Patients About Opioids

Be sure to teach patients the general care needs and precautions related to analgesic therapy for pain (p. 103) in addition to these specific responsibilities for opioids.

Opioids can cause nausea and vomiting. Taking opioids with food rather than on an empty stomach can reduce this problem.

Opioids cause drowsiness. Warn the patient not to drive or operate heavy machinery when taking these drugs. In addition, the patient may feel dizzy or light-headed from a sudden drop in blood pressure. Tell him or her to move slowly when rising or changing positions.

Constipation is a common side effect because opioids slow intestinal movement. Teach the patient to drink at least 3 to 4 L of fluids daily if he or she has no health problem that requires fluid restriction. If the prescriber has ordered a stool softener or laxative, urge the patient to start using these drugs before constipation occurs.

### Life Span Considerations for Opioids

*Pediatric Considerations.*    Opioid drugs are *high-alert medications* that are used for pain control in children of all ages. Dosages are calculated for each child on the basis of the child's age, size (weight in kilograms), health, and pain severity. Identifying pain intensity with a very young child can be difficult but is still needed. For a child who is old enough to talk, use the FACES pain scale (see Figure 7-2) to help determine pain severity. For an infant or child too young to talk, rely on behavior to help determine pain severity such as the behaviors described in the FLACC scale (see Figure 7-3). Infants in pain cry frequently with great intensity. They do not smile, laugh, or show interest in toys and are not comforted by holding, cuddling, rocking, or a pacifier.

A child can have the same side effects as an adult when taking opioids. Constipation is a problem for a child, and the same steps must be taken to avoid it.

Respiratory depression can be a dangerous problem for infants or very young children. When opioids are used with an infant or a small child, it is best to use an apnea monitor and/or pulse oximeter. When these devices are not available, check the patient's rate and depth of respiration at least every 15 minutes. Remember that infants and small children may have a normal respiratory rate between 30 and 40 breaths/minute. A respiratory rate of less than 20 in an infant or small child is cause for concern.

*Considerations for Pregnancy and Breastfeeding.*    Opioids may be prescribed to women during pregnancy. These drugs do cross the placenta and enter the fetus. The fetus can become addicted to opioids and go through withdrawal after birth. If the mother receives long-term opioid therapy or abuses heroin during pregnancy and the drug is discontinued several weeks before birth, the newborn should not

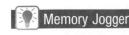
**Memory Jogger**

What is painful for an adult is painful for a child.

have any symptoms of withdrawal. However, if the mother is still receiving long-term opioid therapy or abusing opioid drugs when the baby is born, the newborn will need special care for withdrawal.

When opioids are given to a woman in labor, the baby may have respiratory depression after delivery. Often if an opioid is given intravenously within an hour of delivery, the baby may need a dose of an opioid antagonist such as naloxone (Narcan) after delivery.

Breastfeeding is best avoided when a woman is taking opioid drugs for more than a couple of days. If the mother is unable to stop breastfeeding while taking the drug, teach her the strategies listed in Box 1-1 in Chapter 1, to reduce infant exposure to these drugs.

***Considerations for Older Adults.*** Older adults are often undertreated for pain. One reason for this is that a confused patient may not be able to describe his or her pain level. Observing behaviors and using a pain scale for cognitively impaired adults can be helpful.

In addition to the usual effects of opioids, an older adult is at risk for low vision. The pupil of the older adult does not dilate fully, and less light enters the eye, reducing vision. When the older patient takes an opioid, the pupil is even smaller than usual, reducing vision even more. This problem increases his or her risk for falling. Teach the older adult to increase room lighting to make reading easier and reduce the risk for tripping and falling over objects.

Opioids, especially meperidine (Demerol), can make the chest muscles of older adults tighter, which makes breathing and coughing more difficult. Thus the risk for pneumonia and hypoxia is greater for them. Check the respiratory rate and depth and the oxygen saturation at least every 2 hours. In addition, meperidine causes the buildup of a toxic metabolite in older adults that can result in seizures.

## NONSTEROIDAL ANTI-INFLAMMATORY DRUGS

Nonsteroidal anti-inflammatory drugs (NSAIDs) are one type of nonopioid analgesic. **Nonopioid analgesics** are drugs that reduce a person's perception of pain but are not similar to opium and have little potential for psychologic or physical dependence. NSAIDs can help manage pain associated with inflammation, bone pain, cancer pain, and soft tissue trauma. These drugs act at the tissue where pain starts and do not change a person's perception of pain.

There are many different NSAIDs. They all work in similar ways but vary in cost and some side effects. For example, all NSAIDs except aspirin can cause headaches and kidney problems, but these side effects are more severe in some drugs. For a complete discussion of inflammation and what NSAIDs do at the cell level, see Chapter 8. The listing below describes only the NSAIDs most often prescribed for pain control. Be sure to consult a drug reference for more information about any specific NSAID.

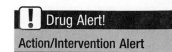

**Drug Alert!**

**Action/Intervention Alert**

If a mother receives an opioid during labor, watch her newborn closely for the first 2 to 4 hours after birth for any sign of respiratory depression.

**Clinical Pitfall**

Avoid the use of meperidine in the older adult.

◄ 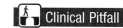-Learning Activity 7-3

### Dosages for Common NSAIDs

| Drug Class | Drug Examples | Dosage |
|---|---|---|
| Salicylic acid | aspirin or ASA (Bayer Aspirin, Bufferin, Ecotrin, Entrophen🍁, many more) | *Adults:* 325-650 mg orally 3-4 times daily<br>*Children:* 10-15 mg/kg orally or rectally every 4-6 hr |
| Propionic acid | ibuprofen (Actiprofen🍁, Advil, Motrin) | *Adults:* 200-800 mg orally every 6-8 hr<br>*Children:* 50-100 mg orally every 6-8 hr |
| | naproxen 🔲 (Aleve, Anaprox, Naprosyn, Naprosyn E🍁, Novo-Naprox🍁, Naxen🍁) | *Adults:* 250-500 mg orally twice daily<br>*Children:* 5 mg/kg orally every 12 hr |
| | oxaprozin (Daypro) | *Adults and children over 6 years old:* 600-1200 mg orally once daily |

*Continued*

### Do Not Confuse

**ketorolac** *with* **Ketalar**

An order for ketorolac can be confused with Ketalar. Ketorolac is an anti-inflammatory drug that can be given orally or parenterally. Ketalar is a type of anesthetic agent.

### Do Not Confuse

**Celebrex** *with* **Celexa**

An order for Celebrex can be confused with Celexa. Celebrex is an anti-inflammatory drug. Celexa is an antidepressant.

### Common Side Effects

**NSAIDs**

Bleeding problems | GI ulcers | Hypertension

### Drug Alert!

**Interaction Alert**

Avoid giving NSAIDs with acetaminophen (Tylenol).

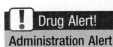

### Drug Alert!

**Administration Alert**

Teach the patient to avoid chewing or crushing an NSAID capsule or enteric-coated NSAID tablet.

---

**Dosages for Common NSAIDs—cont'd**

| Drug Class | Drug Examples | Dosage |
|---|---|---|
| Acetic acid | ketorolac (Toradol) | *Adults:* 10 mg orally every 6 hr; 15-30 mg IV or IM every 6 hr<br>*Children:* 1 mg/kg IM to a maximum of 30 mg or 0.5 mg/kg IV to a maximum of 15 mg daily |
| Cox-2 selective | celecoxib 🔲 (Celebrex) | *Adults:* 100-400 mg orally daily<br>Safety and dosages for children have not been established |

🔲 Top 100 drugs prescribed.

## How NSAIDs Work

NSAIDs reduce pain by suppressing some part of the inflammatory pathway and reducing the amounts of pain-mediating chemicals, especially bradykinin, that are present. As a result, pain is reduced.

*Side Effects.* Most NSAIDs reduce platelet clumping and blood clotting. In fact, aspirin is often prescribed to inhibit platelet aggregation and reduce the risk for heart attack and stroke. Just one dose of aspirin or almost any other NSAID can reduce clotting for up to a week. So, anyone taking NSAIDs is at increased risk for bleeding in response to slight bumps or other injuries.

Other side effects include irritation of the stomach lining and the rest of the GI tract. All NSAIDs except aspirin reduce blood flow to the kidney and slow urine output, which can lead to high blood pressure and kidney damage.

*Adverse Effects.* The most common adverse effect of NSAIDs is the induction of asthma. Allergic reactions also are possible. A person who is sensitive to one NSAID is very likely to be sensitive to all of them.

Excessive aspirin intake can cause salicylate poisoning or toxicity. Signs and symptoms include fever, rapid heart rate, rapid respirations, abdominal pain, nausea, vomiting, confusion, and ringing in the ears (*tinnitus*). Without treatment this condition can lead to acidosis, seizures, coma, and death.

Taking NSAIDs long term at the same time as acetaminophen (Tylenol) increases the risk for kidney and liver damage.

## What To Do *Before* Giving NSAIDs

Be sure to review the general nursing responsibilities related to analgesic therapy for pain (p. 102) in addition to these specific responsibilities for NSAIDs:

Before giving a patient the first dose of an NSAID, always ask whether the patient has had any problems with aspirin or any other over-the-counter NSAID.

Carefully check the order for NSAIDs to be given parenterally. Only ketorolac (Toradol) is approved for IV use.

Ask whether the patient has ever had stomach problems with aspirin or any other NSAID. Give the drug at the time the patient is eating or very shortly after a meal. When possible, have the patient drink a full glass of water or milk with the drug.

Tell the patient not to chew an NSAID capsule or an enteric-coated NSAID because chewing will ruin its stomach-protective properties.

Check the patient's blood pressure because NSAIDs can cause retention of sodium and water, leading to higher blood pressure. If he or she is already taking an angiotensin-converting enzyme (ACE) inhibitor for high blood pressure, the NSAID can reduce its effectiveness.

Ask whether the patient prescribed to take celecoxib (Celebrex) has ever had an allergic reaction to a "sulfa drug" type of antibiotic. Because celecoxib is similar to those antibiotics, an allergic reaction to celecoxib is more likely if the patient is also allergic to sulfa drugs.

## What To Do *After* Giving NSAIDs

Be sure to review the general nursing responsibilities related to analgesic therapy for pain (p. 103) in addition to these specific responsibilities for NSAIDs.

The risk for bleeding increases within several hours after just one NSAID dose. Examine the patient's gums, mucous membranes, and open skin areas (around IV sites) during each shift for bleeding. Look for bruises and tiny purple-red spots. Check urine, stool, or emesis for bright red blood, coffee-ground material, or other indications of bleeding.

Check the patient's blood pressure, breathing pattern, and pulse oximetry hourly after the first dose of an NSAID to determine any sensitivity. Immediately report any breathing difficulty, drop in blood pressure, or decrease of 5% or more in oxygen saturation.

## What To *Teach* Patients About NSAIDs

Be sure to teach patients the general care needs and precautions related to analgesic therapy for pain (p. 103) in addition to these specific responsibilities for NSAIDs.

To avoid GI side effects, teach the patient to always take an NSAID with food or on a full stomach. When possible, he or she should also drink a full glass of water or milk with the drug. Tell the patient not to chew an NSAID capsule or an enteric-coated tablet because chewing will ruin its stomach-protective properties. Teach the patient to examine vomit for obvious blood or the presence of coffee-ground material that may indicate bleeding in the stomach or esophagus. Also teach him or her to check bowel movements for the presence of actual blood or dark, tarry-looking material that would indicate bleeding somewhere in the GI tract and to report these symptoms to the prescriber.

Because NSAIDs reduce blood clotting, teach patients to check their gums daily for bleeding, especially after toothbrushing or flossing. Remind them to inform the dentist about their NSAID use before any dental procedure. If a female patient is still menstruating, warn her that her periods may have heavier blood flow and that her risk for becoming anemic is greater.

Teach the patient taking warfarin (Coumadin) to avoid also taking aspirin and other NSAIDs. Both of these drug types affect blood clotting in different ways, and taking them together places the patient at extreme risk for excessive bleeding and brain hemorrhage.

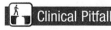
**Clinical Pitfall**

NSAIDs should never be taken with warfarin (Coumadin).

## Life Span Considerations for NSAIDs

*Pediatric Considerations.*   With the exception of ibuprofen, NSAIDs are not recommended for children. Aspirin is to be avoided in children because, if a child with a viral infection is given an NSAID, he or she may develop Reye's syndrome. *Reye's syndrome* is a liver disease that can lead to coma, mental retardation, and death.

*Considerations for Pregnancy and Breastfeeding.*   Most NSAIDs are category C for the first 6 months of pregnancy. The stronger ones, particularly indomethacin and celecoxib, are to be avoided during the last 3 months of pregnancy. Their use at that time can cause a blood vessel important to fetal circulation (the ductus arteriosus) to close, which would impair the oxygen supply to some fetal tissues.

**Clinical Pitfall**

Most NSAIDs should not be given to women during the last 3 months of pregnancy.

*Considerations for Older Adults.*   The older adult is at higher risk for cardiac problems when taking NSAIDs. These drugs cause salt and water retention that can lead to fluid overload and high blood pressure. Both of these problems increase the risk for heart attack and heart failure. Teach older adults taking NSAIDs to carefully monitor weight, pulse, and urine output. Teach about the signs and symptoms of heart failure: weight gain; ankle swelling; and shortness of breath, especially when lying down.

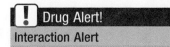
**Drug Alert!**
**Interaction Alert**

Most NSAIDs increase blood pressure and reduce the effects of antihypertensives, especially ACE inhibitors.

## NONOPIOID MISCELLANEOUS PAIN-CONTROL DRUGS

A variety of nonopioid drugs can be used alone or with other pain-control drugs to manage special types of pain. These additional drugs are sometimes termed *adjuvant drugs* because they enhance the pain-control features of other pain drugs. Most have other main uses and are discussed in more detail elsewhere in this text. The issues most important in using these drugs for pain control are included in this section.

### ACETAMINOPHEN

Acetaminophen alone (such as Abenol♦, Atasol♦, Panadol, Tylenol, and many others) can be effective for pain relief. It appears to work in the brain to change the perception of pain, and to a smaller degree it reduces the sensitivity of pain receptors.

Acetaminophen is given orally in tablets, capsules, or liquids and can also be given rectally in a suppository. It is available over-the-counter as a single drug or combined with other substances such as caffeine and aspirin (Excedrin). It also is combined with other pain-control drugs, especially opioids. The usual adult dose is 325 to 650 mg every 3 to 4 hours and should not exceed 4 g/day. For children the usual dose is 7 to 15 mg/kg every 4 hours.

### Important Issues

Because acetaminophen is available without a prescription, many people believe that it has no side effects or adverse effects. However, it can be toxic when taken at high doses or too often. The liver and kidneys can be damaged or destroyed by acetaminophen. Taking this drug with alcohol greatly increases the risk for permanent liver or kidney damage.

Warn patients that many over-the-counter drugs for colds, headache, allergies, and sleep aids also contain acetaminophen, as do a variety of prescribed pain medications. The acetaminophen in these drugs must be figured into the maximum daily dose along with any separate acetaminophen. Remind patients not to drink alcoholic beverages on days when they take acetaminophen or any drug containing acetaminophen.

When acetaminophen overdose occurs, the drug acetylcysteine must be given intravenously as soon as possible as an antidote to prevent liver failure. If acetylcysteine administration is delayed more than 24 hours after an acetaminophen overdose, it will not be effective in saving the liver.

### Life Span Considerations for Acetaminophen

*Pediatric Considerations.*    Acetaminophen is toxic to the liver and kidneys at high doses. *A young child should never receive an adult dose of acetaminophen.* Because acetaminophen comes in liquid forms with different strengths, it is important to teach parents to read labels carefully and not assume that the doses are the same for all liquids. Some liquid forms contain as few as 16 mg/mL, and others may contain as much as 70 mg/mL.

### ANTIDEPRESSANTS

Older and newer antidepressants have been found to reduce some types of chronic pain and cancer pain. The most common antidepressant drugs used for pain control are amitriptyline (Apo-Amitriptyline♦, Elavil), nortriptyline (Pamelor), paroxetine (Paxil), and sertraline (Zoloft). They are usually given orally, and the doses for pain control can be different from those used to treat depression. Antidepressants help increase the amount of natural opioids (endorphins and enkephalins) in the brain and also reduce the depression that can occur with chronic pain. Usually the patient must take one of these drugs for 1 or 2 weeks before he or she feels any relief from pain.

---

**Clinical Pitfall**

Acetaminophen can be toxic to the liver and kidneys and should not be taken by anyone with health problems of these organs.

---

**Drug Alert!**

**Teaching Alert**

Teach parents to read the label on liquid acetaminophen bottles for infants and small children very carefully and ensure that the correct dose is given for the child's size. Teach parents to telephone the nearest pharmacy and talk with the pharmacist to ensure that the dose is correct if they are not confident in their own calculations.

**Important Issues**

The side effects of antidepressants include constipation, dry mouth, urinary retention, sweating, sexual dysfunction, and increased pressure within the eye (*intraocular pressure*). The drugs should not be used for patients who have seizures or cardiac problems because these patients can experience seizures and heart rhythm problems. Teach the patient who is taking antidepressant drugs to call the prescriber if hand tremors develop.

**Life Span Considerations for Antidepressants**

*Pediatric Considerations.*   The use of antidepressants for pain control in children is not recommended except for cancer pain. There has been an increase in suicide attempts in children and adolescents taking these drugs.

*Considerations for Pregnancy and Breastfeeding.*   Most antidepressants are in pregnancy categories B and C. They can be given for pain control during pregnancy if the prescriber and patient believe that the risks to the fetus are offset by the benefits to the mother. However, breastfeeding should be avoided when taking these drugs because the drugs enter breast milk and affect the infant.

*Considerations for Older Adults.*   Antidepressants for pain control should be used carefully in older adults. They can cause heart rhythm problems and may make heart failure worse. Teach older adults taking these drugs to take their pulse at least twice daily and report any persistent changes in rhythm to the prescriber. In addition, the side effect of urinary retention may worsen urinary problems in the older man who also has an enlarged prostate gland. An older adult is more likely to have glaucoma than a younger adult, and the use of antidepressants can make glaucoma worse.

## ANTICONVULSANTS

Certain anticonvulsants (drugs that reduce seizure activity) have been found to reduce some types of chronic pain and cancer pain, especially neuropathic pain (nerve pain with tingling and burning) and migraine headaches. The two most common anticonvulsant drugs used for pain control are gabapentin (Neurontin) and pregabalin (Lyrica). They appear to work by reducing the rate of electrical transmission along sensory nerves and may also affect pain perception. The doses for pain control are often higher than those used to control seizures.

**Important Issues**

Side effects of anticonvulsants include drowsiness, confusion, blurred vision, clumsiness, and muscle aches and weakness. Side effects are worse if the patient also drinks alcohol while using these drugs. Teach the patient not to drive, operate heavy machinery, or engage in activities that require alertness. These effects may become less severe over time.

Both drugs reduce seizure activity. When used to treat seizures, these drugs should not be stopped suddenly because seizures are more likely to occur. Instead the drug doses should be decreased over time. It is not known if seizures could occur when the drug is stopped suddenly in patients taking anticonvulsants for pain control only. To be safe, even when taken just for pain control, teach the patient not to stop these drugs suddenly.

**Life Span Considerations for Anticonvulsants**

*Pediatric Considerations.*   Anticonvulsants may be used in children for pain control. One side effect seen in children but much less often in adults is an increase in aggressive behavior.

*Considerations for Pregnancy and Breastfeeding.*   Anticonvulsants used for pain control are in pregnancy category C. They can be given for pain control during

 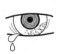

⊖-Learning Activity 7-4 ▶

pregnancy if the prescriber and patient believe that the risks to the fetus are offset by the benefits to the mother. However, breastfeeding should be avoided when taking these drugs because the drugs enter breast milk and affect the infant.

## INSOMNIA

### REVIEW OF RELATED PHYSIOLOGY AND PATHOPHYSIOLOGY

**Sleep** is a natural and necessary periodic state of rest for the mind and body. When we sleep, our bodies rest and restore energy levels. Sleep helps a person recover from illness, cope with stress, and solve problems. During sleep, consciousness is partially or completely lost, the eyes close, body movements decrease, metabolism slows, and responsiveness to external stimuli declines. There are five stages of sleep (Table 7-3). An average sleep cycle is 90 to 110 minutes, and most people have four or five cycles during an 8-hour sleep period.

The amount of sleep a person needs is unique. Some people can get by with 5 to 6 hours of sleep, whereas others need 10 to 11 hours. Most adults need between 7 and 8 hours of sleep per night to function at their best. Sleep needs also vary by age. Infants and children need more sleep (14 to 16 hours per day) than adults. Sleep problems are very common. Typically they include difficulty getting enough sleep, although sleeping too much or at inappropriate times may also be a problem.

Failing to get enough sleep causes sleep debt or sleep deprivation. **Sleep deprivation** is a shortage of quality, undisturbed sleep that reduces physical and mental well-being. Coordination, judgment, reaction time, and social function are all impaired by lack of sleep. Drowsiness interferes with the ability of the brain to concentrate, learn, and remember. Simple tasks seem more difficult to perform, and complex tasks may seem impossible to complete. People become anxious, moody, and impatient and have increased difficulty interacting with others.

Signs of sleep deprivation include falling asleep at the wheel while driving, watching television, or reading a book; sleeping for extra-long periods; difficulty awaking in the morning; irritability during the day; and falling asleep during quiet times of the day. Sleep deprivation may be short term or long term.

Amazingly, the body can make up for lost sleep by sleeping more the next night or on days off from work such as weekends. Catching up on missed sleep is important for the body to recover and restore itself.

**Insomnia** is the inability to go to sleep or remain asleep throughout the night. It is the most common sleep problem. Most people experience acute, short-term insomnia at some time during their lives. People of any age may have insomnia. Symptoms include difficulty falling asleep, waking often during the night or early morning, and not feeling rested after sleep. Many factors may cause a person to have

### Memory Jogger

The five stages of sleep are:
- Stage 1: Drowsiness.
- Stage 2: Light sleep.
- Stages 3 and 4: Deep sleep.
- Stage 5: Rapid eye movement (REM) sleep.

### ? Did You Know?

Sleep deprivation decreases immune function and increases the risk for infection.

### Table **7-3**   Stages of Sleep

| STAGE OF SLEEP | CHARACTERISTICS |
| --- | --- |
| 1—Drowsiness | Person drifts in and out of sleep for around 5-10 minutes and is easily awakened; eyes move very slowly; muscle activity slows. |
| 2—Light sleep | Eye movements stop; brain waves become slower; heart rate and body temperature decrease. |
| 3 and 4—Deep sleep | Slow brain waves (delta waves) appear; by stage 4, brain produces almost all delta waves; there is no eye movement or muscle activity; if awakened, a person feels groggy and disoriented; children may wet the bed, have night terrors, or sleepwalk. |
| 5—REM sleep | Breathing becomes more rapid, irregular, and shallow; eyes jerk rapidly; limb muscles become paralyzed temporarily; heart rate increases; blood pressure increases; males develop erections; dreams occur. |

*REM*, Rapid eye movement.

| Box **7-3** | Causes of Sleep Problems |

**ACUTE SLEEP PROBLEMS**
- Stress (job loss, moving, ending a relationship)
- Jet lag
- Use of stimulants (caffeine, nicotine)
- Use of alcohol
- Noise, light, extreme temperatures
- Minor illnesses (cold, flu)
- Worries (work, school, finances, family)

**CHRONIC SLEEP PROBLEMS**
- Medical conditions (chronic pain, obesity, head injury, cancer, asthma, arthritis, heartburn)
- Mood disorders (depression, anxiety)
- Schedule changes (working nights)
- Other sleep problems (sleep apnea)
- Genetics (some sleep disorders run in families)

insomnia, including lifestyle, environment, psychologic issues, menopause, illness or medical problems, drug therapy, and sleep-related disorders (Box 7-3).

## DRUGS FOR INSOMNIA

The most commonly prescribed sleep drugs are sedatives, a broad group of drugs that promote sleep by acting on signals in the central nervous system (CNS) to produce calm and ease agitation. Sedatives include benzodiazepine receptor agonists, benzodiazepines, antihistamines, and sedating antidepressants.

Benzodiazepine receptor agonists are now the first-line sleep aids to treat insomnia. They are less likely to be addictive but must be carefully monitored by the prescriber because of the possibility of misuse. Benzodiazepines have hypnotic and sedating effects and are mainly used to treat anxiety or stress. They can be habit forming when used for prolonged periods of time (more than 2 to 4 weeks) and are no longer the first-line drugs for insomnia.

Antihistamines are drugs used to treat allergies and allergic reactions. Some, such as diphenhydramine (Allerdryl✿, Benadryl) and dimenhydrate (Dramamine, Gravol✿), have sedating effects and are available over-the-counter to manage insomnia. Sedating antidepressants also have some effect for insomnia.

Generic names, brand names, and dosages of the most commonly prescribed drugs for insomnia are listed in the following table. Be sure to consult a drug reference for information about specific drugs used to treat insomnia.

### Dosages for Common Drugs for Insomnia

| Drug | Dosage |
|---|---|
| *Benzodiazepine Receptor Agonists* | |
| zolpidem (Ambien) | *Adults:* 10 mg orally at bedtime; extended release—12.5 mg at bedtime |
| zaleplon (Sonata) | *Adults:* 10 mg orally at bedtime (dosage range is 5-20 mg) |
| *Benzodiazepines* | |
| flurazepam (Dalmane, Novoflupam✿, Somnol✿) | *Adults:* 15-30 mg orally at bedtime |
| quazepam (Doral) | *Adults:* 7.5-15 mg orally at bedtime |
| triazolam (Gen-Triazolam✿, Halcion, Novotriolam✿) | *Adults:* 0.125-0.25 mg orally at bedtime (maximum dose 0.5 mg) |
| estazolam (ProSom) | *Adults:* 1-2 mg orally at bedtime |
| temazepam 🔲 (Restoril) | *Adults:* 7.5-30 mg orally at bedtime |

*Continued*

**Dosages for Common Drugs for Insomnia—cont'd**

| Drug | Dosage |
| --- | --- |
| *Over-the-Counter Antihistamines* | |
| diphenhydramine (Allerdryl🍁, Benadryl) | *Adults:* 50 mg orally 20-30 min before bedtime<br>*Children (2-12 years):* 1 mg/kg orally 20-30 min before bedtime (maximum dose 50 mg) |
| dimenhydrinate (Dramamine, Gravol🍁, Nauseatol🍁) | *Adults:* 50-100 mg orally<br>*Children 6-12 years:* 25-50 mg orally |
| *Sedating Antidepressants* | |
| trazodone (Desyrel) | *Adults:* 50-100 mg orally at bedtime |
| amitriptyline 🔲 (Apo-Amitriptyline🍁, Elavil) | *Adults:* 10-25 mg orally at bedtime |
| doxepin (Novo-Doxepin🍁, Sinequan, Triadapin🍁) | *Adults:* 25 mg orally at bedtime |

🔲 Top 100 drugs prescribed.

**⇄ Do Not Confuse**

**trazodone** *with* **tramadol**

An order for trazodone can be confused with tramadol. Trazodone is a sedating antidepressant used to treat insomnia, and tramadol is an analgesic used to treat moderate-to–moderately severe pain.

### How Drugs for Insomnia Work

Benzodiazepines such as temazepam (Restoril) and benzodiazepine receptor agonists such as zaleplon (Sonata) relieve insomnia by causing a general depression of the CNS. Antihistamines such as diphenhydramine (Benadryl) and sedating antidepressants such as trazodone (Desyrel) produce drowsiness and mild sedation, which enhances sleep.

#### Intended Responses
- Insomnia is relieved, and sleep is improved.
- Person is sedated, and sleep is induced.
- Length of time to fall asleep is decreased.
- Sleep duration is increased.

***Side Effects.*** Benzodiazepine receptor agonists can cause amnesia, daytime drowsiness, dizziness, and a feeling of "being drugged." Gastrointestinal side effects include nausea, vomiting, and diarrhea. Additional side effects of zaleplon (Sonata) include hallucinations, impaired memory, and impaired psychomotor functions for a brief period of time after the drug dose.

Benzodiazepines may cause confusion, daytime drowsiness, decreased ability to concentrate, dizziness, headache, and lethargy. These drugs can also cause blurred vision, constipation, diarrhea, nausea, and vomiting.

Antihistamines may cause drowsiness, loss of appetite and dry mouth. Other side effects may include dizziness, headache, urinary retention, blurred vision, tinnitus, constipation, nausea, and photosensitivity.

Sedating antidepressant drugs may cause drowsiness, hypotension, and dry mouth. Other side effects may include confusion, dizziness, nightmares, slurred speech, blurred vision, tinnitus, nausea, vomiting, constipation, and diarrhea.

**Common Side Effects**

**Drugs for Insomnia**

Drowsiness    Dizziness    Dry mouth

Headache    GI discomfort

***Adverse Effects.*** Drugs for insomnia are metabolized by the liver and excreted by the kidney. When liver or kidney function is reduced, drug levels can become very high, with more side effects and adverse effects.

A rare adverse effect of any drug for insomnia is a severe allergic reaction that can cause respiratory problems.

Benzodiazepines are potentially addictive. Psychologic and physical dependence can develop within a few weeks or months of regular or repeated use.

### What To Do *Before* Giving Drugs for Insomnia

Obtain a complete list of drugs currently being used by the patient, including herbal supplements and over-the-counter drugs. Ask the patient about usual sleep patterns and assess for possible causes of difficulty with sleeping.

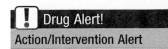

Check the patient's heart rate and rhythm, blood pressure, and respiratory rate. Ask about a history of depression, confusion, falls, and pain. Assess the patient's current mental status.

Ask patients about liver or kidney problems that may affect the metabolism and breakdown of these drugs. Ask all female patients within childbearing years if they are pregnant, breastfeeding, or planning to become pregnant.

### What To Do *After* Giving Drugs for Insomnia

Recheck the patient's vital signs and reassess the level of consciousness. Watch for changes in heart rate, blood pressure, and level of consciousness. Check for orthostatic hypotension, excessive sedation, or confusion, especially in older adults.

Instruct the patient to call for help when getting out of bed and ensure that the call light is within easy reach because these drugs can cause drowsiness and dizziness. Remind the patient to get up or change positions slowly.

### What To *Teach* Patients About Drugs for Insomnia

Tell patients to take these drugs exactly as directed by the prescriber and remind them of the importance of follow-up appointments to monitor the progress of treatment. Remind patients never to take a double dose of these drugs. Tell them to report side effects to the prescriber.

Teach patients taking benzodiazepines about the possibility of becoming dependent on these drugs when they are taken for extended periods of time. Remind them that drugs for insomnia should be taken only for a short period of time (2 to 4 weeks) and only when needed.

Tell patients that drugs for insomnia should not be taken unless there is adequate time to sleep (4 to 8 hours, depending on the sleep drug). Also, teach patients taking zaleplon (Sonata) or zolpidem (Ambien) to go to bed immediately after taking the drug because of its rapid onset of action. Remind them that the amnesia side effect of zaleplon (Sonata) can be avoided if they are able to get 4 or more hours of sleep after taking the drug. Warn patients not to take these drugs on overnight airplane flights of less than 7 to 8 hours because they may experience transient memory loss called *traveler's amnesia*.

Because drugs for insomnia can cause drowsiness and blurred vision, caution patients to avoid driving, operating machines, or performing any activities that require alertness.

Instruct the patient taking an antihistamine about the importance of frequent mouth care, such as oral rinses, to reduce dry mouth.

Caution patients to use sunscreen and wear protective clothing to prevent severe sunburns.

Remind female patients in their childbearing years to notify their prescriber if they become pregnant or plan to become pregnant.

### Life Span Considerations for Drugs for Insomnia

*Pediatric Considerations.*   Antihistamines such as diphenhydramine (Benadryl) can cause an increase in excitement when given to children. (This response, which is opposite of what is expected, is called a *paradoxical response*.)

*Considerations for Pregnancy and Breastfeeding.*   Benzodiazepines (category D/X) should not be taken during pregnancy. Zolpidem (Ambien) is category B/C and is generally considered safe for use during pregnancy, but only if the benefits outweigh the possible side effects. Most insomnia drugs cross the placenta and enter breast milk and can have sedating effects on the fetus or infant.

*Considerations for Older Adults.*   Older adults should be given lower doses of drugs for insomnia because they are more sensitive to the effects of these drugs and more likely to experience side effects. In addition, older adults are at increased risk for falls while taking these drugs.

**! Drug Alert!**
**Action/Intervention Alert**

To better monitor for side effects, assess the level of consciousness before giving a drug for insomnia.

**! Drug Alert!**
**Teaching Alert**

Teach patients taking benzodiazepine receptor agonists to go to bed immediately after taking a dose of these drugs.

**! Drug Alert!**
**Teaching Alert**

Teach patients to be sure that there is adequate time (4 to 8 hours) for sleep before taking a drug for insomnia.

**! Drug Alert!**
**Teaching Alert**

Teach patients taking an insomnia drug to avoid alcohol and other CNS-depressing substances because of the risk for oversedation.

**Clinical Pitfall**

Most drugs for insomnia should not be taken during pregnancy or breastfeeding.

 -Learning Activity 7-5

## NARCOLEPSY

### REVIEW OF RELATED PHYSIOLOGY AND PATHOPHYSIOLOGY

Narcolepsy is a sleep problem with uncontrollable urges to sleep, causing a person to fall asleep at inappropriate times. It is a chronic neurologic disorder in which the brain cannot regulate sleep-wake cycles. This problem tends to occur in patients and families with respiratory illnesses that cause carbon dioxide retention. Sleep episodes caused by narcolepsy can occur at any time during the day, at work, at school, during a conversation, while eating, or while driving or operating machinery. The symptoms of narcolepsy include sudden loss of voluntary muscle tone and reflexes commonly triggered by emotion, a heavy meal, or stress *(cataplexy),* vivid hallucinations during sleep onset or when waking, and brief episodes of total paralysis at the beginning or end of sleep. Not only does a person with narcolepsy fall asleep suddenly, but he or she also frequently wakes up during the night.

### DRUGS FOR NARCOLEPSY

Generic names, brand names, and dosages of the most commonly prescribed drugs for narcolepsy are listed in the following table. Be sure to consult a drug reference for information about any specific drug used to treat narcolepsy.

#### Dosages for Common Drugs for Narcolepsy

| Drug | Dosage |
| --- | --- |
| methylphenidate (Riphenidate✦, Ritalin) | *Adults:* 10 mg orally 2-3 times daily |
| modafinil (Provigil) | *Adults:* 100-200 mg orally; one daily single dose in morning |
| sodium oxybate (Xyrem) | *Adults:* Initial dose 2.25 g orally at bedtime and again 3-4 hr later |

### How Drugs for Narcolepsy Work

Drugs such as methylphenidate (Ritalin) cause increased general CNS stimulation to promote wakefulness and reduce the sudden sleepiness of narcolepsy. Modafinil (Provigil) is a CNS stimulant but appears to be more selective in the brain areas stimulated. Oxybate (Xyrem) increases sedation to ensure a good night's sleep and prevent daytime sleepiness.

### Intended Responses
- Attention span is increased.
- Motor activity and mental alertness during waking hours are increased.
- Fatigue is decreased.
- Episodes of inappropriately falling asleep are decreased.

*Side Effects.* Common side effects of CNS stimulant drugs used for narcolepsy include hyperactivity, insomnia, restlessness, tremor, hypertension, palpitation, tachycardia, and loss of appetite (anorexia). Other side effects include nervousness, headache, upset stomach, diarrhea, mood swings, and depression.

Sodium oxybate (Xyrem) can cause sleepwalking. It should never be used with alcohol because it will dramatically increase CNS effects.

*Adverse Effects.* CNS stimulants may cause seizures. They can also cause abnormal heart rhythms and chest pain.

### What To Do *Before* Giving Drugs for Narcolepsy

Obtain a complete list of drugs currently being used by the patient, including over-the-counter drugs and herbal supplements. Check the patient's blood pressure, heart

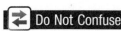
**Memory Jogger**

The three major symptoms of narcolepsy are cataplexy, vivid hallucinations, and total paralysis at the beginning or end of the sleep episode.

**Do Not Confuse**

**Ritalin *with* ritodrine**

An order for Ritalin can be confused with ritodrine. Ritalin is a CNS stimulant sometimes used to treat narcolepsy, and ritodrine is a beta-adrenergic agonist used to manage premature labor.

**Common Side Effects**

**Stimulatory Drugs for Narcolepsy**

| Insomnia | Diarrhea, Upset stomach | Tremors |

rate and rhythm, and respiratory rate. Ask about liver or kidney problems that may affect the metabolism and breakdown of these drugs and may require a reduced dosage. Assess the patient's current level of consciousness and mood.

Ask female patients in their childbearing years if they are pregnant or planning to become pregnant.

### What To Do *After* Giving Drugs for Narcolepsy

Recheck the patient's vital signs every shift and weigh the patient daily. Instruct the patient to call for help when getting out of bed and ensure that the call light is within easy reach because these drugs can cause drowsiness.

Watch for signs and symptoms of allergic reaction such as rash, hives, itching, and difficulty with breathing and swallowing.

Monitor patients on sodium oxybate (Xyrem) for possible sleepwalking. Watch for seizure activity in patients taking CNS stimulants.

### What To *Teach* Patients About Drugs for Narcolepsy

Remind patients to take these drugs exactly as instructed by the prescriber. Tell them about the importance of follow-up appointments to monitor the progress of controlling the narcolepsy. Instruct patients to report side effects and signs of allergic reaction to the prescriber immediately.

Tell patients taking methylphenidate (Ritalin) not to take a missed dose close to bedtime because it may cause difficulty getting to sleep.

Remind female patients taking modafinil (Provigil) that this drug can decrease the effectiveness of birth control pills and that another form of birth control should be used while taking this drug. Tell any woman in childbearing years to notify her prescriber if she becomes pregnant or plans to become pregnant.

Instruct a patient taking modafinil to avoid eating grapefruit and drinking grapefruit juice because it affects the action of this drug.

A patient who is taking sodium oxybate (Xyrem) should have a family member watch him or her for possible sleepwalking. If this occurs, it should be reported to the prescriber.

Instruct patients to take these drugs with food or milk if they cause upset stomach. Because drowsiness, dizziness, and blurred vision can result from using these drugs, caution the patient to avoid driving, operating machines, and performing other activities that require increased alertness. Tell the patient to change positions slowly to keep dizziness to a minimum.

Tell patients to avoid alcohol and other CNS depressants. Remind them to talk with the prescriber before taking any over-the-counter drugs or herbal remedies. Instruct the patient taking methylphenidate (Ritalin) to avoid caffeine-containing drinks while taking this drug.

### Life Span Considerations with Drugs for Narcolepsy

*Pediatric Considerations.*   Methylphenidate can cause slower growth (both height and weight) in children.

*Considerations for Pregnancy and Breastfeeding.*   These drugs are not recommended during pregnancy or breastfeeding.

*Considerations for Older Adults.*   Older adults may need to be started on lower doses of these drugs to avoid adverse effects or side effects. They are at increased risk for changes in thinking patterns and problems with movement.

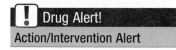

**⚠ Drug Alert!**
**Action/Intervention Alert**

Monitor patients for seizure activity when they also take CNS stimulants.

**⚠ Drug Alert!**
**Teaching Alert**

Remind women taking modafinil (Provigil) to use an additional form of birth control to prevent an unplanned pregnancy.

◄ ⊜-Learning Activity 7-6

## Get Ready for Practice!

### Key Points

- Pain is whatever the patient says it is and exists whenever he or she says it does.
- Acute pain usually triggers the stress response of the body and results in changes in a patient's vital signs; chronic pain often does not.
- Giving pain-control drugs on a regular schedule rather than on a PRN basis is more likely to provide better pain relief.
- A sleeping patient may still have pain. Do not skip a regularly scheduled dose of a drug for pain control just because the patient is sleeping.
- Opioids only alter the perception of pain; they do nothing at the site of the damaged tissue to affect the cause of the pain.
- Physical dependence, addiction, and withdrawal are rare when opioids are taken by a patient who is in pain.
- Use an apnea monitor and pulse oximeter to monitor the breathing effectiveness of an infant or small child receiving opioids.
- Do not give celecoxib (Celebrex) to a patient who is allergic to the sulfa drug type of antibiotics.
- Teach the patient who is taking an antidepressant for pain control to call the prescriber if hand tremors or an irregular heartbeat develops.
- Teach older adults taking antidepressants for pain control to take their pulse at least twice daily and report any persistent changes in rhythm to the prescriber.
- Teach the patient taking anticonvulsants for pain control to avoid stopping the drug suddenly.
- Sleep allows the body to rest and restore energy levels and is essential for a person to recover from illness, cope with stress, and solve problems.
- Sleep deprivation causes negative effects on physical and mental well-being.
- Teach patients taking drugs for insomnia to be sure that there is adequate time for sleep (4 to 8 hours) before taking these drugs.
- Patients taking CNS stimulants must be monitored for signs of seizure activity.
- A family member should be taught to watch the patient taking sodium oxybate (Xyrem) for sleepwalking.

### Additional Learning Resources

**evolve** Go to your Evolve website (http://evolve.elsevier.com/Workman/pharmacology/) for the following FREE learning resources:

- eLearning Activities
- Animations
- Video Clips
- Interactive Review Questions
- Audio Key Points
- Audio Glossary
- Audio Glossary—Spanish-English
- Drug Dosage Calculators
- Patient Teaching Handouts

**SG** Go to your Study Guide for additional learning activities to help you master this chapter content.

### Review Questions

1. Which personal condition or factor can be modified to increase pain tolerance?
   - A. Age or gender
   - B. Pain location
   - C. Fear or anxiety
   - D. Family expectations

2. A patient is reporting pain. Which feature indicates to you that the patient's pain is chronic rather than acute?
   - A. The pain is better in the morning and worse at night.
   - B. The patient is sweating, and blood pressure is elevated.
   - C. The pain limits the ability of the patient to participate in care.
   - D. The patient has difficulty describing the exact nature of the pain.

3. Which drug has the main action of controlling pain by changing the cellular responses at the site of the cause of pain?
   - A. ibuprofen (Advil)
   - B. naloxone (Narcan)
   - C. amitriptyline (Elavil)
   - D. hydromorphone (Dilaudid)

4. Why is morphine categorized in the United States as a schedule II drug rather than a schedule I drug?
   - A. It has a high potential for abuse.
   - B. It has a currently accepted use for treatment.
   - C. It is a synthetic product rather than a naturally occurring substance.
   - D. It contains only small amounts of opioids compared with substances in schedule I.

5. What is the most important action to take after administering any drug for pain?
   - A. Ask the patient whether the pain interferes with sleep.
   - B. Document the patient's response to the medication.
   - C. Ask the patient to rate his or her level of pain relief.
   - D. Remind the patient that dependence is possible.

6. Which side effects or adverse effects are associated with opioid analgesics? (Select all that apply.)
   - A. Constipation
   - B. Slow, shallow respirations
   - C. Aggression
   - D. Insomnia
   - E. Liver failure
   - F. Nausea and vomiting
   - G. Irregular heartbeat

7. A patient taking oxycodone (Percocet) at home has all of the following problems. For which problem should the patient call the prescriber?
   - A. Appetite is absent.
   - B. Pupils are the size of a pinpoint.
   - C. Pain is unrelieved at the current dose.
   - D. Bowel movements have changed color.

8. A patient prescribed amitriptyline (Elavil) asks how this drug can help reduce pain. What is your best response?

   A. "The drug increases the amount of natural endorphins in your brain."
   B. "It binds to receptor sites in the brain and changes your perception of pain."
   C. "It works in the nerve endings and prevents nerve transmission of pain."
   D. "Elavil reduces the tissue damage and inflammation at the injured site."

9. Which precaution should you include when teaching a patient about the proper use of NSAIDs for chronic pain?

   A. "Be sure to drink at least 3 L of fluid each day."
   B. "Take this drug 1 hour before or 2 hours after eating."
   C. "Stop taking the drug 1 week before dental work or surgery."
   D. "Avoid driving or operating dangerous equipment while taking this drug."

10. What is the most important precaution to teach the parents of a 1-year-old child taking acetaminophen (Tylenol) for pain?

    A. "Watch your child closely for slowing of the rate and depth of breathing."
    B. "Be sure to call the prescriber if your child develops tremors of the hand."
    C. "Read the label carefully for the correct amount of liquid drug to give your child."
    D. "Check your child's pain level using the FACES pain scale before and after you give the drug."

11. For which side effect should you be sure to monitor when a patient is taking CNS stimulants for narcolepsy?

    A. Respiratory depression
    B. Temporary amnesia
    C. Seizure activity
    D. Dehydration

12. What factors should you check before giving a drug for insomnia? (Select all that apply.)

    A. Level of consciousness
    B. Handgrip strength
    C. Pupil size
    D. Abdominal distention
    E. Heart rate and rhythm
    F. History of kidney disease
    G. Patient's usual sleeping pattern

13. What should you instruct the patient to do immediately after taking a benzodiazepine receptor agonist?

    A. Go to bed
    B. Drink at least 8 oz of water
    C. Check the pulse for 1 full minute
    D. Listen to soft music to ensure adequate sleep

14. When taking a drug for insomnia, which problem is more likely to occur in an older adult?

    A. Severe constipation
    B. Liver failure
    C. Narcolepsy
    D. Falls

15. An infant is to receive 80 mg of acetaminophen (Tylenol). The liquid you have on hand has a drug concentration of 100 mg/mL.

    a. How many milliliters is the correct dose for this infant? _____ mL
    b. How many milliliters is the correct dose if the liquid has a concentration of 120 mg/5 mL? _____ mL

16. An 80-year-old patient is prescribed to receive hydromorphone (Dilaudid) 1 mg IV. The unit-dose syringe has hydromorphone 4 mg/mL. How many milliliters should you give intravenously? _____ mL

## Critical Thinking Activities

Mr. Green is a 64-year-old man who is 1 day post-op from a total knee replacement. He has a patient-controlled analgesia pump to give him morphine intravenously. He was a heroin addict in his 20s but has been drug-free for more than 30 years. Although he is now in severe pain, Mr. Green is afraid of becoming addicted and is trying to wait as long as he can before he punches in a dose.

1. What type of drug is morphine?

2. What is the major adverse effect of this drug?

3. List three common signs of this adverse effect.

4. Is his history of heroin addiction likely to affect either his current perception of pain or his response to morphine? Why or why not?

5. What should you tell him about addiction?

# Anti-Inflammatory Drugs

## Objectives

*After studying this chapter you should be able to:*

1. Explain how inflammation is different from infection.
2. Describe the basis for the five major signs and symptoms of inflammation.
3. List the names, actions, usual adult dosages, possible side effects, and adverse effects of commonly prescribed corticosteroids.
4. Describe what to do before and after giving corticosteroids.
5. Explain what to teach patients taking corticosteroids, including what to do, what not to do, and when to call the prescriber.
6. Describe life span considerations for corticosteroids.
7. List the names, actions, usual adult dosages, possible side effects, and adverse effects of commonly prescribed nonsteroidal anti-inflammatory drugs (NSAIDs).
8. Describe what to do before and after giving NSAIDs.
9. Explain what to teach patients taking NSAIDs, including what to do, what not to do, and when to call the prescriber.
10. Describe life span considerations for NSAIDs.
11. List the names, actions, usual adult dosages, possible side effects, and adverse reactions of commonly prescribed antihistamines and leukotriene inhibitors.
12. Describe what to do before and after giving antihistamines and leukotriene inhibitors.
13. Explain what to teach patients taking antihistamines or leukotriene inhibitors, including what to do, what not to do, and when to call the prescriber.

## Key Terms

**antihistamines** (ăn-tē-HĬS-tĕ-mēnz) (p. 132) Drugs that reduce inflammation by preventing the inflammatory mediator histamine from binding to its receptor site; same as histamine blockers or histamine antagonists.

**anti-inflammatory drugs** (ăn-tī-ĭn-FLĂM-ĕ-tōr-ē DRŬGZ) (p. 123) A drug that prevents or limits tissue and blood vessel responses to injury or invasion.

**corticosteroids** (kŏr-tĭ-kō-STĔR-ōydz) (p. 123) Drugs similar to natural cortisol that prevent or limit inflammation by slowing or stopping inflammatory mediator production.

**cyclo-oxygenase (COX)** (sī-klō-ŎKS-ĕ-jĕn-ās) (p. 122) An enzyme important in converting body chemicals into mediators of inflammation.

**histamine** (HĬS-tĕ-mēn) (p. 132) A chemical made by the body that binds to receptor sites and causes inflammatory responses.

**infection** (ĭn-FĔK-shŭn) (p. 121) Invasion of the body by microorganisms that disturb the normal environment and cause harm.

**inflammation** (ĭn-flă-MĀ-shŭn) (p. 121) A syndrome of tissue and blood vessel responses to injury or invasion.

**kinins** (KĬN-ĭnz) (p. 130) A group of chemicals made by the body that cause some of the signs and symptoms of inflammation, especially pain.

**leukotriene** (lū-kō-TRĪ-ēn) (p. 130) A chemical made by the body that binds to its receptors and maintains an inflammatory response.

**mediators** (MĒ-dē-ā-tŭrz) (p. 122) Body chemicals such as histamine, leukotriene, prostaglandins, and kinins that cause inflammatory responses.

**nonsteroidal anti-inflammatory drugs (NSAIDs)** (nŏn-stĕr-ŌY-dŭl ăn-tī-ĭn-FLĂM-ĕ-tōr-ē DRŬGZ) (p. 128) Anti-inflammatory drugs that are not similar to cortisol but prevent or limit the tissue and blood vessel responses to injury or invasion by slowing the production of one or more inflammatory mediators.

**prostaglandins** (prŏs-tĕ-GLĂN-dĭnz) (p. 129) A family of chemicals made by the body, some of which cause the signs and symptoms of inflammation.

⊖-Learning Activity 8-1 ►

**Inflammation,** also called the *inflammatory response,* is the normal reactions of tissues and blood vessels in response to injury or invasion. It is nonspecific, which means that the same tissue responses occur with any type of injury or invasion, regardless of the location on the body or what caused the response to start. Thus inflammation triggered by a scald burn to the hand is the same as inflammation triggered by bacteria in the middle ear. The size and severity of the inflammation depends on the intensity, severity, duration, and extent of the injury or invasion. For example, a splinter in the finger triggers inflammation only at the splinter site. A burn injuring 60% of the skin surface triggers inflammation involving the entire body.

Inflammatory responses start tissue actions that cause visible and uncomfortable symptoms. Despite the discomfort, these actions are important in ridding the body of harmful organisms and helping repair damaged tissue. However, if the inflammatory response is excessive, tissue damage may result.

A confusing issue about inflammation is that this process occurs in response to tissue injury and invasion by organisms. An **infection** is an invasion of the body by microorganisms that disturb the normal environment and cause harm. Infection usually occurs with inflammation, but inflammation can occur without infection. Examples of inflammation without infection include sprained joints and blisters. Examples of inflammation caused by noninfectious invasion include hay fever, asthma, and other allergic reactions. Inflammation with infection includes appendicitis, viral hepatitis, and bacterial pneumonia. Therefore inflammation does not always mean that an infection is present.

## REVIEW OF RELATED PHYSIOLOGY AND PATHOPHYSIOLOGY

An inflammatory response is called a "syndrome" because it occurs in a predictable series of steps and stages (Table 8-1). The response is the same, regardless of the triggering event. Responses at the tissue level cause the five main signs and symptoms of inflammation: warmth, redness, swelling, pain, and decreased function.

 Memory Jogger

Infection usually is accompanied by inflammation, but inflammation can occur without infection.

 Memory Jogger

The five main signs and symptoms of inflammation are warmth, redness, swelling, pain, and decreased function.

| Table 8-1 | The Stages of Inflammation | | |
|---|---|---|---|
| **STAGE** | **DURATION** | **ACTIONS** | **SIGNS AND SYMPTOMS** |
| I: Vascular | Begins within minutes after injury or invasion and lasts for hours | White blood cells in the damaged tissues release mediators that do two things: (1) bind to blood vessels, making them dilate and leak, which causes more blood, oxygen, and cells to come to the area and also causes the tissues to swell; and (2) go to the bone marrow and speed up production of more white blood cells. | Redness Swelling Warmth in the area Pain or tenderness in the area Loss of function in the area |
| II: Exudate | Begins hours after injury or invasion and lasts for days | New cells come to the area, releasing many more mediators. Some mediators invade the bloodstream and cause systemic signs and symptoms. | Low-grade fever Increased secretions Achy joints (depending on the extent and severity of the inflammation) |
| III: Tissue repair | Begins at the initial injury but may not be evident until the exudate stage is over; lasts until healing is complete | Structural cells are stimulated to release collagen to form a latticework to use as a base for new tissue growth. Cells are stimulated to divide and form either new tissue just like the damaged tissue or scar tissue. | Tenderness and swelling at the site Skin color change at the site (temporary) |

## STAGE I: VASCULAR

Stage I involves white blood cells (WBCs) and changes in blood vessels. Injured tissues and WBCs in the area release mediators, which are body chemicals such as histamine, leukotriene, prostaglandins, and kinins that cause inflammatory responses. Each type of mediator has different subtypes that affect tissues differently.

Some mediators act on blood vessels in the area of injury or invasion, causing changes. These changes include dilation of the blood vessels and capillary leak (also called *capillary leak syndrome*). These responses cause redness and warmth of the tissues. The increased blood flow brings oxygen, nutrients, and more WBCs to injured tissues.

With capillary leak, blood plasma leaks into the tissues, causing swelling (edema) and pain. The swelling creates a cushion of fluid to prevent more tissue injury. The pain lets the person know that an injury has occurred and leads him or her to protect the area from more harm. Mediators also go to the bone marrow (site of WBC production) and trigger faster WBC production to maintain the inflammation for as long as it is needed.

⊖-Video 8-1: Swelling (Edema) ▶

## STAGE II: EXUDATE

In stage II large numbers of WBCs are created, and an *exudate* (tissue drainage) commonly called *pus* is formed. At this stage the total number of WBCs in the blood can increase up to five times above normal and indicates that an inflammatory response is taking place (see Table 1-6 in Chapter 1 for normal blood cell counts).

During this phase a cascade reaction starts to increase the inflammatory response (Figure 8-1). This action begins by converting fat from broken cell membranes into arachidonic acid, which then enters the cyclo-oxygenase (COX) pathway. Cyclo-oxygenase (COX) is an enzyme important in converting body chemicals into mediators of inflammation that continue the inflammatory response in the tissues. Many anti-inflammatory drugs stop this cascade by preventing COX from converting arachidonic acid into mediators.

## STAGE III: TISSUE REPAIR

Although stage III is completed last, it begins at the time of injury. This process is very important in helping the injured tissue regain function. WBCs secrete chemicals that trigger the remaining healthy cells to divide. So rapid cell division is a part of this stage. In tissues such as the heart that are unable to divide and replace damaged

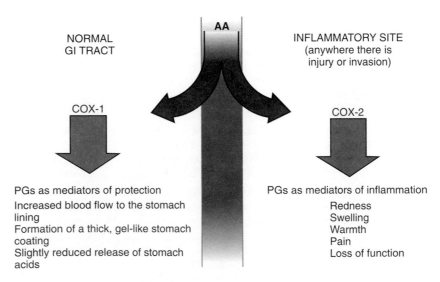

AA = Arachidonic acid   PGs = Prostaglandins
COX-1 = Cyclo-oxygenase 1   COX-2 = Cyclo-oxygenase 2

**FIGURE 8-1** Arachidonic acid cascade and mediator production.

heart cells with new heart cells, WBCs trigger new blood vessel growth and scar tissue formation. Because scar tissue is only a patch and does not behave like normal tissue, loss of function occurs wherever damaged tissues are replaced with scar tissue. How much function is lost depends on how much tissue is replaced by scar tissue rather than by normal tissue. For example, if 25% of the left ventricle of the heart is replaced with scar tissue, the shape of the heart is changed, and the pumping action is reduced because the scar tissue is not heart muscle.

This stage can be harmful if it lasts too long. For example, some diseases cause inflammation in the lungs and trigger scar tissue growth there. If too much scar tissue forms in the lungs, oxygen cannot enter the body, and the person dies of respiratory failure.

Although inflammation is an important protective response, it can cause problems. Inflammation is uncomfortable, reduces function while it is occurring, and can cause tissue damage if it is prolonged. Anti-inflammatory drugs that prevent or limit tissue and blood vessel responses to injury or invasion are prescribed to increase comfort and prevent tissue-damaging complications. These drugs are used as therapy for many common acute problems such as asthma, allergic reactions, and local or systemic irritation. In addition, inflammation appears to play a role in other health problems such as stroke and heart attack. This is one reason why many people are prescribed an aspirin each day to lower their risk for heart attack.

In addition to managing acute inflammatory problems, anti-inflammatory drugs can help manage autoimmune health problems. Autoimmunity is caused by inappropriate inflammatory and immune responses when WBC actions and products are directed against healthy normal cells and tissues. These responses are similar to normal inflammatory responses against invading organisms, but these reactions are now directed against normal body cells.

Examples of autoimmune diseases include systemic lupus erythematosus, polyarteritis nodosa, scleroderma, rheumatoid arthritis, autoimmune hemolytic anemia, rheumatic fever, and Hashimoto's thyroiditis. Anti-inflammatory drugs are commonly used along with symptomatic treatment for autoimmune disorders.

Anti-inflammatory drugs also can help prevent rejection of transplanted organs. Usually the transplanted organ is donated by a person who is not an identical sibling to the *recipient* (person receiving the donated organ). The body considers the donated organ to be foreign material, and the recipient's normal immune system and inflammatory responses will try to destroy and remove it. Some anti-inflammatory drugs, the corticosteroids, are used to suppress these responses so the transplanted organ can continue to function in the recipient's body.

## TYPES OF ANTI-INFLAMMATORY DRUGS

There are many different anti-inflammatory drugs. Some must be prescribed, and others are available over-the-counter. The four main categories of anti-inflammatory drugs include corticosteroids, nonsteroidal anti-inflammatory drugs (NSAIDs), antihistamines, and leukotriene inhibitors.

### CORTICOSTEROIDS

Corticosteroids are drugs similar to natural cortisol that prevent or limit inflammation by slowing or stopping all known pathways of inflammatory mediator production. These drugs are the most powerful of all the drugs used for inflammation.

The cortisol that adrenal glands make has many functions necessary for life. In addition, extra cortisol is secreted during times of stress to help the body maintain important functions even when body systems are overworked. Natural cortisol also helps control inflammatory responses. Corticosteroids may be taken in many ways:
- Orally or parenterally
- By inhalation for asthma and other inflammatory problems of the airways
- Topically for skin problems
- Injected into joints

 **Memory Jogger**

Excess scar tissue formation from prolonged inflammation is more harmful than helpful.

 **Did You Know?**

Some heart attacks are caused by inflammation and infection.

◄ -Learning Activity 8-2

**Memory Jogger**

Types of drugs for treatment of inflammation are:
- Corticosteroids.
- NSAIDs.
- Antihistamines.
- Leukotriene inhibitors.

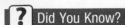 
- Rectally for hemorrhoids
- In drops for eye problems

Chapter 18 discusses the use of inhaled corticosteroids for respiratory problems. Chapter 26 discusses how to place drugs in the eye.

When taken orally or given parenterally, corticosteroids have many side effects and adverse effects. For this reason, corticosteroids are usually prescribed for only a short period of time. However, if the inflammation cannot be controlled with less powerful drugs, they may need to be taken for weeks or months. When needed for long periods of time, the goal is for the patient to take the lowest dose of corticosteroids that will control the inflammation so side effects and complications can be minimized.

There are dozens of different brands and strengths of corticosteroids. They all work the same way and have the same effects. Only those used most commonly are listed in the following table. Be sure to consult a drug handbook for more information about a specific drug.

### Dosages of Common Corticosteroids

| Drugs | Dosages |
|---|---|
| *Oral Corticosteroids* | |
| betamethasone (Betnelan✿, Betnesol✿, Celestone) | 0.5-7 mg orally daily |
| dexamethasone 🔲 (Decadron, Dexasone✿) | 2-20 mg orally daily (dose and schedule depend on the disorder) |
| prednisoLONE 🔲 | 5-40 mg orally daily |
| predniSONE 🔲 (Apo-Prednisone✿) | 5-60 mg orally daily in two doses (⅔ morning, ⅓ evening) |
| *Parenteral Corticosteroids* | |
| cortisone acetate (Cortone✿) | *Adults:* 20-300 mg IM daily<br>*Children:* 1-5 mg/kg IM daily |
| dexamethasone (Decadron, Deronil✿, Dexasone✿, Hexadrol) | *Adults:* 1-80 mg IM or IV daily<br>*Children:* 0.03-0.2 mg/kg IM or IV daily |
| hydrocortisone (Solu-Cortef) | *Adults:* 25-125 mg IM 2-4 times daily<br>*Children:* Dose for children not established |
| methylprednisoLONE (Duralone, Medalone, Solu-Medrol) | *Adults:* 10-60 mg IM or IV 2-4 times daily, depending on disorder<br>*Children:* 0.03-0.5 mg/kg IM or IV daily |
| *Topical Corticosteroids* | |
| hydrocortisone (Ala-Cort, Dermacort, Lanacort)<br>triamcinolone (Aristocort, Kenalog, Oracort, Triderm) | Most topical corticosteroids are available in strengths of 0.05% or 0.1% creams, ointments, and lotions. There is no specific amount of drug prescribed. A thin layer is applied on the affected skin area 2-3 times daily. |

🔲 Top 100 drugs prescribed.

### How Systemic Corticosteroids Work

Corticosteroids decrease the production of all known body chemicals (mediators) that trigger inflammation. They also slow the production of WBCs in the bone marrow. Because WBCs are the source of the mediators that trigger inflammation, the action of corticosteroids on WBCs also helps reduce inflammation. Corticosteroids have main effects and side effects in all cells and tissues.

### Intended Responses

- Swelling at site of inflammation is reduced.
- Redness and pain at site of inflammation are reduced.
- The body area affected by inflammation demonstrates increased function.

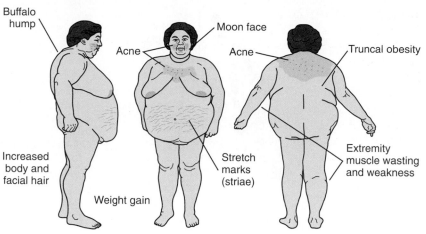

**FIGURE 8-2** Physical changes from long-term corticosteroid therapy, known as a "Cushingoid" appearance.

---

**Box 8-1** Common Side Effects of Systemic Corticosteroids

After 1 week of therapy:
- Acne
- Sodium and fluid retention
- Elevated blood pressure
- Sensation of "nervousness"
- Difficulty sleeping
- Emotional changes, crying easily

Within a month after therapy:
- Weight gain
- Fat redistribution (moon face and "buffalo hump" between the shoulders)
- Increased risk for gastrointestinal ulcers and bleeding
- Fragile skin that bruises easily
- Loss of muscle mass and strength
- Thinning scalp hair
- Increased facial and body hair
- Increased susceptibility to colds and other infections
- Stretch marks

---

***Side Effects.*** Because systemic corticosteroids enter and affect every type of body cell, they have many side effects. The most common are listed in Box 8-1 and shown in Figure 8-2. Most side effects do not occur with just one dose of corticosteroids but may be present as soon as 5 to 7 days after starting drug therapy. Other side effects may not be present for up to a month of therapy. The higher the dose of corticosteroids, the sooner the side effects appear, and the more severe they are. Many side effects change the patient's appearance ("Cushingoid appearance" as shown in Figure 8-2), which may cause distress. The good news is that most of these side effects and body changes return to normal after therapy stops, although it may take a year or longer. Stretch marks shrink but are permanent.

***Adverse Effects.*** Three important adverse effects are adrenal gland suppression, reduced immune function, and delayed wound healing. These can occur in anyone taking systemic corticosteroids for a long period of time. For this reason corticosteroids are taken for systemic inflammation only if the inflammation is severe and cannot be controlled in other ways.

The adrenal glands normally make cortisol. How much cortisol is made each day is determined by how much cortisol is already circulating in the blood. If there are less than normal amounts of cortisol in the blood, the adrenal glands produce and release more cortisol. If there are higher than normal levels of cortisol in the

 **Memory Jogger**

Most long-term side effects of systemic corticosteroid therapy, including those affecting appearance, eventually return to normal after therapy is stopped.

**Common Side Effects**

**Systemic Corticosteroids**

Hypertension    Acne    Insomnia

Nervousness

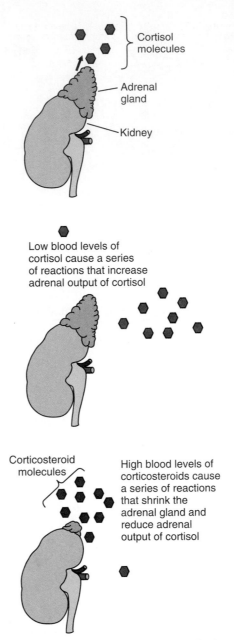

**FIGURE 8-3** Corticosteroid influence on adrenal production of cortisol.

blood, the adrenal glands reduce production of cortisol. When blood levels of cortisol are very high, the adrenal glands stop producing it, and the cells of the adrenal glands *atrophy* (shrink).

To the body, corticosteroid drugs look very much like cortisol. When a person is taking corticosteroids, the blood levels of the drug are high. This high level fools the adrenal glands into stopping their production of cortisol and shrinking (Figure 8-3). These atrophied adrenal glands become a problem if the person suddenly stops taking corticosteroids. The adrenal glands will begin making cortisol again, but this process takes weeks to months. As a result, the person who suddenly stops taking systemic corticosteroids has no circulating cortisol, which is necessary for life, and could die from the effects of *acute adrenal insufficiency*. (Box 8-2 lists the signs and symptoms of acute adrenal insufficiency.) Instead of stopping corticosteroid drugs suddenly when therapy is no longer needed, the patient must slowly decrease the doses over time. This process is called *tapering,* and it allows the adrenal gland cells to gradually resume the process of making cortisol.

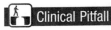 **Clinical Pitfall**

If a patient has been taking a systemic corticosteroid drug for a week or longer, he or she must not suddenly stop taking the drug.

> **Box 8-2** | Signs and Symptoms of Acute Adrenal Insufficiency
>
> - Acute confusion
> - Profound muscle weakness
> - Slow, irregular pulse
> - Hypotension
> - Abdominal pain
> - Nausea and vomiting
> - Salt craving
> - Weight loss
>
> - Low blood glucose levels (hypoglycemia, less than 70 mg/dL)
> - Low serum sodium levels (hyponatremia, less than 130 mEq/L)
> - High serum potassium levels (hyperkalemia, more than 5.5 mEq/L)
> - Low serum cortisol levels (less than 3.0 mcg/dL)

Because systemic corticosteroids reduce WBC numbers and the inflammatory response, the person taking these drugs is at greater risk for infection. When inflammation is reduced, the symptoms of infection may not be obvious. Infection symptoms (fever, redness, pain, pus, or drainage) are caused by the same mediators that cause inflammation. When corticosteroids block their production, an infection may be present but not produce symptoms.

Inflammation begins the process of wound healing. Reducing inflammation with corticosteroids reduces this response and slows cell growth. These actions delay wound healing, which also increases the risk for infection.

### What To Do *Before* Giving Corticosteroids

Check the dose and the specific drug name carefully. *Corticosteroids are not interchangeable because the strength of the drugs varies.* For this reason, drug doses must be recalculated by the prescriber if it is necessary to switch from one corticosteroid to another.

Check for symptoms of infection (for example, fever, drainage, foul-smelling urine, productive cough, or redness around an open skin area) and report any symptoms to the prescriber. Systemic corticosteroids may make an existing infection worse.

Check the patient's blood pressure and weight. Corticosteroids cause sodium and water retention that can lead to high blood pressure (hypertension) and weight gain.

### What To Do *After* Giving Corticosteroids

Check vital signs at least once per shift for changes in blood pressure or temperature elevation. Examine the skin for bruises or tears that indicate that the skin is becoming more fragile. Minimize the use of tape and be very gentle when handling the patient to avoid skin trauma and bleeding. Weigh the patient weekly to monitor for fluid retention.

### What To *Teach* Patients About Corticosteroids

The most important information to teach a patient who is taking systemic corticosteroids is to not stop taking the drug suddenly. If the patient is ill and unable to keep the drug down, he or she should call the prescriber so the drug can be given parenterally. Also tell the patient to wear a medical alert bracelet or to carry a card stating that corticosteroids are taken daily. This allows health care personnel to take steps to prevent adrenal insufficiency if the patient should suddenly become ill or hurt and is unable to communicate.

Tell the patient to take the corticosteroid in the morning or, if the dose is higher, to take two thirds of the dose in the morning and one third before bedtime. This schedule is close to the way the adrenal glands normally release cortisol.

Tell the patient to take corticosteroids with food to help prevent stomach ulcers. Teach him or her to avoid crowds and people who are ill because resistance to infection is decreased.

 **Memory Jogger**

It is possible for an infection to be present without symptoms when a person is taking systemic corticosteroids.

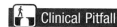 **Clinical Pitfall**

Never substitute one corticosteroid for another because strengths vary.

## Issues with Topical Corticosteroids

Topical corticosteroids are used to relieve itching and skin rashes that occur with skin inflammation. These drugs work like systemic corticosteroids, but their effects are largely confined to the skin area where the drug is applied. They come in creams, ointments, pastes, lotions, foams, and gels of different strengths. The stronger drugs require a prescription; weaker drugs are available over-the-counter.

Topical corticosteroids can be absorbed through the skin and have some systemic effects. Teach the patient to apply only a thin layer just to the areas that need treatment. Topical corticosteroids lower immunity in the area where they are applied. This means that, if there is a skin infection and topical corticosteroids are applied in that area, the infection can spread to surrounding areas more easily. For this reason, do not apply a topical corticosteroid if there is any question that the skin is infected rather than just being irritated or having a rash. Side effects with topical use are rare but can include acne, thinning of the skin in the areas where the drug is applied heavily, and changes in skin color.

## Life Span Considerations for Corticosteroids

***Pediatric Considerations.*** Corticosteroids are prescribed for children who have severe or chronic inflammatory problems. Children are at risk for the same corticosteroid side effects as adults, even stomach ulcers.

***Considerations for Pregnancy and Breastfeeding.*** Severe inflammatory responses during pregnancy can be treated with corticosteroids, although the drug does cross the placenta. Babies born to mothers taking the drug through the last 3 months of pregnancy tend to be smaller than normal. Because this drug group can cross into breast milk, mothers who must take corticosteroids long term are encouraged to stop breast feeding because the baby will have the same side effects as the mother.

***Considerations for Older Adults.*** Corticosteroids cause the same side effects in older adults as they do in younger adults. The increased risk for infection can be very serious in older adults, who may have age-related reduced immune function. The older patient taking systemic corticosteroids must take extra precautions to avoid infection. In addition, because the skin of an older adult is thinner than that of a younger adult, lower strengths of topical corticosteroids should be used. Teach the older adult the importance of using only a thin layer of a topical corticosteroid.

Another side effect of systemic corticosteroid therapy is an increase in blood glucose level. Because the older adult is more likely to have diabetes than a younger adult, this side effect may make controlling diabetes in an older adult much more difficult. For an older adult who has diabetes and also must take a systemic corticosteroid, close follow-up with the prescriber is needed to prevent diabetic complications. Both diet and diabetic drug therapy may need to be changed while the patient is on corticosteroid therapy.

## NONSTEROIDAL ANTI-INFLAMMATORY DRUGS

Nonsteroidal anti-inflammatory drugs (NSAIDs) are anti-inflammatory drugs that are not similar to cortisol but prevent or limit the tissue and blood vessel responses to injury or invasion by slowing the production of one or more inflammatory mediators. They are common in every health care setting and at home. Some of these drugs are available only by prescription; others are available over the counter. NSAIDs usually are taken for pain and inflammation. They are used to treat many health problems, including fever, arthritis and other rheumatologic disorders, gout, systemic lupus erythematosus, pain after surgery, menstrual cramps, and blood clots.

There are many different NSAIDs. They can first be placed into a class on the basis of whether they inhibit the enzyme COX-1 or COX-2. Then they are further separated into groups on the basis of specific chemical makeup. All NSAIDs work

### Clinical Pitfall

Never apply a topical corticosteroid to a skin area that may be infected.

-Learning Activity 8-3 ▶

in similar ways but vary in cost and some side effects. The listings in the following table describe only the most common drugs in each class. Be sure to consult a drug handbook for more information about a specific NSAID.

### Dosages for Common COX-1 Inhibitors

| Drug Class | Drug Examples | Dosage |
|---|---|---|
| Salicylic acid | aspirin (for example, Bayer Aspirin, Bufferin, Ecotrin, Entrophen🍁) | *Adults:* 325-650 mg orally 3-4 times daily<br>*Children:* 80-320 mg orally 3-4 times daily, depending on size |
| Propionic acid | ibuprofen (Advil, Motrin, Actiprofen🍁) | *Adults:* 200-800 mg orally 3-4 times daily<br>*Children:* 50-100 mg orally 3-4 times daily |
| | naproxen  (Aleve, Anaprox, Naprosyn, Naprosyn E🍁, Naprox🍁, Naxen🍁) | *Adults:* 250-500 mg orally twice daily<br>*Children:* 200-600 mg orally once or twice daily |
| | oxaprozin (Daypro) | *Adults:* 600-1800 mg orally once daily<br>*Children:* 600-1200 mg orally once daily |
| Acetic acid | indomethacin (Indameth🍁, Indocid🍁, Indocin, Indochron ER, Nu-Indo🍁) | *Adults/Children:* 50-200 mg orally or by suppository daily |
| | nabumetone (Relafen) | *Adults:* 500-1000 mg orally once or twice daily<br>Dosage not established for children |
| | ketorolac (Toradol) | *Adults:* 10-60 mg orally every 6 hr daily; 15-30 mg IM or IV every 6 hr<br>Dosage not established for multiple doses for children |
| Fenamic acid | mefenamic acid (Ponstel) | *Adults:* 250 mg orally every 6 hr<br>Dosage not established for children |
| | meclofenamic acid (Meclomen) | *Adults:* 50-100 mg orally every 6 hr<br>Dosage not established for children |
| Enolic acid | piroxicam (Apo-Piroxicam🍁, Feldene, Novopirocam🍁) | *Adults:* 20 mg orally once daily<br>Dosage not established for children |

 Top 100 drugs prescribed.

---

### Dosages for Common Cox-2 Inhibitors

| Drugs | Dosages |
|---|---|
| celecoxib (Celebrex)  | *Adults:* 100-400 mg orally daily<br>Dosage not established for children |

 Top 100 drugs prescribed.

> ⇄ **Do Not Confuse**
>
> **ketorolac** *with* **Ketalar**
>
> An order for ketorolac can be confused with Ketalar. The drug ketorolac is an anti-inflammatory drug that can be given orally or parenterally. Ketalar is a type of anesthetic agent.

> ⇄ **Do Not Confuse**
>
> **Celebrex** *with* **Celexa**
>
> An order for Celebrex can be confused with Celexa. Celebrex is an anti-inflammatory drug. Celexa is an antidepressant.

### How NSAIDs Work

The main action of NSAIDs is to inhibit the action of the cyclo-oxygenase (COX) enzyme. As described earlier in the review of physiology and pathophysiology, COX-1 is an enzyme found in many normal cells. Its purpose is to help make many of the different types of prostaglandins inside each cell (see Figure 8-1). **Prostaglandins** are a family of chemicals made by the body, some of which cause the signs and symptoms of inflammation. These prostaglandins have what are called "housekeeping" cell jobs, helping cells and tissues remain healthy and functional. COX-2 is an enzyme found only in inflammatory cells. Its purpose is to help make all the mediators of the inflammatory response, including prostaglandins, leukotriene, and kinins. **Leukotriene** is a chemical made by the body that binds to its receptors and maintains an inflammatory response. **Kinins** are a group of chemicals made by the body that cause some of the signs and symptoms of inflammation, especially pain. The most common one is bradykinin. These mediators are responsible for creating all of the uncomfortable signs and symptoms of inflammation. Most NSAIDs suppress both the COX-1 and COX-2 forms of the enzyme; so production of the helpful housekeeping mediators along with the inflammatory mediators is slowed. This means that these drugs cause side effects that are related to a reduction in the housekeeping mediators.

### Intended Responses
- Redness and pain at the site of inflammation are reduced.
- Swelling and warmth at the site of inflammation are reduced.
- Body function in the area affected by inflammation is increased.
- Fever is reduced.

***Side Effects.***   Because COX-1 NSAIDs reduce the activity of the COX-1 and COX-2 enzymes, some normal healthy cell functions are affected. For example, all COX-1 NSAIDs reduce platelet clumping and blood clotting. In fact, aspirin is often prescribed just for this action. However, just one dose of aspirin or any other COX-1 NSAID can reduce blood clotting for up to a week. Therefore anyone taking a COX-1 NSAID is at increased risk for bleeding in response to slight injuries, surgery, or dental work.

COX-1 NSAIDs can irritate the stomach lining and the rest of the gastrointestinal (GI) tract. The stomach is irritated when the drug touches it directly and again when the drugs are absorbed into the blood. This can lead to development of serious bleeding ulcers and pain in the GI tract.

All the NSAIDs except aspirin can reduce blood flow to the kidney and slow urine output. This action can lead to high blood pressure and kidney damage. In addition, the action of the COX-1 NSAIDs on the kidney is exactly the opposite of the angiotensin-converting enzyme (ACE) inhibitor drugs for high blood pressure and can make them less effective (see Chapter 13).

Because COX-2 NSAIDs mostly suppress the COX-2 pathway (see Figure 8-1), which allows the normal housekeeping functions of the COX-1 pathway to continue, they have fewer side effects than COX-1 NSAIDs. *However, if a patient takes more than the prescribed dose, the side effects are the same as for COX-1 NSAIDs.* These drugs do not affect platelet action and blood clotting, so bruising and gum bleeding are not expected side effects.

***Adverse Effects.***   In addition to possible kidney damage, common adverse effects of NSAIDs are the induction of asthma and allergic reactions. If a person is sensitive to one NSAID, he or she is very likely to be sensitive to all of them.

Taking NSAIDs long term at the same time as acetaminophen (Tylenol) increases the risk for kidney and liver damage. In addition, taking two or more different NSAIDs at the same time increases the side effects and the risk for adverse effects.

Celecoxib (Celebrex) is made from a chemical similar to the sulfa drug type of antibiotic. A patient who is allergic to sulfa drugs is likely to also be allergic to celecoxib.

Another adverse reaction that was responsible for removing two other COX-2 NSAIDs from the market was an increase in heart attacks and strokes among patients taking these drugs. COX-2 NSAIDs appear to increase clot formation in the small arteries of the heart and brain, especially when these arteries are narrowed by atherosclerosis or cigarette smoking. These drugs should be avoided by any patient who has angina or high blood cholesterol levels or who smokes.

The higher the dose of NSAIDs and the longer they are taken, the more likely they are to trigger an adverse effect. Except for low-dose aspirin, most NSAIDs

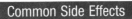

**Common Side Effects**

**NSAIDs**

Bleeding problems

GI ulcers, GI pain

Fluid retention

Hypertension

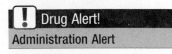

**Drug Alert!**

**Administration Alert**

Avoid giving NSAIDs with acetaminophen (Tylenol).

should not be taken daily for longer than 1 week for common aches and pains. Of course, with chronic diseases such as arthritis, the drugs may need to be taken much longer. When NSAIDs are needed long term, the patient is urged to find the lowest dose that still reduces his or her inflammation and pain.

### What To Do *Before* Giving NSAIDs

Carefully check the order for NSAIDs to be given parenterally. Only ketorolac (Toradol) is approved for IV use.

Before giving celecoxib, ask whether the patient has an allergy to sulfa antibiotics. A patient who is allergic to sulfa drugs is likely to also be allergic to celecoxib.

Always ask the patient whether he or she has had any problems with aspirin or any other over-the-counter NSAID. If the patient reports a previous problem with NSAIDs, do not give this drug without checking with the prescriber.

Give the drug at the time the patient is eating or very shortly after a meal. When possible, have the patient drink a full glass of water or milk with the drug.

Tell the patient not to chew an NSAID capsule or an enteric-coated tablet because it will ruin its stomach-protective properties.

Check the patient's blood pressure because NSAIDs can cause the patient to retain sodium and water, leading to higher blood pressure. If the patient is already taking an ACE inhibitor for high blood pressure, NSAIDs can reduce its effectiveness and make heart failure worse.

### What To Do *After* Giving NSAIDs

Bleeding risk increases within several hours after just one dose of a COX-1 NSAID. Examine the patient's gums, mucous membranes, and open skin areas (around IV sites) during each shift for bleeding. Look for bruises and for pinpoint purple-red spots (petechiae). Check urine, stool, or emesis for bright red blood, coffee-ground material, or other indications of bleeding.

Check the patient's blood pressure, breathing pattern, and pulse oximetry hourly after the first dose of an NSAID in case he or she is sensitive to it. Immediately report any breathing difficulty, drop in blood pressure, or decrease of 5% or more in oxygen saturation. Any of these signs and symptoms may indicate hypersensitivity to the drug.

### What To *Teach* Patients About NSAIDs

To avoid GI side effects, teach the patient to always take an NSAID with food or on a full stomach. Tell the patient not to chew an NSAID capsule or an enteric-coated tablet because doing so will ruin its stomach-protective properties. Teach him or her to check bowel movements for the presence of bright red blood or dark, tarry-looking material that would indicate bleeding somewhere in the GI tract. Tell the patient to immediately report such symptoms to the prescriber.

Because COX-1 NSAIDs reduce blood clotting, teach the patient to check the gums daily for bleeding, especially after toothbrushing or flossing. Tell the patient to let the dentist know that he or she takes NSAIDs before any dental procedure is performed.

Teach the patient not to take aspirin and other NSAIDs when also taking warfarin (Coumadin). Both of these drug types affect blood clotting in different ways, so the patient would be at extreme risk for excessive bleeding and stroke.

*The most important precaution to teach patients taking celecoxib (Celebrex) is to take the drug exactly as prescribed.* At higher doses these drugs also inhibit the COX-1 enzymes, which can make the adverse reactions and side effects the same as for the COX-1 NSAIDs.

Teach patients to weigh themselves at least twice each week in the morning before eating or drinking anything. Instruct them to wear similar clothes each time so the weight is not changed by different types of clothing. Show them how to keep a record of their weight. Instruct them to tell the prescriber about a weight gain of

**Clinical Pitfall**

Do not give celecoxib (Celebrex) to a patient who is allergic to the sulfa drug type of antibiotics.

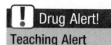

**Drug Alert!**

**Teaching Alert**

Teach the patient to avoid chewing or crushing an NSAID capsule or enteric-coated tablet.

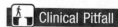

**Clinical Pitfall**

COX-1 NSAIDs should not be taken with warfarin (Coumadin).

more than 3 lb in a week. Also teach them how to check the ankles for swelling (which could mean heart failure, especially if it is present in the morning).

### Life Span Considerations for NSAIDs

*Pediatric Considerations.* With the exception of ibuprofen, NSAIDs are not recommended for children. In particular, aspirin and COX-2 NSAIDs are to be avoided in children. One problem with aspirin is an association with the development of Reye's syndrome, which may occur when aspirin is given to a child who has a viral infection. *Reye's syndrome* is a liver disease that can lead to coma, brain damage, and death.

*Considerations for Pregnancy and Breastfeeding.* Most NSAIDs are in categories C and D. The stronger ones, particularly indomethacin and celecoxib, should be avoided during the last 3 months of pregnancy because they may cause early closure of a blood vessel (the ductus arteriosus) important to fetal circulation and oxygenation.

*Considerations for Older Adults.* The older adult is at higher risk for cardiac problems when taking NSAIDs. These drugs cause salt and water retention that can lead to fluid overload and high blood pressure. Both of these problems increase the risk for heart attack and heart failure. Teach older adults taking NSAIDs to carefully monitor their weight, pulse, and urine output. Teach them the signs and symptoms of heart failure (weight gain; ankle swelling; and shortness of breath, especially when lying down).

⊖-Learning Activity 8-4 ▶

### ANTIHISTAMINES

**Antihistamines,** or histamine antagonists, are drugs that reduce inflammation by preventing the inflammatory mediator histamine from binding to its receptor. **Histamine** is a chemical mediator made by the body that binds to receptor sites and causes changes that lead to inflammatory responses. There are two known types of histamine receptors. $H_1$ receptors are located in blood vessels and respiratory mucous membranes. $H_2$ receptors are located in the stomach lining. When histamine binds to $H_1$ receptors, tissue changes occur, causing blood vessel dilation, swelling, decreased blood pressure, poor heart contractions, narrowed airways, increased mucus production, and the formation of hives on the skin. When histamine binds to $H_2$ receptors, stomach acid production increases, and the risk for stomach ulcers is greatly increased. Drugs that specifically block $H_2$ receptors in the stomach are discussed in Chapter 20.

Histamine is the main mediator of inflammation and capillary leak. Leukotriene, another mediator that binds to a receptor, works with histamine to keep the inflammatory response going once it has started. The drugs used to slow or stop an inflammatory reaction once it has started or to prevent one from starting are the antihistamines and leukotriene blockers. Both are most commonly used for inflammation triggered by allergic reactions such as hives, watery eyes, and runny nose. In addition, one of the antihistamines, diphenhydramine (Benadryl), is given during anaphylaxis and other severe systemic allergic reactions.

Many antihistamines are $H_1$ histamine blockers. Those most commonly prescribed are listed in the following table. Be sure to consult a drug handbook for information about a specific antihistamine.

#### Memory Jogger

Histamine and leukotriene are major mediators of inflammation.

#### ⇄ Do Not Confuse

#### Zyrtec *with* Zyban or Zantac

An order for Zyrtec can be confused with Zyban or Zantac. Zyrtec is an $H_1$ histamine blocker. Zyban (bupropion) is an antidepressant used to help people stop smoking. Zantac (ranitidine) is an $H_2$ histamine blocker used to help heal stomach ulcers and prevent esophageal reflux.

### Dosages for Common Antihistamines

| Drug | Dose |
| --- | --- |
| cetirizine (Zyrtec) 🔟🔟 | *Adults:* 5-10 mg orally daily<br>*Children:* 2.5-5 mg orally daily |
| diphenhydramine (Allerdryl♦, Benadryl) | *Adults/Children:* 12.5-50 mg orally or IV every 6 hr |

### Dosages for Common Antihistamines—cont'd

| Drug | Dose |
| --- | --- |
| loratadine (Claritin) | *Adults:* 10 mg orally daily<br>*Children:* 5 mg orally daily |

**TOP 100** Top 100 drugs prescribed.

## How Antihistamines Work

Antihistamines, or histamine antagonists, bind to $H_1$ histamine receptor sites in mucous membranes of the respiratory tract and in blood vessels, heart muscle, and the skin. This binding prevents the normal histamine of the body from binding to its receptors, thus slowing or stopping the tissue effects of inflammation (Figure 8-4).

### Intended Responses
- Blood vessels do not dilate.
- Swelling is reduced.
- Mucus and other nasal, eye, and respiratory secretions are reduced.
- Narrowed airways widen.
- Hives decrease in size and itchiness.

**Side Effects.**   Most antihistamines cause some degree of drowsiness. In fact, antihistamines may be prescribed (or taken over-the-counter) as a sleep aid. Each one varies in this side effect, and every person reacts differently. For some people even a low dose causes severe drowsiness; for others little or none occurs. Drinking alcohol when taking an antihistamine worsens the side effect of drowsiness.

All antihistamines cause dry mouth and dry throat. The severity depends on which drug is used or prescribed and how the person responds.

These drugs affect the heart as well. Most increase heart rate, and some people may have an irregular heartbeat and high blood pressure while taking the drug.

Eye and vision changes are common. The pupil dilates, and vision blurs. This problem increases an older adult's risk for falling.

Urinary retention can also occur. This is more of a problem in a patient who already has another condition that causes urinary retention such as prostate enlargement.

**Adverse Effects.**   One possible adverse effect of drug therapy with antihistamines is seizures. This is rare at normal doses but common with overdose.

**Common Side Effects**

**$H_1$ Histamine Blockers**

Sleepiness    Dry mouth    Blurred vision

Tachycardia    Urinary retention

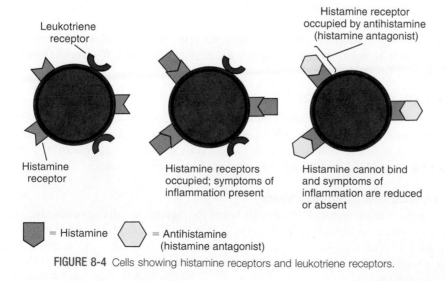

**FIGURE 8-4** Cells showing histamine receptors and leukotriene receptors.

Leukotriene receptor

Histamine receptor

Histamine receptor occupied by antihistamine (histamine antagonist)

Histamine receptors occupied; symptoms of inflammation present

Histamine cannot bind and symptoms of inflammation are reduced or absent

= Histamine     = Antihistamine (histamine antagonist)

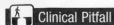

### Clinical Pitfall

Do not give antihistamines to a patient who has glaucoma, prostate enlargement, hypertension, or urinary retention.

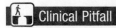

### Clinical Pitfall

Do not give an antihistamine that causes drowsiness to a patient having an acute asthma attack.

### ! Drug Alert!

**Interaction Alert**

When giving an antihistamine to a patient who is also taking opioids, sedatives, muscle relaxants, or barbiturates, avoid giving the antihistamine within 4 hours of these drugs.

For some people the pressure inside the eye *(intraocular pressure)* can become too high while on antihistamines. This is a dangerous situation and can make glaucoma worse or even lead to blindness.

Allergic reactions to antihistamines are very rare but can occur. A patient who has had a bad reaction to one antihistamine may be at risk for allergic reactions to others.

*Antihistamines that induce sedation should not be given during an acute asthma attack.* This is not because the drug causes asthma but because it can make the patient so drowsy that he or she may not be alert enough to work at breathing.

### What To Do *Before* Giving Antihistamines

Ask if the patient is being treated for glaucoma, high blood pressure, or prostate enlargement. Antihistamines are contraindicated for a patient with any of these problems because these drugs could make these conditions worse.

Check to see what other drugs are prescribed for the patient. Opioids, sedatives, muscle relaxants, and barbiturates all increase the drowsy effect of antihistamines. If it is necessary to give an antihistamine to a patient who is taking any of these drug types, it should not be given within 4 hours of these drugs.

### What To Do *After* Giving Antihistamines

Assist the patient whenever he or she is out of bed to prevent falls. Make certain that the call light is within easy reach.

Check the patient's pulse, blood pressure, and respiratory rate at least every 4 hours for the first 8 hours after giving an antihistamine. Notify the prescriber if heart rate becomes irregular, blood pressure changes significantly from the patient's baseline, or respiratory rate falls below 10 breaths/minute and stays low.

### What To *Teach* Patients About Antihistamines

Teach patients to avoid alcoholic drinks when taking antihistamines. Instruct them to avoid driving or operating dangerous or heavy machinery within 6 hours of taking these drugs.

Remind patients that the dry mouth and sore throat sensations caused by antihistamines can be relieved by drinking more water and sucking on mints or hard candy.

Urge the patient to contact the prescriber immediately about vision changes or pain over the eyebrows, which could mean an increase in intraocular pressure.

Teach the male patient who has prostate problems to make sure that he is urinating about as much fluid in a day as he is drinking. Urinary retention can be made worse by antihistamines. If he notices a sudden decrease in urine output or feels an urgent need to urinate and is unable to, he should contact his prescriber.

Remind the patient with asthma not to take antihistamines during an acute asthma attack at home because the drug could cause enough sleepiness to impair the ability to breathe.

### LEUKOTRIENE INHIBITORS

The leukotriene inhibitors are a newer class of drugs used for allergy therapy. Leukotriene is another body chemical that triggers and sustains inflammatory responses. It is found inside many types of WBCs. When it is released, it binds to leukotriene receptors and triggers the symptoms of inflammation (see Figure 8-4).

### How Leukotriene Inhibitors Work

Leukotriene inhibitors work in several ways to prevent an allergy episode. Zileuton (Zyflo) prevents leukotriene production within WBCs. Montelukast (Singulair) and zafirlukast (Accolate) block the leukotriene receptors on cells. As a result of these drugs, a person with allergies has less of an inflammatory response.

### Dosages for Common Leukotriene Inhibitors

| Drug | Dosage |
|---|---|
| montelukast sodium (Singulair) | *Adults:* 10 mg orally daily<br>*Children:* 4 mg orally daily |
| zafirlukast (Accolate) | *Adults:* 20 mg orally twice daily<br>*Children:* 10 mg orally twice daily |
| zileuton (Zyflo CR) | *Adults and children over 12 years:* 1200 mg orally twice daily after morning and evening meals |

### *Intended Responses*
- Swelling of oral, nasal, eye, and respiratory mucous membranes is reduced.
- Secretions are reduced.
- Narrowed airways are opened.

*Side Effects.*  Side effects of therapy with leukotriene inhibitors include headache and abdominal pain.

*Adverse Effects.*  The major adverse effects of leukotriene inhibitors are liver impairment and allergic reactions, including hives and anaphylaxis. Both of these responses are rare.

### What To Do *Before* Giving Leukotriene Inhibitors
Because leukotriene inhibitors, especially zileuton, can cause liver impairment, ask the patient about any previous liver problems or *jaundice* (yellowing of the skin, sclera, or mucous membranes), tenderness in the liver area of the abdomen (right upper quadrant), nausea, or fatigue. Check baseline liver function tests for comparison after the patient has been taking the drug for several months. Table 1-3 lists normal liver function tests.

### What To Do *After* Giving Leukotriene Inhibitors
Regularly assess the patient for signs and symptoms of decreased liver function, including constant fatigue, itchy skin, and yellowing of the skin or sclera.

   Assess the patient taking montelukast (Singulair) for mood changes, especially depression and suicidal thoughts.

### What To *Teach* Patients About Leukotriene Inhibitors
Teach the patient to report any skin yellowing, pain over the liver area, or darkening of the urine to the prescriber.

   Stress to patients taking montelukast (Singulair) to report any depression or thoughts of suicide immediately to the prescriber.

### Life Span Considerations for Leukotriene Inhibitors
*Pediatric Considerations.*  These drugs are prescribed for children who have allergies and inflammation. Care must be taken to calculate drug doses carefully to prevent an accidental overdose.

◄ ⊖-Learning Activity 8-5

---

**⇄ Do Not Confuse**

**Zyflo** *with* **Zyban or Zyrtec**

Zyflo is a leukotriene blocker used to reduce allergic reactions. Zyban is an antidepressant used to help people stop smoking. Zyrtec is an antihistamine also used to reduce inflammation and allergic reactions.

**Common Side Effects**

**Leukotriene Inhibitors**

Headache          Abdominal pain

---

## Get Ready for Practice!

### Key Points

- Inflammation is a general, nonspecific protective response that is helpful if confined to the area of invasion or infection and does not extend beyond the acute phase.
- Teach the patient taking systemic corticosteroids to *never* suddenly stop taking the drug.
- Do not substitute one type of corticosteroid for another.
- Remind patients taking systemic corticosteroids to avoid crowds and people who are ill because the effects of corticosteroids reduce a patient's immunity and resistance to infection.
- Avoid giving an NSAID with acetaminophen or with another NSAID.

- Teach patients to always take an NSAID with food or on a full stomach.
- Teach patients to never take a COX-1 NSAID if they are also taking warfarin (Coumadin).
- Do not give celecoxib (Celebrex) to a patient who is allergic to the sulfa drug type of antibiotics.
- Do not give an antihistamine known to cause drowsiness to a patient having an acute asthma attack.
- Do not give antihistamines to a patient who has glaucoma or an enlarged prostate.
- Drinking alcohol when taking antihistamines increases drowsiness.
- Warn patients who are taking antihistamines at home not to drive or operate heavy machinery within 6 hours of taking these drugs.
- Avoid giving an antihistamine within 4 hours of the time when an opioid, sedative, muscle relaxant, or barbiturate was given to the patient.

## Additional Learning Resources

**evolve** Go to your Evolve website (http://evolve.elsevier.com/Workman/pharmacology/) for the following FREE learning resources:
- eLearning Activities
- Animations
- Video Clips
- Interactive Review Questions
- Audio Key Points
- Audio Glossary
- Audio Glossary—Spanish-English
- Drug Dosage Calculators
- Patient Teaching Handouts

**SG** Go to your Study Guide for additional learning activities to help you master this chapter content.

## Review Questions

1. How do inflammation and infection differ?

   A. There is no true difference between infection and inflammation; the terms are interchangeable.

   B. Infection causes a patient to have a fever, whereas inflammation is never accompanied by increased body temperatures or fever.

   C. Inflammation side effects are minor and do not require drug therapy, whereas infection is serious and does require drug therapy.

   D. Infection is the result of an invasion by disease-causing organisms, whereas inflammation is a result of injury or invasion by non–disease-causing agents or organisms.

2. Which symptoms of inflammation are caused by blood vessel dilation?

   A. Increased production and migration of leukocytes

   B. Phagocytosis and fever

   C. Warmth and redness

   D. Swelling and pain

3. A patient taking 40 mg of prednisone daily for the past 3 months is experiencing the following signs and symptoms. Which ones are most likely related to the prednisone? (Select all that apply.)

   A. Continuous drowsiness

   B. Excessive bruising

   C. Thinning scalp hair

   D. Loss of appetite

   E. Blurred vision

   F. High blood pressure

4. Which question is most important to ask a patient before giving the first dose of a corticosteroid?

   A. Do you have a cold or any other symptoms of infection?

   B. Do you or any members of your family have diabetes?

   C. Have you ever had a rash when taking a corticosteroid?

   D. Have you ever had an allergic reaction to aspirin?

5. A patient who usually takes 40 mg of prednisolone daily has had nausea and vomiting for 12 hours and is still nauseated. What will you tell the patient about the drug therapy?

   A. "Go to the prescriber's office for a parenteral dose of the drug."

   B. "Wait until the next day and then take an extra dose of the drug."

   C. "Take the drug even though you are vomiting because it will be absorbed anyway."

   D. "Avoid taking the drug until you can hold food in your stomach so you won't develop ulcers."

6. For which health problem will you specifically monitor in the older patient taking a corticosteroid?

   A. Sudden hair loss

   B. Irregular heart rate

   C. Difficulty breathing

   D. High blood glucose level

7. Which new symptom in a patient taking celecoxib (Celebrex) requires immediate medical attention?

   A. Headache

   B. Chest pain

   C. Ankle swelling

   D. Increased urine output

8. Which question is most important to ask a patient before giving the first dose of an NSAID?

   A. Do you have a cold or any other symptoms of infection?

   B. Do you or any members of your family have diabetes?

   C. Have you had any recent problems with hair loss?

   D. Have you ever had an allergic reaction to aspirin?

9. You must caution patients who are taking NSAIDs that which health problem may be made worse by NSAIDs?

   A. Urinary incontinence
   B. Hypertension
   C. Constipation
   D. Arthritis

10. Which drug class should a patient who is 8 months pregnant avoid?

    A. Nonsteroidal anti-inflammatory drugs
    B. Antihistamines (histamine antagonists)
    C. Intravenous corticosteroids
    D. Oral corticosteroids

11. A patient who received 20 mg of loratadine (Claritin) for allergy symptoms is now drowsy and talks slowly when asked a direct question, although the patient responds correctly. What is your best action?

    A. Check the patient's mental status and reflexes every 2 hours
    B. Document the response as the only action
    C. Prepare to administer epinephrine
    D. Notify the prescriber

12. The patient prescribed montelukast (Singulair) tells you he has recently been hospitalized for depression. What is your best action?

    A. Ask whether the patient is taking an antidepressant.
    B. Hold the dose and notify the prescriber immediately.
    C. Reassure the patient that depression is common.
    D. Document the report as the only action.

13. Which precaution is important to teach a patient taking antihistamines at home?

    A. Avoid drinking coffee or other beverages containing caffeine
    B. Never take aspirin while taking antihistamines
    C. Do not stop taking antihistamines suddenly
    D. Do not drink alcohol with antihistamines

14. A patient with a severe allergic reaction is prescribed 80 mg of diphenhydramine (Benadryl) by IV push. The vial contains 10 mL of diphenhydramine solution with a concentration of 25 mg/mL. Exactly how many milliliters of diphenhydramine will you give this patient? _____ mL

15. A patient is to receive 40 mg of methylprednisolone (Solu-Medrol) IV in 250 mL of normal saline over the next 4 hours. The administration set has a drop factor of 15 gtts/mL. The vial contains 125 mg of the drug in 5 mL.

    A. How many milliliters will you inject into the 250-mg IV bag? _____ mL
    B. What is the correct flow rate of the IV drip in milliliters per hour and drops per minute? _____ mL/hr; _____ to _____ gtts/min

## Critical Thinking Activities

Mrs. Smith is a 75-year-old woman with osteoarthritis. She has diabetes and moderately high blood pressure. She controls her diabetes with diet alone and is taking furosemide (Lasix), a diuretic, daily for her blood pressure. She is being prescribed celecoxib (Celebrex) 200 mg PO daily for her arthritis.

1. What type of drug is celecoxib?

2. What is the major side effect of this drug?

3. List three common signs of this side effect.

4. List two strategies that you would teach Mrs. Smith to help her identify this problem and know when she should call her prescriber.

## Objectives

*After studying this chapter you should be able to:*

1. List the names, actions, usual adult dosages, possible side effects, and adverse effects of commonly prescribed cell wall synthesis inhibitors and protein synthesis inhibitors.
2. Describe what to do before and after giving cell wall synthesis inhibitors and protein synthesis inhibitors.
3. Explain what to teach patients taking cell wall synthesis inhibitors or protein synthesis inhibitors, including what to do, what not to do, and when to call the prescriber.
4. Describe life span considerations for cell wall synthesis inhibitors and protein synthesis inhibitors.

5. List the names, actions, usual adult dosages, possible side effects, and adverse effects of commonly prescribed sulfonamides, trimethoprim, and fluoroquinolones.
6. Describe what to do before and after giving sulfonamides, trimethoprim, and fluoroquinolones.
7. Explain what to teach patients taking sulfonamides, trimethoprim, or fluoroquinolones, including what to do, what not to do, and when to call the prescriber.
8. Describe life span considerations for sulfonamides, trimethoprim, and fluoroquinolones.

## Key Terms

**antibiotic resistance** (ăn-tī-bī-Ŏ-tĭk rē-ZĬS-tĕns) (p. 161) The ability of a bacterium to resist the effects of antibacterials.

**bactericidal** (băk-tēr-ĭ-SĪD-ŭl) (p. 141) A drug that reduces the number of bacteria by killing them directly.

**bacteriostatic** (băk-tēr-ē-ō-STĂT-ĭk) (p. 141) A drug that reduces the number of bacteria by preventing them from dividing and growing rather than directly killing them.

**drug generation** (DRŬG jĕn-ŭr-Ā-shŭn) (p. 146) Stage of drug development in which later generations are changed slightly to improve their effectiveness or means of administration.

**infection** (ĭn-FĔK-shŭn) (p. 138) Invasion by microorganisms that disturb the normal environment and cause harm or disease.

**nonpathogenic organisms** (nŏn-păth-ō-JĔN-ĭk ŌR-găn-ĭ-zĭmz) (p. 139) Bacteria or other organisms that do not overgrow or cause infection, systemic disease, or tissue damage.

**opportunistic organisms** (ŏp-pŏr-tū-NĬS-tĭk ŌR-găn-ĭ-zĭmz) (p. 139) Bacteria or other organisms that cause infection, systemic disease, or tissue damage only when the immune system is suppressed.

**pathogenic organisms** (păth-ō-JĔN-ĭk ŌR-găn-ĭ-zĭmz) (p. 139) Bacteria or other organisms that cause infection, systemic disease, and tissue damage.

**spectrum of efficacy** (SPĔK-trŭm of ĔF-ĭ-kĕ-sē) (p. 141) A measure of how many different types of bacteria a drug can kill or prevent from growing.

**susceptible organisms** (sŭ-SĔP-tĭ-bŭl ŌR-găn-ĭ-zĭmz) (p. 141) Bacteria or other organisms that either can be killed by or have their reproduction reduced by an antibacterial drug.

**virulence** (VĬR-ŭl-ĕns) (p. 139) The measure of how well bacteria can invade and spread despite a normal immune response.

---

⊖-Learning Activity 9-1 ►

Infection is the single most common reason for drug therapy. An **infection** is an invasion by microorganisms that disturbs the normal environment of the body and cause harm or disease. Infection agents include bacteria, viruses, fungi, protozoa, and other microorganisms. Bacterial infections are the most common cause of disease, sepsis, and death worldwide.

One of the most important advances in health care was the development of drugs to treat bacterial diseases—diseases that had previously led to death or permanent health problems. Before the widespread use of penicillin in the 1940s, death from infection was common. For example, a streptococcal infection such as strep throat could spread in the body and cause heart valve damage or kidney failure. A simple ear infection *(otitis media)* could spread, causing skull bone infection, brain infection, and death. Skin wounds could become infected and eventually cause sepsis (also known as *blood poisoning*). Infections this severe were usually fatal. The death rate from infections dropped dramatically with the use of antibacterial drugs.

## REVIEW OF RELATED PHYSIOLOGY AND PATHOPHYSIOLOGY

Humans interact constantly with different types of bacteria. Some of these bacteria are harmless, and others are or can become pathogenic. **Pathogenic** bacteria cause infection, systemic disease, and tissue damage. Some bacteria are nonpathogenic. **Nonpathogenic** bacteria coexist with us, causing no systemic disease or tissue damage. Indeed, many such bacteria are helpful when kept in check by our immune system. **Opportunistic** bacteria cause disease and tissue damage only in someone whose immune system is not working well. So there are differences in bacteria that make some types more dangerous to humans than others; however, even pathogenic bacteria are not always successful in the infectious process.

Whether or not an infection develops after bacterial invasion depends on how virulent the bacteria are and how well protected the person is by inflammatory responses and immunity. Individual differences in protection from infection could be seen even during the black plague epidemic in the middle ages. Some people became ill and died of the disease; some became ill and recovered; and others, equally exposed, never became ill. So, to understand drug therapy for bacterial infection, you need to know how bacteria cause infection and how people are protected from infection.

## BACTERIAL FEATURES

Bacteria are single cell organisms that have their own genetic material (DNA and genes), cytoplasm, some organelles, and membranes. Unlike human cells, bacterial cells may have several layers of membranes, cell walls, and capsules or coats (Figure 9-1). Just like human cells, bacteria have surface proteins that serve as recognition codes. Different types of bacteria have different shapes such as rodlike, round *(cocci)*, and spiral *(spirochetes)*.

Bacterial types vary in their ability to invade a person and avoid that person's immune and inflammatory responses. The **virulence** of bacteria is a measure of how well they can invade and spread despite a normal immune response. The most virulent bacteria have differences, known as *virulence factors*, that help them be more efficient at infecting a person. For example, some virulence factors are bacterial surface proteins that mimic human cell proteins. This action serves as a decoy and

**Memory Jogger**

*Pathogenic bacteria* are those that can cause damage or tissue disease. *Nonpathogenic bacteria* do not cause disease or damage. *Opportunistic bacteria* cause disease or tissue damage only when the immune system is impaired.

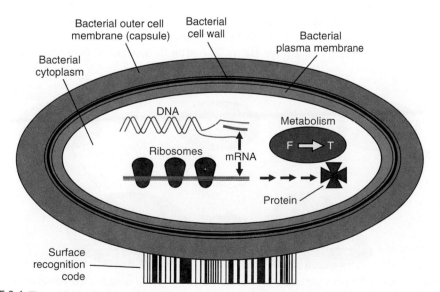

**FIGURE 9-1** The surface of a bacterium, its membrane, and its internal features. $F \rightarrow T$, metabolic conversion of folic acid to thymine.

hides the bacteria from the immune system. Other virulence factors include enzymes that punch holes in human cells, proteins that suppress the immune system, and "sticky" surfaces that keep the bacteria in contact with body cells to allow easier cell infection.

Bacteria are also classified according to whether or not they change color when a dye called *Gram stain* is applied. Those that change color are called *gram-positive*, and those that don't are called *gram-negative*. In general, gram-negative bacteria are more virulent and harder to kill or control because they are surrounded by a protective capsule.

## PROTECTION AGAINST INFECTION

Bacteria enter the body through breaks in the skin, are ingested with food and liquids, are inhaled from the air, and are carried into the body at normal openings by actions such as rubbing the eyes. Barriers to prevent bacterial entry are both general and specific. They exist both on the surface and inside of our bodies.

*General surface protection* prevents bacteria from entering the body and is not targeted to any specific organism. These protections include:

- Intact skin and mucous membranes.
- pH of body secretions.
- Products in saliva, perspiration, tears, and mucus that repel or slow bacterial entry.
- Normal flora on body surfaces and openings.

Normal flora are the nonpathogenic bacteria that we always have on skin, mucous membranes, and in the digestive tract. They provide protection by "crowding out" pathogenic organisms and preventing them from entering the body.

*Specific surface protection* involves making antibodies that can catch and trap bacteria. When the immune system makes an antibody, it does so against specific bacteria that entered the body at an earlier time. For example, if you had a streptococcal infection in the past, you now make antibodies to that strain of streptococcus. These antibodies bind to the bacteria when it appears again and help inactivate or kill it. One type of antibody, immunoglobulin A (IgA), is present in all body secretions. This means that, when a bacterium for which you already make antibodies appears again on your skin, IgA can inactivate or kill it before it enters your body. This is an effective way to protect you from becoming infected with the same organism over and over again.

*General internal protection* is present in all healthy people and does not depend on previous exposure to specific bacteria. White blood cells (WBCs) provide general and specific internal protection against infection. Some WBCs can recognize bacteria when they invade the body because the bacteria have different recognition codes on their surfaces than your own cells have (Figure 9-2). Therefore your WBCs recognize the bacteria as invaders and attack them. The attacks are called *general* because they

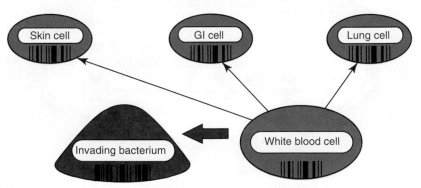

**FIGURE 9-2** A white blood cell compares the surface recognition codes of all four cells and recognizes that three of them are normal body cells but the red one has a different code. It is an invader and must be attacked by the white blood cell. *GI*, Gastrointestinal.

are the same against any type of invader. WBCs are effective at this type of protection and help keep you healthy more often than you are sick.

*Specific internal protection* is something that your body must learn to do. It occurs through WBCs known as *lymphocytes*. There are two main types of lymphocytes: *T lymphocytes (T cells)* and *B lymphocytes (B cells)*. T cells work with general WBCs to recognize invading organisms and keep them from moving all through the body. This gives the B cells time to learn to make antibodies directed against a specific organism. Usually B cells don't make enough antibody at first, so you often become sick from your first exposure to an organism. After that, B cells know how to make the specific antibody and turn on the antibody-making factory whenever you are reexposed to the same organism. Usually there is enough antibody to kill off or get rid of the organisms on reexposure before they have the chance to make you sick.

## ANTIBACTERIAL THERAPY

Despite all of the surface and internal barriers to infection, sometimes bacteria make it past these protections and enter your body where they multiply, damage tissues, and cause disease. Some bacterial infections are minor and can be cured by the immune system. Others are more severe and could cause serious harm and even death. (Usually more virulent bacteria cause more serious infections.) Antibacterial drugs are used to prevent bacteria from spreading infection throughout your body and causing severe damage.

### BACTERICIDAL AND BACTERIOSTATIC DRUGS

Some antibacterial drugs are bactericidal, which means that they kill bacteria directly. Other antibacterial drugs are bacteriostatic, which means that they prevent bacteria from reproducing until the body's own WBCs and antibodies get rid of them. So if a person's immune system is not working well, he or she would benefit from a bactericidal drug and not a bacteriostatic drug.

### SPECTRUM OF EFFICACY

Antibacterial drugs are sometimes described by their spectrum of efficacy, which is a measure of how many different types of bacteria the drug can kill or prevent from growing. Each drug is judged by how many types of bacteria are susceptible to it. Susceptible bacteria are those that either can be killed by a specific antibacterial drug or have their reproduction suppressed by it. A *narrow-spectrum antibacterial drug* is effective against only a few types of bacteria. An *extended-spectrum antibacterial drug* is effective against more types of bacteria. A *broad-spectrum antibacterial drug* is effective against a wide range of bacteria, both gram-positive and gram-negative.

Identifying the type of bacteria causing an infection is important for selecting the appropriate drug to treat the infection. Shape and Gram stain can help in this identification, as can tests that examine bacterial enzymes and genes (although these tests are not in common use). The most common method to identify bacteria is culture and sensitivity (C&S). Culturing bacteria means to transfer it from an infected site and place it in a sterile nutritious broth to grow for 24 to 48 hours. By allowing the bacteria to multiply, more bacteria can be examined microscopically and tested with other procedures for identification. Culturing may be done alone or along with sensitivity testing (which is more expensive). When sensitivity testing is included, discs containing a specific antibacterial drug are placed in the culture with the bacteria. When a drug is effective against the bacteria, the bacteria do not grow in the area where the disc was placed.

A perfect antibacterial drug would kill bacteria and not harm the patient's body in any way. There are no perfect drugs. Because bacteria have some of the same features as human cells (such as DNA and genes, proteins, and cellular metabolism), some of the drug effects on bacteria also have the same effects on your cells. The goal of antibacterial drug therapy is to use a dose that kills or harms the bacteria as

 **Memory Jogger**

WBCs provide general protection against infection.

 **Memory Jogger**

Each antibody is directed against only one type of organism. So, an antibody that works against the chickenpox virus has no effect on a streptococcal bacterium.

 **Memory Jogger**

Bactericidal drugs directly kill bacteria, whereas bacteriostatic drugs stop them from reproducing while the immune system kills the bacteria.

much as possible without serious harm to the patient. However, sometimes, when an infection is life threatening, it may be necessary to use higher doses or combinations of drugs that together have more serious side effects.

## GENERAL ISSUES IN ANTIBACTERIAL THERAPY

Many different drug types are used for antibacterial therapy. Each type has both distinctive and common actions and effects. A discussion of general side effects, adverse effects, and nursing responsibilities for antibacterial drugs follows. Intended responses, specific side effects, adverse effects, and nursing responsibilities are listed with each individual drug class.

The intended response for all antibacterial drugs is the disappearance of signs and symptoms of infection. Body temperature is expected to return to normal; WBC counts are expected to remain between 5000 and 10,000 cells/mm$^3$; and there should be no drainage and redness in the area of infection.

Side effects common to all antibacterial drugs include intestinal disturbances that can range from an increase in the number of bowel movements to severe diarrhea. This is considered an *expected side effect*, not an allergic reaction. The reason these drugs cause diarrhea is that, in addition to killing the infecting bacteria, they also kill some of the normal intestinal flora that help with food digestion and other processes. The normal flora are helpful and nonpathogenic as long as they stay only in the intestinal tract. When their numbers decline, less food is digested and moves out more quickly as diarrhea.

Another side effect resulting from the loss of normal flora in the mouth and vagina is *yeast* infections. In the mouth this is known as *thrush*. Thrush makes food taste bad and can cause gum disease. In the vagina the infection causes a white, cheesy discharge and intense itching.

Adverse effects that are possible with any antibacterial drug include severe allergic reactions and anaphylaxis, especially when the drug is given intravenously (IV). The major symptom of an allergic reaction to an oral drug is a skin rash that may appear days after starting the drug. A more severe allergic reaction to an IV drug is difficulty breathing and shock, which is called *anaphylaxis*. If not recognized and treated quickly, anaphylaxis can lead to vascular collapse, shock, and death.

*Pseudomembranous colitis* is a complication of antibacterial therapy that causes severe inflammation in areas of the colon (large intestine). Other names for this problem include *antibiotic-associated colitis* and *necrotizing colitis*. The cause of the problem is the overgrowth of an intestinal organism called *Clostridium difficile*. This organism is not killed by most antibacterial drugs, and it can take over the patient's intestinal tract when normal flora are killed off. This organism releases a powerful toxin that damages the intestines. The lining of the colon becomes raw and bleeds. Other symptoms include watery diarrhea, the constant feeling of the need to move the bowels, abdominal cramps, low-grade fever, and bloody stools. Patients can lose so much water and so many electrolytes in the watery diarrhea that they become dehydrated. When this problem occurs, the drug should be stopped. Although any antibacterial drug can cause pseudomembranous colitis if it is taken long enough, the more powerful drugs allow it to happen sooner.

*Before giving any antibacterial drug,* ask the patient if he or she has any drug allergies. Notify the prescriber if the patient has an allergy to the drug. If he or she does have an allergy to a drug and is to receive it anyway, check with the prescriber about first giving the patient diphenhydramine and epinephrine to reduce any serious reaction. Place the emergency cart close to the door of the patient's room.

If an order for a culture or C&S test has been made, ensure that the specimen is obtained before drug therapy is started.

Antibacterial drugs often suppress the growth of WBCs in the bone marrow. Check the patient's WBC count before drug therapy begins and use it as a baseline in detecting side effects and gauging the drug's effectiveness. Table 1-6 in Chapter 1 lists the normal values for blood cells.

Also check the patient's vital signs (including temperature) and mental status before starting any antibacterial drug. These too can be used to detect side effects and gauge drug effectiveness.

Many IV antibacterial drugs can interact with other drugs and irritate the tissues. Make sure that the IV infusion is running well and has a good blood return. In addition, either flush the line before giving the antibacterial or use fresh tubing to give it. Double check the recommended infusion rate for the specific drug. Most should be given slowly over at least 30 to 60 minutes. Some may need to be given by slow continuous infusion for 8 hours or longer.

*After giving an antibacterial drug,* ask the patient about the number of daily bowel movements and their character. Although all antibacterial drugs change the normal flora of the intestines and can cause diarrhea, this symptom is also a sign of a more serious problem called *pseudomembranous colitis.* The diarrhea of colitis is more watery and intense.

When giving the first IV dose of an antibacterial drug, check the patient every 15 minutes for any signs or symptoms of an allergic reaction (hives at the IV site, low blood pressure, rapid irregular pulse, swelling of the lips or lower face, the patient feeling a "lump in the throat"). If the patient is having an anaphylactic reaction, your first priority is to prevent any more drug from entering him or her. Stop the drug from infusing but keep the IV access open. If the drug is infusing high into the IV tubing, change the tubing after stopping the drug and do not let any drug remaining in the tubing run into the patient.

Monitor the patient for the effectiveness of the antibacterial drug in treating the infection. Signs and symptoms of a resolving infection include reduced or absent fever; no chills; wound drainage that is no longer thick, foul smelling, brown, green, or yellow; wound edges that are not red and raw-looking; and a WBC count that is in the normal range (see Table 1-6 in Chapter 1).

Check the patient's mouth daily for a white, cottage cheese–like coating on the gums, roof of the mouth, or insides of the cheeks. This substance is an overgrowth of yeast called thrush. Help the patient apply good oral hygiene with toothbrushing and mouthwash at least every shift.

Because many IV antibacterial drugs are irritating to tissues and veins, check the IV site at least every 2 hours for symptoms of phlebitis, which include a change in blood return, any redness or pain, or the feeling of hard or "cordlike" veins above the site. If such problems occur, follow the policy of your agency concerning removal of the IV access.

*Teach patients receiving an antibacterial drug* to take the drug for as long as it was prescribed. Some patients stop taking the drug as soon as they feel better, which can lead to a recurrence of the infection and the development of resistant bacteria.

For all antibacterial therapy, it is important to keep the blood level high enough to affect the bacteria causing the infection. Therefore teach the patient to take the drug evenly throughout a 24-hour day. If the drug is to be taken twice daily, teach the patient to take it every 12 hours. For three times a day, teach the patient to take it every 8 hours. For four times a day, teach the patient to take it every 6 hours. Help the patient plan a schedule that is easy to remember and keeps the drug at the best blood levels.

If a rash or hives develop while taking an antibacterial drug, remind the patient to stop taking the drug and call the prescriber immediately. Explain that this is a sign of drug allergy. Tell the patient to call 911 immediately if he or she has trouble breathing or has the feeling of a "lump in the throat" because these are signs of a more serious allergic reaction.

Teach the patient to check his or her mouth daily for a white, cheesy substance that could indicate an oral yeast infection. Explain that brushing the teeth three to four times daily along with using mouthwash can reduce the risk for this problem. Teach a female patient to also wash her perineum at least twice a day and check for vaginal discharge and itchiness that indicate a vaginal yeast infection. Tell her to report any evidence of a vaginal infection to her prescriber.

 **Memory Jogger**

Signs and symptoms of a severe allergic reaction include hives at the IV site, low blood pressure, rapid irregular pulse, swelling of the lips or lower face, and the patient feeling a "lump in the throat."

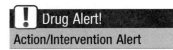 **Drug Alert!**

**Action/Intervention Alert**

If a patient appears to be having anaphylaxis from an IV drug, prevent any more drug from entering the patient but maintain the IV access.

 **Memory Jogger**

Teach patients to take any antibacterial drug exactly as prescribed and for as long as prescribed.

◀ ⊜-Learning Activity 9-2

## TYPES OF ANTIBACTERIAL DRUGS

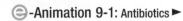

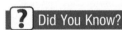
Antibacterial drugs are classified according to how they kill bacteria or how they stop or slow bacterial reproduction. The four major classes of antibacterial drugs are cell wall synthesis inhibitors, protein synthesis inhibitors, metabolism inhibitors, and DNA synthesis inhibitors. Within each class there are several types of drugs. Table 9-1 lists the actions of the different types of antibacterial drugs. Figure 9-3 shows the specific areas of a bacterium that are targeted by different types of antibacterial drugs. The decision to use one type of drug over another is based on whether the bacterium causing the infection is known (by culture and/or sensitivity testing), how serious the infection is, which drugs are known to kill or harm it, how well the patient's immune system is working, the patient's overall health (especially kidney, liver, and bone marrow function), and whether the patient has any known drug allergies.

### PENICILLINS, CEPHALOSPORINS, AND OTHER CELL WALL SYNTHESIS INHIBITORS

The first antibacterial drug developed for general use was penicillin. It was originally a natural product made from bread mold. Some penicillins are still made as a product of mold, and others are made synthetically from chemicals. In addition to penicillin, this drug class includes the cephalosporins, carbapenems, monobactams, and vancomycin. The carbapenems and vancomycin are powerful drugs available only by injection and have serious side effects.

#### How Cell Wall Synthesis Inhibitors Work

Some bacteria have a cell wall, and others do not (see Figures 9-1 and 9-3). Cell wall synthesis inhibitors work against those that do. These drugs kill the susceptible bacteria by preventing them from forming strong, protective cell walls.

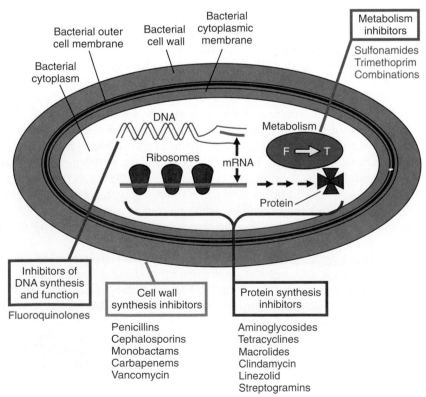

**FIGURE 9-3** Bacterial targets of different types of antibacterial drugs. *F → T*, metabolic conversion of folic acid to thymine.

## Table 9-1  Actions of Antibacterial Agents

| DRUG TYPE | MAJOR ACTIONS | DRUG EXAMPLES |
|---|---|---|
| Cell wall synthesis inhibitors (bactericidal) | Bind to cell wall proteins and prevent them from being incorporated into bacterial cell walls<br>Inhibit the bacterial enzyme needed to cross-link the cell wall components, making the walls loose<br>Activate enzymes called *autolysins* in the bacterial cell walls, which eat holes in the walls, making them leaky | **PENICILLINS**<br>amoxicillin (Amoxil, Amoxicot, Apo-Amoxi🍁, Biomox, Moxilin)<br>amoxicillin; clavulanate potassium (Augmentin, Clavulin🍁)<br>penicillin G benzathine (Bicillin LA)<br>penicillin G (Pfizerpen)<br>penicillin V potassium (Apo-Pen-VK🍁, Nadopen-V🍁, Pen-V, BeePen-VK, Veetids)<br>ticarcillin/clavulanate (Timentin)<br><br>**CEPHALOSPORINS**<br>cefazolin (Ancef, Kefzol)<br>cefdinir (Omnicef)<br>ceftriaxone (Rocephin)<br>cephalexin (Apo-Cephalex🍁, Biocef, Keflex, Keftab, Novo-Lexin🍁, Nu-Cephalex🍁)<br><br>**MONOBACTAMS**<br>aztreonam (Azactam)<br><br>**CARBAPENEMS**<br>ertapenem (Invanz)<br>imipenem/cilastatin (Primaxin)<br>meropenem (Merrem)<br><br>**OTHERS**<br>vancomycin (Vancocin) |
| Protein synthesis inhibitors (bacteriostatic or bactericidal) | Bind to the large (50S) subunit of ribosomes, preventing them from "reading" the mRNA<br>Bind to the small (30S) subunit of ribosomes, preventing them from "reading" the mRNA<br>Bind to the enzyme needed to bring the amino acids into contact with the mRNA and linking them together | **AMINOGLYCOSIDES**<br>amikacin (Amikin)<br>gentamicin (Cidomycin🍁, Garamycin, Gentacidin)<br>streptomycin<br><br>**MACROLIDES**<br>azithromycin 🔲 (Zithromax 🔲, Zmax)<br>clarithromycin (Biaxin)<br>erythromycin (Apo-Erythro🍁, E-Mycin, Erycette, Erymax, Erythromid🍁, Romycin)<br>erythromycin lactobionate (Erythrocin, Lactobionate)<br><br>**TETRACYCLINES**<br>demeclocycline (Declomycin)<br>doxycycline (Adoxa, Apo-Doxy🍁, Atridox, Doryx, Dox-Caps, Doxycin🍁, Monodox, Novodoxyclin🍁, Vibramycin)<br>minocycline (Arestin, Dynacin, Minocin, Vectrin)<br>tetracycline (Ala-Tet, Apo-Tetra🍁, Brodspec, Novotetra🍁, Nu-Tetra🍁, Panmycin, Sumycin, Tetracon)<br><br>**LINCOSAMIDE**<br>clindamycin (Cleocin)<br><br>**OXAZOLIDINONE**<br>linezolid (Zyvox)<br><br>**STREPTOGRAMINS**<br>dalfopristin/quinupristin (Synercid) |

*Continued*

**Table 9-1** | Actions of Antibacterial Agents—cont'd

| DRUG TYPE | MAJOR ACTIONS | DRUG EXAMPLES |
|---|---|---|
| Metabolism inhibitors (bacteriostatic) | Suppress the activity of an enzyme needed to convert other substances (PABA and pteridine) into folic acid in bacteria; as a result, the bacteria do not have enough folic acid to be able to make DNA and grow | **SULFONAMIDES**<br>sulfadiazine sodium<br>sulfisoxazole (Gantrisin, Soxazole🍁, Truxazole)<br><br>**TRIMETHOPRIM**<br>(Primsol, Trimpex)<br><br>**COMBINATION DRUGS**<br>trimethoprim/sulfamethoxazole (Apo-Sulfatrim🍁, Bactrim, Bethaprim, Novo-Trimel🍁, Nu-Cotrimex🍁, Roubac🍁, Septra, Sulfatrim, Uroplus, SMX-TMP) |
| DNA synthesis inhibitors (bactericidal) | Enter bacterial cells and suppress the action of two enzymes (gyrase and topoisomerase) important in allowing the bacteria to make DNA | **FLUOROQUINOLONES**<br>ciprofloxacin (Ciloxan, Cipro)<br>gatifloxacin (Tequin)<br>gemifloxacin (Factive)<br>levofloxacin (Levaquin)<br>lomefloxacin (Maxaquin)<br>moxifloxacin (Avelox)<br>ofloxacin (Floxin) |

**TOP 100** Top 100 drugs prescribed; *DNA,* deoxyribonucleic acid; *mRNA,* messenger ribonucleic acid; *PABA, para*-aminobenzoic acid.

These drugs usually act in at least one of three ways. Think of a cell wall as made up of individual bricks known as penicillin-binding proteins, with mortar between the bricks holding the wall together tightly. One way these drugs interfere with cell walls is that they bind to the bricks, keeping them from being placed in the wall. The second way these drugs work is by preventing the mortar from being made, which results in the bricks just lying loosely on top of each other so the wall is easy to break. The third way these drugs work is by activating an enzyme that punches holes in the wall. So, even though a wall may be formed, it is leaky and does not protect the bacteria.

Cell wall synthesis inhibitors are most effective against bacteria that divide rapidly and are usually found on the skin and mucous membranes, respiratory tract, ear, bone, and blood. Infections for which penicillins, cephalosporins, and other cell wall synthesis inhibitors are prescribed include strep throat, tonsillitis, otitis media, simple urinary tract infections, wound infections, upper and lower respiratory infections, prostatitis, and gonorrhea. They also may be used for sepsis and Lyme disease. The more powerful drugs in this class such as the carbapenems and vancomycin are used for severe infections such as sepsis, endocarditis, abscesses, and infections that involve multiple types of bacteria.

Cell wall synthesis inhibitors have been around longer than other types of antibacterial drugs. Some, especially the cephalosporins, have more than one drug generation. **Drug generation** refers to the stage of development of a drug in which later generations are changed slightly to improve their effectiveness or means of administration. The cephalosporins have four drug generations. Table 9-2 lists the different drugs in each generation and which organisms are most sensitive to them.

The activity of penicillin and some other cell wall synthesis inhibitors can be enhanced when other agents are added to the drug. For example, penicillin can be destroyed by a bacterial enzyme called *beta-lactamase,* which makes bacteria with this enzyme resistant to penicillin. Combining penicillin with clavulanic acid (clavulanate) inhibits this bacterial enzyme and reduces penicillin resistance even though clavulanic acid has little if any antibiotic effect on the bacteria. An agent that improves the activity of imipenem is cilastatin. Without cilastatin, imipenem is rapidly metabolized in the kidney and excreted. Cilastatin slows this metabolism and allows the imipenem to remain in the body longer for better antibacterial action.

**Table 9-2**  **Cephalosporins by Drug Generation**

| DRUG | FEATURES |
|---|---|
| **FIRST GENERATION (EXTENDED SPECTRUM)** | |
| cefazolin (Ancef, Kefzol)<br>cephalexin (Biocef, Keflex)<br>cephradine (Velosef) | Effective against gram-positive bacteria, especially cocci such as streptococcus and staphylococcus bacterial types<br>Somewhat effective against gram-negative bacteria, including *Proteus mirabilis*, *Escherichia coli*, and *Klebsiella* |
| **SECOND GENERATION (BROAD SPECTRUM)** | |
| cefaclor (Ceclor)<br>cefditoren (Spectracef)<br>cefoxitin (Cefoxitin, Mefoxin)<br>cefuroxime (Ceftin, Kefurox, Zinacef)<br>loracarbef (Lorabid) | Effective against gram-negative bacteria<br>Especially effective for gonorrhea, *Enterobacter aerogenes*, *Haemophilus influenza*<br>Not as effective as first generation for gram-positive bacteria |
| **THIRD GENERATION (BROAD SPECTRUM)** | |
| cefdinir (Omnicef)<br>cefixime (Suprax)<br>cefotaxime (Claforan)<br>cefotetan (Cefotan)<br>cefpodoxime (Vantin)<br>ceftazidime (Ceptaz, Fortaz, Tazicef, Tazidime)<br>ceftibuten (Cedax)<br>ceftizoxime (Cefizox)<br>ceftriaxone (Rocephin) | More effective against gram-negative bacteria than either the first- or second-generation drugs<br>Can cross the blood-brain barrier |
| **FOURTH GENERATION (BROAD SPECTRUM)** | |
| cefepime (Maxipime) | Effective against both gram-positive and gram-negative bacteria |

There are many types of cell wall synthesis inhibitors, and within each type there are dozens of different brands and strengths. They all work in similar ways and have similar effects. Only the drugs on the list of the 100 most commonly prescribed and those most often used in acute care settings are listed in the following table. Be sure to consult a drug reference for more information about a specific drug in this class.

### Dosages for Common Cell Wall Synthesis Inhibitors

| Drugs | Dosages |
|---|---|
| *Penicillins* | |
| amoxicillin 🔲 (Amoxil, Amoxicot, Apo-Amoxi🍁, Biomox, Moxilin) | *Adults:* 250-500 mg orally every 8 hr<br>*Children:* 7-8 mg/kg orally every 8 hr |
| amoxicillin/clavulanic acid 🔲 (Augmentin, Clavulin🍁) | *Adults:* 250-500 mg orally every 8 hr<br>*Children:* 10 mg/kg orally every 8 hr |
| penicillin G benzathine (Bicillin LA, Megacillin🍁) | *Adults:* 1.2 million units IM daily<br>*Children:* 300,000-600,000 units IM as a single dose |
| penicillin G (Pfizerpen) | *Adults:* 1-4 million units IV every 6 hr<br>*Children:* 40,000-50,000 units/kg IV every 6 hr |
| penicillin V potassium 🔲 (Apo-Pen-VK🍁, Nadopen-V🍁, Pen-V, VeePen, Pen-VK, Veetids) | *Adults:* 250-500 mg orally every 6 hr<br>*Children:* 8-15 mg/kg orally every 6-8 hr |
| ticarcillin/clavulanic acid (Timentin) | *Adults:* 3 g IV every 4-6 hr<br>*Children:* 50 mg/kg IV every 4-6 hr |

🔲 Top 100 drugs prescribed.

*Continued*

**Dosages for Common Cell Wall Synthesis Inhibitors—cont'd**

| Drugs | Dosages |
|---|---|
| **Cephalosporins** | |
| cefazolin (Ancef, Kefzol) | *Adults:* 500 mg to 1 g IM or IV every 6-8 hr |
| | *Children:* 25-100 mg/kg IM or IV every 6 hr |
| cefdinir  (Omnicef) | *Adults:* 300 mg orally every 12 hr |
| | *Children:* 7 mg/kg orally every 12 hr |
| ceftriaxone (Rocephin) | *Adults:* 1-2 g IM or IV daily |
| | *Children:* 25-50 mg/kg IM or IV every 12 hr |
| cephalexin 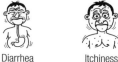 (Apo-Cephalex♦, Biocef, Keflex, Keftab, Novo-Lexin♦, Nu-Cephalex♦) | *Adults:* 250-500 mg orally every 6-12 hr |
| | *Children:* 8-12 mg/kg orally every 6-8 hr |
| **Monobactams** | |
| aztreonam (Azactam) | *Adults:* 500 mg to 2 g IM or IV every 8-12 hr |
| | *Children:* 30 mg/kg IM or IV every 6-8 hr |
| **Carbapenems** | |
| ertapenem (Invanz) | *Adults:* 1 g IV or IM daily |
| | *Children older than 3 months:* 15 mg/kg IV or IM every 12 hr |
| imipenem/cilastatin (Primaxin) | *Adults:* 250 mg-1 g IM or IV every 6-8 hr; 500-750 mg IM every 12 hr |
| | *Children:* 25 mg/kg IM or IV every 6 hr |
| meropenem (Merrem) | *Adults:* 500 mg-1 g IV every 8 hr |
| | *Children:* 10-40 mg/kg IV every 8 hr |
| **Others** | |
| vancomycin (Vancocin) | *Adults:* 500 mg IV every 6 hr |
| | *Children:* 10 mg/kg IV every 6 hr |

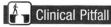 Top 100 drugs prescribed.

---

**Common Side Effects**

**Penicillins and Cephalosporins**

Diarrhea          Itchiness

---

**Common Side Effects**

**Carbapenems and Vancomycin**

Irritation at IV site | Reduced kidney function | Reduced hearing

---

**Drug Alert!**

**Action/Intervention Alert**

Watch closely if a patient who is receiving a cephalosporin is allergic to penicillin. These drugs are similar, and an allergy to one often means an allergy to the other. Remember, diarrhea is *NOT* an allergic reaction.

---

**Clinical Pitfall**

Never give procaine penicillin intravenously.

---

*Side Effects.* Most cell wall synthesis inhibitors have fewer side effects than other types of antibacterial drugs. Part of the reason for this is that human cells have no cell walls, so they are not targeted by these drugs. But remember that all drugs have some side effects. The cell wall synthesis inhibitors are more likely to cause allergic reactions.

The more powerful drugs in this class, especially vancomycin, have more side effects. These include nausea and vomiting, fever, chills, "red man syndrome" (with rash and redness of the face, neck, upper chest, upper back, and arms), pain at the injection site, reduced hearing, and reduced kidney function.

*Adverse Effects.* The carbapenems may cause central nervous system changes, including confusion and seizures.

The cephalosporins, carbapenems, and vancomycin can reduce kidney function. If a patient is being treated with two or more drugs from this class or with an aminoglycoside (discussed later), the risk for kidney damage increases.

**What To Do *Before* Giving Cell Wall Synthesis Inhibitors**

Be sure to review the general nursing responsibilities related to antibacterial therapy (pp. 142-143) in addition to these specific responsibilities before giving a cell wall synthesis inhibitor.

Many people are allergic to cell wall synthesis inhibitors. Ask the patient if he or she has any known drug allergies, especially to the drug prescribed. If a patient is allergic to penicillin, the risk for a cephalosporin allergy is increased.

Oral cephalosporins are poorly absorbed with iron supplements and antacids. If a patient is receiving either of these drugs, the cephalosporin should be given 1 hour before or 4 hours after the dose of iron or antacid.

If a patient will receive IV penicillin, check that the injectable form can be given intravenously. One type of injectable penicillin, procaine penicillin, contains a local anesthetic and is not an IV drug. This drug is milky white rather than clear.

If a patient is to receive a carbapenem, ask whether he or she has ever had seizures. If so, notify the prescriber.

Vancomycin is given only intravenously and has many adverse effects if given too fast. These include low blood pressure; a histamine release that causes dilation of blood vessels and a red appearance to the face, neck, chest, back, and arms (red man syndrome); and cardiac dysrhythmias. To reduce the risk for these problems, vancomycin should be given over at least 60 minutes and never as a bolus or a "push" dose.

**Drug Alert!**
**Administration Alert**

Give IV vancomycin over at least a 60-minute period.

### What To Do *After* Giving Cell Wall Synthesis Inhibitors

Be sure to review the general nursing responsibilities related to antibacterial therapy (p. 143) in addition to these specific responsibilities for what to do after giving cell wall synthesis inhibitors.

Because these drugs are more likely than other antibacterials to cause an allergic reaction, check the patient hourly for the first 4 hours after an oral dose and every 15 to 30 minutes for the first 2 hours after receiving an IV dose.

### What To *Teach* Patients About Cell Wall Synthesis Inhibitors

Be sure to teach patients the general care needs and precautions related to antibacterial therapy (p. 143) in addition to these specific responsibilities for cell wall synthesis inhibitors.

Because oral cephalosporins are poorly absorbed when taken with either iron supplements or antacids, teach patients to take the cephalosporin at least 1 hour before or 4 hours after iron or an antacid.

If a patient is taking a liquid oral form of penicillin or a cephalosporin, instruct him or her to keep the drug tightly closed and refrigerated to prevent loss of drug strength. Teach the patient to shake the suspension well just before measuring the drug.

### Life Span Considerations for Cell Wall Synthesis Inhibitors

*Pediatric Considerations.*   Cell wall synthesis inhibitors are used for infants and children with bacterial infections susceptible to these drugs. One of the most common drugs given to children is amoxicillin for ear infections. The more powerful drugs (carbapenems, monobactams, and vancomycin) are used only for extremely serious infections.

*Considerations for Pregnancy and Breastfeeding.*   Penicillins and most of the cephalosporins are pregnancy category B drugs and can be used to treat infections during pregnancy. The more powerful drugs (carbapenems, monobactams, and vancomycin) are pregnancy category C drugs and are also used, when needed, during pregnancy. All of these drugs pass into breast milk and will affect a nursing infant, possibly causing the infant to develop a drug allergy. These drugs are usually prescribed for only 5 to 14 days, and the breastfeeding mother should be urged to reduce infant exposure to the drug (see Box 1-1 in Chapter 1).

*Considerations for Older Adults.*   The carbapenems and vancomycin can be both *ototoxic* (causing hearing problems) and *nephrotoxic* (causing kidney problems) at higher doses or when taken for many days in a row. Older adults are more sensitive to these problems than younger adults. Be alert for a decrease in hearing or having the patient tell you he or she has a "ringing" in the ears (*tinnitus*). Intake and output should be monitored daily, especially if the patient is also taking another drug known to affect kidney function.

◀ⓔ-Learning Activity 9-3

## AMINOGLYCOSIDES, MACROLIDES, TETRACYCLINES, AND OTHER PROTEIN SYNTHESIS INHIBITORS

The protein synthesis inhibitors are a large class of antibacterial drugs with several main subtypes, including aminoglycosides, macrolides, and tetracyclines. By slowing protein synthesis, these drugs prevent bacteria from performing processes important to their life cycles. All bacteria need to make proteins through the process of protein synthesis. This process starts with a gene that serves as the recipe for how to make a specific protein. Each protein is composed of individual amino acids strung together in a specific order like beads on a string. This recipe is written in the bacterium as a piece of RNA that indicates which amino acids need to be placed in what order to make the correct protein. Molecules known as "ribosomes" read the RNA and are responsible for getting each amino acid into the proper order to make the specific protein (see Figure 9-1). When the amino acids are placed in the proper order, each new one is linked to the previous amino acid to form a protein chain. If any of the pieces and processes needed for protein synthesis are not present or are not working, the bacterium cannot make the protein it needs. As a result, it will either die or not be able to reproduce. Protein synthesis inhibitors work on different parts of this entire process to stop the bacterium from being able to live and reproduce (see Table 9-1).

### How Protein Synthesis Inhibitors Work

*Aminoglycosides* actually go through the cell membrane and enter the bacterium. This process uses a transport system that requires oxygen. After entering, the drug binds to the ribosome, preventing it from "reading" messenger RNA (mRNA) (the recipe) for protein synthesis (see Figure 9-3). As a result, the individual amino acids are not placed in the proper order, and no protein is made. Without these important proteins, bacteria, especially those that use oxygen, usually die.

*Macrolides* also enter the bacterium through the cell membrane but bind to a different site on the ribosomes (see Figure 9-3). The results are the same; no bacterial protein is made, and the bacteria die. So the macrolides are bactericidal to bacteria that have an oxygen-driven transport system. They have no effect on bacteria that do not require oxygen.

*Tetracyclines* also enter the bacterium through the cell membrane. To get inside, they must be brought in by a special transporter on the surface of the bacterium. If a bacterium does not have this transporter, it is not affected by tetracycline. Once inside the bacterium, tetracyclines act in two ways to inhibit protein synthesis. They bind to the ribosome, and they prevent amino acids from being linked together (see Figure 9-3). However, their actions on protein synthesis are usually only bacteriostatic rather than bactericidal.

*Clindamycin* binds to the large part of the ribosome and also prevents the amino acids from linking together. Both of these actions slow bacterial protein synthesis. This drug is usually bacteriostatic but can be bactericidal in high doses. *Linezolid* (Zyvox) binds to all parts of the ribosome and prevents the reading of mRNA, so protein synthesis is inhibited. The current *streptogramin* drug is made up of two chemicals that work together to inhibit protein synthesis at both the beginning and the end of the process.

Each group of protein synthesis inhibitors is described separately in the following table. Within each group the listings include only the drugs on the list of 100 most commonly prescribed drugs and those most often used in acute care settings. Be sure to consult a drug reference for more information about a specific drug in this drug group.

### Dosages of Common Aminoglycosides

| Drug | Dosages |
| --- | --- |
| amikacin (Amikin) | *Adults/Children:* 5 mg/kg IM or IV every 8 hr |
| gentamicin (Cidomycin✤) | *Adults:* 2-3 mg/kg IM or IV every 8 hr<br>*Children:* 2-2.5 mg/kg IM or IV every 8 hr |
| streptomycin | *Adults/Children:* Tuberculosis: 15 mg/kg/day IM once daily (maximum 1 g); 25-35 mg/kg IM 2-3 times weekly (maximum 1.5 g) |

**Do Not Confuse**

**Amikin** *with* **anakinra**

An order for Amikin can be confused with anakinra. Amikin is an antibacterial drug, while anakinra is a biologic agent for rheumatoid arthritis.

**Do Not Confuse**

**gentamicin** *with* **gentian violet**

An order for gentamicin can be confused with gentian violet. The drug gentamicin is an antibacterial drug given intramuscularly or intravenously, whereas gentian violet is a deep purple topical solution for infections of the skin and mucous membranes.

The aminoglycosides are powerful antibacterial drugs given intravenously or intramuscularly that have some uncomfortable side effects and serious adverse effects. They are most commonly used for burns, central nervous system infections, joint and bone infections, intra-abdominal infections, peritonitis, and sepsis. Streptomycin is also used in the treatment of tuberculosis.

## Dosages for Common Macrolides

| Drugs | Dosages |
|---|---|
| azithromycin TOP 100 (Zithromax, Zmax) | *Adults:* 500 mg orally first day, 250 mg orally daily days 2-5<br>*Children:* 10 mg/kg orally first day, 5 mg/kg orally daily days 2-5 |
| clarithromycin (Biaxin) | *Adults:* 250-500 mg orally every 12 hr; extended release 500 mg orally once daily<br>*Children:* 7.5 mg/kg orally every 12 hr |
| erythromycin (Apo Erythro♦, E-mycin, Erycette, Erymax, Erythromid♦, Romycin) | *Adults:* 250-500 mg orally every 6-12 hr<br>*Children:* 5-12 mg/kg orally every 6-12 hr |
| erythromycin lactobionate (Erythrocin Lactobionate) | *Adults/Children:* 4-5 mg/kg IV every 6 hr through continuous slow infusion |

TOP 100 Top 100 drugs prescribed.

The *macrolides* are antibacterial drugs that have extended- to broad-spectrum effects. Depending on the bacteria type and the blood level of drug, they can be bactericidal or bacteriostatic. Usually higher doses are needed for bactericidal effects. These drugs work well against common infections of the skin and mucous membranes and other soft tissues and are prescribed for patients who are allergic to penicillins or cephalosporins. Infections most responsive to macrolides include skin and wound infections, middle ear infections, upper and lower respiratory tract infections, and infections of the genital tract. These drugs are used for Legionnaires' disease, diphtheria, and mycobacterial infections.

## Dosages for Common Tetracyclines

| Drug | Dosage |
|---|---|
| demeclocycline (Declomycin) | *Adults:* 150-300 mg orally every 6-12 hr<br>*Children:* 2-3 mg/kg orally every 6-12 hr |
| doxycycline TOP 100 (Adoxa, Apo-Doxy♦, Atridox, Doryx, Dox-Caps, Doxycin♦, Monodox, Novodoxyclin♦, Vibramycin) | Oral and IV doses:<br>*Adults:* 200 mg first day, then 100-200 mg once or twice daily<br>*Children:* 1 mg/kg first day, then 0.5-1 mg/kg once or twice daily |
| minocycline (Arestin, Dynacin, Minocin, Vectrin) | Oral and IV doses:<br>*Adults:* 200 mg first dose, then 100 mg every 12 hr<br>*Children:* 4 mg/kg first dose, then 2 mg/kg every 12 hr |
| tetracycline (Ala-Tet, Apo-Tetra♦, Brodspec, Novotetra♦, Nu-Tetra♦, Panmycin, Sumycin, Tetracon) | *Adults:* 500 mg orally every 6-12 hr<br>*Children:* 6-9 mg/kg orally every 6 hr |

TOP 100 Top 100 drugs prescribed.

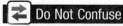 **Do Not Confuse**

**Vibramycin** *with* **ribavirin**

An order for Vibramycin can be confused with ribavirin. Vibramycin is an antibacterial drug, whereas ribavirin is a strong antiviral agent known to cause birth defects.

The *tetracyclines* are broad-spectrum drugs that are bacteriostatic against most of the organisms that are sensitive to penicillins. Because they are only bacteriostatic, tetracyclines should be given only to patients with healthy immune systems. They are often prescribed for patients who are allergic to penicillins or cephalosporins. Infections most responsive to tetracyclines are acne, urinary tract infections, skin and mucous membrane infections, gonorrhea, upper and lower respiratory tract infections, sexually transmitted infections, Rocky Mountain spotted fever, syphilis, Lyme disease, and typhoid fever. In addition, they are used to prevent anthrax after exposure to the bacteria.

**Dosages for Other Protein Synthesis Inhibitors**

| Drug | Dosage |
|---|---|
| *Lincosamides* | |
| clindamycin (Cleocin) | *Adults:* 150-300 mg orally every 6 hr; 300-600 mg IM or IV every 6-8 hr |
| | *Children:* 2-4 mg/kg orally every 6 hr; 20-40 mg IM or IV every 6-8 hr |
| *Oxazolidinones* | |
| linezolid (Zyvox) | Oral and IV doses: |
| | *Adults:* 400-600 mg every 8-12 hr |
| | *Children:* 10 mg/kg every 8-12 hr |
| *Streptogramins* | |
| dalfopristin/quinupristin (Synercid) | *Adults/Children:* 7.5 mg/kg IV (over 60 min) every 8-12 hr |

The three remaining types of protein synthesis inhibitors are very powerful drugs with more severe side effects. These drugs are reserved for treating severe or life-threatening infections that do not respond well to other types of antibacterial drugs. The oxazolidinone and streptogramin classes are usually reserved for treating infections from *vancomycin-resistant enterococcus (VRE)* or *methicillin-resistant Staphylococcus aureus (MRSA)*. They are also used for infected diabetic foot ulcers. The third class, the lincosamides, was previously limited to topical use only (especially for acne) because of the severe side effects. Now oral and parenteral forms of lincosamides are used for severe infections such as pneumonia, peritonitis, cellulitis, abscesses, malaria, and pneumonia caused by *Pneumocystis jiroveci* (formerly *Pneumocystis carinii*). The usual doses for all three drug types may be greatly increased when the infection is life threatening.

**Side Effects.** *Aminoglycosides* often cause nausea, vomiting, rash, lethargy, fever, and increased salivation. They also can increase the number of eosinophils (a type of WBC) in the blood. When given intravenously, these drugs are irritating to the vein.

*Macrolides* have side effects that occur more in the GI tract. They include nausea, vomiting, abdominal pain, diarrhea, loss of appetite, and changes in taste sensation. These drugs greatly increase sun sensitivity *(photosensitivity)*, making serious sunburns possible.

*Tetracycline* side effects include nausea, vomiting, diarrhea, a sore tongue *(glossitis)*, and rash. These drugs greatly increase sun sensitivity to the sun, making serious sunburns possible. Rarely do they cause esophageal irritation and ulcer formation. Tetracycline is more likely than any other antibacterial drug to promote overgrowth of yeast in the mouth and vagina.

*Clindamycin* can cause rash, pain and redness at the injection site (when the drug is given intramuscularly) and thrombophlebitis in the vein where the drug infuses.

*Linezolid* constricts blood vessels and can raise blood pressure in patients who have high blood pressure or who may be taking other blood pressure–raising drugs, foods containing tyramine (such as aged cheese, smoked meats, pickled food, beer, red wine, soy, and sauerkraut), or beverages containing caffeine. Other side effects include nausea, diarrhea, and headaches.

*Streptogramin* side effects include muscle and joint pain, pain and inflammation at the IV site, rash, nausea, and vomiting.

**Adverse Effects.** *Aminoglycosides* are highly toxic to the ears and kidneys, causing hearing loss and reduced kidney function when taken in high doses or for long

**Common Side Effects**

**Aminoglycosides**

Nausea/ Vomiting

Rash

Fever

Lethargy

**Common Side Effects**

**Macrolides**

Nausea/Vomiting, Diarrhea, Loss of appetite

Photosensitivity

**Common Side Effects**

**Tetracyclines**

Nausea/Vomiting, Diarrhea, Sore tongue

Photosensitivity

periods. This is because the tissues that make up the inner ear and the nephrons of the kidney both come from the same tissue layer in the embryo. Because these tissues are similar in structure, both are at risk for damage by the same drugs.

Another adverse effect of these drugs is neuromuscular blockade, which prevents the nerves from fully stimulating muscle contraction. This problem causes muscle weakness with respiratory depression and paralysis of the facial muscles.

*Macrolides* interfere with the metabolism of many drugs. For some such as digoxin, macrolides keep the drug in the blood longer so digoxin side effects occur faster. Macrolides also increase the effects of warfarin (Coumadin), increasing the risk for bleeding. Combining other drugs such as pimozide, astemizole, terfenadine, and ergotamine with a macrolide increases the risk for life-threatening cardiac dysrhythmias.

The effectiveness of oral contraceptives (birth control pills) is reduced while a patient is taking most macrolides. This effect could lead to an unplanned pregnancy.

Parenteral forms of macrolides are irritating to veins and tissues. Symptoms of liver irritation or other problems have also been reported.

*Tetracyclines* can raise pressure inside the brain *(intracranial pressure)*. Symptoms occurring with this adverse reaction include dizziness, blurred vision, confusion, and ringing in the ears *(tinnitus)*.

In high doses tetracyclines can decrease kidney function and increase liver enzyme levels. These problems resolve when the drug is discontinued, but drugs from this class should be used with caution for any patient with reduced liver or kidney function.

*Clindamycin* can reduce liver function and decrease WBC counts. When clindamycin is given too rapidly by IV infusion, shock and cardiac arrest may occur.

*Linezolid* reduces blood cell counts, especially red blood cells and platelets, and causes damage to the optic nerve. Usually these problems occur only in patients who have been taking the drug for longer than 28 days.

*Streptogramin* increases the blood levels of many drugs, which can then lead to adverse effects of these drugs even when the patient is taking them at normal doses.

### What to Do *Before* Giving Protein Synthesis Inhibitors

Be sure to review the general nursing responsibilities related to antibacterial therapy (pp. 142-143) in addition to these specific responsibilities before giving protein synthesis inhibitors.

*Aminoglycosides.*   Check the patient's breathing rate and depth and use it as a baseline to determine whether muscle weakness develops, which could lead to respiratory depression.

Also check the grip strength of both the patient's hands and use it as a baseline to determine whether the patient develops muscle weakness.

Check the patient's current laboratory work, especially blood urea nitrogen (BUN) and serum creatinine levels because aminoglycosides are toxic to the kidneys (see Table 1-5 in Chapter 1). If laboratory values are higher than normal before starting the drug, the risk for kidney damage is greater. Use these data as a baseline to determine whether the patient develops kidney problems while taking aminoglycosides.

Check the patient's hearing using either the ticking watch test or fingernail clicking. To perform the ticking watch test, ask the patient to close his or her eyes. Then hold a ticking watch 3 feet away from one of the patient's ears. As you begin to move the watch slowly toward the patient's ear, ask when the ticking can first be heard. Record the distance from the patient's ear. Repeat the test for the other ear. If a ticking watch is not available, click two fingernails as an alternative method to test hearing. Use these data as a baseline to determine whether the patient's hearing changes after taking the drug.

Make sure that the aminoglycoside is well diluted before giving it intravenously. Give the drugs slowly over 30 to 60 minutes to reduce the risk for vein irritation and adverse cardiac effects.

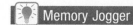 **Memory Jogger**

Drugs that have adverse effects on the kidneys (nephrotoxic) almost always have adverse hearing and balance effects (ototoxic) on the ears.

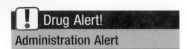

**Drug Alert!**

**Administration Alert**

Only use solutions of erythromycin that were mixed less than 8 hours ago.

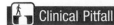

**Clinical Pitfall**

Do not give penicillins at the same time as tetracyclines. Do not mix them together in the same IV bag or run them through the same IV tubing.

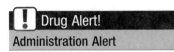

**Drug Alert!**

**Administration Alert**

Mix the parenteral form of strepto-gramins only with dextrose 5% in water.

*Macrolides.* If a patient is prescribed a macrolide, check to see whether he or she is also taking digoxin, warfarin, pimozide, astemizole, terfenadine, or ergotamine. If so, notify the prescriber immediately because macrolides change the metabolism of these drugs, which can cause adverse effects.

When giving these drugs intravenously, infuse them slowly. For example, it is recommended that erythromycin be infused by slow continuous drip over 8 to 12 hours.

*Tetracyclines.* Check whether the patient is receiving a penicillin. Tetracyclines interfere with the action of penicillin. It is important not to give these two drug types at the same time. They should not be mixed together in the same IV bag or run through the same IV tubing.

Food, antacids, and dairy products prevent oral tetracycline from being absorbed. Give drugs from this class 1 hour before or 2 hours after a meal. Do not give with milk. Give the patient a full glass of water to drink with tetracycline capsules or tablets, and urge him or her to drink more fluids throughout the day to prevent irritation to the esophagus.

Check the dosages for doxycycline and minocycline carefully because they are lower than for other tetracyclines and other types of antibacterial drugs.

*Other Protein Synthesis Inhibitors.* Check the patient's current laboratory work, especially BUN and serum creatinine levels because clindamycin, linezolid, and streptogramin are toxic to the kidneys. If these values are higher than normal before starting the drug, the risk for kidney damage is greater.

All three drugs are known to cause vein irritation and phlebitis. Give them slowly over 30 to 60 minutes (or as prescribed) to reduce the risk for vein irritation and cardiac side effects.

When mixing and diluting streptogramins, use only dextrose 5% in water because a precipitate will form in anything else. The IV line used to give these drugs must either be fresh or flushed with only dextrose 5% in water and never with sodium chloride or heparin.

### What To Do *After* Giving Protein Synthesis Inhibitors

Be sure to review the general nursing responsibilities related to antibacterial therapy (p. 143) in addition to these specific responsibilities for what to do after giving protein synthesis inhibitors.

*Aminoglycosides.* Check the patient's hearing daily using the ticking watch test or clicking fingernail test and compare the findings to the patient's hearing before a drug from this class was started.

To determine whether the drug is effective and because aminoglycosides can also *cause* a fever as a side effect, check the patient's temperature every 4 to 8 hours.

Because these drugs are toxic to the kidneys, examine the patient's intake and output record daily to determine if urine output is within 500 mL of the total fluid intake. If blood work was done for kidney function, especially BUN and creatinine levels, compare the values before and after the drug was started (see Table 1-5 in Chapter 1). If the levels rise above the normal range, notify the prescriber.

*Macrolides.* Check the patient's heart rate and rhythm at least every 4 hours during macrolide therapy. If a new change in rhythm develops, check the patient again in 15 minutes. If the change in rhythm persists or recurs, notify the prescriber.

*Tetracyclines.* Tetracyclines increase the effects of warfarin (Coumadin). Check the patient who is also taking warfarin daily for any signs or symptoms of increased bleeding such as bleeding from the gums, presence of bruising or petechiae, oozing of blood around IV insertions or other puncture sites, or the presence of blood in urine or stool.

*Other Protein Synthesis Inhibitors.*   Check the blood pressure of a patient taking linezolid at least every shift. This drug can raise blood pressure, especially in patients who already have high blood pressure or are taking other drugs that also raise blood pressure.

## What To *Teach* Patients About Protein Synthesis Inhibitors

Be sure to teach patients the general care needs and precautions related to antibacterial therapy (p. 143) in addition to these specific ones for protein synthesis inhibitors.

*Macrolides.*   Teach patients to take macrolides with food or within 1 hour of having eaten to reduce some of the intestinal side effects. Also instruct patients not to chew or crush tablets or capsules.

Remind patients taking macrolides to avoid taking other drugs without the prescriber's knowledge.

Teach patients taking either macrolides or tetracyclines to avoid direct sunlight, use sunscreen, and wear protective clothing (including a hat) whenever they are in the sun to prevent a severe sunburn. Remind them to avoid tanning beds and salons.

If the patient also takes warfarin (Coumadin), remind him or her to keep all appointments to check blood clotting. Macrolides, especially erythromycin, increase the effects of warfarin which can greatly increase the risk for bleeding.

Remind any patient taking birth control pills that erythromycin can make them less effective. Teach her to use an additional form of birth control while taking the drug and for one menstrual cycle after completing the drug therapy.

*Tetracyclines.*   Teach patients to drink a full glass of water with the tetracycline capsules or tablets and to drink more fluids throughout the day to prevent irritation to the esophagus.

Food and milk interfere with absorption of oral tetracyclines. Teach the patient to take these drugs 1 hour before or 2 hours after meals and to not take the drug with milk.

*Other Protein Synthesis Inhibitors.*   Teach patients to drink a full glass of water with oral clindamycin and to drink more fluids throughout the day to prevent irritation to the esophagus.

Linezolid can raise blood pressure, sometimes to dangerous levels. When foods containing tyramine are eaten while a patient is taking linezolid, very high blood pressure can result. (Tyramine is a metabolite of the amino acid tyrosine and can cause the release of excess amounts of dopamine, epinephrine, and norepinephrine.) Teach patients to avoid tyramine-containing food such as aged cheese, smoked meats, pickled food, beer, red wine, soy, and sauerkraut while taking this drug.

## Life Span Considerations for Protein Synthesis Inhibitors

*Pediatric Considerations.*   *Aminoglycosides* can cause severe respiratory depression in infants and children. In addition, because infants and children have immature kidney function, the risk for kidney damage is greater.

The use of *tetracyclines* during tooth development in infancy and early childhood can cause a permanent yellow-gray discoloration of the teeth and make the tooth enamel thinner. Therefore these drugs should not be used in children younger than 8 years of age except for anthrax exposure or a serious infection that is not likely to respond to other antibacterial drugs.

*Considerations for Pregnancy and Breastfeeding.*   IV and IM *aminoglycosides* are pregnancy category D drugs (except for gentamicin, which is category C) and should not be given to pregnant women unless the infection is life threatening and the organisms are susceptible only to these drugs. Because these drugs are known to

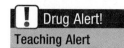

**Drug Alert!**

**Teaching Alert**

Teach patients taking macrolides or tetracyclines to protect themselves from sun exposure because these drugs greatly increase sun sensitivity, even among people with dark skin.

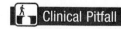

**Clinical Pitfall**

Tetracyclines should not be used in children younger than 8 years of age because it changes tooth enamel in the developing permanent teeth.

cause hearing loss and reduced kidney function, a woman should not breastfeed while taking them.

Most *macrolides* are pregnancy category B drugs and can be taken during pregnancy if needed. These drugs pass into breast milk and affect the infant, often causing colic and diarrhea. Because they are usually prescribed for only 5 to 14 days, teach breastfeeding women to reduce infant exposure to the drug (see Box 1-1 in Chapter 1).

*Tetracyclines* are pregnancy category D drugs. Their use during tooth development in the last half of pregnancy and infancy can cause a permanent yellow-gray discoloration of the teeth and make the tooth enamel thinner. Therefore these drugs should not be used during pregnancy or when breastfeeding except for anthrax exposure or a serious infection that is not likely to respond to other antibacterial drugs.

***Considerations for Older Adults.*** *Aminoglycosides* are both ototoxic and nephrotoxic at higher doses or when taken for many days in a row. Doses are usually lowered for the older adult. In addition, *macrolides* have shown some ototoxicity in older adults who are also taking a high ceiling or "loop" diuretic such as furosemide (Lasix). Be alert for patient reports of reduced hearing or tinnitus. Monitor the intake and output of older adults daily, especially if they are also taking other drugs known to affect kidney function.

## METABOLISM INHIBITORS: SULFONAMIDES AND TRIMETHOPRIM

Metabolism inhibitors, which include sulfonamides and trimethoprim, are bacteriostatic rather than bactericidal. Although classed as antibacterial drugs, metabolism inhibitors can be effective in some infections caused by organisms other than bacteria such as shigellosis, toxoplasmosis, and pneumocystis pneumonia. They are more commonly used to treat urinary tract infections, middle ear infections, pneumonia, and infectious diarrhea. They are also helpful in treating eye, skin, and vaginal infections and infections of the perineum. Sulfonamides and trimethoprim are also available as creams, lotions, eye drops, and ointments.

### How Sulfonamides and Trimethoprim Work

Bacteria need a type of folic acid to be able to make DNA and reproduce. A specific enzyme is needed to convert other substances into folic acid in bacteria. The sulfonamides and trimethoprim prevent that enzyme from converting the other substances into folic acid. As a result, bacteria do not have enough folic acid to make DNA and grow. This does not kill the bacteria; it just limits their ability to reproduce (see Figure 9-3).

The following table focuses on the oral and parenteral forms of these drugs. Be sure to consult a drug reference for more information about a specific drug in this drug group.

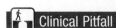
**Clinical Pitfall**

Avoid giving drugs from the aminoglycoside or tetracycline classes to pregnant or breastfeeding women.

*e*-Learning Activity 9-4 ▶

↻ **Do Not Confuse**

**sulfADIAZINE** *with* **sulfiSOXAZOLE**

An order for sulfADIAZINE can be confused with sulfiSOXAZOLE. Although both drugs belong to the sulfonamide class of antibiotics, their dosages are different and they are NOT interchangeable.

### Dosages for Common Sulfonamides, Trimethoprim, and Combination Drugs

| Drug | Dosage |
| --- | --- |
| *Sulfonamides* | |
| sulfADIAZINE sodium | *Adults:* 2-4 g orally first, then 500 mg-1 g orally every 6-8 hr |
| | *Children:* 100 mg orally first, then 30-40 mg/kg orally every 6-8 hr |
| sulfiSOXAZOLE (Gantrisin, Soxazole✦, Truxazole) | *Adults:* 2-4 g orally first, then 1-2 g orally every 6 hr |
| | *Children:* 75 mg orally first, then 30-40 mg/kg orally every 6 hr |
| trimethoprim (Primsol, Trimpex) | *Adults:* 100 mg orally every 12 hr or 200 mg orally daily |
| | *Children:* 5 mg/kg orally every 12 hr |

### Dosages for Common Sulfonamides, Trimethoprim, and Combination Drugs—cont'd

| Drug | Dosage |
| --- | --- |
| *Combination Drugs* | |
| trimethoprim/sulfamethoxazole  (Apo-Sulfatrim , Bactrim, Bactrim DS, Bethaprim, Novo-Trimel , Nu-Cotrimex , Roubac , Septra, Septra DS, Septra IV [only form given parenterally], Sulfatrim, Uroplus, SMZ-TMP) | *Adults:* 1-2 tablets (400 mg sulfamethoxazole and 80 mg trimethoprim) orally every 12 hr<br>DS: 1 tablet (800 mg sulfamethoxazole and 160 mg trimethoprim) orally daily or every 12 hr<br>*Children:* Dose based on trimethoprim content: 3-6 mg/kg orally every 12 hr<br>*IV dosage for adults and children based on trimethoprim content:* 2-2.5 mg/kg trimethoprim IV slow infusion (60 to 90 min) every 6-8 hr |

 Top 100 drugs prescribed.

***Side Effects.***   Common side effects of sulfonamides are headache, fever, rash, and increased sun sensitivity. Serious sunburns are possible while taking drugs from this class. The most common side effects of trimethoprim are headache, nausea, vomiting, and itchiness.

***Adverse Effects.***   The sulfonamides are a type of chemical that can easily turn into crystals. Crystals that form and clump in the kidneys can cause kidney failure or kidney stones.

One of the most serious adverse effects of metabolism inhibitors is suppression of bone marrow cell division. This results in fewer red blood cells *(anemia)* and fewer WBCs. Some patients are affected in this way only slightly. For others the suppression can be so great that they are at risk for infection.

A simple skin rash can occur with metabolism inhibitors, but more serious skin problems are also possible. These include peeling and sloughing, blister formation, and a combination of many types of skin eruptions known as *Stevens-Johnson syndrome.* This problem is serious and can lead to life-threatening losses of fluids and electrolytes.

These drugs can also cause noninfectious hepatitis (liver inflammation). In addition, metabolism inhibitors should be avoided in any person who has a genetic disorder called glucose-6-phosphate dehydrogenase (G6PD) deficiency. In a patient with this health problem the drug causes red blood cells to break. G6PD deficiency is most common among African-American males and males of Mediterranean descent.

### What To Do *Before* Giving Sulfonamides or Trimethoprim

Be sure to review the general nursing responsibilities related to antibacterial therapy (pp. 142-143) in addition to these specific responsibilities before giving a sulfonamide or trimethoprim.

Many people are allergic to sulfonamides. Ask patients about any known drug allergies, especially to sulfa drugs. Notify the prescriber about this issue.

If a patient is African-American or of Mediterranean descent, ask him if he or any member of his family has a genetic blood disorder. If he says yes, ask the prescriber whether a test for G6PD deficiency should be performed before starting the drug.

IV sulfamethoxazole/trimethoprim combination (Septra IV) can interact with other drugs and also can irritate tissues. Make sure that the IV infusion is running well and has a good blood return. This drug must be mixed and diluted only with dextrose 5% in water and should never be given intramuscularly. Either flush the line with dextrose 5% in water before giving the drug or use fresh tubing. Infuse Septra IV over 60 to 90 minutes.

Check the patient's current laboratory work, especially liver function tests, because these drugs are irritating to the liver (see Table 1-3 in Chapter 1).

**Common Side Effects**

**Metabolism Inhibitors**

Headache   Fever   Skin rash, Photosensitivity

 **Cultural Awareness**

Closely watch male patients who are African-American or of Mediterranean descent for anemia and jaundice when they are receiving a metabolism inhibitor.

**Clinical Pitfall**

Never give IV sulfamethoxazole/trimethoprim (Septra IV) by bolus or rapid infusion.

If laboratory values are higher than normal before starting the drug, the risk for liver inflammation is greater. Also check the patient's sclera and skin for yellowing (*jaundice*) because this problem occurs with liver inflammation. Use these data as a baseline to detect developing liver problems in patients taking metabolism inhibitors.

Check the patient's recent laboratory work for counts of WBCs, red blood cells, and platelets (see Table 1-6 in Chapter 1). Check the patient's skin for bruises or petechiae.

Check whether the patient is also taking a thiazide diuretic, especially if he or she is older than age 65. If a thiazide diuretic is also ordered, notify the prescriber because combining these drugs greatly increases the risk for anemia and bleeding.

Give the patient a full glass of water to drink with an oral sulfonamide or trimethoprim. Urge him or her to drink more fluids to prevent crystals from forming in the kidneys.

### What To Do *After* Giving Sulfonamides or Trimethoprim

Be sure to review the general nursing responsibilities related to antibacterial therapy (p. 143) in addition to these specific responsibilities for what to do after giving these drugs.

Offer the patient a full glass of water every 4 hours (day and night) to help prevent crystals from forming in the kidney tubules.

Check the complete blood count every time it is performed to determine whether WBC, red blood cell, and platelet levels have changed (see Table 1-6 in Chapter 1).

Check the patient's skin every shift for rash, blisters, or other skin eruptions that may indicate a drug reaction. Ask whether he or she has noticed any itching or skin changes.

Check the patient daily for yellowing (*jaundice*) of the skin or sclera, which is a symptom of liver problems and red blood cell breakdown (*lysis*). The best places to check are the whites of the eyes closest to the iris, the roof of the mouth, and the skin of the chest. Avoid checking the soles of the feet or palms of the hands, especially in patients with darker skin, because these areas often appear yellow even when the patient is not jaundiced.

### What To *Teach* Patients About Sulfonamides or Trimethoprim

Be sure to teach patients the general care needs and precautions related to antibacterial therapy (p. 143) in addition to these specific responsibilities for sulfonamides and trimethoprim.

Teach patients taking either type of drug from this class to avoid direct sunlight, use sunscreen, and wear protective clothing (including a hat) whenever they are in the sun to prevent a severe sunburn. Remind them to avoid tanning beds and salons.

Teach patients to drink a full glass of water with sulfonamide or trimethoprim tablets and to drink more fluids throughout the day to prevent crystals from forming in the kidneys.

Tell patients to notify the prescriber if yellowing of the skin or eyes, a sore throat, fever, rash, blisters, or multiple bruises develop. All these problems are signs of serious adverse effects.

### Life Span Considerations for Sulfonamides or Trimethoprim

*Pediatric Considerations.*   Infants younger than 2 months of age are likely to become severely jaundiced when taking metabolism inhibitors because free bilirubin levels will rise and brain damage is possible. These drugs are not recommended for infants younger than 2 months of age except for life-threatening toxoplasmosis infections.

*Considerations for Pregnancy and Breastfeeding.*   Metabolism inhibitors are pregnancy category C drugs. Because these drugs can cause severe jaundice in

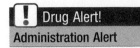
**Drug Alert!**
**Administration Alert**

Give patients a full glass of water to drink with an oral sulfonamide or trimethoprim.

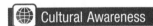
**Cultural Awareness**

In patients with darker skin, check for jaundice on the whites of the eyes closest to the iris and on the roof of the mouth. Do not look at the soles of the feet or palms of the hands.

**Drug Alert!**
**Teaching Alert**

Teach patients taking sulfonamides or trimethoprim to protect themselves from sun exposure because these drugs greatly increase sun sensitivity, even among people with dark skin.

infants, they should be avoided during the last 2 months of pregnancy to reduce the chance that the baby will be born while the mother is taking the drug. For the same reason the breastfeeding mother should use alternate methods of infant feeding during the time that she is taking metabolism inhibitors.

***Considerations for Older Adults.*** Metabolism inhibitors have more intense side effects, especially anemia and an increased risk for bleeding, in people older than age 65. When these drugs are taken by a person who also takes a thiazide diuretic, the risk for bleeding increases greatly.

## DNA SYNTHESIS INHIBITORS: FLUOROQUINOLONES

The major DNA synthesis inhibitors are the fluoroquinolones. These drugs have many uses when taken systemically and in eye drop and ear drop forms. Their most common uses are for skin infections, urinary tract infections, respiratory tract infections, infectious diarrhea, and gonorrhea. Fluoroquinolones also are used to prevent and treat anthrax. Be sure to consult a drug reference for more information about a specific drug in this group.

### How Fluoroquinolones Work

Fluoroquinolones are broad-spectrum antibacterial drugs. They enter bacterial cells and suppress the action of two enzymes important in making bacterial DNA. This action prevents bacteria reproduction. Fluoroquinolones are bactericidal to most bacteria that are sensitive to these drugs.

### Dosages for Common Fluoroquinolones

| Drug | Dosage (Adults Only) |
|---|---|
| ciprofloxacin  (Ciloxan, Cipro, Cipro IV, Cipro XR) | 250-750 mg orally every 12 hr<br>400 mg IV every 12 hr |
| gatifloxacin (Tequin) | 400 mg orally or IV daily |
| gemifloxacin (Factive) | 320 mg orally daily |
| levofloxacin  (Levaquin) | 250-750 mg orally or IV daily |
| lomefloxacin (Maxaquin) | 400 mg orally daily |
| moxifloxacin (Avelox, Avelox IV) | 400 mg orally or IV daily |
| ofloxacin (Floxin) | 200-400 mg orally every 12 hr |

**TOP 100** Top 100 drugs prescribed.

***Side Effects.*** Fluoroquinolone side effects include rash, nausea, headache, abdominal pain, vomiting, dizziness, and changes in taste. One drug, lomefloxacin, increases sun sensitivity, making serious sunburns possible.

These drugs can concentrate in urine, making the urine irritating to tissues. As a result, the patient may have pain or burning of the urethra and nearby tissues during urination. A patient who is incontinent may have skin irritation in the entire perineal area.

***Adverse Effects.*** Fluoroquinolones can cause serious heart dysrhythmias, including prolonged Q-T interval. This serious problem is more common when the patient is also taking other drugs for dysrhythmias (such as amiodarone, quinidine, procainamide, or sotalol) or when he or she also has a low blood potassium level (*hypokalemia*).

The fluoroquinolones may affect the central nervous system, causing seizures, increased pressure inside the brain, tremors, dizziness, confusion, depression, and hallucinations. Some patients have had nightmares while taking these drugs. These effects can occur after just one dose.

Although a simple rash can occur, more serious skin problems are also possible. These include peeling and sloughing, blister formation, and a combination of skin eruptions known as *Stevens-Johnson syndrome*. This problem is serious and can lead to life-threatening losses of fluids and electrolytes.

Development of *peripheral neuropathy* is possible while taking these drugs. Signs and symptoms of this problem include tingling, burning, numbness, and pain in the hands or feet.

Fluoroquinolones increase the blood levels of caffeine and any theophylline-type drug. This response increases the risk for caffeine overdose and serious adverse theophylline effects such as seizures and cardiac arrest.

For a patient with diabetes, these drugs raise or lower blood glucose levels, leading to either *hyperglycemia* or *hypoglycemia*.

A rare adverse effect of fluoroquinolones is the rupture of a tendon, most often in the shoulder, hand, wrist, or heel (Achilles tendon). This complication is most likely to occur in an older patient who is also taking a corticosteroid.

### What To Do *Before* Giving Fluoroquinolones

Be sure to review the general nursing responsibilities related to antibacterial therapy (pp. 142-143) in addition to these specific responsibilities before giving fluoroquinolones.

The oral forms of some fluoroquinolones are poorly absorbed with iron supplements, multivitamins, and antacids. Give fluoroquinolones at least 2 hours before or 4 hours after the dose of a multivitamin, iron, or antacid.

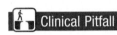

**Clinical Pitfall**

Do not give any fluoroquinolone as a bolus or by intramuscular or subcutaneous routes.

Check whether the patient also takes amiodarone, quinidine, procainamide, or sotalol. If so, notify the prescriber immediately because taking any of these drugs with fluoroquinolones can lead to serious dysrhythmias.

Check whether the patient also takes any type of theophylline. When these two drugs are taken together, the risk for seizures and cardiac arrest increases.

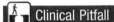

**Clinical Pitfall**

Do not use sterile water to mix or dilute IV forms of fluoroquinolones.

When mixing or diluting parenteral forms of this drug, use only sterile dextrose 5% in water, normal saline, lactated Ringer's, or 5% sodium bicarbonate. Do not use sterile water.

Give patients a full glass of water to drink with oral fluoroquinolone capsules or tablets and urge them to drink more fluids throughout the day. This action prevents forming a very concentrated amount of drug in the urine that can irritate the urethra and perineum. Even the parenteral forms of the drug can concentrate in the urine. Make sure that patients receiving the drug by IV infusion also have a good fluid intake.

### What To Do *After* Giving Fluoroquinolones

Be sure to review the general nursing responsibilities related to antibacterial therapy (p. 143) in addition to these specific responsibilities for what to do after giving fluoroquinolones.

Check the patient's heart rate and rhythm at least every 4 hours during therapy. If a new change in rhythm develops, check the patient again in 15 minutes. If the change persists or recurs, notify the prescriber.

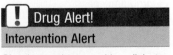

**Intervention Alert**

Check patients with diabetes often for hypoglycemia or hyperglycemia because fluoroquinolones can cause quick changes in blood glucose levels.

For a patient who also has diabetes, check the blood glucose level even more often than usual. Check him or her every 2 hours for signs and symptoms of *hypoglycemia* (cool, clammy skin; sweating; anxiety; hunger; double vision; tachycardia) and *hyperglycemia* (warm, dry skin; flushed appearance; rapid, deep respirations; nausea; abdominal cramps).

### What To *Teach* Patients About Fluoroquinolones

Be sure to teach patients the general care needs and precautions related to antibacterial therapy (p. 143) in addition to these specific responsibilities for fluoroquinolones.

Because oral fluoroquinolones are poorly absorbed when taken with vitamin supplements, iron supplements, or antacids, teach patients to take the fluoroquinolone at least 2 hours before or 4 hours after taking a multivitamin, iron supplement, or antacid.

Warn patients to carefully limit the amount of coffee and other caffeine-containing food or drinks because too much caffeine can lead to heart dysrhythmias and seizures. Tell patients that if they begin to have hand tremors, stop all caffeine-containing drinks or foods and notify the prescriber immediately.

Remind patients who also take warfarin (Coumadin) to keep all appointments to check blood clotting. Fluoroquinolones increase warfarin levels and the risk for bleeding.

Teach patients to drink a full glass of water with oral fluoroquinolone capsules or tablets and to drink more fluids throughout the day to prevent the forming of a very concentrated amount of drug in the urine that can irritate the urethra and perineum.

Teach patients how to check their pulse and remind them to check it twice each day. Tell them to notify the prescriber if their pulse becomes irregular, if palpitations occur, or if they become dizzy.

Tell patients to stop taking the drug and see the prescriber as soon as possible if pain or swelling in a tendon or joint occurs. The risk for a tendon rupture is increased while taking the drug and for about 1 month after the drug is stopped.

Sun sensitivity greatly increases the risk for sunburn, even for people who have dark skin. Teach patients to avoid direct sunlight, use sunscreen, and wear protective clothing (including a hat) whenever they are in the sun to prevent severe sunburn. Remind them to avoid tanning beds and salons.

### Life Span Considerations for Fluoroquinolones

*Pediatric Considerations.*   The use of fluoroquinolones in infants and children younger than 18 years of age is not recommended unless the infection is life threatening and not sensitive to other drugs. Fluoroquinolones can damage bones, joints, muscles, tendons, and other soft tissues when given to patients who are still growing.

*Considerations for Pregnancy and Breastfeeding.*   Fluoroquinolones are pregnancy category C drugs that increase the incidence for bone, joint, and tendon defects. These drugs should not be used during pregnancy. The breastfeeding mother should use alternate methods of infant feeding during the time that she is taking fluoroquinolones.

*Considerations for Older Adults.*   Tendon rupture is seen more often in older adults taking fluoroquinolones. The tendons most often affected are in the shoulder, hand, wrist, and Achilles tendon at the heel. Taking corticosteroids at the same time as a fluoroquinolone increases the risk, but tendon rupture can occur when taking fluoroquinolones alone. Tendon rupture also can occur up to 1 month after the drug has been stopped. If the patient has pain or inflammation of a tendon or around a joint, he or she should stop the drug, stop moving or exercising that joint, and see the prescriber as soon as possible.

## ANTIBACTERIAL DRUG RESISTANCE

When antibacterials are overused, prescribed for conditions not responsive to these drugs, or taken improperly, drug-resistant strains of bacteria may develop. **Antibiotic resistance** is the ability of a bacterium to resist the effects of antibacterial drugs. Bacteria that can either be killed by antibacterials or have their reproduction suppressed are called *susceptible* organisms. Those that are neither killed nor suppressed by antibacterial drugs are called *resistant* organisms. Some bacteria are resistant to one type of antibacterial drug but susceptible to other types. The concern now is that many bacteria species and strains that were once susceptible to many types of antibacterial drugs are becoming resistant to most types. When a bacterium becomes resistant to three or more different types of antibacterial drugs, it is called a *superbug* or a *multiple drug–resistant (MDR) organism.* The fear is that common bacteria that

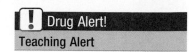

**! Drug Alert!**
**Teaching Alert**

Warn patients to stop drinking all caffeine-containing drinks or foods if hand tremors occur.

**! Drug Alert!**
**Teaching Alert**

Teach patients taking fluoroquinolones to protect themselves from sun exposure because these drugs greatly increase sun sensitivity, even among people with dark skin.

◄ ⊖-Learning Activity 9-5

**Memory Jogger**

When antibacterial drug resistance develops, the bacteria are resistant to the drug, but the patient is not resistant to the drug. This means that if the patient should later develop an infection with a bacterium that is susceptible to the drug, the patient can then take that drug and it will be effective.

**Memory Jogger**

MRSA is spread easily by person-to-person contact.

**Memory Jogger**

Patients most at risk for HA-MRSA are older adults; those with a history of prolonged antibiotic therapy; and those who are immunosuppressed, have an indwelling catheter, use IV drugs, and have had invasive procedures or recently been hospitalized, especially in an ICU.

**Memory Jogger**

CA-MRSA is transmitted by direct contact from person to person; skin contact with contaminated linen, sports equipment, and clothing; and sharing cosmetics or personal care items (for example, shavers, hairbrushes).

are not particularly hard to treat will become superbugs and cause "superinfections" that are difficult or impossible to control or cure. Several families of bacteria have already become more resistant to antibacterial therapy. The infections caused by these bacteria cost more to treat, increase the lengths of hospital stays, and lead to higher death rates. In addition, the drugs used against MDR bacteria are more powerful and often cause more side effects than standard antibacterial drugs.

## EXAMPLES OF MDR ORGANISMS

### Methicillin Resistant *Staphylococcus aureus*

*Staphylococcus aureus* is a common bacterium found on the skin, nose, and perineum of about 30% of adults in the United States. *S. aureus* that is present on intact skin or mucous membranes is usually not infectious when their numbers can be controlled with good hygiene measures. However, when skin is not intact, *S. aureus* can cause minor skin infections such as boils or conjunctivitis (pink eye). These minor infections can heal without drug therapy or usually respond to antibacterial drugs. If *S. aureus* enters deeper wounds, surgical incisions, the lungs, or the bloodstream, more serious infections result that require aggressive antibacterial therapy. Such infections historically have responded to penicillin.

However, within the last 40 years more *S. aureus* infections are not responding to methicillin or any other penicillin-based drug. These strains are known as *methicillin-resistant Staphylococcus aureus (MRSA)*. The incidence of MRSA infections is rapidly increasing in hospitals, especially in critical care areas. The incidence in intensive care units (ICUs) is now 50% of all patients. This type of MRSA is known as *hospital-acquired MRSA* or *HA-MRSA*. HA-MRSA is usually multidrug resistant and is a superbug that is easily spread from person to person by skin contact with infected drainage.

In addition to skin sites, the organism often invades hospitalized patients through indwelling catheters, vascular access lines, and endotracheal tubes. It is susceptible to only a few antibacterial drugs such as vancomycin (Lyphocin, Vancocin) and linezolid (Zyvox). HA-MRSA pneumonia, abscesses, or bacteremia can quickly lead to sepsis and death.

Although methicillin resistance first developed in the acute care setting, MRSA can now be found in nonhospital health care settings (such as nursing homes, clinics, dialysis centers, and physician offices) and nonhealth care communal settings (such as schools, day-care facilities, dormitories, camps, and correctional facilities). First discovered in the 1990s, these infections are known as *community-acquired MRSA* or *CA-MRSA*. CA-MRSA, although resistant to methicillin, usually still responds to ciprofloxacin, clindamycin, gentamicin, and trimethoprim antibiotics.

CA-MRSA is transmitted by direct contact from person to person; by skin contact with contaminated linen, sports equipment, and clothing; and by sharing cosmetics or personal care items (for example, shavers, hairbrushes). The organism divides more rapidly in warm and moist conditions, making locker rooms and other communal bathing areas or group living situations common sites of contamination. Recommendations for preventing the spread of CA-MRSA in the home when one family member is colonized or infected include:

- Good daily personal hygiene for all family members.
- Not sharing towels or bed linens with an infected person.
- Cleaning the infected person's environment daily and, when soiled with wound drainage, using a 1:10 concentration of liquid laundry bleach to water.
- Using paper towels rather than cloth towels for drying hands after hand washing.
- Washing hands with soap and water before leaving the home environment.
- Using disposable gloves when contact with body fluids from an infected person is expected.
- Washing hands with soap and water after any physical contact with an infected person.

### Other Organisms of Disease Resulting from Multidrug Resistance

Although MRSA is receiving much attention, other organisms are also becoming drug resistant and causing infections that are more difficult to treat. MDR tuberculosis is on the rise as is gonorrhea. Because these diseases are more difficult to treat effectively, they are more likely to be spread from person to person than infections that are susceptible to antibacterial drug therapy. The organism *Streptococcus pneumoniae*, a common cause of meningitis and pneumonia, has become increasingly drug resistant. VRE is an intestinal organism that can cause serious infections when it moves from the intestinal tract to other body areas. Other infections, infestations, or diseases that no longer respond well to anti-infective drugs include typhoid fever, malaria, and even head lice.

## Get Ready for Practice!

### Key Points

- Gram-negative bacteria are harder to kill or control with antibacterial drugs because they have a protective capsule that limits the effects of drugs.
- Diarrhea is an expected side effect of therapy with most antibacterial drugs.
- Check the patient's vital signs (including temperature) and mental status before starting an antibacterial drug.
- Check to determine which solutions can be used to dilute a particular IV antibacterial drug and which solutions or drugs should be avoided with that drug.
- For drugs that are toxic to the ears and hearing (ototoxic) such as vancomycin and the aminoglycosides, check the patient's hearing with the ticking watch test or the clicking fingernail test before therapy begins.
- For drugs that cause heart rhythm disturbances such as macrolides and fluoroquinolones (whether given alone or with other drugs), check the patient's heart rate for rhythm and quality for a full minute before giving the first dose of the drug.
- For drugs that increase the effects of warfarin (and the patient is also taking warfarin) such as macrolides, tetracyclines, streptogramins, and fluoroquinolones, check the patient's most recent international normalized ratio (INR) before giving the first dose of the drug.
- Give antibacterial drugs on a schedule that evenly spaces them throughout 24 hours.
- Do not give (and teach patients not to take) cephalosporins, tetracyclines, or fluoroquinolones with antacids, multiple vitamins, or iron supplements.
- For the patient taking warfarin and a macrolide, tetracycline, streptogramin, or fluoroquinolone, check the patient daily for any signs or symptoms of increased bleeding.
- Drugs that have adverse effects on the kidneys (nephrotoxic) almost always have adverse effects on the ears for hearing and balance (ototoxic).
- Urge the patient taking any antibacterial drug to stop the drug and inform the prescriber if a rash or other skin eruption develops.
- Warn patients to immediately call 911 if they begin to have difficulty breathing, a rapid irregular pulse, swelling of the face or neck, or the feeling of a "lump in the throat."
- Teach patients taking macrolides to take the drug with food or within 1 hour of having eaten.
- Teach patients taking macrolides, tetracyclines, sulfonamides, or a fluoroquinolones that these drugs can cause severe sunburn, even for patients with dark skin.
- Warn women taking macrolides, especially erythromycin, that these drugs reduce the effectiveness of birth control pills. Women should use an additional method of birth control while taking the drug and for one menstrual cycle after drug therapy is completed.
- Drug types that should be avoided during pregnancy, while breastfeeding, and with infants or children unless the infection is life threatening include aminoglycosides, tetracyclines, sulfonamides, and fluoroquinolones.
- Even a patient who has never taken an antibacterial drug can have an infection with bacteria that is resistant to antibacterial drug therapy.

### Additional Learning Resources

**evolve** Go to your Evolve website (http://evolve.elsevier.com/Workman/pharmacology/) for the following FREE learning resources:
- eLearning Activities
- Animations
- Video Clips
- Interactive Review Questions
- Audio Key Points
- Audio Glossary
- Audio Glossary—Spanish-English
- Drug Dosage Calculators
- Patient Teaching Handouts

**SG** Go to your Study Guide for additional learning activities to help you master this chapter content.

### Review Questions

1. Which antibacterial drug kills bacteria by binding to cell wall proteins and preventing them from being incorporated into bacterial cell walls?

   A. levofloxacin (Levaquin)
   B. minocycline (Vectrin)
   C. vancomycin (Vancocin)
   D. gentamicin

2. A patient who has been taking tetracycline for a week tells you that a cheesy white substance on the gums and roof of the mouth has appeared. What is your best suggestion?

   A. "Drink at least 3 L of water each day and avoid all dairy products while you are on this drug."
   B. "Go immediately to the emergency room because this is a sign of a serious allergic reaction."
   C. "Stop taking the drug and notify your prescriber because this is a sign of the beginning of an allergic reaction."
   D. "Brush your teeth at least three times a day and use mouthwash to help clear this yeast infection."

3. A patient who developed a wound infection with MRSA after surgery is being discharged to home and is prescribed a cell wall synthesis inhibitor for 10 days. Which statement made by the patient indicates correct understanding of this drug therapy?

   A. "If my temperature is normal for 3 days in a row, the infection is gone, and I can stop taking my medicine."
   B. "If my temperature goes above 100° F for 2 days, I should take twice as much medicine."
   C. "When my incision stops draining, I will no longer need to take the medication."
   D. "Even if I feel completely well, I should take the medication until it is gone."

4. Which action is most important to implement for a 72-year-old patient receiving amikacin (Amikin)?

   A. Assess urine output every shift
   B. Check the patient's hematocrit and hemoglobin levels daily
   C. Teach the patient to wear sunscreen, long sleeves, and a hat when outdoors
   D. Give the drug 1 hour before meals or 2 hours after meals and never with milk

5. Which drug is a fluoroquinolone?

   A. ticarcillin (Ticar)
   B. ciprofloxacin (Cipro)
   C. ceftriaxone (Rocephin)
   D. doxycycline (Vibramycin)

6. When you check on a patient receiving Tequin IV 15 minutes after the drug was started, the patient tells you, "I can't swallow, my chest hurts, and I feel like something bad is going to happen, but I don't know what." What do you do next?

   A. Discontinue the IV
   B. Notify the prescriber
   C. Stop the drug infusion
   D. Check the arms, chest, and back for hives or a rash

7. Which precaution is most important to teach a patient taking trimethoprim/sulfamethoxazole (Septra)?

   A. "Be sure to report any joint or muscle pain to your prescriber."
   B. "Drink at least 4 L of fluid each day that you are taking this drug."
   C. "Avoid coffee and other caffeine-containing drinks while taking this drug."
   D. "Avoid alcoholic beverages while you are taking this drug and for 1 month after you finish taking it."

8. Which drugs should be avoided for infants and children unless an infection is so severe that it is life threatening? (Select all that apply.)

   A. amoxicillin (Amoxil)
   B. ceftriaxone (Rocephin)
   C. erythromycin (Erymax)
   D. levofloxacin (Levaquin)
   E. minocycline (Minocin)
   F. sulfisoxazole (Gantrisin)

9. Your patient is to receive ticarcillin (Ticar) 3 g by IV piggyback. The solution you have is ticarcillin 200 mg/mL. How many milliliters will you add to the piggyback bag to make a dose of 3 g?_____ mL

10. Your patient is to receive linezolid (Zyvox) 300 mg orally. You have on hand linezolid tablets of 600 mg/tablet. How many tablets will you give for a 300-mg dose? _____ tablet(s)

## Critical Thinking Activities

The patient is a 52-year-old woman with diabetes who has cellulitis from a scrape to her right shin. The prescriber orders cefazolin (Kefzol) 1 g IV to be given immediately. Then the patient will be sent home on an oral dose. When you ask her if she is allergic to any antibacterial drugs, she tells you that she gets a rash and has a hard time breathing with penicillin. The IV infusion is started. About 5 minutes after the drug has started infusing, she tells you that she is dizzy, scared, and having a hard time catching her breath. You see that her lips are dusky and her pulse is rapid and thready.

1. What is the most likely cause of this reaction?

2. What should you do with the IV?

3. What type of drug is cefazolin?

4. What is the explanation for this reaction to cefazolin?

# Anti-Infectives: Antiviral Drugs

## Objectives

*After studying this chapter you should be able to:*

1. List the names, actions, usual adult dosages, possible side effects, and adverse effects of antiviral drugs.
2. Describe what to do before and after giving antiviral drugs.
3. Explain what to teach patients taking antiviral drugs, including what to do, what not to do, and when to call the prescriber.
4. Describe life span considerations for antiviral drugs.
5. List the names, actions, usual adult dosages, possible side effects, and adverse effects of antiretroviral drugs.
6. Describe what to do before and after giving antiretroviral drugs.
7. Explain what to teach patients taking antiretroviral drugs, including what to do, what not to do, and when to call the prescriber.
8. Describe life span considerations for antiretroviral drugs.

## Key Terms

**acquired immune deficiency syndrome (AIDS)**
(ă-KWĪ-ŭrd ĭ-MYŪN dĕ-FĬSH-ĕn-sē SĬN-drōm) (p. 175) The most severe form of immune deficiency disease caused by HIV infection.

**common virus** (KŎ-mŭn VĪ-rŭs) (p. 166) A virus that uses either DNA or RNA as its genetic material and has a relatively low efficiency of cellular infection. A nonretrovirus.

**efficiency of infection** (ĕ-FĬSH-ĕn-sē of ĭn-FĔK-shŭn) (p. 166) The ease with which a specific type of organism causes disease through infection.

**host** (HŌST) (p. 165) A person infected by a virus (or other organism) whose cells allow viral reproduction.

**human immune deficiency virus (HIV)** (HYŪ-mŭn ĭm-MYŪN dĕ-FĬSH-ĕn-sē VĪ-rŭs) (p. 175) The most common retrovirus known to cause disease among humans. It is the organism known to cause HIV disease and AIDS.

**opportunistic infections** (ŏp-pŭr-tū-NĬS-tĭk ĭn-FĔK-shŭnz) (p. 176) Infections caused by organisms that are present as part of the normal environment and kept in check by normal

immune function. They occur only in people whose immune systems are not working properly.

**retrovirus** (RĔ-trō-vī-rŭs) (p. 175) A special virus that always uses RNA as its genetic material and carries with it the enzymes reverse transcriptase, integrase, and protease, which allow high-efficiency infection.

**teratogen** (tĕ-RĂ-tō-jĕn) (p. 173) An agent that can cause birth defects.

**viral load** (VĪ-rŭl LŌD) (p. 177) The number of viral particles in a blood sample, which indicates the degree of viral infection.

**virulence** (VĬR-ŭ-lĕns) (p. 167) The measure of how well a microorganism can invade and persist in growing, even when the person's body is trying to destroy or eliminate it.

**virus** (VĪ-rŭs) (p. 165) An intracellular, submicroscopic parasite.

**virustatic** (vī-rŭ-STĂ-tĭk) (p. 168) Drug actions that reduce the number of viruses present by preventing them from reproducing and growing.

◄ⓔ-Learning Activity 10-1

As discussed in Chapter 9, one of most common reasons for drug therapy is the development of infection. An *infection* is an invasion of the body by microorganisms that disturb the normal environment and cause harm or disease. This chapter focuses on viral infections and the drugs used to prevent or control them.

## VIRAL INFECTION

**Viruses** are intracellular, submicroscopic parasites that must infect a living host cell to reproduce. A **host** is the person infected by a virus whose cells allow viral

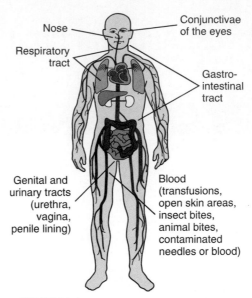

FIGURE 10-1 Common entry sites for viruses.

reproduction. They are extremely small microorganisms that can be seen only with powerful electron microscopes. When they infect a living cell in just the right way, the resources, energy, and machinery of that living cell are used to make new viruses. Because they are so small, viruses can more easily enter the body than bacteria and funguses can. Usually viruses enter through mucous membranes in the nose, conjunctiva of the eye, respiratory tract, digestive tract, and genital or urinary tract (Figure 10-1). They can also enter through broken skin, and they can be injected into the body in blood or blood products.

There are two basic types of viruses: *common viruses* (nonretroviruses) and *retroviruses*. Likewise there are two basic categories of antiviral drugs: those that work against some common viruses *(antiviral drugs)* and those that have some effect against retroviruses *(antiretrovirals).* Common viruses are discussed in this section; retroviruses are discussed later in this chapter.

## REVIEW OF RELATED PHYSIOLOGY AND PATHOPHYSIOLOGY FOR COMMON VIRUSES

A **common virus** is a nonretrovirus that uses either DNA or RNA as its genetic material and has a relatively low efficiency of cellular infection. (**Efficiency of infection** is the ease with which an organism causes disease through infection.) This means that most common viruses must invade the body in large numbers to cause disease. These viruses are responsible for common infections such as chickenpox, shingles, measles, mumps, herpes, warts, hepatitis, and the common cold. The basic anatomy of a common virus is shown in Figure 10-2.

For viruses to cause disease after they enter the body, they must actually enter cells and use the reproductive machinery of the cell to make more viruses that then leave the cell to infect more cells. So becoming sick with a viral disease requires that many cells be infected by common viruses. Inside the body viruses can be destroyed or removed by the immune system. A healthy person will not become ill from most viruses unless the number of invading viruses overwhelms the normal protections. Figure 10-3 shows the cycle of infection for common viruses.

Viruses that enter the body and survive must next find a susceptible cell and bind to its surface. Some viruses cross the plasma membrane of the cell directly, whereas others first bind to a receptor that helps the virus across the membrane. Once inside the cell, the virus must insert its genetic material into the nucleus of the cell and connect it to the genetic material of the cell. Then viral genes direct the host

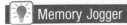

**Did You Know?**

Viruses are not capable of self-reproduction.

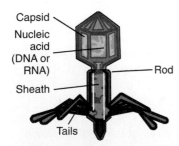

FIGURE 10-2 The basic anatomy of a common virus.

**Memory Jogger**

Most common viruses must enter the body in large numbers for infection to result in disease because these viruses have a low efficiency of infection.

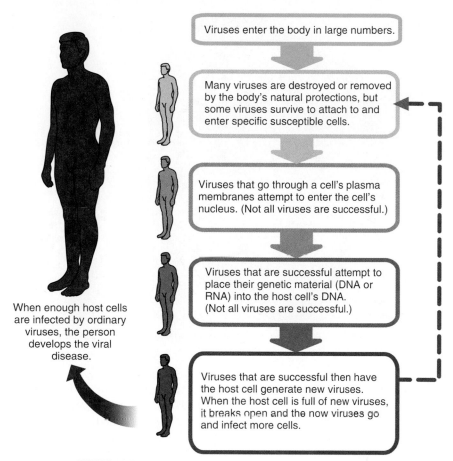

**FIGURE 10-3** Steps in the cycle of infection for common viruses.

cell to make more viruses. These new viruses fill the cell and eventually break out of it to infect new host cells (Figure 10-4). When enough host cells are infected, the person becomes ill with the specific disease caused by the virus.

Viral infections are not cured but are self-limiting, meaning that in a person with a healthy immune system the illness only lasts for so long. If a person's immune system is working properly, the body fights off the infection by itself. If the immune system is weak or if the body has other health problems, the person may die from the effects of the disease.

Most people become ill with a specific viral disease only once because the body learns how to improve protection against that virus. This means that specific viral destruction or removal is much more efficient when a person is reexposed to a virus that once caused illness. Most of this learned protection is provided by antibodies formed against the virus. For example, at the same time a person first develops chickenpox, some of his or her white blood cells (WBCs) learn to make antibodies to the chickenpox virus. This is why the disease lasts only 5 to 10 days instead of months. Then at the next exposure to the chickenpox virus, the body can produce more antibodies to attack, destroy, remove, or inactivate the virus before enough cells are infected to produce chickenpox again.

Some common viruses are stronger than others, with more **virulence** (the measure of how well a microorganism can invade and persist in growing, even when the person's body is trying to destroy or eliminate it). One of the most virulent viruses is the hepatitis B virus (HBV). Others, such as the virus group that cause the common cold, are less virulent. The ease with which a virus causes disease is called the *efficiency of infection.* For disease to occur, many more less virulent viruses are needed, or the host has to be more susceptible to the infection. When more viruses are required for disease to result, the efficiency of infection for that virus is low. If

 **Memory Jogger**

Most people develop a disease caused by a specific viral infection only once. After the first experience with the disease, they become immune to further infections from the same virus.

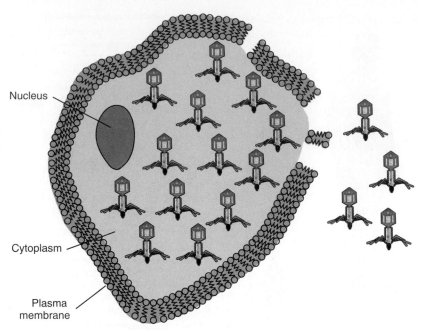

**FIGURE 10-4** An infected cell generates new viruses and then opens the cell and sends newly generated viruses out to infect more host cells.

**Memory Jogger**

The more virulent a virus is, the fewer viruses are needed to cause infection and disease. The efficiency of infection is higher.

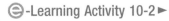-Learning Activity 10-2 ▶

**Memory Jogger**

Antiviral drugs do not kill viruses; they only suppress their reproduction and growth.

**Memory Jogger**

Signs and symptoms of a severe allergic reaction include hives at the IV site; low blood pressure; rapid, irregular pulse; swelling of the lips or lower face; and the patient feeling a lump in the throat.

fewer viruses are required to cause an infection to develop into a disease, the efficiency of infection is high.

Despite barriers to infection, sometimes viruses make it into the body where they infect cells, multiply, damage tissue, and cause disease. Some infections are minor (such as the common cold) and can be limited by the immune system. Others are more severe (such as hepatitis B), and could cause serious harm and even death. Antiviral drugs are used to control such infections by preventing viruses from spreading infection all through the body and causing severe damage.

## GENERAL ISSUES IN ANTIVIRAL THERAPY

An important concept to remember for all antiviral drugs is that they are only virustatic. **Virustatic** drugs reduce the number of viruses by preventing them from reproducing and growing. They are not *virucidal* and cannot kill the virus. By keeping the number of viruses low, antiviral drugs allow the natural defenses of the body to destroy, eliminate, or inactivate them.

Drugs that are effective against common viruses do not have specific categories and may have more than one mechanism of action. Some antivirals suppress viral reproduction. Others prevent the virus from opening its coat and allowing the genetic material to be released. The exact mechanism of action of still other antivirals is not known.

Allergic reactions are possible with any antiviral drug. The allergy may be mild and annoying or severe and life threatening *(anaphylaxis)*. More serious reactions occur when antiviral drugs are given intravenously.

Intended responses for antiviral drugs include:
- The duration or intensity of an existing viral disease is shortened.
- Reactivation of a dormant viral infection is prevented.
- A viral infection is prevented from multiplying to the point that a disease results.

*Before giving an antiviral drug,* ask whether the patient has any drug allergies. If so, notify the prescriber before giving the drug.

*After giving the first dose of an IV antiviral drug,* check the patient every 15 minutes for signs or symptoms of an allergic reaction (hives at the IV site; low blood pressure; rapid, irregular pulse; swelling of the lips or lower face; the patient feeling a lump in the throat). If the patient is having an anaphylactic reaction, your first action is to prevent any more drug from entering him or her. Stop the drug from infusing but keep the IV access. If the drug is infusing high into the IV tubing, change the tubing after stopping the drug and do not let any drug left in the tubing run into the patient.

Inspect the IV site at the beginning of the infusion, halfway through the infusion, and at the end of the infusion and document your findings. If redness is present or the patient reports discomfort at the site, slow the infusion and check for a blood return. Look for any redness or pain or the feeling of hard or cordlike veins above the site. If any of these problems occur, follow the policy of your facility for removing the IV line.

*Teach patients receiving antiviral drugs* the importance of taking the drug long enough to ensure suppression of viral reproduction. If the patient stops taking the drug as soon as he or she feels better, symptoms of infection may recur, and resistant viruses may develop. Teach the patient to take antiviral drugs exactly as prescribed and for as long as prescribed.

For all antiviral therapy it is important to keep the blood level high enough to affect the viruses causing the infection. So it is best for the patient to take the drug evenly throughout a 24-hour day. If the drug should be taken twice daily, teach the patient to take it every 12 hours. For three times a day, teach the patient to take it every 8 hours. Help the patient plan an easy-to-remember schedule that keeps the drug at the best blood levels.

> **! Drug Alert!**
> **Action/Intervention Alert**
>
> If the patient appears to be having anaphylaxis from an IV drug, prevent more drug from entering the patient but maintain IV access.

> **! Drug Alert!**
> **Teaching Alert**
>
> Teach patients to take antiviral drugs exactly as prescribed and for as long as prescribed.

◄ ⊖-**Animation 10-1:** Antivirals

## TYPES OF ANTIVIRAL DRUGS

### Dosages for Common Antiviral Drugs

| Drug | Dose Ranges |
|---|---|
| acyclovir (Apo-Acyclovir🍁, Avirax🍁, Zovirax) | *Adults:* 5-10 mg/kg IV every 8 hr; 200 mg orally 5 times daily (genital herpes)<br>*Children:* 10-20 mg/kg IV every 8 hr; 400-800 mg orally 4 times daily (chickenpox) |
| amantadine (Symmetrel, Endantadine🍁) | *Adults/Children over 10 years:* 100 mg orally twice daily or 200 mg orally once daily<br>*Adults over 65 years:* 100 mg orally once daily<br>*Children under 10 years:* 2.5 mg/kg orally every 12 hr |
| ribavirin (Copegus, Rebetol, RibaPak, Ribasphere, RibaTab, Virazole) | *Adults/Children over 75 kg:* 600 mg orally every 12 hr<br>*Children 60-75 kg:* 400-600 mg orally every 12 hr; other oral dosing is weight dependent<br>*Aerosol administration:* 20 mg/mL for respiratory syncytial virus at 12-18 hr/day delivers an average of 190 mcg/L of air |
| oseltamivir (Tamiflu) | *Adults/Children over 40 kg:* 75 mg orally every 12 hr for 5 days (dosage adjusted downward by weight for children less than 40 kg) |
| rimantadine (Flumadine) | *Adults/Children over 10 years:* 100 mg orally twice daily<br>*Adults over 65 years:* 100 mg orally once daily<br>*Children under 10 years:* 5 mg/kg orally once daily (maximum 150 mg) |
| valacyclovir (Valtrex) | *Adults/Children:* 1-2 g orally every 8-12 hr |
| zanamivir (Relenza) | *Adults/Children over 7 years:* Two oral inhalations (one 5-mg blister per inhalation for a total dosage of 10 mg) every 12 hr for 5 days |

> **⮂ Do Not Confuse**
> **Zovirax** *with* **Zyvox**
>
> An order for Zovirax can be confused with Zyvox. Zovirax is an antiviral drug, whereas Zyvox is an antibacterial drug used to treat methicillin-resistant *Staphylococcus aureus* (MRSA).

> **⮂ Do Not Confuse**
> **Valtrex** *with* **Valcyte**
>
> An order for Valtrex can be confused with Valcyte. Valtrex is an oral antiviral drug use to treat herpes simplex, varicella zoster, cytomegalovirus, and Epstein-Barr viruses. Valcyte is a drug for cytomegalovirus retinitis for patients with AIDS.

## ACYCLOVIR AND VALACYCLOVIR

Acyclovir and valacyclovir are related drugs. At the cell level valacyclovir is converted to acyclovir when it is metabolized.

### How Acyclovir and Valacyclovir Work

Acyclovir and valacyclovir slow viral reproduction by forming "counterfeit" DNA bases and inhibiting the enzymes needed to complete the formation of viral DNA chains. These drugs are most effective against Epstein-Barr virus, cytomegalovirus, herpes simplex virus types 1 and 2, and varicella-zoster virus. Table 10-1 lists diseases caused by these viruses. The dosages and length of therapy for these drugs depend on which virus is causing the infection, the severity of the infection, and the health of the patient's immune system. Other related drugs with actions similar to those of acyclovir include famciclovir and penciclovir.

***Side Effects.*** Common side effects of both of these drugs are headaches, dizziness, and nausea and vomiting. Less common side effects are rash, muscle aches, and a sense of not feeling well *(malaise).*

***Adverse Effects.*** Pain and irritation at the injection site may occur with IV acyclovir, especially when the drug is given rapidly.

Both drugs can reduce kidney function and lead to kidney damage and failure. This problem is caused by the drugs precipitating in the kidney tubules, which is most likely to occur when the patient is not well hydrated.

### What To Do *Before* Giving Acyclovir or Valacyclovir

Be sure to review the general nursing responsibilities related to antiviral therapy (p. 168) in addition to these specific responsibilities before giving acyclovir or valacyclovir.

| Common Side Effects |
| :--- |
| **Acyclovir and Valacyclovir** |

| Headache | Dizziness | Nausea/Vomiting |

---

### Table 10-1 Diseases Caused by Specific Viruses

| VIRUS | DISEASE |
| :--- | :--- |
| Cytomegalovirus (CMV) | Mononucleosis<br>Serious eye infections (retinitis) in people who are immunosuppressed |
| Epstein-Barr virus (EBV) | Chronic fatigue syndrome<br>Some types of lymphoma<br>Whole body infection in newborns and people with severe immunosuppression |
| Hantavirus (HV) | Hantavirus pulmonary syndrome (HPS) |
| Hepatitis A virus (HAV) | Hepatitis A |
| Hepatitis B virus (HBV) | Acute hepatitis B<br>Chronic hepatitis B<br>Liver failure<br>Liver cancer |
| Hepatitis C virus (HCV) | Chronic hepatitis C<br>Liver failure |
| Herpes simplex virus type 1 (HSV1) | Cold sores<br>Whole body infection in newborns and people with severe immunosuppression |
| Herpes simplex virus type 2 (HSV2) | Genital herpes infections |
| Respiratory syncytial virus (RSV) | Severe respiratory infection in infants, young children, and adults over 80 years |
| Varicella-zoster virus (VZV) | Chickenpox<br>Shingles |
| West Nile virus (WNV) | Severe infection causes central nervous system symptoms similar to those of encephalitis or meningitis |

Check whether the patient takes phenytoin (Dilantin) or another drug for seizure control. Acyclovir and valacyclovir reduce the effectiveness of phenytoin, and the prescriber may need to adjust the phenytoin dosage to prevent seizures while the patient is on antiviral therapy.

Ask whether the patient has an allergy to acyclovir. If so, notify the prescriber. Valacyclovir should not be given to any patient with a known allergy to acyclovir.

Make sure that the IV infusion is running well and has a good blood return. Dilute parenteral acyclovir to the proper concentration with only sterile water for injection. Inspect the drug for discoloration or particles.

Acyclovir can interact with other drugs in the tubing. Either flush the line before giving acyclovir or use fresh tubing for the infusion.

Administer the drug slowly over 60 minutes to avoid kidney problems and reduce the risk for irritation at the injection site.

### What To Do *After* Giving Acyclovir or Valacyclovir

Be sure to review the general nursing responsibilities related to antiviral therapy (pp. 168-169) in addition to these specific responsibilities after giving acyclovir or valacyclovir.

Give the patient a full glass of water to drink with oral doses and urge him or her to drink more fluids throughout the day to keep these drugs from precipitating in the kidneys. This is even more important if the patient also takes other drugs that can damage the kidney.

### What To *Teach* Patients About Acyclovir or Valacyclovir

Be sure to teach patients the general care needs and precautions related to antiviral therapy (p. 169) in addition to the specific ones for acyclovir or valacyclovir. Teach patients to drink a full glass of water with each dose of the drug and to drink at least 3 L of fluid daily.

### Life Span Considerations for Acyclovir or Valacyclovir

*Pediatric Considerations.* Oral dosages of these drugs for children older than 2 years of age are very similar to the dosages for adults.

*Considerations for Pregnancy and Breastfeeding.* Both acyclovir and valacyclovir are pregnancy category B drugs. The benefits of the use of acyclovir or valacyclovir during pregnancy should be weighed against any possible risks. These drugs appear in breast milk and can enter the infant during breastfeeding. Teach breastfeeding mothers to reduce the infant's exposure to these drugs (see Box 1-1 in Chapter 1).

*Considerations for Older Adults.* Dizziness, agitation, and confusion may occur as side effects. Older adults are at greater risk for these effects as a result of age-related changes in kidney function and may require more frequent monitoring of kidney function tests (see Table 1-5 in Chapter 1). These changes increase the time that acyclovir and valacyclovir remain in the body, increasing the risk for side effects. Teach older patients to avoid driving or operating heavy equipment until they know how these drugs may affect them.

## AMANTADINE AND RIMANTADINE

### How Amantadine and Rimantadine Work

Amantadine is an oral drug that prevents viral infection by blocking the opening of the external coating of the influenza A virus and stopping the release of viral particles into respiratory epithelial cells. These actions prevent infection and also inhibit viral replication in infected cells. Currently it is used to treat influenza A.

Rimantadine is similar in chemical structure and action to amantadine and also is used to treat influenza A. However, it tends to concentrate more in respiratory

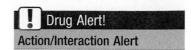

**Drug Alert!**
**Action/Interaction Alert**

Acyclovir and valacyclovir reduce the effectiveness of phenytoin (Dilantin) for seizure control.

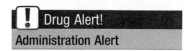

**Drug Alert!**
**Administration Alert**

Administer IV acyclovir as an infusion over 60 minutes.

**Drug Alert!**
**Action/Intervention Alert**

Ensure that patients taking acyclovir or valacyclovir drink at least 3 L of fluid daily.

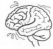

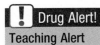
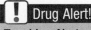

tissues and less in the brain than amantadine. As a result, it has fewer nervous system side effects.

***Side Effects.*** The most common side effects of amantadine (and to a lesser extent rimantadine) include dizziness, blurred vision, dry mouth, hallucinations, and orthostatic (postural) hypotension. Less common side effects include depression and an irregular or fast heart rate.

***Adverse Effects.*** Amantadine affects the central nervous system and may worsen glaucoma and urinary retention. It should not be taken by patients who have either of these problems. Patients who have psychiatric disorders may have an increased risk for suicidal thoughts while taking this drug. These adverse effects have been seen with rimantadine only at very high doses.

### What To Do *Before* Giving Amantadine or Rimantadine

Be sure to review the general nursing responsibilities related to antiviral therapy (p. 168) in addition to these specific responsibilities before giving amantadine or rimantadine.

Ask whether the patient has an allergy to amantadine. If so, notify the prescriber. Rimantadine should not be prescribed for a patient who is allergic to amantadine.

Ask whether the patient has glaucoma or a problem with urinary retention, especially whether male patients have an enlarged prostate gland. Also check whether the patient has any known psychiatric problems, especially severe depression, or has attempted suicide in the past. If the patient has any of these problems, notify the prescriber before administering the drug.

### What To *Teach* Patients About Amantadine or Rimantadine

Be sure to teach patients the general care needs and precautions related to antiviral therapy (p. 169) in addition to the specific ones for amantadine or rimantadine.

Teach patients to not stand or sit up quickly because this may lower blood pressure rapidly, causing dizziness and an increased risk for falls. Also instruct them to hold onto railings when going up or down steps.

Tell the patient and family to report to the prescriber immediately any worsening of depression or thoughts of suicide.

### Life Span Considerations for Amantadine or Rimantadine

***Considerations for Pregnancy and Breastfeeding.*** Amantadine and rimantadine are pregnancy category C drugs and appear in breast milk. Therefore it is not recommended that either of these drugs be used during the first trimester of pregnancy or by women who are breastfeeding.

***Considerations for Older Adults.*** The dosage of either drug should be reduced for patients older than age 65. Both drugs can worsen heart failure and increase edema formation. Teach older adults taking either amantadine or rimantadine to weigh themselves daily and notify the prescriber if they have gained more than 3 lbs in 2 days. Also teach older patients to measure their pulse at least once daily and notify the prescriber if it becomes more irregular or is hard to find.

## RIBAVIRIN

### How Ribavirin Works

Ribavirin is a "counterfeit" base that suppresses viral action and reproduction by unknown mechanisms. It is effective at suppressing many viruses; however, because of its severe side effects and adverse effects, it is most commonly used for viral infections that do not respond to other antiviral agents. These may include Hantavirus and hepatitis A, hepatitis C, respiratory syncytial, and West Nile viruses, among other more rare viruses. This drug is most often used to treat respiratory syncytial virus infection in children and chronic hepatitis C infection in combination with interferon.

*Side Effects.* Ribavirin has many side effects. The most common include nausea, vomiting, diarrhea, fever, and headache. Additional side effects include rash, conjunctivitis, muscle pain, fatigue, dizziness, runny nose, and injection site pain or irritation (parenteral form).

*Adverse Effects. Ribavirin is a potent drug with many adverse effects, and its use is limited to patients who have severe viral infections for which no other drugs are effective. A major adverse effect is that ribavirin is a* teratogen, *an agent that can cause birth defects. It should not be given to pregnant or breastfeeding women. It should not be handled or inhaled by anyone who is pregnant.*

This drug can suppress the bone marrow production of red blood cells (RBCs) and WBCs, especially when it is used along with interferon therapy. As a result, the patient can be anemic and at risk for infection.

With prolonged use ribavirin can impair the function of the liver, kidneys, heart, and ears. In addition, it may lead to some forms of cancer.

### What To Do *Before* Giving Ribavirin

Be sure to review the general nursing responsibilities related to antiviral therapy (p. 168) in addition to these specific ones before giving ribavirin.

Check the patient's heart rate, rhythm, and pulse quality. Also check lung function by assessing the rate and depth of respiratory effort, breath sounds, pulse oximetry, color of skin and mucous membranes, and level of consciousness. Assess kidney function by checking the most recent 24-hour intake and output and comparing the amount of urine excreted with the amount of fluids consumed. Also check the patient's current kidney tests, especially the blood urea nitrogen (BUN) and serum creatinine levels. (See Table 1-5 in Chapter 1 for a listing of normal values.) If the values are higher than normal before starting the drug, the risk for kidney damage is greater. Assess liver function by checking for yellowing *(jaundice)* of the skin, palate, or whites of the eyes and by checking liver function tests. (See Table 1-3 in Chapter 1 for a listing of normal values.) Check the patient's hearing by performing either the "ticking watch" test or the clicking fingernail test (both described in Chapter 9). Use these data as a baseline to detect changes that may result from adverse drug effects.

Because ribavirin often suppresses the growth of bone marrow cells, check the patient's most recent WBC and RBC counts before drug therapy begins. Use these data as a baseline in determining the presence of side effects and whether or not the drug is effective against the infection. (See Table 1-6 in Chapter 1 for a listing of normal values for blood cells.)

Check the patient's vital signs (including temperature and mental status) before starting ribavirin. Use this information as a baseline to determine whether any side effect or adverse effect is present and whether the drug therapy is effective against the infection.

Ribavirin can interact with didanosine (Videx), a drug used in the treatment of human immune deficiency virus (HIV). When ribavirin is used with didanosine, severe liver problems and death from liver failure can result.

When administering aerosolized ribavirin, use only the SPAG-2 aerosol generator. Read the instruction manual before using this instrument. Prepare the aerosolized form of the drug using sterile technique and following the manufacturer's directions for preparation and dilution.

Antacids interfere with absorption of oral ribavirin. Administer the ribavirin at least 1 hour before or 2 hours after an antacid has been given.

**Clinical Pitfall**

Do not permit anyone who is pregnant or breastfeeding to administer ribavirin, handle it, care for a patient taking it, or enter the room of a patient receiving the aerosolized form.

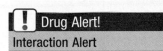

**Drug Alert!**

**Interaction Alert**

Ribavirin should not be given to anyone who is also receiving didanosine.

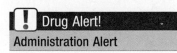

**Drug Alert!**

**Administration Alert**

Administer ribavirin at least 1 hour before or 2 hours after an antacid.

**Common Side Effects**
**Oseltamivir**

Nausea/ Vomiting; Diarrhea    Dizziness    Headache

**Common Side Effects**
**Zanamivir**

  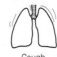

Nausea; Diarrhea    Headache    Cough

### What To Do *After* Giving Ribavirin

Be sure to review the general nursing responsibilities related to antiviral therapy (pp. 168-169) in addition to these specific ones after giving ribavirin.

Monitor the patient closely for any sign of side effects or organ toxicity. Check laboratory values daily for WBC and RBC counts, bilirubin level, liver enzyme levels, and BUN and creatinine levels. Compare urine output with fluid intake. Check hearing daily. Document all changes and notify the prescriber.

### What To *Teach* Patients About Ribavirin

Be sure to teach patients the general care needs and precautions related to antiviral therapy (p. 169) in addition to these specific ones for ribavirin.

Most patients who are taking ribavirin out of the acute care environment are being treated for hepatitis C and are on drug therapy with interferon. In this situation the drug is taken in its oral form.

Teach patients to take ribavirin 1 hour before or 2 hours after taking an antacid because antacids interfere with ribavirin absorption.

Teach patients to contact their prescriber as soon as possible if symptoms of allergy or other adverse effects develop.

### Life Span Considerations with Ribavirin

*Considerations for Pregnancy and Breastfeeding.* This drug is pregnancy category X. It should never be given to a woman who is pregnant because it can cause birth defects. If a woman of childbearing age who is sexually active is prescribed ribavirin, she must use two forms of contraception. Male patients taking this drug whose partners are pregnant should use condoms to prevent exposure of the pregnant women to the drug. Pregnant women living in the household of a person taking ribavirin should not touch the drug.

*Considerations for Older Adults.* Ribavirin should be administered cautiously to older adults. These patients are more likely to have age-related changes in major organs and are at greater risk for organ toxicities. The older adult may be started at a lower drug dosage. Older patients taking ribavirin have a much greater risk for anemia than younger patients. Aerosolized ribavirin is not indicated for older adults.

## OSELTAMIVIR AND ZANAMIVIR

### How Oseltamivir and Zanamivir Work

Oseltamivir and zanamivir work by inhibiting the enzyme neuraminidase, which is needed to spread viral particles in the respiratory tract. They are effective for prevention and treatment of influenzas A and B, swine influenza, and avian influenza. For effective treatment oseltamivir must be taken within 12 to 48 hours, and zanamivir must be taken within 12 to 36 hours of the onset of the first influenza symptoms. These drugs shorten the duration and reduce the severity of influenza. They can also prevent influenza from developing after exposure to the virus.

*Side Effects.* Oseltamivir is an oral drug taken as a liquid (suspension) or capsule. The most common side effects are nausea and vomiting, diarrhea, dizziness, and headache.

Zanamivir is an inhaled drug with effects of nausea, cough, diarrhea, headache, and nasal congestion.

*Adverse Effects.* Specific adverse effects of oseltamivir are rare but include worsening hyperglycemia in diabetes and elevation of liver enzyme levels. Specific adverse effects of zanamivir are rare but include breathing problems, confusion, and seizures.

### What To *Teach* Patients About Oseltamivir or Zanamivir

Be sure to teach the patient the general care needs and precautions related to antiviral therapy (p. 169) in addition to these specific ones for oseltamivir or zanamivir.

| Box 10-1 | Preparation of Oseltamivir Oral Suspension |

- Shake the bottle for about 5 to 10 seconds before each use to mix the drug evenly.
- Open the bottle by pushing down and turning the cap at the same time.
- Push the plunger of the measuring device completely down to the tip.
- Insert the tip of the measuring device firmly into the opening on the top of the bottle.
- Turn the bottle (with the measuring device attached) upside down.
- Pull back on the plunger slowly until the amount of drug prescribed fills the measuring device to the correct marking. (Some larger doses may need to be measured using the measuring device twice.)
- Turn the bottle (with the measuring device attached) right-side up and slowly remove the measuring device.
- Place the liquid directly into your mouth from the measuring device; *do not mix it with any other liquids.*
- Replace the cap on the bottle and close tightly.
- Remove the plunger from the rest of the device and rinse both parts under warm running tap water. Allow the parts to air dry before using them again.

Because most patients prescribed either oseltamivir or zanamivir will be taking it at home, teach them how to take these drugs properly.

Teach patients and families that, if an adverse effect occurs, they should stop taking the drug and notify the prescriber as soon as possible.

Teach patients prescribed oseltamivir suspension about the proper way to mix it and take it. This drug comes with its own mixing device and measuring device. Box 10-1 describes the steps for mixing and taking oseltamivir.

Teach patients taking zanamivir how to use an inhaler (see Box 18-2 in Chapter 18). For this drug, remind the patient *not* to use a spacer. If the patient takes other drugs by inhalation for another breathing problem such as asthma or chronic obstructive pulmonary disease, teach him or her to use the bronchodilator *before* using the zanamivir inhaler and to wait at least 5 minutes before using the zanamivir inhaler.

## RETROVIRAL INFECTION

### REVIEW OF RELATED PHYSIOLOGY AND PATHOPHYSIOLOGY

A retrovirus is a special virus that always uses RNA as its genetic material and carries with it the enzymes reverse transcriptase, integrase, and protease, which allow high efficiency of cellular infection. This means that disease may result even when low levels of retroviruses enter the body. The human immune deficiency virus (HIV) is a retrovirus that attacks the immune system of an infected person, eventually causing him or her to have little or no immune protection. The most severe form of immune deficiency disease caused by HIV infection is known as acquired immune deficiency syndrome (AIDS).

HIV has an outer layer with special "docking proteins," known as *gp41* and *gp120*, that help the virus enter cells with receptors for these proteins (Figure 10-5). Inside, the virus has its genetic material along with the enzymes reverse transcriptase and integrase. One of the cells that has receptors for the docking proteins is the *CD4+ cell, helper/inducer T cell,* or *T4 cell.* This cell directs immune system defenses and regulates the activity of all immune system cells. If HIV enters a CD4+ T cell, it can then create more virus particles.

After entering a host cell, HIV must get its genetic material into the DNA of the host cell. DNA is the genetic material of the human cell. The genetic material of HIV is RNA. To infect and take over a human cell, the genetic material must be the same. HIV carries the enzyme *reverse transcriptase.* This enzyme converts the RNA of HIV into DNA, making the viral genetic material the same as human DNA. Then HIV uses the enzyme *integrase* to insert its DNA into the human DNA of the CD4+ T cell. This action completes the infection of the CD4+ T cell.

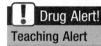

**Drug Alert!**

**Teaching Alert**

Teach patients who take other drugs by inhalation for another breathing problem to use the bronchodilator at least 5 minutes *before* using the zanamivir inhaler.

-Learning Activity 10-3

 **Did You Know?**

Everyone with AIDS has HIV infection but not everyone with HIV infection has AIDS.

**Memory Jogger**

The main cell type infected and destroyed by HIV infection is the CD4+ cell (helper/inducer T cell).

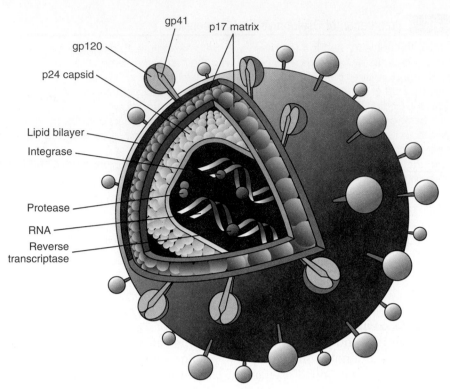

gp41

p17 matrix

gp120

p24 capsid

Lipid bilayer

Integrase

Protease

RNA

Reverse transcriptase

**FIGURE 10-5** The components of the human immune deficiency retrovirus.

**Memory Jogger**

CD4+ T cells are the "generals" of the immune system army. When they are infected and destroyed, the person is immune deficient and cannot successfully fight off other infections.

⊖-Learning Activity 10-4 ▶

**Memory Jogger**

The six classes of antiretroviral drugs are:
- Nucleoside analog reverse transcriptase inhibitors (NRTIs).
- Non-nucleoside analog reverse transcriptase inhibitors (NNRTIs).
- Protease inhibitors (PIs).
- Fusion inhibitors.
- Entry inhibitors.
- Integrase inhibitors.

HIV particles are made in the infected CD4+ T cell using the machinery of the host cell. The new virus particle is made in the form of one long protein strand. The strand is clipped with chemical scissors called *HIV protease* into several small pieces. These pieces are formed into a new finished viral particle. The new virus particle then fuses with the membrane of the infected cell and buds off, able to infect other CD4+ T cells (Figure 10-6).

In early HIV infection the immune system can attack and destroy the newly created viral particles. With time the number of HIV particles overwhelms the immune system. As the CD4+ T-cell level drops, the patient is at risk for bacterial, fungal, and viral infections and some cancers. Opportunistic infections are caused by organisms that are present as part of the normal environment and kept in check by normal immune function. In a person with AIDS the immune system is extremely suppressed. T-cell count falls, viral load rises, and without treatment the patient dies relatively quickly of opportunistic infections or cancer.

## GENERAL ISSUES IN ANTIRETROVIRAL THERAPY

The six classes of antiretroviral drugs are nucleoside analog reverse transcriptase inhibitors (NRTIs), non-nucleoside analog reverse transcriptase inhibitors (NNRTIs), protease inhibitors (PIs), fusion inhibitors, entry inhibitors, and integrase inhibitors.

A patient with HIV infection or AIDS receives drugs from several classes in regimens called *cocktails* because HIV is not affected by any individual antiretroviral drug alone. This approach is termed *highly active antiretroviral therapy (HAART)*. Antiretroviral drugs are virustatic and do not kill the virus. Different types of HAART drugs are available as combination tablets containing two or three drugs. This reduces the number of individual drugs that a patient may have to take.

An important issue with HAART is the development of drug-resistant mutations in the HIV organism. When resistance develops, viral replication is no longer suppressed by the drugs. Several factors contribute to the development of drug resistance to HAART, with the most important being missed drug doses. When doses

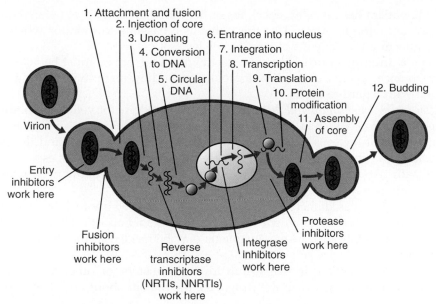

1. Attachment and fusion
2. Injection of core
3. Uncoating
4. Conversion to DNA
5. Circular DNA
6. Entrance into nucleus
7. Integration
8. Transcription
9. Translation
10. Protein modification
11. Assembly of core
12. Budding

Virion

Entry inhibitors work here

Fusion inhibitors work here

Reverse transcriptase inhibitors (NRTIs, NNRTIs) work here

Integrase inhibitors work here

Protease inhibitors work here

**FIGURE 10-6** Sites in the life cycle of the human immune deficiency virus (HIV) in which different antiretroviral drugs work. *NRTI,* nucleoside analog reverse transcriptase inhibitor; *NNRTI,* non-nucleoside analog reverse transcriptase inhibitor.

are missed, the blood concentrations become lower than that needed to inhibit viral replication, allowing the virus to replicate and produce new viruses that are resistant to the drugs being used.

Any antiretroviral drug can cause an allergic reaction. It may be minor, with a rash appearing days after starting the drug. The major symptoms of a severe allergic reaction *(anaphylaxis)* are tightness in the chest with trouble breathing; low blood pressure; hives around the injection site; swelling of the face, mouth, and throat; weak, thready pulse; and a sense that something bad is happening. If not recognized and treated quickly, anaphylaxis can lead to vascular collapse, shock, and death.

Two common adverse effects of the antiretrovirals are liver toxicity and worsening hyperglycemia.

Most antiretroviral drugs interact with other drugs and food. These interactions can cause serious adverse effects and can change the activity of drugs.

Intended responses with antiretroviral therapy focus on the results of suppression of viral reproduction. These responses include:

- **Viral load** (the number of viral particles in a blood sample, which indicates the degree of viral infection) is reduced.
- Immune function is improved, as evidenced by higher CD4+ cell count; higher CD4+ to CD8+ ratio.
- The patient has fewer episodes of opportunistic infections.

*Before giving an antiretroviral drug,* obtain a list of all other drugs that the patient takes because antiretrovirals interact with many other drugs. Check with the pharmacist for possible interactions and the need to consult the prescriber about dosage or changing the patient's other drugs.

Ask the patient about previous allergic reactions to drugs. If a drug allergy has occurred, determine which drug or drugs caused it, the specific reactions the patient had, and how the problem was treated. Notify the prescriber of previous allergic reactions to drugs and make sure that this information is documented in the patient's chart.

Because antiretroviral therapy can lead to liver toxicity, make sure that the patient does not have a liver problem before starting these drugs. Check the patient's most recent laboratory values for liver problems (elevated liver enzyme levels). (See Table 1-3 in Chapter 1 for a listing of normal values.)

 **Clinical Pitfall**

Do not delay, skip, or reduce HAART doses.

 **Memory Jogger**

Signs and symptoms of an anaphylactic reaction to a drug are tightness in the chest with trouble breathing; low blood pressure; hives around the IV site; swelling of the face, mouth, and throat; weak, thready pulse; and a sense that something bad is happening.

 **Drug Alert!**

**Interaction Alert**

Before giving antiretroviral drugs, ask the patient about *all* other drugs or supplements that he or she takes and then check with the pharmacist to avoid a possible drug interaction.

⊖-Learning Activity 10-5 ▶

If the patient has diabetes, check his or her blood glucose level before administering an antiretroviral drug. Use this value as a baseline to monitor whether the drug is affecting the patient's blood glucose level.

Some antiretroviral drugs must be taken with food; others must be taken on an empty stomach. Check a drug reference to determine how an individual drug should be given with regard to meals.

*After giving an antiretroviral drug,* check the patient daily for yellowing of the skin or sclera *(jaundice),* which is a symptom of liver problems. The best places to check are the whites of the eyes closest to the iris, the roof of the mouth, and the skin of the chest. Avoid checking the soles of the feet or palms of the hands, especially in a patient with darker skin, because these areas often appear yellow even when the patient is not jaundiced.

If the patient has diabetes, check blood glucose levels more often and assess fasting blood glucose levels whenever they are ordered. Report higher-than-normal levels to the prescriber because adjustments may be needed in the dosages of antidiabetic drugs.

Check the patient's skin every shift for rash, blisters, or other skin eruptions that may indicate a reaction to the drug. Ask the patient about any itching or skin changes.

*Teach patients receiving antiretroviral therapy* the importance of taking their drugs exactly as prescribed to maintain the effectiveness of HAART drugs. Even a few missed doses per month can promote drug resistance.

Remind patients that antiretroviral drugs do not kill the virus or cure the disease. These drugs only help reduce the number of viruses in the body; the person will still have HIV disease.

Teach patients to follow the manufacturer's directions for whether a specific drug should be taken with food or on an empty stomach.

Warn patients taking antiretrovirals to tell all health care providers that they are taking these drugs because of the potential for drug interactions. Teach patients not to take any over-the-counter drug or herbal supplement without consulting the antiretroviral prescriber. These interactions may:

- Reduce the effectiveness of the antiretroviral drug.
- Reduce the effectiveness of the other drug.
- Lead to serious and life-threatening responses.

Tell patients to notify the prescriber if they develop yellowing of the skin or eyes, darkening of the urine, or lightening of the stools. These problems are signs of liver toxicity, a serious adverse effect of these drugs.

Teach women that many antiretroviral drugs, especially when taken in combination as part of HAART, reduce the effectiveness of birth control pills. Tell patients to use an additional form of birth control to prevent an unplanned pregnancy.

Considerations for pregnancy and breastfeeding include that most antiretroviral drugs for HAART are recommended to be taken by pregnant women who are known to be HIV positive because the virus can cross the placenta and infect the fetus. When these drugs are taken as prescribed, they can reduce the chances of fetal infection. The woman who is HIV positive should not breastfeed because the virus can be transferred from the mother to the infant in breast milk.

## TYPES OF ANTIRETROVIRAL DRUGS

### NUCLEOSIDE ANALOG REVERSE TRANSCRIPTASE INHIBITORS

#### How NRTIs Work

Nucleoside analog reverse transcriptase inhibitors (NRTIs) are similar to bases that form DNA. These drugs are converted in the infected cell to counterfeit bases and compete with the actual bases that are placed into DNA by reverse transcriptase. They inhibit reverse transcriptase and viral DNA synthesis, slowing viral reproduction. (See Figure 10-6 for where these drugs work to disrupt HIV reproduction.)

## Dosages for Common NRTIs

| Drug | Dosage |
|---|---|
| abacavir (Ziagen) | *Adults:* 300 mg orally twice daily or 600 mg orally once daily<br>*Children:* 8 mg/kg orally twice daily |
| didanosine (ddI, Videx) | *Adults/Children over 60 kg:* 125-200 mg orally twice daily |
| didanosine (Videx EC) | *Adults/Children over 60 kg:* 400 mg orally once daily |
| emtricitabine (Emtriva) | *Adults:* 200 mg tablet or 240 mg solution orally daily<br>*Children:* 6 mg/kg, up to 240 mg (24 mL) orally daily |
| lamivudine (Epivir, Epivir-HPV, 3TC) | *Adults:* 300 mg orally daily<br>*Children:* 4 mg/kg orally every 12 hr (maximum of 150 mg) |
| stavudine (d4T, Zerit) | *Adults:* 40 mg orally twice daily<br>*Children less than 60 kg:* 0.5-1 mg/kg orally every 12 hr |
| tenofovir (Viread) | *Adults:* 300 mg orally daily<br>*Children:* Safe dosages have not been established |
| zidovudine (Apo-Zidovudine✦, Azidothymidine, AZT, Novo-AZT✦, Retrovir) | *Adults/Children over 30 kg:* 300 mg orally twice daily<br>*Children less than 30 kg:* 9 mg/kg orally twice daily |

*Side Effects.* Common side effects of NRTIs are nausea, headache, and increased digestive upsets when eating fatty or fried foods. Each NRTI may have more side effects. Be sure to consult a drug reference for side effects of each specific drug.

*Adverse Effects.* The two most common adverse effects of NRTIs are liver toxicity and peripheral neuropathy with long-term use.

Abacavir is more likely to cause hypersensitivity reactions within the first 4 weeks. This response starts with flulike symptoms and progresses to life-threatening hypersensitivity.

### What To *Teach* Patients About NRTIs

Be sure to teach patients the general care needs and precautions related to antiretroviral therapy (p. 178) in addition to these specific ones for NRTIs.

Teach patients to avoid fatty foods and fried foods. These foods can cause digestive upsets and lead to pancreatitis when combined with NRTIs.

After long-term use patients often develop peripheral neuropathy with reduced sensation. Teach patients who have reduced sensation to prevent injury. Loss of sensation increases the patient's risk for injury because he or she may not be aware of excessive heat, cold, or pressure. The risk for injury to the feet is very high. In addition, falls are more likely because the patient cannot feel changes in terrain and because of orthostatic hypotension. Box 10-2 lists important tips to teach the patient with peripheral neuropathy.

Teach patients taking abacavir to stop the drug and notify the prescriber if flulike symptoms occur. Warn them that, if this response occurs, to never take the drug again.

### Life Span Considerations for NRTIs

*Pediatric Considerations.* Children of any age who are HIV positive should take NRTIs as part of HAART. Dosages for small children are usually based on weight.

*Considerations for Pregnancy and Breastfeeding.* NRTIs increase the risk for lactic acidosis in pregnant women. Lactic acidosis is the buildup of lactic acid in muscle and other tissues when not enough oxygen is present to allow metabolism to occur normally. Signs and symptoms of lactic acidosis are muscle aches; tiredness and difficulty remaining awake; abdominal pain; hypotension; and a slow, irregular heartbeat. Other considerations for pregnancy and breastfeeding are listed in the General Issues section on p. 178.

**Do Not Confuse**

**lamivudine** *with* **lamotrigine**

An order for lamivudine can be confused with lamotrigine. lamivudine is an antiretroviral drug, whereas lamotrigine is a drug used to control seizures.

**Do Not Confuse**

**Retrovir** *with* **ritonavir**

An order for Retrovir can be confused with ritonavir. Retrovir is an antiretroviral drug from the NRTI class, whereas ritonavir is an antiretroviral drug from the protease inhibitor class.

**Common Side Effects**

**NRTIs**

Nausea, Intolerance to fatty foods    Headache

**Drug Alert!**

**Teaching Alert**

Warn patients taking abacavir to stop the drug if flulike symptoms develop, to report the response to the prescriber, and to never restart taking the drug.

| Box 10-2 | Patient Teaching Guide for Peripheral Neuropathy |
| --- | --- |

- Protect feet and other body areas where sensation is reduced (for example, do not walk around in bare feet or stocking feet. Always wear shoes with protective soles).
- Be sure that shoes are long enough and wide enough to prevent creating sores or blisters.
- Provide a long break-in period for new shoes; do not wear new shoes for longer than 2 hours at a time.
- Avoid pointed-toe shoes and shoes with heels higher than 2 inches.
- Inspect your feet daily (with a mirror) for open areas or redness.
- Avoid temperature extremes; wear warm clothing in the winter, especially over hands, feet, and ears.
- Test water temperature with a thermometer when washing dishes or bathing. Use warm water rather than hot water (less than 110° F)
- Use potholders when cooking.
- Use gloves when washing dishes or gardening.
- Do not eat foods that are "steaming hot"; allow them to cool before placing them in your mouth.
- Eat foods that are high in fiber (such as fruit, whole-grain cereals, and vegetables) to prevent constipation.
- Drink 2 to 3 L of fluid (nonalcoholic) daily unless your health care provider has told you to restrict fluid intake.
- Get up from a lying or sitting position slowly. If you feel dizzy, sit back down until the dizziness fades before you walk, especially before using stairs.
- Look at your feet and the floor or ground where you are walking to assess how the ground, floor, or step changes to prevent tripping or falling.
- Avoid using area rugs, especially those that slide easily.
- Use handrails when going up or down steps.

***Considerations for Older Adults.***  Peripheral neuropathy develops more quickly in the older adult taking NRTIs and greatly increases the risk for falls and other injuries. Be sure to teach older adults the tips in Box 10-2 to prevent injuries related to neuropathy.

## NON-NUCLEOSIDE ANALOG REVERSE TRANSCRIPTASE INHIBITORS

### How NNRTIs Work

Non-nucleoside analog reverse transcriptase inhibitors (NNRTIs) inhibit the action of the enzyme reverse transcriptase by binding directly to the enzyme, preventing it from converting viral RNA to DNA. As a result, viral reproduction is suppressed. Figure 10-6 shows where these drugs work to disrupt HIV reproduction.

### Dosages for Common NNRTIs

| Drug | Dosage |
| --- | --- |
| delavirdine (Rescriptor) | *Adults:* 400 mg orally three times daily<br>*Children:* Safe dosages have not been established |
| etravirine (Intelence) | *Adults:* 200 mg orally twice daily<br>*Children:* Safe dosages have not been established |
| efavirenz (Sustiva) | *Adults/Children over 40 kg:* 600 mg orally once daily<br>*Children 10 to 39 kg:* 200-300 mg orally once daily at bedtime |
| nevirapine (Viramune) | *Adults:* 200 mg orally daily for first 14 days, then 200 mg orally twice daily<br>*Children:* Dosages for young children based on total body surface area |

**Memory Jogger**

The generic names for the common NNRTIs usually have "*vir*" in the *middle* of the name (for example, efavirenz).

***Side Effects.***  Common side effects of NNRTIs are rash, nausea and vomiting, headache, and abdominal pain. Additional side effects with these drugs are difficulty sleeping and vivid dreams or nightmares. Each individual NNRTI may have more side effects. Be sure to consult a drug reference for side effects associated with each specific drug.

*Adverse Effects.*  The two most common adverse effects with NNRTIs are anemia and liver toxicity.

## What To *Teach* Patients About NNRTIs

Be sure to teach patients the general care needs and precautions related to antiretroviral therapy (p. 178) in addition to these specific ones for NNRTIs.

Tell patients to notify their prescriber if they develop a sore throat, fever, different types of rashes, blisters, or multiple bruises. These problems are signs of serious adverse effects of drugs from this class.

Teach patients to take the drug at least 1 hour before or 2 hours after taking an antacid. Antacids inhibit the absorption of drugs in the NNRTI class.

Remind patients to keep all appointments for blood tests because NNRTIs can cause anemia.

The herbal supplement St. John's wort greatly reduces the effectiveness of NNRTIs.

## Life Span Considerations for NNRTIs

*Pediatric Considerations.*  Children of any age who are HIV positive should take NNRTIs as part of HAART. Anemia is more likely to occur in children.

*Considerations for Pregnancy and Breastfeeding.*  Etravirine and nevirapine are pregnancy category B drugs and may be taken at any stage of pregnancy. Neither delavirdine nor efavirenz should be taken during pregnancy. Other considerations for pregnancy and breastfeeding are listed in the General Issues section on p. 178.

*Considerations for Older Adults.*  Older adults are more likely to be taking other drugs that could interact with an NNRTI. Remind the patient to tell all health care providers about all drugs he or she takes. Also teach older adults how to take their pulse and assess it for irregularities. Remind the patient to report new irregularities to the prescriber.

## PROTEASE INHIBITORS

### How Protease Inhibitors Work

Protease inhibitors (PIs) prevent viral replication and release of viral particles. HIV produces its proteins, including those needed to move viral particles out of the host cell, in one long strand. For the proteins to be active, this large protein must be broken down into separate smaller proteins through the action of the viral enzyme HIV protease. When PIs are taken into an HIV-infected cell, they make the protease enzyme work on the drug rather than on the initial large protein. Thus active proteins are not produced, and viral particles cannot leave the cell to infect other cells. (See Figure 10-6 for where these drugs work to disrupt HIV reproduction.)

### Dosages for Common Protease Inhibitors

| Drug | Dosage |
|---|---|
| atazanavir (Reyataz) | *Adults:* 300 mg orally daily<br>*Children:* 7 mg/kg orally daily |
| darunavir (Prezista) | *Adults:* 800 mg orally twice daily<br>*Children over 40 kg:* 600 mg orally every 12 hr<br>*Children under 40 kg:* 450 mg orally every 12 hr |
| fosamprenavir (Lexiva) | *Adults:* 700 mg orally twice daily<br>*Children:* 18 mg/kg orally twice daily |
| indinavir (Crixivan) | *Adults:* 800 mg orally every 8 hr<br>*Children:* 500 mg/m² orally every 8 hr |
| nelfinavir (Viracept) | *Adults/Children older than 12 years:* 1250 mg orally every 12 hr<br>or 750 mg orally every 8 hr |

*Continued*

---

**Common Side Effects**

**NNRTIs**

Rash   Nausea/Vomiting,   Headache
Abdominal pain

---

**(!) Drug Alert!**

**Teaching Alert**

Teach patients taking NNRTIs to avoid St. John's wort.

---

**(!) Drug Alert!**

**Action/Intervention Alert**

Assess a child taking an NNRTI for indications of anemia: low RBC count, low hemoglobin levels, pallor or cyanosis, fatigue, increased heart rate and respiratory rate, decreased blood pressure.

---

 **Do Not Confuse**

**Viracept** *with* **Viramune**

An order for Viracept can be confused with Viramune. Viracept is an antiretroviral drug from the PI class, whereas Viramune is an antiretroviral drug from the NNRTI class.

---

 **Do Not Confuse**

**ritonavir** *with* **Retrovir**

An order for ritonavir can be confused with Retrovir. Ritonavir is an antiretroviral drug from the PI class, whereas Retrovir is an antiretroviral drug from the NRTI class.

**Memory Jogger**

The generic names for the common PIs usually have "*-avir*" at the *end* of the name (for example, indinavir).

---

**Common Side Effects**

**Protease Inhibitors**

Headache   Diarrhea;   Insomnia
Abdominal
weight gain

Depression

---

 **Drug Alert!**

**Interaction Alert**

Reyataz, Prezista, Lexiva, and Invirase *must* be given with ritonavir, which causes a drug-drug interaction that results in *higher* blood levels and effectiveness.

---

**Drug Alert!**

**Teaching Alert**

Teach patients taking PIs to avoid taking St. John's wort.

---

**Dosages for Common Protease Inhibitors—cont'd**

| Drug | Dosage |
|------|--------|
| ritonavir (Norvir) | *Adults:* 600 mg orally every 12 hr<br>*Children:* 350-400 mg/m² orally every 12 hr |
| saquinavir (Invirase) | *Adults/Children older than 16 years:* 1000 mg orally every 12 hr<br>*Children younger than 16 years:* 33 mg/kg orally every 8 hr |

*Side Effects.* Common side effects of PIs are headache, diarrhea, depression, difficulty sleeping, and abdominal weight gain. Each drug may have more side effects. Be sure to consult a drug reference for side effects of each specific drug.

*Adverse Effects.* The most common adverse effect of PIs is liver toxicity. They also increase lipid levels, leading to hyperlipidemia, atherosclerosis, and pancreatitis.

PIs should be used cautiously in anyone who has hemophilia. They can induce uncontrolled bleeding in these patients.

Atazanavir and ritonavir can impair electrical conduction in the heart and lead to heart block, especially in a person who has an abnormally slow heart rate.

Darunavir and fosamprenavir both contain sulfa and should not be used for patients who have allergies to sulfa drugs.

### What To *Teach* Patients About Protease Inhibitors

Be sure to teach patients the general care needs and precautions related to antiretroviral therapy (p. 178) in addition to these specific ones for PIs.

Warn patients not to crush or chew capsules because these actions may cause the drug to be absorbed too rapidly and increase the risk for side effects.

Teach patients taking atazanavir or ritonavir to check their pulse for a full minute at least twice daily. They should report any changes in heart rate or regularity to the prescriber.

An herbal supplement that greatly reduces the effectiveness of PIs is St. John's wort. Warn patients to not take St. John's wort while on HIV therapy that includes any of the PIs.

### Life Span Considerations for Protease Inhibitors

*Pediatric Considerations.* HIV-positive children over the age of 6 years take PIs as part of HAART. Dosages for older children are nearly the same as for adults. For children younger than 6 years of age and infants, the optimal dosages are unknown.

*Considerations for Older Adults.* Older adults are more likely to be taking other drugs that could interact with PIs, especially cardiac drugs and lipid-lowering drugs. Remind the patient to tell all health care providers about all drugs that he or she takes. Teach older adults how to check their pulse for irregularities. Remind them to report new irregularities to the prescriber.

### FUSION INHIBITORS

The only drug in this category is enfuvirtide (Fuzeon). The usual dosage is 90 mg subcutaneously twice daily. It is used with other drugs as part of a HAART regimen.

### How Fusion Inhibitors Work

Fusion inhibitors block the viral docking protein (gp41) from fusing with the host cell. Without fusion, infection of new cells does not occur. (See Figure 10-6 for where these drugs work to disrupt HIV reproduction.)

*Side Effects.* The most common side effect of enfuvirtide is an injection site reaction (itching, warmth, swelling, bump formation, skin hardening). Other common side effects are constipation, trouble sleeping, depression, and muscle aches.

***Adverse Effects.*** Adverse effects are peripheral neuropathy with pain and numbness of the hands and feet (most common), increased respiratory infections (including pneumonia), and liver toxicity.

## What To *Teach* Patients About Enfuvirtide

Be sure to teach the patient the general care needs and precautions related to antiretroviral therapy (p. 178) in addition to these specific ones for enfuvirtide.

The most important aspect of enfuvirtide therapy to teach patients is how to safely self-inject the drug. A 1-month supply of the drug is available in a kit that contains single-use vials, vials of sterile water for injection, preparation syringes, administration syringes, alcohol wipes, and instruction guides. Teach the patient how to prepare the drug correctly, draw it up, inject it, dispose of the needle, and store it following the instruction guide.

Teach patients the manifestations of respiratory infection (cough; shortness of breath; fever; mucus production or a change in the color of mucus from clear to yellow, green, or brown). Instruct them to report these symptoms immediately to the prescriber.

Teach patients to store unmixed vials of drug and water at room temperature, between 59° F and 86° F and to store the mixed drug and water vial in a refrigerator between 36° F and 46° F for up to 24 hours. Unused mixed drug should be discarded after 24 hours.

Teach patients to assess injection sites daily for signs of infection or reactions. Remind them that, if an injection site reaction occurs, they should not use that site again until it heals and the skin is normal. Instruct patients to report an injection site infection to the prescriber and to not reuse that site until the infection has completely cleared and the skin has healed.

Like the NRTIs, after long-term use of enfuvirtide, patients often develop peripheral neuropathy with reduced sensation. See What To Teach Patients About NRTIs (p. 178) for information regarding this problem.

## Life Span Considerations for Enfuvirtide

***Pediatric Considerations.*** Drug dosages for children 6 years of age and older are based on weight (2 mg/kg) and are given subcutaneously twice daily up to a maximum dose of 90 mg twice daily. Dosages for children younger than 6 years of age have not been established.

Injection site infections occur more often in adolescents. Teach adolescents the proper skin cleansing techniques and how to prevent contamination of the drug and needle.

***Considerations for Pregnancy and Breastfeeding.*** Enfuvirtide is a pregnancy category B drug given in combination with other antiretrovirals during pregnancy. Enfuvirtide therapy should begin during the second trimester.

***Considerations for Older Adults.*** Some older adults have vision or mobility problems that make self-administration of enfuvirtide more difficult. Assess the older patient's ability to prepare the drug, draw up the correct dosage, and reach an appropriate injection site. Include a family member or other responsible person when teaching about drug preparation and administration.

## ENTRY INHIBITORS

The major drug in this category is maraviroc (Selzentry). The usual dosage range for an adult is 150 to 600 mg orally twice daily.

### How Entry Inhibitors Work

Entry inhibitors prevent cellular infection by blocking the CCR5 receptor on CD4+ T cells. (See Figure 10-6 for where these drugs work to disrupt HIV reproduction.) Because this drug is not effective against all HIV subtypes, the patient must first

**Common Side Effects**

**Enfuvirtide**

 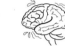 

Injection site  Constipation  Insomnia
reaction

 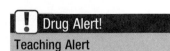

Muscle aches  Depression

---

**! Drug Alert!**

**Teaching Alert**

Teach patients how to prepare, administer, and store enfuvirtide.

## Common Side Effects

### Maraviroc

Muscle aches, Pains  Diarrhea  Dizziness

Insomnia  Cough

be tested to ensure that his or her HIV infection is likely to respond to this therapy.

*Side Effects.* Common side effects of maraviroc include muscle aches and pains, cough, diarrhea, dizziness, and trouble sleeping. Other less common side effects include rhinitis, sinusitis, depression, and numbness or tingling of the hands and feet.

*Adverse Effects.* The most common adverse effects of maraviroc are hypotension and liver toxicity.

### What To *Teach* Patients About Maraviroc

Be sure to teach patients the general care needs and precautions related to antiretroviral therapy (p. 178) in addition to these specific ones for maraviroc.

Warn patients not to crush or chew capsules because these actions may cause the drug to be absorbed too rapidly and increase the risk for side effects.

Teach patients about safety and low blood pressure and to change positions slowly. When they are getting out of bed, teach them to sit on the side of the bed for a few minutes and then slowly move to a standing position. If they become dizzy, they should sit back down again for a few more minutes. Tell them to use handrails when going up or down steps and to avoid driving or operating heavy equipment while dizzy.

### Life Span Considerations for Maraviroc

*Pediatric Considerations.* Maraviroc is not approved for use in children under the age of 16.

*Considerations for Pregnancy and Breastfeeding.* Maraviroc is a pregnancy category B drug. When the patient's viruses are identified as being sensitive to this drug, it may be started in combination with other antiretrovirals during the second trimester of pregnancy.

*Considerations for Older Adults.* Older adults are more likely to develop orthostatic hypotension with maraviroc and increase the risk for falls. Box 10-3 lists precautions to help prevent falls. Stress the need to change positions slowly and use handrails when going up or down steps. Also warn older adults to not drive or operate heavy equipment until they know how maraviroc affects them.

### INTEGRASE INHIBITORS

The major drug in this category is raltegravir (Isentress). The usual dosage for an adult is 400 mg orally twice daily. It is usually prescribed for people who have HIV

---

| Box **10-3** | Fall Precautions |

- Check blood pressure in the lying, sitting, and standing positions.
- Check muscle strength in legs.
- Orient the patient to the environment.
- Remind the patient to call for help before getting out of bed or a chair.
- Help the patient to get out of bed or a chair.
- Provide or remind the patient to use a walker or cane for ambulating.
- Help the incontinent patient to toilet every 1 to 2 hours.
- Clean up spills in the patient's environment immediately.
- Provide adequate lighting at all times, especially at night.
- Keep the call light within reach and ensure that the patient can use it.
- Place the bed in the lowest position with the brakes locked.
- Place objects that the patient needs within reach.
- Ensure that adequate handrails are present in the patient's room, bathroom, and hall.
- Encourage family members or significant others to stay with the patient.

disease, are already taking HAART, and are beginning to have increased viral load. The safety and effectiveness of this drug in children have not yet been established.

### How Integrase Inhibitors Work

Integrase inhibitors prevent HIV infection by inhibiting the enzyme integrase, which is needed to allow insertion of viral DNA into the DNA of the human host cell. Without this action viral proteins are not made, and viral replication is inhibited. (See Figure 10-6 for where these drugs work to disrupt HIV reproduction.)

*Side Effects.* The most common side effect of raltegravir is diarrhea. Other side effects may include dizziness, headache, nausea and vomiting, and abdominal pain.

*Adverse Effects.* Adverse effects of raltegravir include anemia, hyperglycemia, and muscle pain and weakness *(rhabdomyolysis)*. Although rare, muscle problems occur more often among patients who also take other drugs that can cause rhabdomyolysis (for example, "statin" type of lipid-lowering drug).

### What To *Teach* Patients About Raltegravir

Be sure to teach patients the general care needs and precautions related to antiretroviral therapy (p. 178) in addition to these specific ones for raltegravir.

Tell patients not to crush or chew raltegravir tablets and to take the drug with food to reduce GI side effects.

Teach patients to report any persistent muscle pain or weakness to the prescriber as soon as possible.

Tell patients to report increased fatigue, paleness, and increased heart rate or shortness of breath to the prescriber. These are symptoms of anemia.

### Life Span Considerations for Raltegravir

*Pediatric Considerations.* Raltegravir is not approved for use in children under the age of 16.

*Considerations for Pregnancy and Breastfeeding.* Raltegravir is a pregnancy category C drug. It should not be used during pregnancy if the patient's viral load indicates that her traditional HAART therapy is effective.

*Considerations for Older Adults.* Older adults are more likely to be taking a "statin" type of lipid-lowering drug, which increases the risk for muscle weakness. Older adults may have loss of muscle mass and strength as a result of the aging process. These conditions increase the risk for falls. Implement the precautions listed in Box 10-3 to help reduce this risk.

◄ ⊖-Learning Activity 10-6

---

| Common Side Effects |
| --- |
| **Raltegravir** |

| Diarrhea, Nausea/ Vomiting, Abdominal pain | Dizziness | Headache |

**⚠ Drug Alert!**

**Interaction Alert**

When raltegravir is taken with any of the "statin" type of lipid-lowering drugs, muscle problems are more likely to occur.

---

## Get Ready for Practice!

### Key Points

- Viruses are tiny intracellular parasites that are not capable of self-reproduction and must infect a living cell to reproduce.
- Most common viruses have a relatively low efficiency of cellular infection and must invade the body in large numbers to cause disease.
- A retrovirus, specifically HIV, is virulent with a high efficiency of infection.
- Antiviral and antiretroviral drugs do not kill viruses; they only suppress viral reproduction and growth. They are virustatic rather than virucidal.

- Teach patients taking antiviral or antiretroviral drugs to take them exactly as prescribed and for as long as prescribed and to not stop therapy just because they feel better.
- Women should not breastfeed while taking an antiviral or antiretroviral drug.
- Ribavirin is highly teratogenic, which means that it can cause birth defects. Do not allow a pregnant or breastfeeding woman to touch ribavirin or care for a patient taking it.
- Antiretroviral therapy is most effective when given in multiple combinations of drugs known as highly active antiretroviral therapy (HAART).

- Most antiretroviral drugs have interactions with other drugs and herbals.
- Warn women that antiretroviral drugs in HAART can reduce the effectiveness of oral contraceptives. Suggest using an additional method of birth control during HAART.
- HAART drugs can cause hyperglycemia and make diabetes worse.
- Some PIs are to be taken with food, and others must be taken on an empty stomach.
- Maraviroc and raltegravir are not approved for use in children under 16 years of age.
- Maraviroc can cause severe orthostatic hypotension and increase the risk for falls. Teach patients how to prevent falls.

## Additional Learning Resources

**evolve** Go to your Evolve website (http://evolve.elsevier.com/Workman/pharmacology/) for the following FREE learning resources:
- eLearning Activities
- Animations
- Video Clips
- Interactive Review Questions
- Audio Key Points
- Audio Glossary
- Audio Glossary—Spanish-English
- Drug Dosage Calculators
- Patient Teaching Handouts

**SG** Go to your Study Guide for additional learning activities to help you master this chapter content.

## Review Questions

1. A patient is to receive ribavirin (Virazole) by aerosol inhalation. Which precaution is the most important for you to implement?
   A. Wearing gloves while preparing the drug
   B. Administering oxygen right before giving the drug
   C. Ensuring that no pregnant woman enters the room during the aerosol treatment
   D. Using sterile isopropyl alcohol to dilute the drug rather than using sterile water

2. Which question should you ask the patient before giving a first dose of amantadine (Symmetrel)?
   A. "Do you have glaucoma or prostate enlargement?"
   B. "Have you ever had an allergic reaction to a sulfa drug?"
   C. "Have you gained or lost more than 10 lbs in the past month?"
   D. "Are you taking any other drugs for heart problems or high blood pressure?"

3. A patient is prescribed valacyclovir (Valtrex) 1 g orally every 8 hours for a herpes outbreak. Which statement by the patient indicates the need for more teaching?
   A. "I will take this drug until it is gone even if my blisters go away sooner."
   B. "I will take two tablets in the morning and one tablet before I go to bed."

   C. "I will drink lots of water while I am taking this drug to prevent kidney problems."
   D. "I will be sure to abstain from sexual intercourse until I am finished taking this drug."

4. Which of these antiviral drugs should be avoided during the first trimester of pregnancy?
   A. acyclovir (Zovirax)
   B. amantadine (Symmetrel)
   C. oseltamivir (Tamiflu)
   D. zanamivir (Relenza)

5. How does raltegravir (Isentress) suppress HIV reproduction?
   A. Enters HIV and binds its RNA so tightly that the virus cannot replicate
   B. Coats the outer surface of the virus, preventing nutrients from entering and resulting in viral death
   C. Inhibits the enzyme integrase, preventing the synthesis of viral proteins needed for reproduction
   D. Prevents HIV from joining to the receptors of the host cell so the virus does not enter the host cell and use its machinery to reproduce

6. What is the most important question for you to ask a patient before administering the first dose of darunavir (Prezista)?
   A. "When did you last eat or drink?"
   B. "Do you have glaucoma or prostate enlargement?"
   C. "Have you ever had an allergic reaction to a sulfa drug?"
   D. "Have you gained or lost more than 10 lbs in the past month?"

7. A patient on HAART that includes nevirapine (Viramune) has the following side effects. For which one should the patient notify the prescriber immediately?
   A. Nausea
   B. 2-lb weight loss
   C. Clay-colored stools
   D. Dizziness on standing

8. Which antiretroviral drug is not approved for use in children?
   A. abacavir (Ziagen)
   B. saquinavir (Invirase)
   C. maraviroc (Selzentry)
   D. delavirdine (Intelence)

9. A patient is prescribed 300 mg of ribavirin oral suspension. You have ribavirin oral suspension at a concentration of 50 mg/mL. How many milliliters will you give? _____ mL

10. A patient is prescribed 45 mg of enfuvirtide by subcutaneous injection. You have a premixed solution of enfuvirtide at a concentration of 90 mg/mL. How many milliliters will you draw up and inject? _____ mL

## Critical Thinking Activities

The patient is an 8-year-old girl with HIV whose birth mother died of AIDS when the child was a toddler. She has been adopted and is doing well on HAART. She is about to go to camp for a week and has come for a required camp checkup. The camp forms request a list of all drugs that she is taking so the camp nurse can administer them. Her adopted mother asks that the information about her disease and drugs not be listed so no one at the camp will learn of the child's illness. The mother states, "Surely this won't be a problem just for a week."

1. Is the mother's concern about keeping the disease confidential realistic? Provide a rationale for this response.

2. Is there any harm in the child not receiving HAART for 1 week? Provide a rationale for this response.

3. How should you address this mother's request?

# Anti-Infectives: Antitubercular and Antifungal Drugs

℮volve

http://evolve.elsevier.com/Workman/pharmacology/

## Objectives

*After studying this chapter you should be able to:*

1. List the names, actions, usual adult dosages, possible side effects, and adverse effects of the four first-line drugs used to treat tuberculosis.
2. Describe what to do before and after giving antituberculosis drugs.
3. Explain what to teach patients taking antituberculosis drugs, including what to do, what not to do, and when to call the prescriber.
4. Describe life span considerations for antituberculosis drugs.
5. List the names, actions, usual adult dosages, possible side effects, and adverse effects of antifungal drugs.
6. Describe what do before and after giving antifungal drugs.
7. Explain what to teach patients taking antifungal drugs, including what to do, what not to do, and when to call the prescriber.
8. Describe life span considerations for antifungal drugs.

## Key Terms

**aerosol transmission** (ĂR-ō-sŏl trănz-MĬSH-ŭn) (p. 188) Transfer of bacteria-filled droplets through the air when a person with active tuberculosis coughs, laughs, sneezes, whistles, or sings.

**cavity or cavitation** (KĂV-ĭ-tē or kăv-ĭ-TĀ-shŭn) (p. 190) An area of tissue destruction and cell death caused by growth of the tuberculosis organism.

**fungicidal** (fŭn-jĭ-SĪ-dŭl) (p. 196) Having the ability to kill a fungus.

**fungistatic** (fŭn-jĭ-STĂT-ĭk) (p. 196) Having the ability to suppress fungal reproduction and growth.

**fungus** (FŬN-gĭs) (p. 195) A simple organism with one or more cells (such as yeasts, molds, and mushrooms) that reproduces by spores, has walled cells, and can live peacefully with humans or infect humans and cause disease.

**primary TB lesion** (PRĪ-măr-ē LĒ-zhŭn) (p. 188) Small pocket of tuberculosis bacteria that forms after initial infection and causes inflammation that creates an exudate.

**secondary TB** (SĔK-ŭn-dăr-ē) (p. 190) A reactivation of tuberculosis in a previously infected person whose primary lesions never completely resolved.

**tuberculosis (TB)** (tū-bŭr-kyū-LŌ-sĭs) (p. 188) A highly communicable disease caused by *Mycobacterium tuberculosis*.

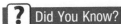 **-Learning Activity 11-1** ▶

## TUBERCULOSIS

### REVIEW OF RELATED PHYSIOLOGY AND PATHOPHYSIOLOGY

**Tuberculosis (TB)** is a highly communicable disease caused by *Mycobacterium tuberculosis*, which is a very slow–growing bacteria. TB is the most common bacterial infection worldwide. It spreads by **aerosol transmission**, which is transfer of bacteria-filled droplets through the air when a person with active TB coughs, laughs, sneezes, whistles, or sings. These droplets may then be inhaled by others (Figure 11-1). Far more people are infected with the bacteria and overcome the infection than actually develop active TB.

Once inhaled, the bacteria multiply freely when they reach a susceptible site in the lungs (bronchi or alveoli) and form a primary TB lesion. These initial or **primary TB lesions** are small pockets of tuberculosis bacteria that form after initial infection and cause inflammation that creates an exudate. The lesion is surrounded by macrophages (a type of white blood cell [WBC]), causing an inflammatory response

> **? Did You Know?**
>
> TB is the most common bacterial infection worldwide.

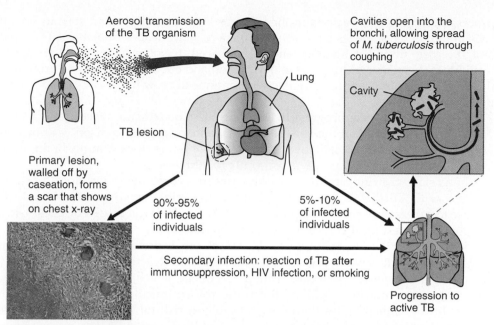

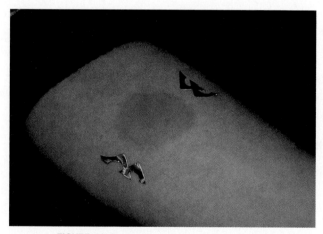

**FIGURE 11-1** Primary TB infection with progression to secondary infection and active disease. *HIV,* Human immune deficiency virus; *TB,* tuberculosis.

**FIGURE 11-2** A positive tuberculosis skin test.

known as *pneumonitis.* During this time many people who have an intact immune system develop immunity to the TB organism, and further growth of bacteria is controlled by confining it to the primary lesions. These lesions "wall off" the organism with scar tissue and WBCs, a process called *caseation* (see Figure 11-1). They usually resolve, leaving little or no residual bacteria, and may show on chest x-ray as a scar. Only a small percentage of people initially infected with the bacteria ever develop active TB.

Immune responses develop 2 to 10 weeks after the first infection with a TB organism and can be detected by a positive reaction to an intradermal TB skin test (Figure 11-2). A skin test is positive when a reddened area of 10 mm or more that is much harder than the surrounding soft tissue *(induration)* forms around the injection site. Initial infection may be so small that it does not appear on a chest x-ray. Thus most people who are exposed to TB will have a positive TB skin test but never fully develop the disease. Remember that once a TB skin test is positive, it will always be positive unless the immune system is very suppressed.

When a person is heavily exposed (often by repeated close contact with a person who has undiagnosed active TB) and has less resistance to the infection, the infection

**Memory Jogger**

A positive TB skin test means that the person has been infected with the bacteria at some point in his or her life but does not mean that he or she has active disease that can be spread to others.

process may progress. Bacteria in the primary lesions multiply and start to kill off cells in the center of the lesion, turning it into a *necrotic* (dead tissue) mass. The mass and the area around it liquefies and is destroyed, forming a cavity. A TB cavity (cavitation) is an area of lung tissue destruction and cell death caused by growth of the TB organism (see Figure 11-1). Bacteria continue to grow in the cavity and spread into new lung areas.

TB lesions also may progress by entering the bloodstream. Once in the blood, TB can spread throughout the body and damage many organs (a disorder known as *miliary TB*). Although TB can develop in any body tissue (for example, brain, liver, kidney, bone marrow), it usually affects only the lungs.

TB is slow-growing, and it may take years for symptoms to develop. A person infected with TB that is progressing beyond the initial stage cannot spread the disease to others until active symptoms occur. Active TB is diagnosed by chest x-ray, blood assay to test for the TB organism, and sputum culture.

Secondary TB is reactivation of the disease in a previously infected person whose primary lesions never completely resolved. Reactivation is more likely when immune defenses are weak. Without treatment, which includes drug therapy, rest, and proper nutrition, active TB can destroy so much lung tissue that death occurs. In the United States the people at greatest risk for development of active TB are:

- Those in constant, frequent contact with a person with active untreated TB.
- Those with immune dysfunction or human immune deficiency virus (HIV) infection.
- Those who live in crowded areas such as long-term care facilities, prisons, and mental health facilities.
- Older adults and homeless people.
- Abusers of injection drugs or alcohol.
- Lower socioeconomic groups.
- Foreign immigrants (especially from Mexico, the Philippines, and Vietnam).

**Memory Jogger**

Symptoms of active TB include a persistent productive cough, weight loss, poor appetite, night sweats, bloody sputum, shortness of breath, fever, aching chest pain that occurs with the cough, and chills.

**Clinical Pitfall**

Drug therapy will not control TB unless it is continued for at least 6 months.

**Memory Jogger**

Strict adherence to the prescribed drug regimen is crucial for controlling TB.

## TYPES OF DRUGS FOR TUBERCULOSIS

### FIRST-LINE ANTITUBERCULAR DRUGS

The risk of TB transmission is reduced after an infectious person has received first-line anti-TB drug therapy for 2 to 3 weeks and clinical improvement occurs. However, even with initial improvement, drug therapy must continue for at least 6 months to control the disease.

Because the TB organism is slow growing, many common antibacterial drugs are not effective in controlling or killing it. Combination drug therapy is the most effective method of treating TB and preventing transmission. Therapy continues until the disease is under control. The use of multidrug regimens destroys organisms as quickly as possible and reduces the emergence of drug-resistant organisms. Current first-line therapy for TB uses isoniazid, rifampin, pyrazinamide, and ethambutol in different combinations and schedules. Figure 11-3 shows the probable sites of action for these drugs. Some are now available in two- or even three-drug combinations. Variations of these first-line drugs along with other drug types are used when the patient does not tolerate the standard first-line therapy. Control of TB depends on strict adherence to drug therapy. This issue often is a problem for people who have no insurance or limited finances and for homeless people.

#### How First-Line Antitubercular Drugs Work

Figure 11-3 shows where each of the first-line TB drugs works. With the exception of ethambutol, these drugs can be either *bactericidal* (kills the bacteria) or *bacteriostatic* (only suppresses bacterial growth), depending on the drug concentration within an infected site and the susceptibility of the organism.

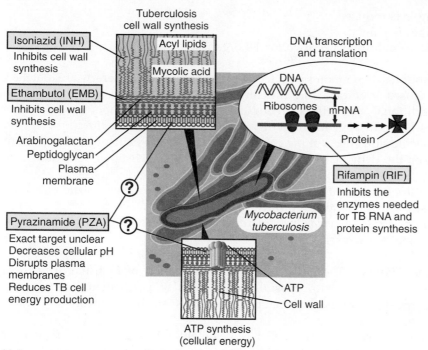

**FIGURE 11-3** Probable sites of drug activity against the TB organism. *ATP*, Adenosine triphosphate; *TB*, tuberculosis.

*Isoniazid* works by inhibiting several enzymes important to mycobacteria metabolism and reproduction. It is able to inhibit these enzymes even when TB is dormant (in an inactive state).

*Rifampin* prevents reproduction of the TB organism by binding to the enzyme that allows RNA to be transcribed from DNA. Without this enzyme, TB cannot make the proteins needed to reproduce.

*Pyrazinamide* has an unknown mechanism of action but does reduce the pH of the intracellular fluid of WBCs in which the TB bacillus resides. The lower pH inhibits TB reproduction most effectively in the early stages of the disease.

*Ethambutol* suppresses the reproduction of TB bacteria by an unknown mechanism. It is only bacteriostatic and must be used in combination with other TB drugs. It is most effective when the TB bacillus is actively dividing.

## Dosages for Common First-Line Antitubercular Drugs

| Drug | Dosage |
|------|--------|
| isoniazid (INH, Isotamine❦, Laniazid, Nydrazid, PMS-Isoniazid❦) | *Adults:* 5 mg/kg (maximum 300 mg) orally daily or 15 mg/kg (maximum 900 mg) orally twice each week<br>*Children/Infants:* 10-15 mg/kg orally once daily |
| rifampin (RIF, Rifadin, Rimactane, Rofact❦) | *Adults:* 10 mg/kg (maximum 600 mg) orally daily or twice each week<br>*Children:* 10-20 mg/kg (maximum 300 mg) orally once daily or twice each week |
| pyrazinamide (PZA, PMS-Pyrazinamide❦, Tebrazid❦) | *Adults:* 15-30 mg/kg (maximum 2 g) orally daily or 50-70 mg/kg (maximum 4 g) orally twice each week<br>*Children:* 15-30 mg/kg (maximum 2 g) orally daily |
| ethambutol (EMB, Etibi❦, Myambutol) | *Adults:* 15-25 mg/kg (maximum 2.5 g) orally daily or 50 mg/kg (maximum 4 g) orally twice each week for the first 2 months of therapy<br>*Children:* 15-25 mg/kg (maximum 2.5 g) orally daily |

### Intended Responses
- Cough is reduced.
- Sputum production is reduced.

- Fatigue is reduced.
- Weight is gained.
- Sputum culture is negative for TB organisms.

***Side Effects.*** Common side effects of first-line TB drug therapy are diarrhea, headache, nausea, vomiting, and difficulty sleeping.

Additional side effects of *isoniazid* include breast tenderness or enlargement (in men), loss of appetite, difficulty concentrating, and sore throat.

Specific side effects of *rifampin* include abdominal pain and urinary retention. In addition, the drug stains the skin, urine, tears, and all other secretions a reddish-orange color. It can also stain soft contact lenses.

Additional side effects of *pyrazinamide* include muscle aches and pains, acne, and increased sensitivity to sun or ultraviolet light.

*Pyrazinamide* and *ethambutol* increase the formation of uric acid, which can cause gout or make it worse.

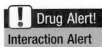 **Memory Jogger**

Peripheral neuropathy from isoniazid therapy is caused by a deficiency of the B complex vitamins and can be prevented by increasing the intake of these vitamins during drug therapy.

***Adverse Effects.*** The most common adverse effect of first-line drug therapy for TB is liver toxicity, with possible progression to permanent liver damage. This risk is greatly increased if the patient drinks alcoholic beverages while taking the drugs.

First-line drug therapy for TB has the potential to interact with many other drugs and herbal supplements. The interactions can be complex and serious.

*Isoniazid* can cause peripheral neuropathy with loss of sensation, especially in the hands and feet. This effect occurs most often in malnourished patients, those with diabetes, and alcoholics.

The intravenous (IV) form of *rifampin* contains a sulfite preservative that can cause hypersensitivity reactions in patients allergic to sulfite preservatives (which are not the same as "sulfa" drugs), such as sodium metabisulfite or potassium metabisulfite. Rifampin also may cause anemia.

*Ethambutol* at high doses can cause optic neuritis vision changes that include reduced color vision, blurred vision, and reduced visual fields. This problem can lead to blindness. When the problem is discovered early, the eye problems are usually reversed when the drug is stopped.

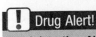 **Drug Alert!**

**Interaction Alert**

First-line anti-TB drugs interact with many drugs and herbal supplements. Before giving a TB drug, ask the patient about *all* other drugs or supplements that he or she takes; then check with the pharmacist to avoid a possible drug interaction.

**Drug Alert!**

**Administration Alert**

When giving pyrazinamide or ethambutol, have the patient drink a full glass of water to help excrete uric acid crystals faster and prevent them from precipitating in joints or the kidneys.

### What To Do *Before* Giving First-Line Antitubercular Drugs

Because of the potential interactions with many other drugs, obtain a list of all drugs the patient takes. Check with the pharmacist for possible interactions. Notify the prescriber about any identified interactions before giving TB drugs.

Because drugs for TB can lead to liver toxicity, make sure that the patient has no liver problems before starting this therapy. Check the patient's most recent laboratory values for evidence of liver problems (such as elevated liver enzymes). (Refer to Table 1-3 in Chapter 1 for a listing of normal values.)

Ask male patients whether they have an enlarged prostate. Ask all patients whether they have any problem that causes urine retention. If so, report this problem to the prescriber before giving TB drugs.

Before giving *IV rifampin*, ask whether the patient has a known allergy to sulfite preservatives. If so, notify the prescriber before giving IV rifampin.

Because rifampin can lead to anemia, check for anemia before starting this drug. Check the patient's most recent laboratory values for anemia (low red blood cell [RBC] count, low hemoglobin level). (Refer to Table 1-6 in Chapter 1 for a listing of normal values.)

Before giving *pyrazinamide* or *ethambutol*, ask whether the patient has ever had gout. If so, other precautions need to be taken. For example, the patient should drink a full glass of water with the drug and drink at least 3000 mL of water daily.

Before giving the first dose of *ethambutol*, assess the patient's vision and document your findings in the patient's chart. Use this information to determine whether vision changes are occurring during therapy.

Patients who have memory or compliance problems or who are homeless may benefit from directly observed therapy (DOT), in which the nurse or other health care provider watches the patient swallow the drugs. This practice contributes to more treatment successes, fewer relapses, and less drug resistance.

### What To Do *After* Giving First-Line Antitubercular Drugs

For IV drug forms, check the patient's vital signs and respiratory status at least every 15 minutes for the first hour. Tell the patient to immediately report any shortness of breath or change in breathing.

Check the patient daily for yellowing (*jaundice*) of the skin or sclera, which is a symptom of liver problems. The best places to check are the whites of the eyes closest to the iris, the roof of the mouth, and the chest. Avoid checking the soles of the feet or palms of the hands, especially in patients with darker skin, because these areas often normally appear yellow.

Check the complete blood count every time it is performed to determine whether RBC or platelet levels have changed. Ask whether the patient feels more tired since therapy began. In addition, check the patient's skin for increased bruising or petechiae.

If a patient has diabetes, check blood glucose levels more frequently and assess fasting blood glucose levels or levels of hemoglobin $A_{1c}$ whenever they are ordered. Report higher than normal levels to the prescriber for adjustments in the dosages of antidiabetic drugs.

Check intake and output. If a patient's urine output is 1000 mL less than he or she is drinking or if other symptoms of urinary retention are present (enlarged bladder, lower abdominal discomfort), notify the prescriber.

Urge patients to drink plenty of water throughout the day and night. Ask about any pain in the joints (especially the big toe, foot, or ankle) and check for any joint swelling.

### What To *Teach* Patients About First-Line Antitubercular Drugs

Teach patients to keep a supply of the prescribed drugs on hand at all times. Remind them that the disease is usually no longer contagious after drugs have been taken for 2 to 3 consecutive weeks and clinical improvement is seen. However, *stress that the patient must continue taking the drugs for 6 months or longer, exactly as prescribed.*

Explain that alcoholic beverages should be avoided throughout the entire drug therapy period. Many TB drugs, especially taken together, are toxic to the liver. This effect is increased by alcohol. In addition, when the patient is intoxicated, he or she is less likely to remember to take the prescribed drugs or to use precautions to prevent TB spread.

Tell patients to notify their prescriber if yellowing of the skin or eyes, darkening of the urine, or lightening of the stools develops. These problems are signs of liver toxicity.

Tell patients that TB drugs may cause nausea. To help prevent it, suggest taking the daily dose at bedtime.

Teach patients who develop loss of sensation how to prevent injury and falls. (Refer to Box 10-3 in Chapter 10.)

Teach patients with diabetes to check their blood glucose level as often as prescribed and to notify their prescriber if the level is consistently out of the target range. The prescriber may need to change the antidiabetic drug dosage, schedule, or drug type.

*Isoniazid* can raise blood pressure to dangerous levels when taken with caffeine. Teach patients taking it to avoid coffee, tea (including green tea), chocolate, colas, and any other forms of caffeinated drinks or "stay-awake" pills.

Teach patients taking *rifampin* to expect the drug to stain the skin, urine, and all other secretions. These will have a reddish-orange tinge but will be clear to normal within a few weeks after the drug is discontinued. Soft contact lenses used at this time will become permanently stained.

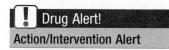

**Drug Alert!**

**Action/Intervention Alert**

Observe the patient receiving IV rifampin for signs and symptoms of sensitivity to the preservative. Check vital signs and respiratory status at least every 15 minutes for the first hour.

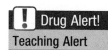

**Drug Alert!**

**Teaching Alert**

Teach all patients on TB drug therapy to avoid alcoholic beverages for the entire therapy period.

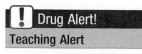

**Drug Alert!**

**Teaching Alert**

Teach patients taking isoniazid to avoid coffee, tea (including green tea), chocolate, colas, and any other forms of caffeinated drinks or "stay-awake" pills.

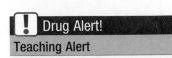

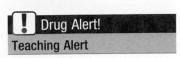

*Rifampin* decreases the effectiveness of oral contraceptives, and an unplanned pregnancy could result. Teach women using oral contraceptives to use an additional method of contraception while taking this drug and for 1 month after stopping it.

Teach patients to drink at least 8 oz of water when taking these drugs and increase fluid intake to at least 3 L of water daily. Tell them to drink water throughout the day and at least one full glass of water during the night.

A TB drug regimen increases sun sensitivity (*photosensitivity*) and can cause a severe sunburn, even among patients with darker skin. Teach patients to wear protective clothing, a hat, and sunscreen when going outdoors in the sunlight.

Remind patients taking *ethambutol* to notify their prescriber immediately if any change in vision develops. Patients who have glaucoma or cataracts should be followed by an ophthalmologist during ethambutol therapy.

Warn patients to tell all other health care providers that they are taking first-line drugs for TB because of the potential for drug interactions. Warn patients to not take any over-the-counter drug without checking with the prescriber of the TB drugs. Interactions may:

- Reduce the effectiveness of rifampin.
- Reduce the effectiveness of the other drug.
- Lead to serious and life-threatening responses (for example, cardiac dysrhythmias, seizures).

### Life Span Considerations for First-Line Antitubercular Drugs

*Pediatric Considerations.*   With the exception of ethambutol, infants and children of any age who have active TB should take first-line anti-TB drugs. Dosages for larger children and adolescents are nearly the same as for adults.

*Considerations for Pregnancy and Breastfeeding.*   First-line anti-TB drugs are approved for treatment of active TB in pregnant women. This therapy is not approved for prevention of TB during pregnancy. The risk for liver toxicity is higher when taking TB drug therapy during pregnancy, and close monitoring of liver function is needed. In addition, the pregnant woman needs higher doses of a B-complex vitamin supplement when taking isoniazid.

First-line anti-TB drugs appear in breast milk. When possible, breastfeeding should be avoided. If breastfeeding continues during TB therapy, teach the breastfeeding mother to reduce infant exposure to these drugs. (Refer to Box 1-1 in Chapter 1.) In addition, the breastfed infant should receive supplementation with B-complex vitamins.

*Considerations for Older Adults.*   The risk for liver toxicity is higher among older adults taking drugs for TB. Teach them to assess the skin and whites of the eyes daily for any sign of yellowing. Also instruct them to report persistent darkening of the urine or lightening of the stools to the prescriber.

Older adults are more likely to be taking other drugs that interact with TB drugs, especially antihypertensives, cardiac drugs, and lipid-lowering drugs. Be sure that the prescriber is aware of these other drugs and works with the pharmacist to ensure that the patient receives the appropriate dosages for the effectiveness of his or her total drug therapy.

Although gout can occur at any age, it is more common among older adults. In addition, older adults are more likely to have other health problems that require fluid restriction (such as heart failure).

Older adults may have some degree of cataract formation in one or both eyes. This condition makes visual assessment for optic neuritis more difficult. Older adults taking ethambutol should be followed monthly by an ophthalmologist during therapy.

ⓔ-Learning Activity 11-2 ▶

## FUNGAL INFECTIONS

### REVIEW OF RELATED PHYSIOLOGY AND PATHOPHYSIOLOGY

A **fungus** is a simple organism with one or more cells (such as yeasts, molds, and mushrooms) that reproduces by spores, has walled cells, and can either live peacefully with humans or infect humans and cause disease. Fungi have a thick, tough cell wall and a plasma membrane that is made of materials different from bacterial cell walls (Figure 11-4).

Fungi live in places that are moist and dark. There are more than 100,000 different kinds of fungi, some of which are harmless and can be used as food. Others can cause infection and disease.

Fungi are found almost everywhere, especially in soil. Because of their tough cell walls, they can live easily on human skin and mucous membrane surfaces and are not completely removed by usual bathing. Some types such as *Candida* are part of normal skin flora that do not cause problems unless they overgrow or enter the body. Table 11-1 lists types of fungi and the health problems they can cause.

Without treatment, fungal infections remain and can become widespread, especially in people whose immune systems are not healthy. Superficial fungal infections are uncomfortable and change the appearance and function of the infected skin area. When fungal infections enter the body by inhalation or through breaks in the skin, deep fungal infections can result. With deep fungal infection, function in the affected organ is reduced, and the organ can be destroyed.

### TYPES OF ANTIFUNGAL DRUGS

The thick fungal cell walls make fungi resistant to many anti-infective drugs. In addition, fungal DNA is similar to human DNA, and antifungal drugs often have more side effects than other types of anti-infective drugs.

#### DRUGS FOR SUPERFICIAL FUNGAL INFECTIONS

Treatment of superficial fungal infections of the skin or mucous membranes involves topical application of antifungal drugs. These are usually the same types of drugs used to treat deeper fungal infections but are prepared as creams, lotions, ointments, powders, oral lozenges, and vaginal suppositories. Topical drugs are successful at clearing fungal infections that are not severe in patients with healthy immune systems. An exception is fungal infection of the fingernails or toenails. Because the

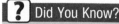 **Did You Know?**

The mushrooms on your pizza are a type of fungus.

 **Memory Jogger**

Deep fungal infections require systemic therapy. Superficial fungal infections may be cured with topical antifungal therapy.

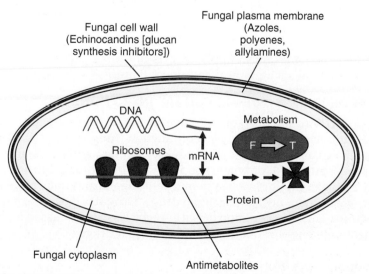

**FIGURE 11-4** Sites of antifungal drug activity. $F \rightarrow T$, metabolic conversion of folic acid to thymine.

### Table 11-1 Diseases Caused by Specific Fungal Infections

| FUNGUS | DISEASE |
|---|---|
| Aspergillus | Allergic reactions<br>Sinus infections<br>Opportunistic infections in immunocompromised patients:<br>    Deep infections of any organ<br>    Widespread or disseminated infection (aspergillosis) |
| Blastomycosis | Skin infections<br>Pneumonia and pulmonary infection<br>Opportunistic infections in immunocompromised patients:<br>    Deep infections of any organ<br>    Widespread or disseminated infection |
| Candida | "Yeast" infections, candidiasis:<br>    Vaginitis<br>    Thrush<br>    Irritated skin in skinfold areas<br>Fingernail and toenail infections<br>Opportunistic infections in immunocompromised patients:<br>    Deep infections of any organ<br>    Widespread or disseminated infection |
| Coccidioidomycosis | Pulmonary infections<br>Widespread disseminated infection (may be fatal during pregnancy)<br>Opportunistic infections |
| Cryptococcosis | Skin infections<br>Pneumonia<br>Meningitis<br>Opportunistic infections |
| Dermatomycosis (Tinea) | Ringworm infections:<br>    Tinea capitis (scalp)<br>    Tinea corporis (body)<br>    Tinea cruris (groin, "jock itch")<br>    Tinea manus (hand)<br>    Tinea pedis (athlete's foot)<br>    Tinea unguium (fingernails, toenails) |
| Histoplasma | Histoplasmosis:<br>    Pulmonary infections<br>    Eye infections<br>Opportunistic infections in immunocompromised patients:<br>    Deep infections of any organ<br>    Widespread or disseminated infection |

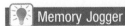

**Memory Jogger**

Superficial fungal infections of the skin or mucous membranes are treated with topical application of antifungal drugs.

**Memory Jogger**

The major classes of antifungal drugs are:
- Azoles.
- Polyenes.
- Allylamines.
- Antimetabolites.
- Echinocandins.

fungus is under the nail, topical application is not often successful. Box 11-1 lists points to teach patients using topical antifungal therapy.

## DRUGS FOR DEEP OR SYSTEMIC FUNGAL INFECTIONS

When fungal infections are deep or extensive, systemic drugs are needed to kill the fungi (fungistatic action) or slow their reproduction (fungistatic action). The classes of antifungal drugs are the azoles, polyenes, allylamines, antimetabolites, and echinocandins. (See Figure 11-4 for where specific types of antifungal drugs work to kill or disrupt the growth of fungi.) All systemic antifungal drugs have more side effects and adverse effects than most antibacterial drugs. Drug dosages vary, depending on infection severity. The most common drugs in each class are discussed in this chapter. Consult a drug reference for other specific antifungal drugs.

### How Antifungal Drugs Work

To reproduce and live, fungal cells must keep their plasma membranes and cell walls intact. Membranes are made up of phospholipids and ergosterol as shown in

| Box 11-1 | Patient Teaching Tips for Topical Antifungal Agents |

**GENERAL**
- Report any indication of an allergic reaction (new redness, swelling, blisters, or drainage) to the prescriber.
- Immediately after applying the drug, wash your hands to remove all traces of it.
- Avoid getting any antifungal drug in your eye. If the drug does get into your eye, wash the eye with large amounts of warm, running tap water and notify the prescriber.
- Use the drug exactly as prescribed and for as long as prescribed to ensure that the infection is cured.

**POWDERS**
- Ensure that the skin area is clean and completely dry before applying the powder.
- Hold your breath while applying to prevent inhaling the drug.
- For the foot area, be sure to apply the powder between and under your toes. Wear clean cotton socks (night and day). Change the socks at least twice daily.
- For the groin area, wear clean, close-fitting (but not tight) cotton underwear (briefs or panties).

**SKIN CREAMS, LOTIONS, OINTMENTS**
- Ensure that the skin area is clean and dry before applying the drug.
- Be careful to apply it only to the skin that has the infection. Keep it away from the surrounding skin.
- Apply a thin coating as often as prescribed.
- Wash and dry the area right before reapplying the next dose.
- Loosely cover the area to prevent spreading the drug to other body areas, clothing, or furniture.

**ORAL LOZENGES**
- Brush your teeth and tongue before using the tablet or troche.
- Let the tablet or troche completely dissolve in your mouth.
- Clean your toothbrush daily by running it through the dishwasher or soaking it in a solution of 1 part household bleach with 9 parts water. After using bleach, rinse the toothbrush thoroughly.

**VAGINAL CREAMS OR SUPPOSITORIES**
- Place creams or suppositories just before going to bed to help keep them within the vagina longer.
- Wash your hands before inserting the drug.
- Insert the suppository (rounded end first) into the vagina as far as you can with your finger.
- Insert a full applicator of the cream as far into the vagina as is comfortable.
- Wash the applicator and your hands with warm, soapy water; rinse well; and dry.
- A sanitary napkin can be worn to protect your clothing and the bed from drug leakage.
- Avoid sexual intercourse during the treatment period. If you do have intercourse, the drug can create holes in a condom or damage a diaphragm and increase your risk for an unplanned pregnancy. In addition, you could spread the infection or become reinfected.
- Use the drug on consecutive days for as long as prescribed.

Figure 11-5. Ergosterol is a fat (lipid) similar to the cholesterol that is part of human cell plasma membranes. The azoles, polyenes, and allylamines either prevent the fungus from making ergosterol or bind to the ergosterol and prevent it from being properly placed in the fungal membrane. As a result, the fungal membranes are leaky and damage the fungus and prevent its reproduction. In some cases the membranes can leak so much that enough changes take place inside the fungal cell to kill the fungus (drug is fungicidal).

*Antimetabolites* work by entering the fungal cell and acting as a "counterfeit" DNA base. When flucytosine is part of fungal cell DNA, it prevents fungal proteins needed for reproduction and growth from being made.

The *echinocandins* are also called *glucan synthesis inhibitors*. Fungi have a tough cell wall for protection (see Figure 11-4) that is different from the plasma

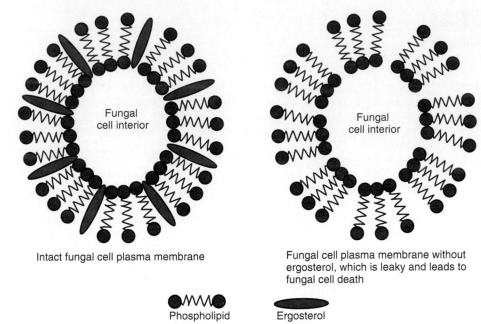

Intact fungal cell plasma membrane

Fungal cell plasma membrane without ergosterol, which is leaky and leads to fungal cell death

Phospholipid          Ergosterol

**FIGURE 11-5** Intact fungal cell plasma membrane (left) and the effects of azoles, polyenes, and allylamines on fungal cell membranes (right).

membrane. This wall is made up of many substances that serve as "bricks" in the cell wall; glucan, which serves as "mortar" in the cell wall, holds the bricks tightly in place. Echinocandins stop fungal production of glucan so the mortar is thin and weak. This makes the entire fungal cell wall weak and not able to protect the fungal cell.

## Dosages for Common Antifungal Drugs

| Drug | Dosage |
|------|--------|
| *Azoles* | |
| fluconazole (Diflucan) | *Adults:* 200-400 mg orally or 200-800 mg IV daily<br>*Children:* 6-12 mg/kg orally or IV daily |
| ketoconazole (Extina, Nizoral) | *Adults:* 200-400 mg orally once daily<br>*Children:* 3.3-6.6 mg/kg orally once daily |
| posaconazole (Noxafil) | *Adults:* 400 mg orally twice or 200 mg 3 times daily<br>*Children:* Safe and effective use not established |
| voriconazole (Vfend) | *Adults/Children:* 6-12 mg/kg IV loading dose, then<br>    4 mg IV every 12 hr; 200-400 mg orally every 12 hr |
| *Polyenes* | |
| amphotericin B "classic" ❶<br>    (Amphocin, Fungizone) | *Adults/Children:* Dosage varies with type of infection,<br>    seriousness of infection, and patient tolerance;<br>    IV dosage not to exceed 1.5 mg/kg daily |
| amphotericin B lipid<br>    formulations ❶ (Abelcet,<br>    AmBisome, Amphotec) | *Adults/Children:* Dosage varies with type of infection,<br>    seriousness of infection, and patient tolerance;<br>    IV dosage not to exceed 4-6 mg/kg daily |
| *Allylamines* | |
| terbinafine (Lamisil) | *Adults/Children over 35 kg:* 250 mg orally daily<br>*Children 25 to 35 kg:* 187.5 mg orally daily<br>*Children less than 25 kg:* 125-mg oral granules |
| *Antimetabolites* | |
| flucytosine (Ancobon) | *Adults/Children:* 12.5-40 mg/kg orally every 6 hr |
| *Echinocandins* | |
| anidulafungin (Eraxis) | *Adults:* 200 mg IV loading dose; then 100 mg IV daily<br>*Children:* 1.5 mg/kg IV loading dose, then 0.75 mg/<br>    kg IV daily |

⇄ **Do Not Confuse**

**Lamisil** *with* **Lamictal**

An order for Lamisil can be confused with Lamictal. Lamisil is an antifungal drug, whereas Lamictal is an anticonvulsant prescribed for seizure disorders and certain psychiatric problems.

## Dosages for Common Antifungal Drugs—cont'd

| Drug | Dosage |
|------|--------|
| caspofungin (Cancidas) | *Adults:* 70 mg IV loading dose, then 50 mg IV daily<br>*Children:* 70 mg/m² IV loading dose; then 50 mg/m²<br>IV daily |
| micafungin (Mycamine) | *Adults:* 50 mg IV daily (prophylaxis); 100-150 mg IV<br>daily (treatment) |

❶ High-alert drug.

***Intended Responses.***   The intended response to successful antifungal drug therapy is the eradication of the infection and normal function of all tissues and organs.

***Side Effects.***   Common side effects of most antifungal drugs are changes in how food tastes, diarrhea, headache, nausea, and vomiting. Many patients taking a drug for several weeks report hair thinning. Drugs given intravenously may cause pain and redness at the injection site. Ketoconazole and voriconazole increase sun sensitivity and can lead to a severe sunburn.

***Adverse Effects.***   Antifungal drugs have many possible adverse effects, including anemia, liver toxicity, low serum potassium levels *(hypokalemia),* severe rashes, abnormal heart rhythms, and reduced kidney function. Most occur only at high doses or in patients with other health problems.

Skin irritation and rashes can occur with systemic antifungal therapy. Rashes may be severe with many types of lesions *(Stevens-Johnson syndrome).* If the rashes become widespread with crusting, fever, and tissue necrosis, the condition can be life threatening.

Antifungal drugs have the potential to interact with many other drugs and herbal supplements. These interactions can be complex and serious.

*Terbinafine* (Lamisil) and *flucytosine* (Ancobon) can reduce WBC counts and increase the risk for infection.

The *azoles* and *amphotericin B* are all excreted by the kidney and can cause renal insufficiency. When renal insufficiency is present, the drugs are retained longer and are then more likely to cause additional severe side effects and adverse effects. If the patient is being treated with an additional drug that also impairs the kidney, the risk for kidney damage increases.

*Flucytosine* (Ancobon) and the *echinocandins* can cause peripheral neuropathy with loss of sensation. The degree of sensation loss is related to how long the nerve-damaging drugs are used. It is not known if the loss is reversible over time after therapy is stopped.

At very high doses the *azoles* may cause cardiac dysrhythmias, especially prolonged QT and torsades de pointes, a condition of unusual ventricular tachycardia. In addition, the drugs can interfere with cardiac drugs that are prescribed to control abnormal heart rhythms.

The *echinocandins* can increase the rate of clot formation, which increases the risk for deep vein thrombosis (DVT). DVT is most likely to occur in veins of the lower legs and pelvis. Symptoms of DVT in an extremity include swelling, warmth, and pain or discomfort.

*Amphotericin B* has more adverse reactions than other antifungal drugs. For this reason systemic therapy with amphotericin B is used only for serious, life-threatening fungal infections. Common adverse effects of systemic amphotericin B include fever and chills that are so severe that this drug has been nicknamed "shake and bake." The drug dilates blood vessels, causing widespread skin flushing (known as *red man syndrome*). Hypotension and shock may occur as a result of blood vessel dilation. In addition, allergic reactions are possible, including anaphylaxis. Amphotericin B has a long half-life (15 days), and adverse effects may be present for weeks to months after the drug has been stopped.

**Common Side Effects**

**Antifungal Drugs**

Taste changes,   Headache   Hair loss
Diarrhea,
Nausea/
Vomiting

 **Memory Jogger**

Antifungal drugs should be used with caution in patients who have kidney failure, liver disease, heart failure, or severe dysrhythmias.

**Memory Jogger**

Amphotericin B causes renal insufficiency in *all* patients receiving it.

 **Memory Jogger**

All patients receiving amphotericin B develop side effects, and most develop serious adverse effects. Monitor these patients very carefully because they are very sick.

## What To Do *Before* Giving Antifungal Drugs

Because of potential interactions with many other drugs, obtain a list of all other drugs the patient takes. Check with the pharmacist for possible interactions and the need to consult with the prescriber about dosage changes.

Because antifungal drugs may cause anemia and liver toxicity, make sure that the patient is not anemic and has no liver problems before starting these drugs. Check the patient's most recent laboratory values for anemia (low RBC count, low hemoglobin level) and liver problems (elevated liver enzyme levels). (Refer to Table 1-6 and Table 1-3 in Chapter 1 for a listing of normal values.)

Check the patient's current laboratory work, especially blood urea nitrogen (BUN) and serum creatinine levels, because these drugs can cause kidney impairment. (Refer to Table 1-5 in Chapter 1 for a listing of normal values.) If these values are higher than normal before starting the drug, the risk for kidney damage is greater. Use these values as a baseline to determine whether the patient develops any kidney problems while taking an antifungal drug.

Some of the antifungal drugs should be taken with meals, whereas others should be taken on an empty stomach. Carefully plan the dosing schedule around meals. If a drug is to be taken with a meal, consider the time when meals are brought to the unit. If a drug is to be taken on an empty stomach, make sure that it is given 1 hour before or at least 2 hours after a meal.

The activity of *azole* antifungal drugs can be reduced by grapefruit juice in large quantities. Do not administer an azole with grapefruit juice and limit the patient's grapefruit juice intake to no more than 24 oz per day. In addition, *ketoconazole* should not be given with drugs that reduce gastric acid such as proton pump inhibitors or histamine blockers because the drug is activated by stomach acids.

For *amphotericin B*, a test dose (1 mg IV over 20 to 30 minutes) is recommended because hypersensitivity is common. Check and recheck the exact dose to be administered each time the drug is given. Usually the first dose of amphotericin B is much smaller than the daily maintenance doses. After the first dose the drug is given either daily or every other day using gradually increasing doses.

Many health care providers prescribe premedication with specific drugs to counteract the side effects of amphotericin B. These drugs may include acetaminophen or ibuprofen to prevent or reduce fever, antihistamines (for example, diphenhydramine), IV corticosteroids (for example, hydrocortisone) to reduce blood vessel dilation, and meperidine (Demerol) to reduce or prevent excessive chills and shaking (*rigors*). Check the order to determine whether these drugs should be given in advance, and administer them at the appropriate time.

Parenteral amphotericin B must be used as soon as it is mixed. Administer the drug *slowly*, regardless of the dose.

## What To Do *After* Giving Antifungal Drugs

When giving the first IV dose of an antifungal drug, check the patient every 15 minutes for any signs or symptoms of an allergic reaction (hives at the IV site, low blood pressure, rapid irregular pulse, swelling of the lips or lower face, the patient feeling a lump in the throat). If the patient is having an anaphylactic reaction, your first action is to prevent any more drug from entering him or her. Stop the drug from infusing but keep the IV access. If the drug is infusing high into the IV tubing, change the tubing after stopping the drug and do not let any drug left in the tubing run into the patient.

Check the patient's skin every shift for rash, blisters, or other skin eruption that may indicate a reaction to the drug. Ask the patient about any itching or skin changes.

Check the patient daily for yellowing (*jaundice*) of the skin or sclera, which is a symptom of liver problems. The best places to check are the whites of the eyes closest to the iris, the roof of the mouth, and the skin of the chest. Avoid checking the soles of the feet or palms of the hands, especially in patients with darker skin, because these areas often appear yellow even when the patient is not jaundiced.

Check the patient's apical pulse for a full minute at least twice daily. Check whether there is a change in heart rate or regularity, document any changes, and notify the prescriber.

Check the patient's laboratory values, especially WBC counts, RBC counts, platelets, blood hematocrit, hemoglobin, BUN, creatinine, and potassium levels, every time they are taken. Compare these values with those obtained before drug therapy was started. If the potassium level is lower than 3.5 mEq/L (3.5 mmol/L) or if kidney function test values are rising, notify the prescriber. Examine the patient's intake and output record daily to determine if urine output is within 500 mL of the total fluid intake. Notify the prescriber if the WBC, RBC, or platelet counts are low.

With *terbinafine* or *flucytosine*, check the patient every shift for any signs of a new infection (for example, the presence of fever, drainage, foul-smelling urine, productive cough, or redness around an open skin area) and report any symptoms to the prescriber.

With *echinocandins*, check the patient's calves daily for signs of DVT (swelling, warmth, and pain or discomfort). If present, check the opposite calf and notify the prescriber. Do not massage any part of the legs. Urge the patient to perform calf-pumping exercises and to avoid keeping the legs in a position with either the knees or hips bent (flexed). Also urge him or her to drink at least 3 L of water daily unless another health problem requires fluid restriction.

With *amphotericin B*, check the patient's blood pressure at least every hour while the drug is infusing because the drug causes blood vessel dilation with hypotension. This can become severe enough to induce shock. Check for other symptoms of shock (pulse oximetry reading below 90%, rapid heart rate, rapid and shallow respirations, decreased urine output, change in level of consciousness). If shock symptoms are present or if blood pressure drops more than 15 mm Hg below the patient's normal level, call the Rapid Response Team and notify the prescriber immediately.

Expected side effects that usually occur during (or shortly after) the infusion with conventional IV amphotericin B include headache, chills, fever, rigors, flushing, hypotension, nausea, and vomiting. *Unlike other parenteral drugs, further slowing of the IV rate does not prevent these effects.* Assess the patient hourly for these side effects. Administer drugs as prescribed to reduce them. Even if these effects occur, it is important to attempt to administer the entire prescribed dose of amphotericin B because the infection is often life threatening.

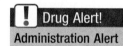

**Drug Alert!**

**Administration Alert**

Check the IV site during amphotericin B administration at least every 2 hours for a change in blood return, any redness or pain, or the feeling of hard or "cordlike" veins above the site. If such problems occur, follow the policy of your facility about removing the IV access.

## What To *Teach* Patients About Antifungal Drugs

Warn patients taking antifungal drugs to tell all other health care providers that they are taking them because of the potential for drug interactions. Also warn patients to not take any over-the-counter drugs without consulting the prescriber of the antifungal drug. Interactions may:

- Reduce the effectiveness of the antifungal drug.
- Reduce the effectiveness of the other drug.
- Lead to serious and life-threatening responses.

Work with patients to make sure that they understand whether the drug is to be taken with a meal or on an empty stomach. Remind patients to avoid or minimize drinking grapefruit juice while taking an azole.

Teach patients to check their pulse for irregularities. Remind them to report new irregularities, rates faster than 100 beats per minute at rest, or rates slower than 50 beats to their prescriber.

Tell patients to notify their prescriber if they develop yellowing of the skin or eyes, darkening of the urine, or lightening of the stools. These problems are signs of liver toxicity.

Tell patients to check weekly for increased fatigue, paleness, and increased heart rate or shortness of breath. These are symptoms of anemia and should be reported to their prescriber.

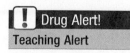

**Drug Alert!**

**Teaching Alert**

Teach patients taking an azole to check their pulse daily and to report new irregularities, rates faster than 100, or rates lower than 50 to the prescriber.

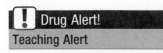

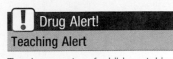

Teach patients to check their entire skin surface at least once daily for any rashes, blisters, or other skin changes. If skin changes occur, patients should notify their prescriber immediately.

Teach patients taking either *ketoconazole* or *voriconazole* to avoid direct sunlight, use sunscreen, and wear protective clothing (including a hat) whenever they are in the sun to prevent a severe sunburn. In addition, tell them to avoid tanning beds and salons.

Teach patients taking *terbinafine* or *flucytosine* for more than 1 week to avoid crowds and people who are ill because resistance to infection is now decreased. Also remind them to notify their prescriber at the first sign of an infection.

### Life Span Considerations for Antifungal Drugs

***Pediatric Considerations.***    The safety and effectiveness of many systemic antifungal drugs have not been established. However, they are used cautiously in infants and children with severe fungal infections.

Children are prescribed terbinafine for ringworm of the scalp. Terbinafine is provided as granules that are packaged in single-dose packets to be sprinkled on a spoonful of pudding or other soft, nonacidic food. Tell the child to swallow the entire spoonful without chewing.

The risk for low platelet counts and bleeding appears to be increased in infants receiving flucytosine.

***Considerations for Pregnancy and Breastfeeding.***    Antifungal drugs are not recommended during pregnancy unless the fungal infection is serious or life threatening. Breastfeeding is not recommended during antifungal therapy.

***Considerations for Older Adults.***    Older adults are more likely to have some degree of renal insufficiency and can develop kidney problems more quickly while taking antifungal drugs. Maintain strict intake and output records for the older adult. If daily urine output drops to less than 1 L, notify the prescriber immediately.

Older adults are more likely to be taking other drugs that could interact with antifungal drugs, especially cardiac drugs and warfarin (Coumadin). Remind patients to tell all health care providers about all drugs they are taking. Also teach older adults how to check their pulse for irregularities. Remind them to report new irregularities to their prescriber.

The risk for drug-induced liver toxicity is higher among older adults. Teach these patients to check the skin and whites of the eyes daily for any sign of yellowing. Also instruct them to report persistent darkening of the urine or lightening of the stools to their prescriber.

With *amphotericin B,* older adults may develop neurologic reactions more often. These reactions include abnormal thinking, agitation, anxiety, cerebral vascular accident, coma, confusion, depression, blurred vision, dizziness, drowsiness, hallucinations, hearing loss, and peripheral neuropathy. Assess older adults every shift for the presence of any of these changes.

With *echinocandins,* older adults are at greater risk for DVT. Apply antiembolism stockings or venous sequential compression devices as prescribed. Assist patients in passive or active range-of-motion exercises for the legs and calf-pumping exercises. If the patient's condition permits, assist him or her to get out of bed and ambulate several times daily. Administer anticoagulants as prescribed and encourage patients to drink plenty of water. Assess patients daily for swelling, pain, or tenderness in the lower legs. Document positive findings and notify the prescriber.

ℰ-Learning Activity 11-3 ►

# Get Ready for Practice!

## Key Points

- TB is spread by the airborne route, which allows droplets containing the bacteria to be exhaled when a person with active TB coughs, laughs, sneezes, whistles, or sings.
- For active TB to be controlled, the patient must adhere to combination anti-TB therapy for at least 6 months, even when symptoms are no longer present.
- A positive TB skin test never becomes negative again, even after treatment has successfully controlled or eradicated the TB organism.
- All first-line drugs for TB can cause liver toxicity.
- All systemic antifungal drugs have more side effects and adverse effects than most antibacterial drugs.
- The most common adverse effect of antifungal therapy is anemia.
- Amphotericin B and the echinocandins are IV drugs that are usually given only in the in-patient setting. Patients receiving these drugs are usually very ill.
- Teach patients to limit intake of grapefruit juice to less than 24 oz daily while taking an azole and to not take the drug with grapefruit juice.
- Treatment with systemic amphotericin B is reserved for severe or life-threatening fungal infections.
- Amphotericin B has a long half-life (15 days), which means that side effects and adverse effects may be present for days to weeks after the drug has been stopped.
- Premedication may be prescribed before administration of amphotericin B to counteract the side effects of the drug.
- Do not administer amphotericin B at the same time as any blood product because the expected side effects of the drug may mask a transfusion reaction.

## Additional Learning Resources

**evolve** Go to your Evolve website (http://evolve.elsevier.com/Workman/pharmacology/) for the following FREE learning resources:
- eLearning Activities
- Animations
- Video Clips
- Interactive Review Questions
- Audio Key Points
- Audio Glossary
- Audio Glossary—Spanish-English
- Drug Dosage Calculators
- Patient Teaching Handouts

**SG** Go to your Study Guide for additional learning activities to help you master this chapter content.

## Review Questions

1. Which side effect is common to all the first-line antitubercular drugs?
   - A. Liver toxicity
   - B. Blurred vision
   - C. Reddish-orange urine
   - D. Excessive daytime drowsiness

2. You are about to give the first IV dose of rifampin (RIF, Rifadin, Rimactane) to the patient. Which action is *most important* to perform before administering the drug?
   - A. Obtaining an accurate weight and blood pressure
   - B. Checking the patient's most recent liver enzyme and bilirubin levels
   - C. Asking whether the patient has a known allergy to sulfite preservatives
   - D. Asking how recently the patient has used either St. John's wort or green tea

3. Which precaution is *most important* to teach a patient who has been prescribed the four first-line anti-TB drugs?
   - A. "Do not drive or operate heavy machinery while taking these drugs."
   - B. "Take these drugs at night to prevent nausea and vomiting."
   - C. "Do not drink alcoholic beverages while on these drugs."
   - D. "Be sure to take these drugs with food."

4. A 78-year-old patient who is prescribed pyrazinamide and ethambutol (Myambutol) for active TB also has gout. What adjustments will the patient's condition require?
   - A. Gout is not affected by TB drug therapy, and no adjustments are needed.
   - B. The prescribed therapy will improve gout and reduce the need for drug therapy to treat gout.
   - C. The prescribed therapy increases the risk for gout attacks, and the patient should increase his or her intake of water.
   - D. The drugs for treatment of gout interact with the drugs for TB, and the patient must not take the gout drugs within 2 hours of taking the TB drugs.

5. Which antifungal drug causes some degree of renal insufficiency in *everyone* who receives it?
   - A. amphotericin B (Amphocin)
   - B. terbinafine (Lamisil)
   - C. caspofungin (Cancidas)
   - D. fluconazole (Diflucan)

6. Which laboratory value in a 76-year-old woman on systemic fluconazole (Diflucan) therapy will you report immediately to the prescriber?
   - A. Hematocrit of 38%
   - B. Bilirubin of 0.4 mg/dL
   - C. Potassium of 2.2 mEq/L
   - D. Blood urea nitrogen (BUN) of 12.2 mg/dL

7. A patient is taking ketoconazole (Nizoral) for prevention of a fungal infection after a bone marrow transplant. Which statement made by the patient indicates the need for more teaching?
   - A. "I will stop taking the drug if I should become pregnant."
   - B. "I will stay in the sun as much as possible to avoid catching an infection."

C. "I will avoid drinking alcoholic beverages during the time I am on this therapy."

D. "If I miss a dose, I will take it as soon as I remember it and not wait until the next day."

8. Which specific action is most important to perform for an older adult who is receiving antifungal therapy with an echinocandin?

   A. Testing the blood glucose level more frequently

   B. Removing dentures before administering the oral solution

   C. Administering the drug with a meal to prevent nausea and vomiting

   D. Assessing the calves daily for pain, swelling, warmth, and tenderness

9. A patient who weighs 100 kg is prescribed 15 mg/kg of ethambutol (EMB, Myambutol) daily. The ethambutol tablets contain 100 mg of the drug. How many milligrams per day will be given to the patient? How many tablets will be given to the patient?

   A. _____ mg/day

   B. _____ tablet(s)

10. A patient is to receive 200 mg of fluconazole (Diflucan) by IV piggyback over the next hour. The piggyback bag containing the fluconazole has a total of 60 mL of fluid, and the drop factor of the administration set is 20 gtts/mL. How many drops per minute ensure that 200 mg of fluconazole is delivered in 1 hour? _____ drops/min

## Critical Thinking Activities

The patient is a 62-year-old nurse who works at a prison clinic/hospital. She has type 2 diabetes, hypertension, and a gastric ulcer. Her usual prescribed drugs include losartan (Cozaar), omeprazole (Prilosec), and metformin (Glucophage). She is confirmed to have active TB. Her prescribed drug regimen for the first 2 months includes:

Isoniazid (Nydrazid) 250 mg PO daily
Rifampin (Rifadin) 500 mg PO daily
Pyrazinamide 750 mg PO daily
Ethambutol (Myambutol) 750 mg PO daily

1. Are there any issues or special considerations for the prescribed TB drug therapy and the patient's other drug regimen?

2. Is this patient a candidate for directly observed therapy (DOT)? Why or why not?

# Drugs That Affect Urine Output

## Objectives

*After studying this chapter you should be able to:*

1. List the common names, actions, usual adult dosages, possible side effects, and adverse effects of diuretic drugs.
2. Describe what to do before and after giving diuretic drugs.
3. Explain what to teach patients taking diuretic drugs, including what to do, what not to do, and when to call the prescriber.
4. Describe life span considerations for diuretic drugs.
5. List the common names, actions, usual adult dosages, possible side effects, and adverse effects

6. of drugs for overactive bladder and benign prostatic hyperplasia.
6. Describe what to do before and after giving drugs for overactive bladder and benign prostatic hyperplasia.
7. Explain what to teach patients taking drugs for overactive bladder and benign prostatic hyperplasia, including what to do, what not to do, and when to call the prescriber.
8. Describe life span considerations for drugs for overactive bladder and benign prostatic hyperplasia.

## Key Terms

**androgens** (ĂN-drō-jěnz) (p. 217) The group of male sex hormones that includes testosterone.

**benign prostatic hyperplasia (BPH)** (bě-NĪN prō-STĂT-ĭk hī-pŭr-PLĂ-zhě) (p. 217) Enlargement of the prostate gland caused by an increased number of cells in the gland. Formerly known as benign prostatic hypertrophy.

**detrusor muscle** (dē-TRŪ-zŭr MŬS-ŭl) (p. 214) The layer of involuntary muscle in the bladder wall; during urination it contracts to squeeze urine out of the bladder into the urethra.

**diuretics** (dī-ŭr-ĔT-ĭks) (p. 205) Drugs that help rid the body of excess water and salt (sodium).

**excretion** (ěks-KRĒ-shŭn) (p. 206) A general term for removal of substances from the body.

**loop diuretic** (LŪP dī-ŭr-ĔT-ĭk) (p. 210) Diuretic that acts on the ascending loop of Henle in the kidney. It is used primarily to treat hypertension and edema often caused by congestive heart failure or renal insufficiency.

**natriuretic diuretic** (nă-trē-yŭ-RĒ-tĭk dī-ŭr-ĔT-ĭk) (p. 208) Diuretic that causes the excretion of sodium and water in the urine.

**nephron** (NĚF-rŏn) (p. 206) The filtering unit of the kidney.

**nocturia** (nŏk-TŪR-ē-ă) (p. 218) Increased urination at night.

**overactive bladder (OAB)** (ō-vŭr-ĂK-tĭv BLĂ-dŭr) (p. 214) A problem with bladder function that causes a sudden urge to urinate and can even lead to the involuntary loss of urine (incontinence).

**potassium-sparing diuretic** (pō-TĂS-ē-ŭm SPĂR-ĭng dī-ŭr-ĔT-ĭk) (p. 213) A drug that blocks exchange of sodium for potassium and hydrogen ions in the distal tubule, leading to increased sodium and chloride excretion without increased potassium excretion.

**prostate gland** (PRŎS-tāt GLĂND) (p. 217) A walnut-size male sex gland that surrounds the upper part of the urethra and secretes substances into seminal fluid.

**renal tubules** (RĒ-nŭl TŪB-yŭlz) (p. 206) Microscopic chemical factories in the kidneys that manufacture urine from filtered blood serum while also conserving essential nutrients and other substances.

**thiazide diuretic** (THĪ-ŭ-zīd dī-ŭr-ĔT-ĭk) (p. 208) A drug that slows down or turns off the salt pumps in the nephron tube furthest away from the capillaries and causes more sodium, potassium, and water to stay in the urine and leave the body through urination. It is used primarily in the treatment of hypertension.

◀ ⊖-Learning Activity 12-1

## DIURETICS

Diuretics are drugs that help rid the body of excess water and sodium by increasing a person's urine output. People often call these drugs "water pills" because they cause the body to lose water. Diuretics may work on the kidneys directly, or they may increase blood flow to the kidney. Either way, these drugs cause a person to urinate more and lose water from the body.

## REVIEW OF RELATED PHYSIOLOGY AND PATHOPHYSIOLOGY

Urine is made from the blood. Blood travels to the kidney where there are millions of small tubes called **nephrons**, which are the filtering units of the kidneys (Figure 12-1). Each nephron has a collection of capillaries at the beginning of the nephron. Whole blood flows into these capillaries, which are leaky to water and small particles such as sugar, salt (sodium), potassium and chloride but do not leak cells, proteins, and large particles. When whole blood goes through capillaries, the water and small particles leave the capillaries and go into the nephrons. The blood cells, proteins, and large particles go directly back into the blood.

The purpose of the nephrons is to act like a "washing machine" and take out all the waste products (such as urea and ammonia) and extra water, sodium, and potassium, keeping the blood "clean." In healthy kidneys about 100 mL (3 to 4 oz) of water (and small particles) enters the nephron tubules each minute. If nothing happened to this 100 mL of water, everyone would have a urine output of 6000 mL (6 qt or 6 L) every hour, which is too much water for the body to lose. To prevent this much water from being lost along with the waste products, places along the nephron tube **(renal tubules)** draw out most of the water and the helpful particles but keep the waste products in the urine. The cleaned water and helpful particles are put back into the blood by *reabsorption*. The waste products and excess sodium and potassium stay in the urine along with just enough water to allow them to be urinated out from the body **(excretion)**. In this way a person loses waste products and excess particles without losing too much water.

The places in the nephron tubes that allow water, sodium, and potassium to be pulled out from the urine and put back into the blood have special "pumps" that remove the sodium and potassium. Because of the rule "where sodium goes, water follows," the pulling of sodium from the urine pulls water along with it. This process allows us to make only about 1 mL of urine each minute. The urine collects in the bladder until it is ready to be eliminated through urination. Most people have a urine output of about 2400 mL (nearly 2.5 quarts) each day. The amount of urine output increases when a person's fluid intake increases and decreases when fluid intake

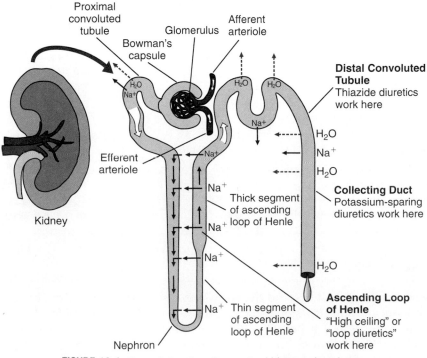

**FIGURE 12-1** Sites of diuretic action on the kidney and nephrons.

decreases. To clean the blood properly, a person needs to take in enough fluid to ensure that he or she urinates at least 400 mL each day.

Since the action of diuretics leads to increased urine output, patients taking these drugs are at increased risk for *dehydration,* a condition caused by the loss of too much water from the body. Signs and symptoms of dehydration to watch for include:

- Increased pulse rate with a "thready" pulse that may be hard to feel.
- Low blood pressure (hypotension).
- Thirst.
- Sunken appearance to the eyeballs.
- Dry mouth with thick, sticky coating on tongue.
- Skin "tenting" on the forehead or chest (gently pinch up a section of skin on the forehead or chest, release it, and see how long it takes for the "tent" you made to go away).
- Constipation.
- Decreased urine output (less than 30 mL/hr) with urine that is dark and strong smelling.

Diuretics are used most often to treat problems when the body is retaining too much water, too much sodium, or too much potassium. They are often prescribed for people who have the following health problems:

- High blood pressure (hypertension)
- Heart failure
- Kidney disease
- Liver disease (cirrhosis)

## GENERAL ISSUES IN DIURETIC THERAPY

There are several classes of diuretic drugs that have different, as well as common, actions and effects. Nursing responsibilities for these common actions and effects are listed in the following paragraphs. Specific nursing responsibilities are listed in the discussions of each individual class of diuretics.

*Before giving any diuretic drug,* always obtain a complete list of drugs that the patient is currently taking, including over-the-counter and herbal preparations. Obtain baselines for weight, blood pressure, and heart rate for comparison after giving a diuretic drug. If blood pressure is low (less than 90/60 mm Hg), ask the prescriber if the patient should receive the drug. Also check the latest set of blood electrolyte levels and notify the prescriber of any abnormal values. Ask patients about their usual urine output pattern.

Make certain that the patient does not have a problem with a blockage in any area of the urinary system (for example, an enlarged prostate that interferes with urine flow). Giving diuretics to a person with a blockage can cause backflow of urine into the kidney and damage it.

Give scheduled doses in the morning to avoid loss of sleep because of the patient's need to urinate. Make sure that the patient has a urinal or other collection device to measure urine output.

*After giving any diuretic drug,* be sure to recheck and continue to monitor blood pressure and heart rate at least once every 8 hours because rapid water loss decreases blood volume and lowers blood pressure. Monitor for signs of orthostatic hypotension such as dizziness or light-headedness. Ensure that the call light is within easy reach and instruct patients to call for help getting out of bed. Assist patients to change positions slowly. Have them sit on the side of the bed for 1 to 2 minutes before getting up and then stand up slowly.

Keep a record of urine output because increased urine output is an expected response to all diuretic drugs. Obtain daily weights at the same time each day, using the same scale and with the patient wearing the same or similar clothing.

Continue to monitor blood electrolyte levels for any changes that may result from the diuretic drug. The most important electrolytes to monitor are potassium and sodium.

**Memory Jogger**

The rule "where sodium goes, water follows" works with sodium-excreting diuretics in the kidney. When sodium moves into the nephron tubules, water follows and is excreted in the urine.

◄ ⊖-Learning Activity 12-2

**Memory Jogger**

Diuretics do *not* cure health problems, and the drugs may need to be taken daily for the rest of a patient's life.

◄ ⊖-Learning Activity 12-3

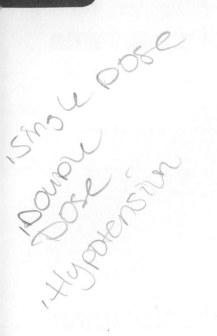

*Teach patients receiving a diuretic drug* to take it exactly as ordered by the prescriber. Tell them to take these drugs according to a schedule that will least affect daily activities. For example, they should take single doses of diuretics early in the day to avoid having to awaken during the night to urinate. If a patient is taking more than one dose per day, the last dose should be taken no later than 6:00 PM to avoid frequent nighttime urination and disruption of sleep and rest. Tell them *never* to double the dose the next day if a dose is missed.

Tell patients about the signs of hypotension (for example, dizziness, light-headedness). Because of the risk for hypotension, remind them to change positions slowly. Instruct patients on the proper techniques for checking their blood pressure and heart rate. Tell them to notify the prescriber if their heart rate is lower than 60 or higher than 100 beats per minute. If blood pressure is less than 90/60 mm Hg or they experience the symptoms of hypotension, they should notify their prescriber.

After discharge, teach patients to weigh themselves every day using the same scale and wearing the same or similar clothing. Instruct them to keep a record of their daily weights. Remind them to drink the same amount of fluid as they urinate each day.

## TYPES OF DIURETICS

There are two types of diuretics. The most commonly used diuretics are called **natriuretic diuretics.** They slow down or turn off the sodium (salt) pumps in the nephrons and make a person excrete more sodium. They include:

- Thiazide diuretics.
- Loop diuretics.
- Potassium-sparing diuretics.

The second type of diuretics is osmotic diuretics such as mannitol (Osmitrol), which increase the blood flow to the kidneys. These drugs are used only in critical situations. Consult a critical care resource for a discussion of their use.

Carbonic anhydrase inhibitors are another class of drugs that are sometimes used for diuresis. These drugs are primarily used for treatment of glaucoma and are discussed in Chapter 26.

### THIAZIDE DIURETICS

#### How Thiazide Diuretics Work

**Thiazide diuretics** slow down or turn off the salt pumps in the nephron tube furthest away from the capillaries (see Figure 12-1). They cause more sodium, potassium, and water to stay in the urine and leave the body through urination. This action reduces blood volume and lowers blood pressure. Commonly prescribed thiazide diuretics are listed in the following table. Be sure to consult a drug handbook for more information about a specific thiazide diuretic.

**Dosages for Common Thiazide Diuretics**

| Drug | Dosage |
|---|---|
| chlorothiazide (Diuril) | *Adults:* PO—250 mg orally every 6-12 hr to decrease body water; 250-1000 mg orally daily to reduce blood pressure<br>*Adults:* IV—250 mg every 6-12 hr to decrease body water; 500-1000 mg IV in single or 2 divided doses per day to lower blood pressure<br>*Children:* Dose based on weight and determined by prescriber |
| hydrochlorothiazide 💯 (Apo-Hydro🍁, Microzide, Novo-Hydrazide🍁, Oretic) | *Adults:* 25-100 mg orally once or twice daily<br>*Children:* Dose based on weight and determined by prescriber |

💯 Top 100 drugs prescribed.

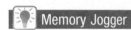

**Memory Jogger**

The three major types of natriuretic diuretics are thiazide, loop, and potassium-sparing.

🄴-Animation 12-1: Diuretics ▶

**Dosages for Common Thiazide Diuretics—cont'd**

| Drug | Dosage |
|------|--------|
| metolazone (Zaroxolyn) | *Adults:* 5-20 mg orally once daily to decrease body water; 2.5-5 mg orally once daily to decrease blood pressure<br>*Children:* Dose determined by prescriber |

### Intended Responses
- Urine output is increased.
- Urine is lighter in color.
- Blood pressure is lower.

***Side Effects.***   The side effects of thiazide diuretics increase with higher blood levels of these drugs. At lower doses side effects are less common. Potential side effects of thiazide diuretics include fluid and electrolyte imbalances such as decreased blood volume, potassium (hypokalemia), sodium (hyponatremia), chloride (hypochloremia), and magnesium (hypomagnesemia) and increased calcium (hypercalcemia) and urea (hyperuremia). Because of decreased blood volume, blood pressure drops faster when the patient moves from a sitting or lying position to a standing position, causing some dizziness or light-headedness *(postural hypotension)*. When postural hypotension is severe, the patient could faint and fall.

A decreased potassium level may result in dry mouth, increased thirst, irregular heartbeat, mood changes, muscle cramps, nausea, vomiting, fatigue or weakness, and weak pulses.

Decreased sodium level may lead to confusion, convulsions, decreased mental activity, irritability, muscle cramps, and unusual fatigue or weakness.

Less common side effects include decreased sexual ability, diarrhea, increased sensitivity of skin to sunlight *(photosensitivity)*, loss of appetite, and upset stomach.

Rare side effects may include black and tarry stools, blood in urine or stools, cough and hoarseness, fever or chills, joint pain, lower back or side pain, painful or difficult urination, skin rash or hives, unusual bleeding or bruising, and yellow eyes or skin.

***Adverse Effects.***   Adverse effects of thiazide diuretics include "passing out" or falling when changing positions, muscle weakness, and blurred vision.

### What To Do *Before* Giving Thiazide Diuretics
Be sure to review the general nursing responsibilities related to diuretic therapy (p. 207) in addition to these specific responsibilities before giving thiazide diuretics.

Check the most recent serum potassium level. If it is below 3.5 mEq/L or 3.5 mmol/L, inform the prescriber. Patients who have low blood potassium levels may develop life-threatening abnormal heart rhythms.

Ask patients about prior allergic reactions to thiazide diuretics. Ask women in their childbearing years if they are pregnant, plan to become pregnant, or are breast-feeding because thiazide diuretics should not be used with these patients.

### What To Do *After* Giving Thiazide Diuretics
Be sure to review the general nursing responsibilities related to diuretic therapy (p. 207) in addition to these specific responsibilities after giving thiazide diuretics.

Keep track of the patient's blood electrolyte levels, including potassium. Watch for signs of decreased potassium, including abnormal heart rhythms, muscle cramps, constipation, and changes in reflexes. Table 12-1 provides a summary of normal electrolyte levels.

**Common Side Effects**

**Thiazide Diuretics**

  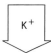

Dizziness, Light-headedness    Hypotension    Hypokalemia

Na⁺

Hyponatremia

**Drug Alert!**

**Administration Alert**

Check the apical pulse of a patient receiving a thiazide diuretic for a full minute to determine whether the rhythm is regular.

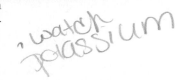
*watch potassium*

Table **12-1**  Normal Blood Electrolyte Values

| ELECTROLYTE | NORMAL VALUE RANGE FOR ADULTS |
|---|---|
| Sodium | 136-145 mEq/L |
| Potassium | 3.5-5.1 mEq/L |
| Chloride | 98-107 mEq/L |
| Calcium | 8.6-10.0 mg/dL |
| Magnesium | 1.5-2.5 mEq/L<br>1.8-3.0 mg/dL |
| Bicarbonate | *Arterial:* 21-28 mEq/L<br>*Venous:* 22-29 mEq/L |
| Creatinine | *Males:* 0.6-1.3 mg/dL<br>*Females:* 0.5-1.0 mg/dL |
| Blood urea nitrogen | 5-20 mg/dL |

### What To *Teach* Patients About Thiazide Diuretics

Be sure to teach patients about general issues related to diuretic therapy (p. 208) in addition to these specific teaching points.

Teach patients the signs of decreased body potassium levels and remind them to report side effects such as muscle weakness or cramps, sudden decrease in urination, and irregular heartbeat to the prescriber. Tell them to take all prescribed potassium pills or liquid. Tell them to take the drug with food if stomach upset occurs.

### Life Span Considerations for Thiazide Diuretics

*Pediatric Considerations.*   Dosage of diuretic drugs is based on weight in children. Side effects in children are the same as in adults. Thiazide diuretics should be used with caution when infants have jaundice because the drugs worsen the condition.

*Considerations for Pregnancy and Breastfeeding.*   Thiazide diuretics are pregnancy category B drugs and should be avoided during pregnancy because they may cause side effects in the newborn, including jaundice and low potassium levels. These drugs have been shown to cause birth defects in animals. They should also be avoided during breastfeeding because they pass into breast milk. Their action may decrease the flow of breast milk.

*Considerations for Older Adults.*   Dizziness or light-headedness and signs of low potassium levels may be more likely in older adults because they are more sensitive to the effects of thiazide diuretics. This greatly increases the older adult's risk for falls. Teach them to change positions slowly and to always use the handrails when going up or down stairs.

### LOOP DIURETICS

#### How Loop Diuretics Work

Loop diuretics (also called "high-ceiling" diuretics) slow down or turn off the sodium pumps in the nephron tube in a place different from thiazide diuretic action. They cause more sodium, potassium, and water to stay in the urine and leave the body through urination (see Figure 12-1). Loop diuretics are the most powerful diuretics. Although this power can be helpful, it also means that the *side effects are more severe* because there is greater water, sodium, and potassium loss. Another difference between loop diuretics and thiazide diuretics is that loop diuretics cause patients to lose calcium in the urine.

Commonly prescribed loop diuretics are listed in the following table. Be sure to consult a drug handbook for more information about a specific loop diuretic.

### Clinical Pitfall

If a patient forgets to take a thiazide diuretic, a double dose should *not* be taken the next day.

### Clinical Pitfall

Thiazide diuretics should *not* be given during pregnancy or to breastfeeding mothers because they cause side effects, pass into breast milk, and may cause a decrease in the flow of breast milk.

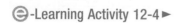-Learning Activity 12-4 ▶

**Dosages for Common Loop Diuretics**

| Drug | Dosage |
|---|---|
| furosemide  (Furoside🍁, Lasix, Lasix Special🍁, Novosemide🍁, Urotol🍁) | *Adults:* PO—20-80 mg daily; prescriber may increase dose as needed<br>*Adults:* IV or IM—20-40 mg; prescriber may increase dose every 2 hours as needed; after dose is working, it is injected IV or IM 1 to 2 times daily<br>*Children:* PO—2 mg/kg daily; prescriber may increase dose every 6-8 hr as needed<br>*Children:* IV or IM—1 mg/kg; prescriber may increase dose every 2 hr as needed<br>*Special Considerations:*<br>Can be given IV slowly, no more than 4 mg/min<br>For very high blood pressure in adults, 40-200 mg may be given IV |
| bumetanide (Bumex) | *Adults:* PO—0.5-2 mg daily; prescriber may increase dose as needed<br>*Adults:* IM or IV—0.5-1 mg every 2-3 hr as needed<br>*Children:* Dose must be determined by prescriber |
| ethacrynic acid (Edecrin) | *Adults:* PO—50-200 mg daily; single or divided doses<br>*Adults:* IV—50 mg every 2-6 hr as needed<br>*Children:* PO—25 mg daily; prescriber may increase dose as needed<br>*Children:* IV—1 mg/kg |
| torsemide (Demadex) | *Adults:* 10-20 mg orally or IV once daily; may increase up to 200 mg daily as needed |

 Top 100 drugs prescribed.

## Intended Responses
- Urine output is increased.
- Urine is lighter in color.
- Blood pressure is lower.

***Side Effects.*** Among the more common side effects of loop diuretics is dizziness or light-headedness when the patient moves from a sitting or lying position to a standing position. This occurs because blood pressure drops in response to the loss of fluid from the blood vessels *(postural hypotension)*.

Blood levels of potassium and sodium decrease *(hypokalemia, hyponatremia)* with loop diuretics. Signs and symptoms of low potassium include dry mouth, increased thirst, irregular heartbeat, mental and mood changes, muscle cramps or muscle pain, nausea, vomiting, fatigue, weakness, and weak pulses. Signs and symptoms of low sodium include confusion, convulsions, decreased mental activity, irritability, muscle cramps, and unusual fatigue or weakness.

Less common side effects include blurred vision, stomach pain or cramps, headache, and redness or pain at the injection site for injectable forms of these drugs. An additional side effect of furosemide is increased sensitivity of skin to sunlight *(photosensitivity)*, possibly with skin rash, itching, redness, or severe sunburn. Ethacrynic acid may cause confusion, diarrhea, loss of appetite, and nervousness. Blurred vision, chest pain, and premature ejaculation or difficulty maintaining an erection may occur with bumetanide.

***Adverse Effects.*** Fainting or falling when changing positions, muscle weakness, and irregular heart rhythms can occur.

Loop diuretics can be *ototoxic* (cause hearing loss from damage to the auditory [ear] tissues). Ototoxicity is reversible when the drug is discontinued, and it becomes worse when the patient is taking other ototoxic drugs such as aminoglycoside antibiotics (for example, gentamicin) while taking a loop diuretic. Hearing loss can occur

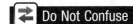

**Do Not Confuse**

**Lasix** *with* **Luvox**

An order for Lasix can be mistaken for Luvox. Lasix is a loop diuretic; Luvox is an antidepressant.

**Common Side Effects**

**Loop Diuretics**

  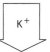

Dizziness, Light-headedness   Hypotension   Hypokalemia

Hyponatremia

when these drugs are given too rapidly by IV and/or in very high doses. The hearing loss is usually temporary.

High blood glucose (hyperglycemia) levels can also occur. Patients with diabetes must check their blood sugar (glucose) levels regularly.

### What To Do *Before* Giving Loop Diuretics

Be sure to review the general nursing responsibilities related to diuretic therapy (p. 207) in addition to these specific responsibilities before giving loop diuretics.

Check the most recent serum potassium level. If it is below 3.5 mEq/L or 3.5 mmol/L, be sure to inform the prescriber. Check to see if the patient is scheduled to receive a potassium supplement. If the potassium level is low, the prescriber may want to order an extra dose of potassium. Check the serum sodium level. If it is below 135 mEq/L or 135 mmol/L, inform the prescriber.

Check the patient's prescribed drugs to determine whether another drug is also ototoxic. If you find that the patient is taking two or more ototoxic drugs, inform the prescriber.

If the drug is to be given intravenously, always check the IV site for patency and signs of inflammation or infection.

### What To Do *After* Giving Loop Diuretics

Be sure to review the general nursing responsibilities related to diuretic therapy (p. 207) in addition to these specific responsibilities after giving loop diuretics.

Monitor serum potassium levels and report low values (less than 3.5 mEq/L or 3.5 mmol/L) to the prescriber. Give prescribed potassium supplements as ordered. Continue to monitor patients for any signs of hearing loss.

Frequently check and record urine output. Regularly empty urine collection devices. Check IV sites for patency at least every 8 hours and monitor for signs of phlebitis or infection (for example, redness, swelling, warmth).

### What To *Teach* Patients About Loop Diuretics

Be sure to teach patients about the general issues related to diuretic therapy (p. 208) in addition to these specific teaching points about loop diuretics.

Remind patients that increased urine output can occur rapidly after an IV injection of loop diuretics. Make sure that the patient understands that urine output can increase dramatically within an hour of taking a loop diuretic, increasing the risk for unexpected or uncontrolled urination (incontinence).

Instruct patients to limit alcohol intake while taking loop diuretics. Alcohol increases the chance of dizziness, light-headedness, and fainting.

Instruct patients to report any decrease in hearing or "ringing" in the ears (*tinnitus*) to the prescriber because this may be the first indication of damage to the ear or hearing.

Tell patients who develop skin sensitivity with furosemide to stay out of direct sunlight, wear protective clothing, and use sun block products with a skin protection factor of at least 15. Remind them not to use sunlamps or tanning beds.

Because loop diuretics cause loss of potassium, the prescriber may want the patient to eat foods that contain potassium. Tell patients to be sure to take any prescribed potassium pills or liquid. Teach them to take it with food or drink to prevent stomach irritation.

### Life Span Considerations for Loop Diuretics

*Pediatric Considerations.*   Side effects of these drugs in children are expected to be the same as in adults. The dosage of furosemide is based on weight; however, some loop diuretic dosages must be determined individually by the prescriber.

*Considerations for Pregnancy and Breastfeeding.*   Loop diuretics are pregnancy category B drugs and should not be given to women who are pregnant or breastfeeding. Animal studies have shown these drugs to cause fetal harm. Furosemide passes into breast milk and should not be used while breastfeeding.

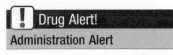

**Drug Alert!**

**Administration Alert**

Give IV doses of furosemide (Lasix) slowly at a rate of 20 mg per minute to avoid ototoxicity.

**Drug Alert!**

**Teaching Alert**

Teach patients that diuresis (increased urine output) can occur rapidly after IV administration of a loop diuretic and may lead to incontinence.

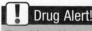

**Drug Alert!**

**Teaching Alert**

Teach patients taking loop diuretics about foods that contain potassium such as bananas, oranges, or citrus fruit juices.

*Considerations for Older Adults.*   Older adults are more sensitive to the effects of loop diuretics and are more likely to develop dizziness and light-headedness, which increases their risk for falls. They are also more likely to develop blood clots and signs of low blood potassium. Teach them to report new-onset muscle weakness to the prescriber. Older adults are more likely to have tinnitus and hearing loss with these drugs. Teach them to note whether they are having more difficulty hearing what is said and whether they need to set the volume higher on the radio or television.

## POTASSIUM-SPARING DIURETICS

### How Potassium-Sparing Diuretics Work

Potassium-sparing diuretics slow the sodium pumps so more sodium and water are excreted as urine, but these drugs do not increase the loss of potassium. In fact, these drugs prevent potassium loss in the urine and cause more potassium to be returned to the blood. They work in a place in the nephron tubes different from the action of other diuretics (see Figure 12-1).

Commonly prescribed potassium-sparing diuretics are listed in the following table. Be sure to consult a drug handbook for more information on a specific potassium-sparing diuretic.

### Dosages for Common Potassium-Sparing Diuretics

| Drug | Dosage |
|------|--------|
| spironolactone [TOP 100] (Aldactone, Novospiroton🍁) | *Adults:* 25-200 mg orally daily divided into 2-4 doses to decrease body water, prescriber may increase dose as needed; 50-100 mg orally daily in a single dose or 2-4 divided doses to decrease blood pressure; 25-100 mg orally daily in single doses or 2-4 divided doses to treat low potassium levels<br>*Children:* 1-3 mg/kg orally daily in a single dose or 2-4 divided doses |
| triamterene (Dyrenium) | *Adults:* 100 mg orally twice daily; prescriber may gradually increase dose<br>*Children:* 2-4 mg/kg daily or every other day, divided into equal small doses; prescriber may increase dose as needed |
| amiloride (Midamor) | *Adults:* 5-10 mg orally once daily<br>*Children:* Dose must be determined by prescriber |

[TOP 100] Top 100 drugs prescribed.

*handwritten margin note:* ↑sodium decrease

### Intended Responses
- Urine output is increased.
- Urine is lighter in color.
- Blood pressure is lower.
- Serum potassium level stays within the normal range (3.5 to 5.0 mEq/L).

*Side Effects.*   Blood pressure drops faster when the patient who is taking potassium-sparing diuretics moves from a sitting or lying position to a standing position, causing some dizziness or light-headedness (postural hypotension). Patient falls are more likely.

Blood levels of sodium decrease (hyponatremia). Symptoms of low sodium level include drowsiness, dry mouth, increased thirst, lack of energy, and muscle weakness.

Other common side effects of potassium-sparing diuretics include nausea, vomiting, stomach cramps, and diarrhea.

Women may develop *hirsutism* (facial hair), irregular menstrual cycles, and deepening of the voice. Men may have trouble getting or keeping an erection. Both men and women may develop breast enlargement (*gynecomastia* in men).

Triamterene may cause the skin to become more sensitive to sunlight (*photosensitivity*), possibly with skin rash, itching, redness, or severe sunburn.

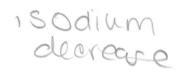

**Common Side Effects**
**Potassium-Sparing Diuretics**

Hypotension   Hyponatremia   Vomiting, Diarrhea

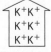

Hyperkalemia

*Adverse Effects.*    Fainting or falling when changing positions may occur because of the decrease in blood volume and blood pressure.

Because these drugs "spare" potassium, the patient is at risk for increased potassium levels (hyperkalemia). A life-threatening side effect of high potassium level is development of an irregular heartbeat *(dysrhythmia)*. Symptoms of a high potassium level include confusion; irregular heartbeat; nervousness; numbness or tingling in hands, feet, or lips; shortness of breath or difficulty breathing; unusual fatigue or weakness; and weakness or a heavy feeling in the legs.

### What To Do *Before* Giving Potassium-Sparing Diuretics

Be sure to review the general nursing responsibilities related to diuretic therapy (p. 207) in addition to these specific responsibilities before giving potassium-sparing diuretics.

Check the most recent serum electrolyte levels. If the potassium level is above 5 mEq/L or 5 mmol/L or the sodium level is below 135 mEq/L or 135 mmol/L, inform the prescriber.

### What To Do *After* Giving Potassium-Sparing Diuretics

Be sure to review the general nursing responsibilities related to diuretic therapy (p. 207) in addition to these specific responsibilities after giving potassium-sparing diuretics.

Monitor the patient for signs and symptoms of high potassium (for example, dry mouth, increased thirst, irregular heartbeat, mood changes, muscle cramps, nausea, vomiting, fatigue or weakness, and weak pulses), and low sodium levels (including confusion, convulsions, decreased mental activity, irritability, muscle cramps, and unusual fatigue or weakness).

### What To *Teach* Patients About Potassium-Sparing Diuretics

Be sure to teach patients the general issues related to diuretic therapy (p. 208) in addition to these specific teaching points for potassium-sparing diuretics.

Also teach patients to avoid eating excessive amounts of high-potassium foods such as meats, dairy products, dried fruits, bananas, cantaloupe, kiwi, oranges, avocados, broccoli, dried beans or peas, lima beans, soybeans, or spinach.

### Life Span Considerations for Potassium-Sparing Diuretics

*Pediatric Considerations.*    Safe use of these drugs has not been established or researched in children, but side effects are expected to be the same as in adults.

*Considerations for Pregnancy and Breastfeeding.*    Safe use of potassium-sparing diuretics during pregnancy and breastfeeding has not been established. These drugs pass into breast milk, but no problems have been noted in breastfeeding infants. Spironolactone is a pregnancy category D drug. Triamterene and amiloride are pregnancy category B drugs.

*Considerations for Older Adults.*    Older adults are more sensitive to the action of potassium-sparing diuretics and more likely to experience side effects.

## OVERACTIVE BLADDER

An **overactive bladder (OAB)** is caused by sudden, involuntary contraction of the muscle in the bladder wall, which causes a sudden, unstoppable need to urinate. Drugs for OAB are used to treat the symptoms of this disorder.

### REVIEW OF RELATED PHYSIOLOGY AND PATHOPHYSIOLOGY

In people with OAB the layered, smooth muscle that surrounds the bladder (**detrusor muscle**) contracts spastically, sometimes without a known cause. This results in

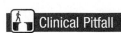

**Clinical Pitfall**

Do *not* give potassium supplements, salt substitutes, or angiotensin-converting enzyme inhibitors to patients taking potassium-sparing diuretics because these drugs can increase the risk of developing high-to–extremely high blood potassium levels.

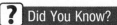

**Did You Know?**

Most salt substitutes are made by replacing sodium with potassium. Therefore salt substitutes should be avoided while taking a potassium-sparing diuretic.

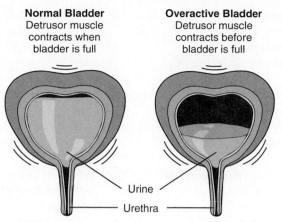

**Normal Bladder**
Detrusor muscle
contracts when
bladder is full

**Overactive Bladder**
Detrusor muscle
contracts before
bladder is full

Urine

Urethra

**FIGURE 12-2**   Pathophysiology of overactive bladder.

continuous high bladder pressure and the urgent need to urinate, also known as *urgency* (Figure 12-2). Normally the detrusor muscle contracts and relaxes in response to the amount of urine in the bladder and the initiation of urination.

People with OAB often have urgency at inconvenient and unpredictable times and sometimes lose control before reaching a toilet *(incontinence).* Thus OAB interferes with work, daily routine, intimacy, and sexual function; causes embarrassment; and can diminish self-esteem and quality of life. OAB is fairly common in older adults.

Treatments for OAB include pelvic muscle exercises such as *Kegel exercises,* behavioral therapies such as bladder training, and medications such as urinary antispasmodics.

## TYPES OF DRUGS FOR OVERACTIVE BLADDER

### URINARY ANTISPASMODICS

#### How Urinary Antispasmodics Work

Drugs for OAB (urinary antispasmodics) are prescribed to treat and improve symptoms, including frequent urination, urgency of urination, and urinary incontinence. These drugs decrease the spasms of the detrusor muscle.

Commonly prescribed drugs for OAB are listed in the following table. Be sure to consult a drug handbook for more information about a specific drug for OAB.

> **Memory Jogger**
>
> Kegel exercises (contracting and relaxing pelvic floor muscles) can strengthen and improve muscle tone to help control urinary incontinence.

◄ -Learning Activity 12-5

#### Dosages for Common Urinary Antispasmodics

| Drug | Dosage |
|---|---|
| oxybutynin (Ditropan) | *Adults/Adolescents:* 5 mg orally 2-3 times daily (do not exceed 20 mg/day); extended release (XL)—5 mg daily (do not exceed 30 mg/day)<br>*Children over 5 years:* 5 mg orally 2-3 times daily (do not exceed 15 mg/day) |
| oxybutynin transdermal system patch (Oxytrol; Gelnique) | *Adults:* 3.9 mg/day applied transdermally every 3-4 days; remove old patch before applying a new one; Gelnique—topical packet 100 mg daily; apply to abdomen, upper arms/shoulders, or thighs |
| tolterodine (Detrol, Detrol LA) | *Adults:* 2 mg orally twice daily; 4 mg orally once daily (Detrol LA) |
| solifenacin (VESIcare) | *Adults:* 5 mg orally once daily |
| darifenacin (Enablex) | *Adults:* 7.5 mg orally once daily; may increase to 15 mg once daily after 2 weeks |
| trospium chloride (Sanctura, Sanctura XR) | *Adults:* 20 mg orally twice daily 1 hr before meals; 60 mg once daily 1 hr before breakfast (Sanctura XR) |

**Common Side Effects**

**Urinary Antispasmodics**

Headache    Dizziness,    Constipation
             Light-
             headedness

Dry mouth    Dry eyes

*Intended Responses*
- Urinary frequency is decreased.
- Urinary urgency is decreased.
- Urinary incontinence is decreased.

*Side Effects.*   Frequent side effects of drugs for OAB include dry mouth, dry eyes, headache, dizziness, and constipation.

Other less common side effects include nausea, drowsiness, blurred vision, and dyspepsia (heartburn).

*Adverse Effects.*   Adverse effects of these drugs include chest pain, fast or irregular heart rate, shortness of breath, swelling (edema) and rapid weight gain, confusion, and hallucinations. In addition, these drugs may cause decreased urination or no urine output and painful or difficult urination.

Signs of an allergic reaction include rash (hives); difficulty breathing; and swelling of face, lips, tongue, or throat.

Patients may be at increased risk for heatstroke during exercise or hot weather because these drugs decrease perspiration (sweating).

### What To Do *Before* Giving Urinary Antispasmodics

Before giving drugs for OAB, be sure to ask patients for a complete list of current drugs, including over-the-counter and herbal drugs. Also ask about allergies.

Check the patient's blood pressure and heart rate. Assess heart rate for any irregularities. Obtain a baseline weight and assess for edema.

Ask patients about their symptoms associated with OAB. Ask about usual urinary pattern and urine output.

Check patients for history of liver disease, kidney disease, or glaucoma because drugs for OAB often worsen these problems.

Ask women of childbearing age if they are pregnant, planning to become pregnant, or breastfeeding; it is not known how these drugs affect the fetus or infant.

### What To Do *After* Giving Urinary Antispasmodics

After giving drugs for OAB, recheck blood pressure and heart rate. Report increased or irregular heart rhythms to the prescriber.

Weigh patients daily and assess for swelling. Report weight gain (more than 2 pounds per day) or increased edema to the prescriber.

Monitor patients for urinary urgency, frequency, difficulty urinating, or incontinence. Keep track of fluid intake and output.

### What To *Teach* Patients About Urinary Antispasmodics

Teach patients to take these drugs on an empty stomach with water. If they experience stomach upset, the drugs may be given with milk or food.

Instruct patients not to crush, chew, break, or open extended-release or long-acting capsules. Tell them to swallow the capsule whole because these drugs are made to release the medication slowly into the body. When the capsules are opened in any way, the drug is released all at once. This may cause an initial overdose with more side effects and prevents the drug from being effective throughout the day.

If a dose is missed, teach patients to take it as soon as possible. If it is almost time for the next dose, they should skip the missed dose and take the drug at the next scheduled time. Tell them not to take extra pills to make up for the missed dose.

Remind patients to avoid becoming overheated or dehydrated during exercise or hot weather. These drugs may decrease sweating, placing patients at risk for heatstroke.

Because of the visual side effects of OAB drugs, teach patients to avoid driving or any other activities that require clear vision and mental alertness until they know how the drugs will affect them.

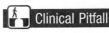 **Clinical Pitfall**

Patients taking drugs for OAB are at risk for heatstroke during exercise or hot weather.

Teach patients to avoid consuming alcohol within 2 hours of these drugs because side effects such as drowsiness are increased. They should drink alcohol only when they do not plan to drive or operate dangerous equipment.

Tell patients to contact their prescriber if urinary symptoms do not improve or if they become worse while taking these drugs.

Instruct patients using the transdermal patch system to apply a new patch to their skin every 3 to 4 days (as prescribed). The patch should be applied to a different clean, dry, and smooth area and pressed firmly to ensure that it stays in place. Teach patients to report skin redness, itchiness, or irritation to the prescriber.

### Life Span Considerations for Urinary Antispasmodics

*Considerations for Pregnancy and Breastfeeding.*  OAB drugs are pregnancy category C drugs except for oxybutynin, which is a pregnancy category B drug. They are not recommended for use with pregnant or breastfeeding women.

*Considerations for Older Adults.*   Older adults may be more sensitive to the effects of these drugs and may need to be prescribed lower drug doses.

> **! Drug Alert!**
> **Teaching Alert**
>
> Teach patients using the transdermal patch system to remove the old patch before applying a new one.

◄ⓔ-Learning Activity 12-6

## BENIGN PROSTATIC HYPERPLASIA

### REVIEW OF RELATED PHYSIOLOGY AND PATHOPHYSIOLOGY

The prostate gland is a walnut-sized male sex gland that surrounds the upper part of the urethra and secretes substances into seminal fluid (Figure 12-3). These secretions improve the chance of pregnancy with intercourse by increasing the amount of seminal fluid, improving sperm movement, and reducing acidity in the vagina. The activity and size of the prostate gland depend on the presence of testosterone, the main androgen secreted by the testes and adrenal glands. (Androgens are a group of male sex hormones that includes testosterone, dihydrotestosterone [DHT], and androstenedione.) The prostate gland has testosterone receptors in the nucleus of each cell that bind circulating testosterone. When bound, these receptors trigger the genes for prostate cell growth and activity.

Many men older than age 50 have benign prostatic hyperplasia (BPH), which is enlargement of the prostate gland as a result of increased numbers of cells in the gland. Although the amount of circulating testosterone decreases with age, the number of testosterone receptors in the prostate gland *increases*. Then even small amounts of testosterone, especially DHT, are more likely to bind with receptors and eventually cause the prostate gland to enlarge.

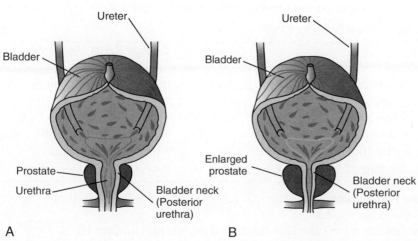

**FIGURE 12-3 A,** Normal prostate gland. **B,** Enlarged prostate gland showing the narrowing of the urethra, decreasing urine flow.

-Learning Activity 12-7 ►

Because of its location, when the prostate enlarges, it squeezes the urethra, narrowing it and decreasing urine flow from the bladder (see Figure 12-3).

Symptoms of BPH are:
- Increased frequency of urination.
- Nocturia (increased urination at night).
- Difficulty in starting (hesitancy) and continuing urination.
- Reduced force and size of the urine stream.
- The feeling of incomplete bladder emptying.
- Dribbling after urinating.

Signs and symptoms of BPH are the same as for prostate cancer. Any man with symptoms of BPH should be seen by his physician to rule out prostate cancer.

The symptoms of prostate enlargement are uncomfortable and can interfere with adequate sleep and rest. Often urine stays in the bladder much longer than normal, leading to urinary tract infection. With rapid or severe enlargement, the bladder can become completely blocked, with urine backing up into the ureters and kidneys, leading to kidney damage or failure. With severe blockage surgery is needed. When symptoms are mild to moderate, drug therapy can reduce prostate pressure and improve urine flow.

## TYPES OF DRUGS FOR BENIGN PROSTATIC HYPERPLASIA

### DHT INHIBITORS AND SELECTIVE ALPHA-1 BLOCKERS

The two main categories of drugs to treat prostate enlargement are DHT inhibitors and selective alpha-1 blockers. Because the actions of these two drug types differ, they can be used alone or together to improve urine flow.

#### How Drugs for Benign Prostatic Hyperplasia Work

DHT inhibitors work directly on the prostate gland. They are a "counterfeit" drug that looks like testosterone and binds to the enzyme that normally converts testosterone to DHT, its most powerful form. This counterfeit drug cannot be converted to DHT; and, while it is bound to the enzyme, the enzyme is not available to convert the real testosterone to DHT. With much less DHT in the prostate, the cells in the prostate gland do not receive the signal to grow. As a result, the gland shrinks and puts less pressure on the urethra, allowing better urine flow.

Selective alpha-1 blockers act to relax smooth muscle tissue in the prostate gland, neck of the bladder, and urethra. These smooth muscles contain alpha-1 adrenergic receptors. When the receptors are activated, the smooth muscle constricts, tightening the prostate, which increases the pressure and squeezes the urethra. Smooth muscle in the bladder neck and urethra also contract and make the urethra narrower. When these receptors are bound with selective alpha-1 blockers, the smooth muscle relaxes, placing less pressure on the urethra and improving urine flow.

#### Dosages for Common Drugs for BPH

| Drug | Dosage (Adult Men Only) |
| --- | --- |
| *DHT Inhibitors* | |
| dutasteride (Avodart) | 0.5 mg orally once daily |
| finasteride (Proscar) | 5 mg orally once daily |
| *Selective Alpha-1 Blockers* | |
| alfuzosin (Uroxatral, Xatral♦) | 10 mg orally once daily |
| silodosin (Rapaflo) | 8 mg orally once daily |
| tamsulosin (Flomax, Novo-Tamsulosin♦) | 0.4-0.8 mg orally once daily |

#### Intended Responses
- Pressure is decreased.
- Urine flow from the bladder through the urethra is improved.
- BPH symptoms (frequency, difficulty starting or stopping the urine stream, dribbling, excessive nighttime urination, feeling of incomplete bladder emptying) are decreased.

*Side Effects.*   The most common side effect of drugs for BPH is a decreased interest in sexual activity (decreased libido).

Side effects for DHT inhibitors also include erectile dysfunction, decreased seminal fluid, and reduced fertility. Other side effects for some men are a slowing of hair loss from the scalp and in some cases scalp hair regrowth.

Selective alpha-1 blockers may lower blood pressure, especially when changing positions (orthostatic hypotension), causing dizziness or light-headedness. Other side effects may include back pain and runny or stuffy nose.

*Adverse Effects.*   Drugs for BPH are metabolized by the liver. If the patient's liver is impaired, the drug is excreted more slowly, and higher blood levels could result. Higher blood levels lead to more severe side effects. Patients with liver impairment should be prescribed lower dosages of these drugs.

DHT inhibitors can adversely affect other hormone or sex tissues. Breast changes such as enlargement, lumps, pain, or fluids leaking from the nipple can occur. Any of these changes or pain in the testicles is a reason to stop the drug.

DHT inhibitors can cause birth defects when taken or handled by a pregnant woman. Women who are pregnant or who may become pregnant should avoid handling the tablets or capsules, especially if they are crushed or broken. Because these drugs enter the seminal fluid of men who take them, men should wear a condom when having sex with a woman who is pregnant or may become pregnant.

Alpha-1 blockers are excreted by the kidneys. Patients who have renal impairment retain the drug longer and have more severe hypotension. Although these drugs are not toxic to the kidney *(nephrotoxic)*, they should not be taken by patients who have severe renal impairment or kidney failure.

Tamsulosin is made from a sulfonamide and may cause an allergic reaction in patients who are allergic to sulfa drugs.

All of the alpha-1 blockers can interact with many other drugs and herbal supplements, especially antihypertensives, cardiac drugs, and drugs for erectile dysfunction. The interactions can be complex and serious.

Alpha-1 blockers have been associated with a problem called *floppy iris syndrome* during cataract surgery. With this problem the iris does not respond as expected to drugs that dilate or constrict it and can collapse toward the surgical site. Although this is not a reason to stop the drug, the surgeon performing cataract surgery must take special steps to prevent a floppy iris from causing complications.

## What To Do *Before* Giving Drugs for BPH

The signs and symptoms of BPH are the same as for prostate cancer. Before a drug for BPH is taken, the patient should have a digital rectal examination by his prescriber and have his blood tested for prostate-specific antigen (PSA) levels to rule out prostate cancer.

Because liver impairment can increase the blood level of the drugs for BPH, make sure that the patient does not have a liver problem before starting these drugs. Check the patient's most recent laboratory values for liver problems (elevated liver enzymes). (See Table 1-3 for a listing of normal values.)

Because alpha-1 blockers may cause orthostatic hypotension, take the patient's blood pressure in the lying, sitting, and standing positions.

If a patient will be taking tamsulosin, ask whether he has ever had an allergic reaction to sulfa drugs. If he has had such a reaction, report this to the prescriber.

## What To Do *After* Giving Drugs for BPH

Assess the patient for orthostatic (postural) hypotension and related problems (dizziness, light-headedness), especially after the first dose. Remind the patient to call for assistance when getting out of bed.

## What To *Teach* Patients About Drugs for BPH

Remind patients to continue their annual prevention and early detection practices for prostate cancer. These include a digital rectal examination and blood PSA levels.

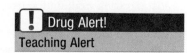

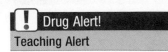

**Drug Alert!**

**Teaching Alert**

Instruct patients who take a DHT inhibitor with saw palmetto (*Serenoa repens*) or soy isoflavones to notify the prescriber if any unusual side effects occur.

Caution men taking DHT inhibitors to make sure that women who are or may become pregnant do not come into contact with the drug or handle it. Methods for men to reduce exposure to women include:

- Wearing a condom during sexual intercourse.
- Not donating blood (which could be given to a pregnant woman).

Some common herbal preparations have an action similar to that of DHT inhibitors. They include saw palmetto (*Serenoa repens*) and soy isoflavones. If a man takes a DHT inhibitor with one of these substances, it is possible that it could increase the intended responses of the drug, including side effects.

Teach patients taking alpha-1 blockers to change positions slowly, especially when rising to a standing position, because a rapid drop in blood pressure can cause dizziness. Although this problem is more likely to occur when a patient first takes an alpha blocker, it can occur at any time, especially if he is dehydrated or taking drugs for hypertension, erectile dysfunction drugs, or cardiac drugs such as beta blockers or calcium channel blockers. Warn patients to avoid driving or operating dangerous equipment until they know how the drugs will affect them.

Warn patients taking alpha-1 blockers to tell all other health care providers that they are taking this drug because of the potential for drug interactions. Also warn them not to take over-the-counter drugs without checking with their prescriber.

Remind patients taking an alpha-1 blocker to inform their surgeon that they are taking this drug when cataract surgery is being planned.

### Life Span Considerations for Drugs for BPH

*Pediatric Considerations.*  DHT inhibitors and selective alpha-1 blockers should not be administered to children or adolescents.

*Considerations for Pregnancy and Breastfeeding.*  DHT inhibitors (pregnancy category X) are teratogens and can cause birth defects, especially in male fetuses. Women who are pregnant, may become pregnant, or are breastfeeding should not take these drugs or handle them if the tablet or capsule is crushed or broken. Although selective alpha-1 blockers are pregnancy category B drugs, they are used *only* to treat BPH in men and are not indicated for women, regardless of pregnancy or breastfeeding status.

*Considerations for Older Adults.*  Drugs for BPH are more commonly prescribed for older men. Prostate cancer is much more common in this age-group. Ensure that older men taking drugs for BPH understand the need to have annual prostate cancer screening.

The risk for orthostatic (postural) hypotension is higher in older patients taking alpha-1 blockers than in younger adults, especially with the first dose. Monitor older adults carefully for severe hypotension.

## Get Ready for Practice!

### Key Points

- Most diuretics work on the nephrons in the kidneys to increase urine output.
- Diuretics are prescribed to treat hypertension, heart failure, kidney disease, and liver disease.
- The two major types of diuretics are natriuretic diuretics (thiazide, loop, and potassium-sparing), and osmotic diuretics.
- The most common side effects of diuretics are dizziness and light-headedness related to hypotension.
- Patients taking potassium-sparing diuretics should be taught to avoid use of salt substitutes because these substitutes are made with potassium instead of sodium.
- Unless a patient is on a fluid restriction, be sure that fluid intake closely matches the urine output in a patient taking diuretics.

- Monitor patients taking diuretics for signs and symptoms of dehydration.
- Monitor electrolytes carefully when a patient is taking a diuretic.
- Check the blood pressure of a patient who is taking diuretics at least once per shift, even if it is not ordered.
- OAB is caused by spastic contractions of the detrusor muscle.
- People with OAB often experience urgency and leakage of urine (incontinence).
- Drugs for OAB decrease detrusor muscle spasms and relive symptoms.
- Patients taking OAB drugs are at risk for heatstroke.
- An enlarged prostate squeezes the urethra, narrowing it and decreasing urine flow from the bladder.
- Because BPH and prostate cancer have similar symptoms, all men being treated for BPH should be screened for prostate cancer annually.
- Women who are pregnant, may become pregnant, or are breastfeeding should neither take DHT inhibitors nor handle these drugs if the tablet or capsule is crushed or broken.
- Orthostatic hypotension may occur with selective alpha-1 blocker therapy, especially with the first dose.

## Additional Learning Resources

**evolve** Go to your Evolve website (http://evolve.elsevier.com/Workman/pharmacology/) for the following FREE learning resources:
- eLearning Activities
- Animations
- Video Clips
- Interactive Review Questions
- Audio Key Points
- Audio Glossary
- Audio Glossary—Spanish-English
- Drug Dosage Calculators
- Patient Teaching Handouts

**SG** Go to your Study Guide for additional learning activities to help you master this chapter content.

## Review Questions

1. What are the two most common side effects of loop diuretics such as furosemide (Lasix)?

   A. Stomach pain and cramps
   B. Skin rashes and sensitivity to sunlight
   C. Dizziness and light-headedness
   D. Diarrhea and loss of appetite

2. Before giving a thiazide diuretic such as hydrochlorothiazide (Hydrodiuril), which laboratory value must you be sure to check?

   A. Sodium
   B. Calcium
   C. Creatinine
   D. Potassium

3. A patient prescribed a thiazide diuretic for hypertension reports light-headedness after taking the drug. To ensure the safety of the patient, what action do you take?

   A. Keep the patient on bed rest.
   B. Notify the prescriber immediately.
   C. Make sure that all four side rails are in an upright position.
   D. Instruct the patient to call for help before getting out of bed.

4. An 80-year-old patient prescribed furosemide tells you that she hears a "ringing" sound in her ears. What is your best action?

   A. Reassure the patient that this is an expected action of the drug.
   B. Document the finding as the only action.
   C. Hold the drug and notify the prescriber.
   D. Refer the patient for a hearing test.

5. A patient prescribed oxybutynin (Ditropan) asks you about the reason for taking the drug. What is your best response?

   A. "It will increase spasms in your bladder and improve urination."
   B. "It will decrease spasms in your bladder and decrease urinary incontinence."
   C. "It will completely cure your problem with incontinence."
   D. "It will allow you to urinate only two or three times a day."

6. Which action is most important after administering silodosin (Rapaflo) to a patient?

   A. Reminding the patient to change positions slowly
   B. Elevating the head of the bed to at least 45 degrees
   C. Checking the patient's liver function tests for elevated enzyme levels
   D. Warning the patient that the action of improved urine flow is rapid and incontinence can occur

7. Which precaution is most important to teach a patient prescribed tamsulosin (Flomax) for treatment of BPH?

   A. Avoid donating blood.
   B. Be sure to have annual prostate cancer screenings.
   C. Do not take this drug if you are allergic to "sulfa" drugs.
   D. Do not drink alcoholic beverages while taking this drug.

8. What must you teach a woman being discharged after delivering a baby about using drugs for overactive bladder?

   A. "These drugs pose no harm to your child."
   B. "Use the transdermal patch system if you plan to breastfeed."
   C. "These drugs are not recommended while you are breastfeeding."
   D. "Animal research has found that drugs for overactive bladder are safe to use."

9. A patient is to be given furosemide 60 mg IV push. The drug comes in a 10-mL vial with a concentration of 10 mg/mL. How many milliliters will be drawn up in a syringe to give this patient? _____ mL

10. A patient with BPH is prescribed 0.8 mg of tamsulosin (Flomax) daily. The drug comes in 0.4-mg capsules. How many capsules will you teach the patient to take? _____ capsule(s)

## Critical Thinking Activities

Mr. James is a 65-year-old man with type 2 diabetes, hypertension, and mild heart failure. He has been taking hydrochlorothiazide (HCTZ) 25 mg by mouth twice a day to control his high blood pressure and heart failure for the past 2 years. When admitted to the hospital, Mr. James reports the following symptoms: dizziness when he first gets up every morning, fatigue, weakness, increased thirst and dry mouth, and occasional muscle cramps.

1. Which electrolyte should be checked right away?

2. What strategy should you teach Mr. James for coping with the dizziness?

3. What drug do you anticipate the physician will prescribe?

4. What diet changes will you be sure to teach Mr. James to prevent most of these symptoms from recurring?

# Drugs for Hypertension

## Objectives

*After studying this chapter you should be able to:*

1. Explain how antihypertensive drugs lower blood pressure.
2. List the common names, actions, usual adult dosages, possible side effects, and adverse effects of angiotensin-converting enzyme (ACE) inhibitors and angiotensin II receptor antagonists.
3. Describe what to do before and after giving ACE inhibitors and angiotensin II receptor antagonists.
4. Explain what to teach patients taking ACE inhibitors and angiotensin II receptor antagonists, including what to do, what not to do, and when to call the prescriber.
5. Describe life span considerations for ACE inhibitors and angiotensin II receptor antagonists.
6. List the common names, actions, usual adult dosages, possible side effects, and adverse effects for calcium

channel blockers, beta blockers, alpha blockers, alpha-beta blockers, central-acting adrenergic drugs, and direct vasodilators.

7. Describe what to do before and after giving calcium channel blockers, beta blockers, alpha blockers, alpha-beta blockers, central-acting adrenergic drugs, and direct vasodilators.
8. Explain what to teach patients taking calcium channel blockers, beta blockers, alpha blockers, alpha-beta blockers, central-acting adrenergic drugs, and direct vasodilators, including what to do, what not to do, and when to call the prescriber.
9. Describe life span considerations for calcium channel blockers, beta blockers, alpha blockers, alpha-beta blockers, central-acting adrenergic drugs, and direct vasodilators.

## Key Terms

**ACE inhibitor** (ĂS ĭn-HĬB-ĭ-tŭr) (p. 228) A drug that lowers blood pressure; ACE stands for angiotensin-converting enzyme.

**alpha blocker** (ĂL-fĕ BLŎ-kŭr) (p. 228) A drug that opposes the excitatory effects of norepinephrine released from sympathetic nerve endings at alpha receptors and causes vasodilation and a decrease in blood pressure. Also called alpha-adrenergic blocking agents.

**alpha-beta blocker** (ĂL-fĕ BĀ-tĕ BLŎ-kŭr) (p. 228) Drugs that combine the effects of alpha blockers and beta blockers.

**angioedema** (ăn-jē-ō-ĕ-DĒ-mĕ) (p. 231) Diffuse swelling of the face, including the eyes, lips, and tongue. May progress to swelling of the trachea (airway), which is life threatening.

**angiotensin II receptor antagonist** (ăn-jē-ō-TĔN-sĭn TŪ rē-SĔP-tŭr ăn-TĂG-ō-nĭst) (p. 228) Angiotensin II receptor antagonists, or angiotensin receptor blockers, are a group of drugs that modulate the renin-angiotensin-aldosterone system and lower blood pressure.

**antihypertensive** (ăn-tē-hī-pŭr-TĔN-sĭv) (p. 225) A substance or drug that lowers blood pressure.

**arteriosclerosis** (ăr-TĔR-ē-ō-sklĕ-RŌ-sĭs) (p. 225) Hardening of the arterial walls.

**atherosclerosis** (ĂTH-ŭr-ō-sklĕ-RŌ-sĭs) (p. 225) Clogging, narrowing, and hardening of the large arteries and medium-size blood vessels of the body, which can lead to stroke, heart attack, and eye and kidney problems.

**beta blocker (beta adrenergic blocker)** (BĀ-tĕ ăd-rĕn-ŬR-jĭk BLŎ-kŭr) (p. 228) A drug that limits the activity of epinephrine (a hormone that increases blood pressure); beta blockers reduce the heart rate and the force of muscle contraction, thereby reducing the oxygen demand of the heart muscle.

**blood pressure** (BLŬD PRĔ-shŭr) (p. 224) The force of blood pushing against the walls of the arteries as it flows through them.

**calcium channel blocker** (KĂL-sē-ŭm CHĂ-nĕl BLŎ-kŭr) (p. 228) A drug that slows the movement of calcium into the cells of the heart and blood vessels, relaxing blood vessels and reducing the workload of the heart.

**central-acting adrenergic agents** (SĔN-trŭl ĂK-tĭng ăd-rĕn-ŬR-jĭk Ā-jĕnts) (p. 228) Drugs that lower blood pressure by stimulating alpha receptors in the brain, which open peripheral arteries and ease blood flow.

**diastolic blood pressure** (dī-ĕ-STŎL-ĭk BLŬD PRĔSH-ŭr) (p. 224) Blood pressure when the heart is resting between beats.

**direct vasodilators** (dī-RĔKT văz-ō-DĪ-lā-tŭrz) (p. 228) Drugs that act directly on the smooth muscle of small arteries, causing these arteries to expand (dilate).

**diuretic** (dī-ŭr-ĔT-ĭk) (p. 228) Drug that eliminates excess water and salt from the body.

**hypertension** (hī-pŭr-TĔN-shŭn) (p. 224) Arterial disease in which chronic high blood pressure is the primary symptom. Abnormally elevated blood pressure.

**hypertensive crisis** (hī-pŭr-TĔN-sĭv KRĪ-sĭs) (p. 224) Dangerously high and life-threatening blood pressure of acute onset.

**hypotension** (hī-pō-TĔN-shŭn) (p. 224) Low blood pressure.

**orthostatic hypotension** (ōr-thō-STĂT-ĭk hī-pō-TĔN-shŭn) (p. 227) Also called postural hypotension. A reduction of systolic blood pressure of at least 20 mm Hg or diastolic pressure of at least 10 mm Hg within 3 minutes of standing.

**primary (essential) hypertension** (PRĪ-mār-ē ĕs-SĔN-chŭl hī-pŭr-TĔN-shŭn) (p. 225) Hypertension for which there is no known cause but that is associated with risk factors; 85% to 90% of cases of hypertension are of this type.

**secondary hypertension** (SĔK-ŭn-dār-ē hī-pŭr-TĔN-shŭn) (p. 225) Hypertension caused by specific disease states and drugs.

**systolic blood pressure** (sĭs-STŎL-ĭk BLŬD PRĔSH-ŭr) (p. 224) Blood pressure when the heart contracts.

**vasodilator** (văz-ō-DĪ-lā-tŭr) (p. 244) Any drug that relaxes blood vessel walls.

---

 -Learning Activity 13-1 ►

 **Memory Jogger**

Hypertension is a systolic blood pressure greater than 140 mm Hg and/or a diastolic blood pressure greater than 90 mm Hg.

**Clinical Pitfall**

When hypertension is not treated, the following health problems may result:
- Arteriosclerosis (atherosclerosis)
- Heart attack (myocardial infarction)
- Stroke (cerebrovascular accident, brain attack)
- Enlarged heart (cardiomyopathy)
- Kidney damage (may lead to end-stage kidney disease)
- Blindness

## OVERVIEW

**Blood pressure** is the force of blood pushing against the walls of the arteries as the blood flows through them. Everyone's blood pressure goes up and down during a 24-hour period. Blood pressure goes up when you are active and down when you are resting or sleeping. When blood pressure remains abnormally high, it is called **hypertension.** Often people are unaware of having high blood pressure because there are no specific symptoms. Sudden, dangerously high, and life-threatening blood pressure is called **hypertensive crisis.** Low blood pressure is called **hypotension.**

Blood pressure measurements include two numbers. The higher number is called the **systolic blood pressure.** It represents pressure of blood against the artery walls when the heart contracts. The lower number is called the **diastolic blood pressure.** It represents pressure of blood against the artery walls when the heart relaxes. A sphygmomanometer and stethoscope are used to measure blood pressure. In some settings automatic blood pressure monitoring machines are used.

As people age, they are more likely to develop hypertension. *Hypertension* is defined by the American Heart Association as a systolic blood pressure (SBP) greater than or equal to 140 mm Hg and/or a diastolic blood pressure (DBP) greater than or equal to 90 mm Hg in people who do not have diabetes. There are four classifications for blood pressure: normal, prehypertension, stage 1 hypertension, and stage 2 hypertension (Table 13-1). In the United States alone there are around 50 million people with hypertension.

-Learning Activity 13-2 ►

| Table **13-1** | Blood Pressure Classification | |
|---|---|---|
| **CLASSIFICATION** | **BLOOD PRESSURE MEASUREMENT** | **BLOOD PRESSURE READING** |
| Normal | Systolic and diastolic | <120 mm Hg <br> <80 mm Hg |
| Prehypertension | Systolic or diastolic | 120-139 mm Hg <br> 80-89 mm Hg |
| Stage 1 hypertension | Systolic or diastolic | 140-159 mm Hg <br> 90-99 mm Hg |
| Stage 2 hypertension | Systolic or diastolic | >160 mm Hg <br> >100 mm Hg |

From Joint National Committee. (2003). *The Seventh Report of the Joint National Committee on Prevention, Detection, Evaluation, and Treatment of High Blood Pressure.* NIH Publication No. 03-5233. Bethesda, MD: National Heart, Lung, and Blood Institute.

Box 13-1  Lifestyle Changes for Treating Hypertension

- Decrease salt (sodium) intake.
- Decrease fat intake.
- Lose weight.
- Exercise regularly.
- Quit smoking.
- Decrease alcohol intake (not more than two alcohol drinks per day).
- Decrease and manage stress.

Several risk factors have been associated with developing high blood pressure. Some, such as smoking, being overweight, and being physically inactive can be changed. Others, such as age, gender, family history, and race cannot be changed. Yet other risk factors (for example, diabetes and hyperlipidemia) can be controlled with drugs. Use of oral contraceptives (birth control pills) increases the risk for hypertension in younger women, whereas being postmenopausal increases the risk for older women. Treatment of hypertension includes lifestyle changes (Box 13-1) and drugs that lower blood pressure (antihypertensives).

## REVIEW OF RELATED PHYSIOLOGY AND PATHOPHYSIOLOGY

### ARTERIOSCLEROSIS AND ATHEROSCLEROSIS

Arteriosclerosis is the hardening of the arterial walls. High blood pressure causes arterial walls to thicken and harden. With atherosclerosis plaques are formed inside the walls of arteries (Figure 13-1). As arterial walls harden and thicken, the arteries become narrow. Narrowed arteries decrease blood flow so body organs and tissues may not receive enough blood. Narrowed arteries can also result in the formation of clots that block the flow of blood. Reduced or blocked blood flow to the heart can cause a heart attack, whereas reduced or blocked blood flow to the brain can cause a stroke.

High blood pressure also makes the heart work much harder to pump blood to the lungs and body. Over time the extra work can cause the heart muscle to thicken and stretch. This can lead to an enlarged heart (*cardiomyopathy*) and heart failure.

High blood pressure can affect the ability of the kidneys to remove body wastes from the blood by hardening, thickening, and narrowing the arteries to the kidneys. This causes less blood flow to the kidneys and less filtering of waste products, which then build up in the blood. As kidney function becomes worse, kidney failure, including end-stage kidney disease (ESKD), can occur. When the kidneys fail, a patient needs either dialysis or a kidney transplant.

The two main types of hypertension are primary (essential) hypertension and secondary hypertension. *Primary hypertension* has no known cause. *Secondary hypertension* is caused by other diseases and drugs that raise blood pressure.

### PRIMARY (ESSENTIAL) HYPERTENSION

Primary hypertension is the most common form of high blood pressure, accounting for 85% to 90% of cases. Although it has no known cause, it is associated with certain risk factors (Table 13-2). A contributing factor may be the changes that occur in the arteries as people age. With increasing age blood pressure rises, large arteries become stiffer, and smaller arteries may become partly blocked. Examples of other factors that play a part in developing high blood pressure include smoking, an unhealthy diet (too much fat, salt, and alcohol), stress, obesity, and changes in the kidneys.

### SECONDARY HYPERTENSION

Secondary hypertension, the less common form of high blood pressure, is the result of other health problems or drugs. Examples of disorders that can cause this type of hypertension include partial blockages of the arteries to the kidneys (atherosclerosis)

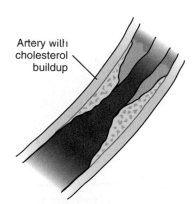

Artery with cholesterol buildup

**FIGURE 13-1** Atherosclerosis.

**?  Did You Know?**

About 25% of patients who are on kidney dialysis have kidney failure that was caused by hypertension.

**Table 13-2** Causes of Hypertension

| TYPE OF HYPERTENSION | CAUSES | |
|---|---|---|
| Primary (essential) hypertension | Cause is unknown<br>Associated risk factors:<br>    Family history<br>    High sodium intake<br>    High calorie intake<br>    Physical inactivity<br>    Excessive alcohol intake<br>    Low potassium intake | |
| Secondary hypertension | Specific diseases:<br>    Renal vascular disease<br>    Primary aldosteronism<br>    Pheochromocytoma<br>    Cushing's disease<br>    Coarctation of the aorta<br>    Brain tumors<br>    Encephalitis<br>    Psychiatric disturbances<br>    Pregnancy<br>    Sleep apnea | Medications:<br>    Estrogen (oral contraceptives)<br>    Glucocorticoids<br>    Mineralocorticoids<br>    Sympathomimetics |

From Ignatavicius D, Workman L: *Medical-surgical nursing: patient-centered collaborative care,* 6th edition, 2010, St Louis, Saunders.

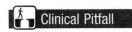

**Clinical Pitfall**

A patient with high blood pressure should *not* take over-the-counter allergy and cold drugs that contain phenylephrine.

-Learning Activity 13-3 ▶

and diseases that damage the kidneys such as infections and diabetes. Tumors of the adrenal glands, which sit on top of the kidneys, and sleep apnea may cause secondary hypertension (see Table 13-2).

Drugs that cause secondary hypertension include nonsteroidal anti-inflammatory drugs (NSAIDs) and corticosteroids. Other drugs that may result in high blood pressure include over-the-counter allergy and cold drugs that contain phenylephrine or pseudoephedrine.

## GENERAL ISSUES FOR ANTIHYPERTENSIVE THERAPY

Antihypertensive drugs are prescribed to control and manage high blood pressure. Awareness and treatment of hypertension are very important because, when left untreated, it can cause diseases that damage the heart and arteries, kidneys, and brain. Untreated hypertension also decreases life expectancy in adults. Treating the cause of secondary hypertension can cure the problem. Managing primary hypertension is a lifelong process and usually requires that patients continue with lifestyle changes and drugs for the rest of their lives. The Seventh Report of the Joint National Committee on Prevention, Detection, Evaluation, and Treatment of High Blood Pressure provides current guidelines for prescribing drugs to decrease blood pressure (Box 13-2).

There are many classes of antihypertensive drugs that have both different and common actions and effects. Nursing responsibilities for the common actions and effects are listed in the following discussion. Specific nursing responsibilities are discussed with each individual class of drugs.

*Before giving any antihypertensive drug,* always obtain a complete list of drugs that the patient is currently using, including herbal and over-the-counter drugs.

Obtain a baseline set of vital signs. If the patient's blood pressure is low (less than 90/60 mm Hg) or the heart rate is low (less than 60 beats per minute), notify the prescriber and ask if the patient should receive the drug. Ask the patient about signs and symptoms such as dizziness, light-headedness, or headaches.

Ask women of childbearing years if they are pregnant, planning to become pregnant, or breastfeeding because some of these drugs can harm the fetus directly or reduce blood pressure in the fetus.

| Box 13-2 | Guidelines for Prescribing Antihypertensive Drugs |

- Thiazide diuretics should be used for most patients with uncomplicated hypertension, either alone or in combination with other drugs.
- Most patients with hypertension require two or more antihypertensive drugs to achieve blood pressure control (less than 140/90 mm Hg or less than 130/80 mm Hg in patients with diabetes or chronic kidney disease).
- If blood pressure exceeds the goal by more than 20/10 mm Hg above the goal blood pressure, the prescriber should consider therapy with two drugs, one of which is a thiazide diuretic.
- Motivation of patients improves control of blood pressure. Motivation improves when the patient has had positive experiences with and trusts the prescriber.

From U.S. Department of Health and Human Services, National Institutes of Health, National Heart, Lung, and Blood Institute, National High Blood Pressure Education Program: *The Seventh Report of the Joint National Committee on Prevention, Detection, Evaluation, and Treatment of High Blood Pressure.* NIH Publication No. 04-5230. August 2004. Available online at http://www.nhlbi.nih.gov/guidelines/hypertension/jnc7full.pdf. Accessed 8/3/09.

*After giving any antihypertensive drug,* recheck and continue to monitor the patient's vital signs every 4 to 8 hours. Ask the patient about dizziness or light-headedness because these are signs of hypotension. If these symptoms occur, check the patient's blood pressure and heart rate while lying down, sitting, and standing (orthostatic vital signs). Notify the prescriber of positive orthostatic vital signs. Orthostatic hypotension is said to occur if, within 3 minutes of standing, systolic pressure drops by at least 20 mm Hg, diastolic pressure drops by at least 10 mm Hg, or heart rate increases more than 20 beats per minute. Tell the patient to call for help when getting out of bed and make sure the call light is within easy reach. Help the patient change positions slowly.

*Teach patients receiving antihypertensive drugs* the proper techniques for checking their blood pressure and heart rates. Tell them to keep a daily record. Remind patients about the symptoms of hypotension and tell them to change positions slowly. Patients experiencing these symptoms should be instructed not to drive, operate machines, or do anything that is dangerous until they know how the drug will affect them.

Instruct patients to keep all follow-up appointments with their prescriber to monitor blood pressure and side effects of antihypertensive drugs. Tell them to take all prescribed doses as directed. If a dose is missed and the next dose is not due for over 4 hours, instruct patients to take the dose as soon as possible. If the next dose is due in less than 4 hours, tell patients to skip the missed dose and return to the regular dosing schedule. Remind patients to never take double doses of antihypertensive drugs.

Remind patients to notify the prescriber for any signs of hypotension or chest pain. Tell them to consult with their prescriber before taking over-the-counter drugs.

Talk with patients about lifestyle changes that will also help manage hypertension. Possible changes include weight loss, exercise, stress reduction, smoking cessation, and a low-salt, low-fat diet.

Remind patients that these drugs will help to control, *not* cure, high blood pressure and that they may take these drugs for the rest of their lives. Stress the importance of controlling high blood pressure to prevent other serious health problems such as heart failure, kidney disease, and vascular diseases.

Instruct patients taking antihypertensive drugs to obtain and wear a medical alert bracelet that states the drug, dose, and diagnosis.

## TYPES OF ANTIHYPERTENSIVE DRUGS

Several types of drugs are used to control hypertension. They may be used alone or in combination with other drugs. Antihypertensive drugs have several classes:

 **Memory Jogger**

Orthostatic hypotension criteria:
- Decreased SBP of 20 mm Hg or more
- Decreased DBP of 10 mm Hg or more
- Increased heart rate of 20 beats per minute or more

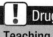 **Drug Alert!**

**Teaching Alert**

Teach patients to take missed doses as soon as possible; but, if it's almost time for the next dose, skip the missed dose and return to the regular dosing schedule.

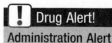 **Drug Alert!**

**Administration Alert**

Patients with hypertension should *not* take over-the-counter drugs (such as drugs for appetite control, asthma, colds, and hay fever) without asking their prescriber.

- Diuretics—drugs that eliminate excess water and salt from the body (see Chapter 12).
- Angiotensin-converting enzyme (ACE) inhibitors—drugs that lower blood pressure. For people with diabetes, especially those with protein (albumin) in their urine, ACE inhibitors also help slow kidney damage.
- Angiotensin II receptor antagonists—drugs that change the action of the renin-angiotensin-aldosterone system. These drugs block the activation of angiotensin II type 1 receptors. Angiotensin II receptor antagonists are mainly used in the treatment of hypertension when the patient is intolerant of ACE inhibitor therapy. These drugs are also called *angiotensin receptor blockers (ARBs).*
- Calcium channel blockers—drugs that slow the movement of calcium into the cells of the heart and blood vessels. This in turn relaxes the blood vessels, increases the supply of oxygen-rich blood to the heart, and reduces the workload of the heart.
- Beta blockers (beta-adrenergic blockers)—drugs that limit the activity of epinephrine (a hormone that increases blood pressure). Beta blockers reduce the heart rate and force of contraction, leading to decreased oxygen demand by the heart muscle.
- Alpha blockers—drugs that oppose the excitatory effects of norepinephrine released from sympathetic nerve endings at alpha receptors and cause blood vessel relaxation and vasodilation, leading to a decrease in blood pressure. These drugs are also called alpha-adrenergic blocking agents.
- Alpha-beta blockers—drugs that combine the effects of alpha and beta blockers.
- Central-acting adrenergic agents—drugs that lower blood pressure by stimulating alpha receptors in the brain, which widen (dilate) peripheral arteries and ease blood flow. Central alpha agonists such as clonidine are usually prescribed when all other antihypertensive medications have failed. For treating hypertension these drugs are usually administered in combination with a diuretic.
- Direct vasodilators—drugs that act directly on the smooth muscle of small arteries, causing these arteries to expand (dilate).

## DIURETICS

Diuretics control blood pressure by eliminating excess salt and water from the body. Those most commonly used include loop, thiazide, and potassium-sparing diuretics (see Chapter 12).

### How Diuretics Work

Most diuretics help the kidneys get rid of excess salt and water from body tissues and blood, reducing swelling. A decrease in body fluids lowers blood pressure. Some of these drugs relax arteries, which also lowers blood pressure. Diuretics are often the first-choice drugs for high blood pressure and are usually part of a multidrug plan to manage this condition. Thiazide diuretics are commonly the first prescribed drug for uncomplicated hypertension. They are relatively inexpensive and may be prescribed alone or in combination with other antihypertensive drugs. See Chapter 12 for additional information on the use of diuretic drugs.

**Memory Jogger**

The types of diuretics used to treat hypertension are thiazide, loop, and potassium-sparing.

### *Intended Responses*
- Urine output is increased.
- Volume in the blood vessels is decreased.
- Excess salt in the body is decreased.
- Blood vessels are dilated.
- Blood pressure is lowered.

*Side Effects.* The most common side effects of diuretics include dizziness, light-headedness, postural hypotension, decreased potassium level *(hypokalemia),* and decreased sodium level *(hyponatremia).*

*Adverse Effects.* Adverse effects of diuretics include "passing out" or falling when changing positions, muscle weakness, and blurred vision.

### What To Do *Before* Giving Diuretics

Be sure to review the general nursing responsibilities related to antihypertensive therapy (p. 226) in addition to these specific responsibilities before giving diuretics.

Check the most recent serum potassium level. If it is below 3.5 mEq/L or 3.5 mmol/L, inform the prescriber.

Ask all patients about any allergic reactions to thiazide drugs.

### What To Do *After* Giving Diuretics

Be sure to review the general nursing responsibilities related to antihypertensive therapy (p. 227) in addition to these specific responsibilities after giving diuretics.

Be sure to monitor the patient's urine output and blood pressure to determine the effectiveness of the drug therapy. Watch for signs of ototoxicity with administration of intravenous (IV) furosemide. Monitor blood electrolytes, especially potassium. Watch for signs of low or high potassium levels.

### What To *Teach* Patients About Diuretics

Be sure to teach patients about general issues and precautions related to antihypertensive therapy (p. 227) in addition to these specific teaching points for diuretics.

Teach patients to keep a record of daily weights. Instruct them to weigh in every day at the same time, using the same scale and wearing the same or similar clothing.

Remind patients to report side effects such as muscle weakness or cramps, sudden decrease in urination, and irregular heartbeat to the prescriber. These may be symptoms of hypokalemia.

Instruct patients to be sure to take any potassium pills or liquids that are ordered and to drink the same amount of fluid as they urinate. Teach patients about foods that are rich in potassium such as bananas, raisins, and green leafy vegetables.

See Chapter 12 for additional information on thiazide, loop, and potassium-sparing diuretics.

## ANGIOTENSIN-CONVERTING ENZYME INHIBITORS

### How ACE Inhibitors Work

ACE inhibitors block production of substances that constrict (narrow) blood vessels (Figure 13-2). They also help decrease the buildup of water and salt in the blood and body tissues. The exact way that these drugs work is not known. They block an enzyme in the body that is necessary for production of angiotensin II (a substance that causes blood vessels to tighten or constrict). The result is that blood vessels relax and blood pressure is decreased. This also decreases heart workload and increases the blood flow and oxygen to the heart and other organs.

These drugs are often given to patients with health problems such as heart failure, kidney disease, and diabetes. ACE inhibitors are often prescribed *along with* diuretics to control hypertension, and combined ACE inhibitor/diuretic drug forms are available. For example, lisinopril/hydrochlorothiazide (Prinzide, Zestoretic) is often prescribed for the management of hypertension; lisinopril is an ACE inhibitor, and hydrochlorothiazide is a diuretic.

Usually the first doses of an ACE inhibitor are lower when the patient is also taking a diuretic or has renal (kidney) impairment. Be sure to consult a drug reference book for information on any specific ACE inhibitor.

  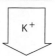
 **Memory Jogger**

The generic names for ACE inhibitors end in *"-pril"* (for example, enalapril).

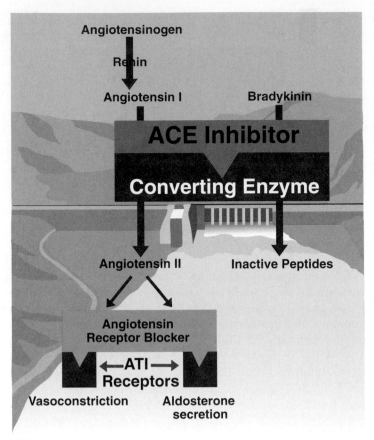

**FIGURE 13-2** Function of ACE inhibitors and angiotensin II receptor antagonists.

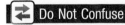 **Do Not Confuse**

**Accupril** *with* **Aciphex**

An order for Accupril may be confused with Aciphex. Accupril is an ACE inhibitor, whereas Aciphex is a proton pump inhibitor used for healing gastrointestinal ulcers.

**Do Not Confuse**

**Zestril** *with* **Zetia**

An order for Zestril may be confused with Zetia. Zestril is an ACE inhibitor, whereas Zetia is a cholesterol-lowering drug.

## Dosages for Common ACE Inhibitors

| Drug | Dosage |
| --- | --- |
| captopril (Capoten, Novo-Captopril🍁) | *Adults:* 12.5-50 mg orally 2-3 times daily |
| enalapril 🔟 (Vasotec) | *Adults:* 2.5-40 mg orally daily as single dose or 2 divided doses |
| lisinopril 🔟 (Prinivil, Zestril) | *Adults:* 10-40 mg orally once daily |
| perindopril (Aceon) | *Adults:* 4-16 mg orally daily as single dose or 2 divided doses |
| quinapril (Accupril 🔟) | *Adults:* 10-80 mg orally daily as single dose or 2 divided doses |
| ramipril (Altace) | *Adults:* 2.5-20 mg orally once daily as single dose or 2 divided doses |
| trandolapril (Mavik) | *Adults:* 1-4 mg orally once daily; in African-American patients begin with 2 mg daily |

🔟 Top 100 prescribed drugs.

### Intended Responses
- Production of angiotensin II is decreased.
- Vasodilation of blood vessels is increased.
- Excess tissue water and salt are decreased.
- Blood pressure is lowered.
- Workload on the heart is decreased.

***Side Effects.*** The more common side effects of ACE inhibitors include hypotension; protein in the urine; taste disturbances; increased blood potassium level *(hyperkalemia)*; headache; and persistent, dry cough. If one ACE inhibitor causes a cough, it is likely that others will also, and the patient will need to be prescribed another type

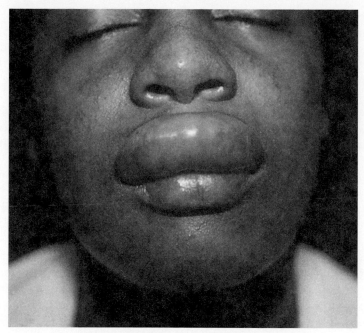

FIGURE 13-3 Angioedema.

of antihypertensive drug. Less common side effects include diarrhea, nausea, and unusual fatigue.

***Adverse Effects.*** Adverse effects include fever and chills; hoarseness; swelling in the face, hands, or feet; trouble swallowing or breathing; stomach pain; chest pain; rashes and itching skin; and yellow eyes or skin. Some patients also develop dizziness, light-headedness, or fainting.

Allergic reactions and kidney failure are serious but rare adverse effects with ACE inhibitors.

Angioedema is a diffuse swelling of the eyes, lips, and tongue (Figure 13-3). It may occur with allergic reactions to these drugs and may be life threatening. Swelling of the trachea (windpipe/airway) can interfere with breathing, a life-threatening event. Angioedema can occur months or even years after ACE inhibitor therapy is started.

Neutropenia (decreased leukocytes in the blood) may occur, increasing the risk for infections. Infections may develop in the throat, intestinal tract, other mucous membranes, or the skin. Symptoms of neutropenia include any signs of infection such as chills, fever, or sore throat.

Some ACE inhibitors (for example, enalapril, quinapril, and ramipril) cause increased sun sensitivity (photosensitivity).

### What To Do *Before* Giving ACE Inhibitors

Be sure to review the general nursing responsibilities related to antihypertensive therapy (p. 226) in addition to these specific responsibilities before giving ACE inhibitors.

Ask about any allergies to drugs, foods, preservatives, and dyes, because more people develop allergies with ACE inhibitors than with any other drug for blood pressure. Ask patients if they are also taking diuretics to control blood pressure because ACE inhibitors enhance the blood pressure–lowering effects of diuretics.

### What To Do *After* Giving ACE Inhibitors

Be sure to review the general nursing responsibilities related to antihypertensive therapy (p. 227) in addition to these specific responsibilities after giving ACE inhibitors.

**Common Side Effects**
**ACE Inhibitors**

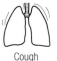  

Cough    Hypotension    Taste disturbances

Hyperkalemia    Headache

**!** **Drug Alert!**
**Administration Alert**

If a patient taking an ACE inhibitor develops a persistent, dry cough, the prescriber should be notified, and the drug discontinued.

**!** **Drug Alert!**
**Action/Intervention Alert**

Monitor patients for angioedema, which is a serious adverse effect of ACE inhibitors.

**!** **Drug Alert!**
**Interaction Alert**

ACE inhibitors may increase the effect of decreased blood pressure in patients who are also taking diuretics. ACE inhibitors and potassium-sparing diuretics cause much higher increases in blood potassium levels.

Check patients' blood potassium level because these drugs reduce the excretion of potassium. This is even more important if the patient is also prescribed a potassium-sparing diuretic. Keep track of urine output and weight. Kidney failure is a rare but serious adverse effect of these drugs.

Check for any signs or symptoms of allergic reactions or infections.

### What To *Teach* Patients About ACE Inhibitors

Be sure to teach patients about general issues and precautions related to antihypertensive therapy (p. 227) in addition to these specific teaching points for ACE inhibitors.

Tell patients to take this drug at the same time every day. Captopril (Capoten) should be taken 1 hour before eating or on an empty stomach.

Tell patients not to drink alcohol until they talk with their prescriber because ACE inhibitors can increase the low blood pressure effect and the risk for dizziness or fainting.

Teach patients to avoid salt substitutes. Salt substitutes contain potassium, and a side effect of ACE inhibitors is increased blood potassium level (hyperkalemia).

Instruct patients to report any side effects of ACE inhibitors to their prescriber. Tell patients to go to the emergency room immediately to report any facial swelling because this is a sign of angioedema, a life-threatening adverse reaction. Remind patients that angioedema can occur even months to years after beginning to take these drugs.

Teach patients taking enalapril (Vasotec), quinapril (Accupril), or ramipril (Altace) to limit direct sunlight, wear protective clothing, and use sunscreens because sun sensitivity (photosensitivity) is a side effect of these drugs.

### Life Span Considerations for ACE Inhibitors

*Pediatric Considerations.* Children are more sensitive to the effects of ACE inhibitors for blood pressure. They are at higher risk of having severe side effects from the drugs. Before giving these drugs to children, parents should discuss the benefits and risks with their pediatric cardiologist.

*Considerations for Pregnancy and Breastfeeding.* ACE inhibitors are pregnancy category D and can cause birth defects. They are not prescribed for women who are pregnant or are thinking about becoming pregnant. Lisinopril is pregnancy category C during the first trimester and pregnancy category D during the second and third trimesters. These drugs pass into breast milk and should not be used while breastfeeding because they can lower blood pressure and lead to kidney damage in the infant.

*Considerations for Older Adults.* Older adults are at greater risk for postural hypotension when taking ACE inhibitors because of the cardiovascular changes associated with aging. Teach patients to not stand or sit up quickly because this may lower blood pressure rapidly, causing dizziness and an increased risk for falls. Also instruct them to hold onto railings when going up or down steps.

### ANGIOTENSIN II RECEPTOR ANTAGONISTS

#### How Angiotensin II Receptor Antagonists Work

Angiotensin II receptor antagonists block the effects of angiotensin II (vasoconstriction, sodium and water retention) by directly blocking the binding of angiotensin II to angiotensin II type 1 receptors.

These drugs may be given in combination with diuretics. Losartan combined with the thiazide diuretic hydrochlorothiazide (Hyzaar) is often prescribed to control high blood pressure. Lower doses of angiotensin II receptor antagonists are used when a patient is taking a diuretic or has renal (kidney) or hepatic (liver) impairment. These drugs are inactivated by the liver and excreted from the body by the kidney. Patients who have impairment of either of these organs may have higher blood levels of the drugs and are at greater risk for side effects or adverse effects. Be sure to

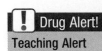

**Drug Alert!**

**Teaching Alert**

Tell patients who are taking ACE inhibitors that drinking alcohol can increase the low blood pressure effect and the risk of dizziness or fainting.

**Clinical Pitfall**

ACE inhibitors should *not* be prescribed for women who are pregnant. They can cause low blood pressure, severe kidney failure, increased potassium, and even death in a newborn when used after the first trimester of pregnancy.

⊖-Learning Activity 13-4 ▶

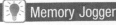

**Memory Jogger**

The generic names for angiotensin II receptor antagonists end in "*-sartan*" (for example, valsartan)

consult a drug reference book for additional information on any angiotensin II receptor antagonist.

### Dosages for Common Angiotensin-II Receptor Antagonists

| Drug | Dosage |
|------|--------|
| losartan 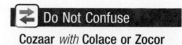 (Cozaar) | *Adults:* 25-100 mg orally daily as a single dose or in 2 divided doses |
| valsartan (Diovan) | *Adults:* 80-320 mg orally once daily |
| irbesartan (Avapro) | *Adults:* 150-300 mg orally once daily |
| candesartan (Atacand) | *Adults:* 16-32 mg orally once daily |
| telmisartan (Micardis) | *Adults:* 20-80 mg orally once daily |
| eprosartan (Teveten) | *Adults:* 400-800 mg orally once daily or in 2 divided doses |

Top 100 drugs prescribed.

### Intended Responses
- Vasodilation of blood vessels is increased.
- Excess body water and salt are decreased.
- Blood pressure is lowered.
- Workload on the heart is decreased.

***Side Effects.*** There are few documented side effects from angiotensin II receptor antagonists. Side effects include dizziness, fatigue, headache, hypotension, diarrhea, and high blood potassium levels (hyperkalemia).

***Adverse Effects.*** Adverse effects are rare but include kidney failure and life-threatening angioedema (swelling of the face, eyes, lips, tongue, and trachea that can interfere with breathing) (see Figure 13-3).

An additional rare adverse effect is liver toxicity or drug-induced hepatitis. These drugs should not be given to patients who have known liver problems.

### What To Do *Before* Giving Angiotensin II Receptor Antagonists
Be sure to review the general nursing responsibilities related to antihypertensive therapy (p. 226) in addition to these specific responsibilities before giving angiotensin II receptor antagonists.

Check blood urea nitrogen (BUN) and creatinine levels for preexisting kidney disease because these drugs are excreted by the kidneys. Ask whether the patient has any kidney or liver problems because these drugs can worsen liver disease.

### What To Do *After* Giving Angiotensin II Receptor Antagonists
Be sure to review the general nursing responsibilities related to antihypertensive therapy (p. 227) in addition to these specific responsibilities after giving angiotensin II receptor antagonists.

Look for any swelling of the face, including the eyes, lips, or tongue (signs of angioedema). Report this immediately to the prescriber. Do not administer the drug to the patient again because this is a life-threatening adverse reaction. Check the urine output and weight. Report decreased urine output or weight gain to the prescriber.

Check laboratory values for any changes in the blood potassium level because these drugs reduce potassium excretion by the kidneys. If the potassium level is higher than 5.5 mEq/L, notify the prescriber. Assess heart rate and rhythm, especially for a slow rate. If the patient has a heart monitor, assess for an increasing height of T waves—a sign of high potassium level. Check bowel sounds every shift. Increased bowel sounds and diarrhea are associated with high potassium levels.

### What To *Teach* Patients About Angiotensin II Receptor Antagonists
Be sure to teach patients about general issues and precautions related to antihypertensive therapy (p. 227) in addition to these specific teaching points for angiotensin II receptor antagonists.

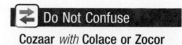

**Do Not Confuse**

**Cozaar** *with* **Colace or Zocor**

An order for Cozaar may be confused with Colace or Zocor. Cozaar is an angiotensin II receptor antagonist used to decrease blood pressure. Colace is a stool softener, and Zocor is a drug used to decrease blood lipids (fats).

**Common Side Effects**

**Angiotensin II Receptor Antagonists**

Dizziness, Light-headedness  Headache  Hypotension

Diarrhea  Hyperkalemia

**Clinical Pitfall**

Report any swelling of the face, eyes, lips, or tongue to the prescriber immediately. These are signs of life-threatening angioedema. Do *not* administer the drug to the patient again because this is a life-threatening adverse reaction.

Remind patients to get up slowly to prevent dizziness and falls. Alcohol use, standing for long periods, exercise, and hot weather may contribute to hypotension.

Instruct female patients to talk with their prescriber if they are taking an angiotensin II receptor antagonist drug and plan to become pregnant. These drugs can cause harm to the fetus.

Tell patients to go to the emergency department immediately to report any facial swelling because this is a sign of angioedema, a life-threatening adverse reaction. Remind them that angioedema can occur months to years after beginning to take these drugs. Teach them that, if this happens, they should avoid taking this drug ever again.

### Life Span Considerations for Angiotensin II Receptor Antagonists

*Pediatric Considerations.* Safe use of these drugs in children under the age of 18 has not been researched or established.

*Considerations for Pregnancy and Breastfeeding.* Angiotensin II receptor antagonists are pregnancy category C during the first trimester and pregnancy category D during the second and third trimesters. They should not be taken during the second or third trimesters of pregnancy. Valsartan is pregnancy category D during all trimesters. These drugs can interfere with fetal blood pressure control and kidney function. They have been associated with problems in fetal kidney and skull development. It is not known if they pass into breast milk. A woman who plans to breastfeed should not use these drugs.

### CALCIUM CHANNEL BLOCKERS

#### How Calcium Channel Blockers Work

Calcium channel blockers block calcium from entering the muscle cells of the heart and arteries. Blocking calcium causes a decrease in the contraction of the heart and also dilates (widens) the arteries. Widening the arteries causes a decrease in blood pressure and reduces the workload of the heart.

⊜-Animation 13-1: Calcium ▶ Channel Blockers

When these drugs are prescribed for older patients or patients with hepatic (liver) or renal (kidney) impairment, initial lower doses are used. Be sure to consult a drug reference book for information on any calcium channel blocker drug.

#### Dosages for Common Calcium Channel Blockers

| Drug | Dosage |
| --- | --- |
| amlodipine 🔲 (Norvasc) | *Adults:* 2.5-10 mg orally once daily |
| diltiazem 🔲 (Cardizem) | *Adults:* 30-120 mg orally 3-4 times daily, or 60-120 mg twice daily as SR capsules, or 180-240 mg once daily as XR/CD capsules; do not exceed 360 mg/day<br>IV: 0.25 mg/kg; may repeat after 15 min with dose of 0.35 mg/kg<br>IV infusion: 5-15 mg/hr |
| felodipine (Plendil) | *Adults:* 2.5-10 mg orally daily |
| niCARdipine (Cardene) | *Adults:* 20 mg orally 3 times daily. May be given as 30-60 mg twice daily as SR capsules<br>IV infusion: 5-15 mg/hr |
| NIFEdipine (Adalat, Novo-Nifedin♣, Nu-Nifedin♣, Procardia, Procardia XL) | *Adults:* 10-30 mg orally 3 times daily, do not exceed 180 mg daily; CC/XL—initially 30-60 mg daily, titrate upward as necessary and do not exceed 90 mg daily<br>*Note: Do **not** give immediate-release capsules sublingually* |
| verapamil 🔲 (Calan, Isoptin, NovoVerapamil♣, Nu-Verap♣) | *Adults:* 80-120 mg orally 3 times daily<br>*Children:* 4-8 mg/kg orally daily in 3 divided doses |

🔲 Top 100 drugs prescribed.

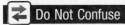

### Do Not Confuse

#### niCARdipine *with* NIFEdipine

An order for niCARdipine may be confused with NIFEdipine. Both are calcium channel blockers.

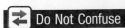

### Do Not Confuse

#### Norvasc *with* Navane

An order for Norvasc may be confused with Navane. Norvasc is a calcium channel blocker, whereas Navane is an antipsychotic drug used for schizophrenia and other psychotic disorders.

*Intended Responses*
- Heart contraction is decreased.
- Artery dilation (widening) is increased.
- Heart workload is decreased.
- Blood pressure is lowered.
- Blood flow and oxygen to the heart are increased.

*Side Effects.*  The most common side effects of these drugs are constipation, nausea, headache, flushing, rash, edema (legs), hypotension, drowsiness, and dizziness.

Gingival hyperplasia (overgrowth of gum tissue) is a rare side effect that may occur in children. Gynecomastia (development of the enlarged male breasts) may also occur with rare unusual secretion of milk when taking verapamil.

*Adverse Effects.*  Dysrhythmias may occur with calcium channel blockers, including irregular, rapid, pounding, or excessively slow heart rhythms (less than 50 beats per minute).

Patients with heart failure symptoms may worsen with verapamil and diltiazem because of the increased abilities of the drugs to reduce the strength and rate of heart contraction.

*Stevens-Johnson syndrome* (erythema multiforme) is a potentially lethal skin disorder resulting from an allergic reaction to drugs, infections, or illness. It causes damage to blood vessels of the skin. Symptoms include many different types of skin lesions (Figure 13-4), itching, fever, joint aching, and generally feeling ill.

Rare but serious adverse effects include difficulty breathing; irregular, rapid, or pounding heart rhythm; slow heart rate (<50 beats per minute); bleeding; chest pain; and vision problems (difficulty seeing).

### What To Do *Before* Giving Calcium Channel Blockers

Be sure to review the general nursing responsibilities related to antihypertensive therapy (p. 226) in addition to these specific responsibilities before giving calcium channel blockers.

Find out if the patient has any health problems that may be affected by these drugs such as heart failure, blood vessel disease, and liver or kidney disease.

### What To Do *After* Giving Calcium Channel Blockers

Be sure to review the general nursing responsibilities related to antihypertensive therapy (p. 227) in addition to these specific responsibilities after giving calcium channel blockers.

---

## Common Side Effects
### Calcium Channel Blockers

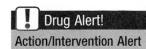

Hypotension       Constipation;       Headache
                     Nausea

Dizziness,
Light-
headedness

---

### ! Drug Alert!
#### Action/Intervention Alert

Calcium channel blockers can cause a severe skin disorder called Stevens-Johnson syndrome. Always check the patient for skin lesions, itching, fever, and achy joints.

---

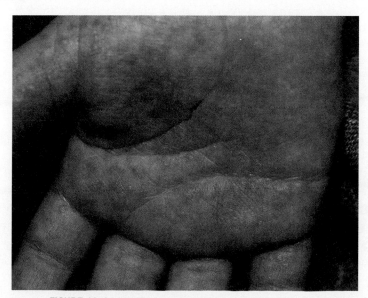

**FIGURE 13-4** Hand lesions of Stevens-Johnson syndrome.

Report irregular heart rhythms to the prescriber. Watch for side effects or adverse effects of these drugs. If a patient develops skin lesions, itching, fever, and achy joints, report this to the prescriber at once because these are signs of Stevens-Johnson syndrome and allergic reaction to the drug.

### What To *Teach* Patients About Calcium Channel Blockers

Be sure to teach patients about general issues and precautions related to antihypertensive therapy (p. 227) in addition to these specific teaching points for calcium channel blockers.

Remind patients to get up and change positions slowly to decrease dizziness. Explain that exercising in hot weather can cause dizziness and low blood pressure.

Explain that, if the patient should suddenly stop taking these drugs after taking them for several weeks, hypertension may return. The prescriber can advise the patient on how to gradually stop taking the drug.

### Life Span Considerations for Calcium Channel Blockers

*Pediatric Considerations.* Safe use of calcium channel blockers in children has not been researched. Before using these drugs with children, parents should discuss risks and benefits with the prescriber.

*Considerations for Pregnancy and Breastfeeding.* Calcium channel blockers are pregnancy category C. Their effects have not been tested in human pregnancy. In studies of laboratory animals, birth defects and stillborns have occurred. Women should consult with their prescriber and pediatrician before using these drugs during pregnancy. Some calcium channel blockers pass into breast milk. Women who wish to breastfeed while taking these drugs should discuss this with their prescriber.

*Considerations for Older Adults.* Older adults may be especially sensitive to the effects of calcium channel blocking agents. This may increase the chance of side effects during treatment. A lower starting dose may be required.

⊖-Learning Activity 13-5 ▶

### BETA BLOCKERS

#### How Beta Blockers Work

Beta blockers block the effects of epinephrine (adrenaline) on the heart (Figure 13-5). They decrease the heart rate and force of heart contractions, which leads to decreased blood pressure. As a result the heart does not work as hard and requires less oxygen.

Beta blockers are classified as cardioselective and noncardioselective. *Cardioselective* drugs work only on the cardiovascular system. *Noncardioselective* drugs have effects on all of the organs and systems of the body (systemic effects).

When beta blockers are prescribed for a patient with kidney damage, a lower dose of the drug is prescribed, or the time between doses is increased. An older adult may also be started on a lower drug dose. Be sure to consult a drug reference book for information about a specific beta blocker.

> 💡 **Memory Jogger**
>
> The generic names of beta blockers end with "*-olol*" (for example, metoprolol).

#### Dosages for Common Beta Blockers for Hypertension

| Drug | Dosage |
| --- | --- |
| acebutolol ❶ (Monitan✽, Sectral)—selective | *Adults:* 400-1200 mg orally daily in 2 divided doses |
| atenolol 🔝❶ (Apo-Atenolol✽, Novo-Atenol✽, Tenormin)—selective | *Adults:* 25-200 mg orally once daily |
| betaxolol ❶ (Kerlone)—selective | *Adults:* 10-20 mg orally once daily |
| bisoprolol ❶ (Zebeta)—selective | *Adults:* 2.5-20 mg orally once daily |
| labetalol ❶ (Normodyne, Trandate)—nonselective | *Adults:* PO: 100-400 mg orally twice daily<br>*Adults:* IV: 20 mg initially; additional doses of 40-80 mg may be given every 10 min as needed; do not exceed 300-mg total dosage |

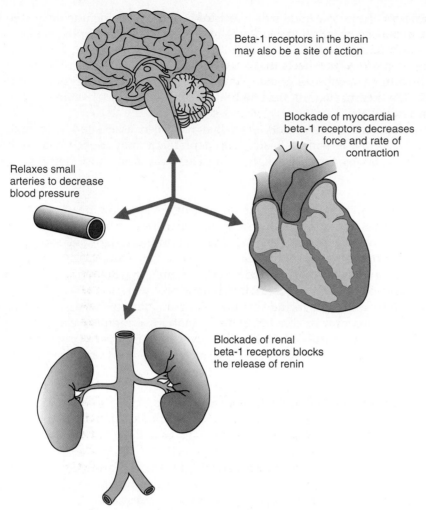

Beta-1 receptors in the brain may also be a site of action

Blockade of myocardial beta-1 receptors decreases force and rate of contraction

Relaxes small arteries to decrease blood pressure

Blockade of renal beta-1 receptors blocks the release of renin

**FIGURE 13-5** Potential sites of action for beta blockers.

## Dosages for Common Beta Blockers for Hypertension—cont'd

| Drug | Dosage |
|------|--------|
| metoprolol **TOP 100** ❶ (Betaloc♣, Lopresor♣, Lopressor, Nu-Metop♣, Toprol XL)—selective | *Adults:* PO: 100-450 mg orally once daily or in 2 divided doses; extended-release forms should be given once daily<br>*Adults:* IV: 5 mg every 2 min for 3 doses followed by oral dosing |
| nadolol ❶ (Corgard)—nonselective | *Adults:* 40-320 mg orally once daily |
| propranolol ❶ (Detensol♣, Inderal, NovoPranol♣)—nonselective | *Adults:* 40-120 mg orally twice daily; extended action form—80-120 mg once daily<br>*Children:* 0.5-l mg/kg orally daily in 2-4 divided doses; may increase as needed (usual range 2-4 mg/kg daily in 2 divided doses) |
| timolol ❶ (Apo-Timol♣, Blocadren, Novo-Timol♣)—nonselective | *Adults:* 10-30 mg orally twice daily |

**TOP 100** Top 100 drugs prescribed; ❶ High-alert drug.

### Intended Responses
- Heart rate is decreased.
- Force of heart contraction is decreased.
- Work of heart is decreased.
- Blood pressure is lowered.

⇄ **Do Not Confuse**

**Inderal** *with* **Adderall**

An order for Inderal may be confused with Adderall. Inderal is a noncardioselective beta blocker, whereas Adderall is a stimulant used for narcolepsy and attention deficit disorder in children.

⇄ **Do Not Confuse**

**Toprol XL** *with* **Topamax**

An order for Toprol XL may be confused with Topamax. Toprol XL is an extended-release form of metoprolol, a cardioselective beta blocker. Topamax is a central nervous system anticonvulsant.

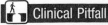 
*Side Effects.* Fairly common side effects of beta blockers include decreased sexual ability, dizziness or light-headedness, drowsiness, trouble sleeping *(insomnia),* and fatigue or weakness.

Less common side effects that must be reported to the prescriber include difficulty breathing or wheezing; cold hands or feet; mental depression; shortness of breath; slow heart rate (less than 50 beats per minute); and swelling in the ankles, feet, or lower legs.

Depression is another side effect that has been associated with taking beta blockers. A patient with a history of depression may notice that it becomes worse while taking these drugs. Beta blockers may also cause depression for the first time.

*Adverse Effects.* Signs of drug overdose include very slow heart rate, chest pain, severe dizziness or fainting, fast or irregular heart rate, difficulty breathing, bluish-colored fingernails and palms, and seizures. Report these signs and symptoms to the prescriber at once.

Adverse effects may also include "passing out" or falling when changing positions related to orthostatic (postural) hypotension.

Other adverse effects include back or joint pain, dark urine, dizziness or fainting when getting up, fever or sore throat, hallucinations, irregular heart rate, skin rash, unusual bleeding or bruising, and yellow eyes or skin. These drugs can affect the blood glucose level of a patient with diabetes and may cause hypoglycemia or hyperglycemia.

### What To Do *Before* Giving Beta Blockers

Be sure to review the general nursing responsibilities related to antihypertensive therapy (p. 226) in addition to these specific responsibilities before giving beta blockers.

For patients with diabetes, check blood glucose levels regularly. Beta blockers can mask signs of hypoglycemia such as rapid heart rate, making it difficult to recognize and treat. Ask patients about a history of depression.

### What To Do *After* Giving Beta Blockers

Be sure to review the general nursing responsibilities related to antihypertensive therapy (p. 227) in addition to these specific responsibilities after giving beta blockers.

If the heart rate is less than 60 beats per minute, notify the prescriber. Continue to monitor blood glucose in patients with diabetes because these drugs can mask the signs of hypoglycemia. Watch for signs and symptoms of depression.

### What To *Teach* Patients About Beta Blockers

Be sure to teach patients about general issues and precautions related to antihypertensive therapy (p. 227) in addition to these specific teaching points for beta blockers.

Teach patients to not stand or sit up quickly because this may lower blood pressure rapidly, causing dizziness and an increased risk for falls. Also instruct them to hold onto railings when going up or down steps.

Remind patients to check with the prescriber before stopping a beta blocker. It may be necessary to gradually decrease the daily dose of the drug. Suddenly stopping beta blockers can increase the risk of a heart attack.

Have patients notify their prescriber for any weight gain or increase in shortness of breath. These are signs of worsening heart failure.

Tell patients to always inform their prescriber that they are taking a beta blocker before any form of surgical or emergency treatment. Patients should also inform health care providers about beta blocker use before medical tests and allergy shots. These drugs can affect the results of medical tests and can cause serious reactions with allergy shots.

Tell patients that any chest pain experienced during activity should be reported to their prescriber so safe activity levels may be discussed.

Beta blockers can cause increased sensitivity to sunlight and cold. Tell patients to stay out of direct sunlight, use a sun block skin protector, and wear protective clothing. Advise patients to dress warmly during cold weather because decreased blood flow to the hands increases the risk for frostbite.

Teach patients that these drugs can cause new-onset depression or worsen existing depression.

### Life Span Considerations for Beta Blockers

***Pediatric Considerations.***  Use of beta blockers in children has not been researched. Although there is no evidence that risks from using beta blockers are different from those in adults, parents should discuss the risks and benefits with a pediatric cardiologist before a child begins taking these drugs.

***Considerations for Pregnancy and Breastfeeding.***  Most beta blockers are pregnancy category C and should not be used during pregnancy unless absolutely necessary. Atenolol is pregnancy category D and acebutolol is pregnancy category B. These drugs are excreted in breast milk. No adverse effects on infants have been documented, but the possibility of slowed heart rate and lowered blood pressure exists. Women who are breastfeeding should consult with their prescriber about continued use of these drugs.

***Considerations for Older Adults.***  Older adults are prescribed lower doses of beta blockers because they have a higher rate and intensity of side effects such as dizziness. A side effect of beta blockers that is more likely to occur in older adults is mental confusion. Teach family members to watch for this change and report it to the prescriber. These drugs may also decrease the patient's ability to tolerate cool temperatures. Teach him or her to dress warmly in cool weather and to wear hats and gloves when outdoors.

## ALPHA BLOCKERS

### How Alpha Blockers Work

Alpha blockers block receptors in arteries and smooth muscle. This relaxes the blood vessels and leads to an increase in blood flow and a lower blood pressure (Figure 13-6). Be sure to consult a drug reference book for information about any specific alpha blocker.

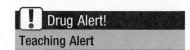

**Drug Alert!**
**Teaching Alert**

Teach patients that beta blockers can cause new-onset depression or worsen existing depression.

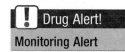

**Drug Alert!**
**Monitoring Alert**

Monitor older adults who have been prescribed beta blockers for mental confusion or changes in level of consciousness.

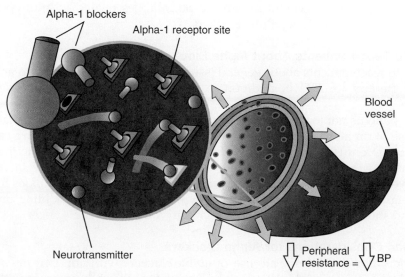

Alpha-1 blockers

Alpha-1 receptor site

Blood vessel

Neurotransmitter

Peripheral resistance = BP

**FIGURE 13-6** Alpha-1 blockers fill alpha-1 receptor sites, preventing neurotransmitters from binding. With fewer receptors being stimulated, vasoconstriction is prevented or reversed and blood pressure is lowered. *BP,* Blood pressure.

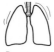
### Dosages for Common Alpha Blockers

| Drug | Dosage |
|---|---|
| doxazosin (Cardura) | *Adults:* 1-16 mg orally once daily |
| prazosin (Minipress) | *Adults:* 1-5 mg orally 2-3 times daily; do not exceed 20 mg daily<br>*Children:* 20-400 mcg/kg orally daily in 2-3 divided doses; do not exceed 7 mg/dose or 15 mg daily |
| terazosin (Hytrin) | *Adults:* 1-10 mg orally daily in 1 or 2 divided doses |

### *Intended Responses*
- Artery relaxation and dilation (widening) are increased.
- Blood flow is increased.
- Blood pressure is lowered.

***Side Effects.*** The most common side effects of alpha blockers are dizziness, drowsiness, fatigue, headache, nervousness, irritability, stuffy or runny nose, nausea, pain in the arms and legs, hypotension, and weakness.

Less common side effects include depression, abnormal or blurred vision, dyspnea, chest pain, palpitations, decreased sexual function, and rash.

A side effect of prazosin and terazosin is first-dose orthostatic hypotension because initially the patient is more sensitive to the blood pressure–lowering effects. As patients continue to take these drugs, they become less sensitive and have fewer problems with hypotension.

***Adverse Effects.*** Alpha blockers can lower blood pressure more than is desired and cause side effects. Life-threatening effects are rare. Adverse effects to report to the prescriber include fainting; shortness of breath or difficulty breathing; fast, pounding, or irregular heart rhythm; chest pain; and swollen feet, ankles, or wrists.

### What To Do *Before* Giving Alpha Blockers
Be sure to review the general nursing responsibilities related to antihypertensive therapy (p. 226) in addition to these specific responsibilities before giving alpha blockers.

Ask male patients if they are taking any phosphodiesterase type 5 inhibitor erectile dysfunction drugs (e.g., sildenafil [Viagra], tadalafil [Cialis], or vardenafil [Levitra]).

### What To Do *After* Giving Alpha Blockers
Be sure to review the general nursing responsibilities related to antihypertensive therapy (p. 227) after giving alpha blockers.

### What To *Teach* Patients About Alpha Blockers
Be sure to teach patients about general issues and precautions related to antihypertensive therapy (p. 227) in addition to these specific teaching points for alpha blockers.

Tell patients not to drive or use machines for at least 24 hours after taking the first dose of an alpha blocker because a sudden drop in blood pressure can cause dizziness or confusion. Remind them to get up slowly, especially during the middle of the night.

Have patients weigh themselves twice a week and check their ankles for swelling. Weight gain and ankle swelling are signs that the body is holding onto extra fluid and should be reported to the prescriber.

### Life Span Considerations for Alpha Blockers
***Pediatric Considerations.*** Safe use of alpha blockers with children has not been established. Parents should discuss the risks and benefits of these drugs with a pediatric cardiologist.

*Considerations for Pregnancy and Breastfeeding.* Alpha blockers are pregnancy category C drugs. The effect of these drugs on pregnancy has not been researched or fully understood. Women who are pregnant or planning to become pregnant should inform their prescriber. Alpha blockers pass into breast milk; mothers who wish to breastfeed should discuss this with their prescriber and pediatrician. It may be necessary to avoid breastfeeding while taking these drugs.

*Considerations for Older Adults.* Older adults experience a higher frequency and stronger side effects of alpha blockers, especially hypotension, confusion, and increased risk for falling. They often need lower doses of these drugs.

## ALPHA-BETA BLOCKERS

### How Alpha-Beta Blockers Work
Alpha-beta blockers combine the effects of alpha blockers and beta blockers. They relax blood vessels like alpha blockers, and they slow the heart rate and decrease the force of heart contractions like beta blockers. These actions result in lower blood pressure. Be sure to consult a drug reference book for information on any specific alpha-beta blocker drug.

### Dosages for Common Alpha-Beta Blockers

| Drug | Dosage |
| --- | --- |
| carvedilol ❶ (Coreg) | *Adults:* 6.25-25 mg orally twice daily |
| labetalol HCL ❶ (Normodyne, Trandate) | *Adults:* PO: 100 mg orally twice daily (usual dosage range is 400-800 mg daily in 2-3 divided doses) <br> *Adults:* IV: 20 mg (0.25 mg/kg) initially |

❶ High-alert drug.

### Intended Responses
- Artery relaxation and dilation (widening) are increased.
- Heart rate is decreased.
- Force of heart contraction is decreased.
- Heart workload is decreased.
- Blood pressure is lowered.
- Blood flow and oxygen to the heart are increased.

*Side Effects.* Common side effects of alpha-beta blockers include dizziness, fatigue, weakness, orthostatic hypotension, diarrhea, impotence, and increased blood glucose levels (hyperglycemia).

Less common side effects include anxiety, depression, drowsiness, insomnia, memory loss, mental status changes, nausea, constipation, decreased sex drive, itching and rash, back pain, muscle cramps, and paresthesia.

*Adverse Effects.* Suddenly stopping alpha-beta blockers can cause life-threatening heart dysrhythmias, hypertension, or chest pain. Bradycardia, heart failure, and pulmonary edema can also occur.

Other adverse effects of these drugs may include yellow skin or eyes, swelling in the feet or ankles, weight gain, wheezing or trouble breathing, cold hands or feet, and difficulty sleeping.

### What To Do *Before* Giving Alpha-Beta Blockers
Be sure to review the general nursing responsibilities related to antihypertensive therapy (p. 226) in addition to these specific responsibilities before giving alpha-beta blockers.

Obtain a baseline weight. Use this information to compare for changes after therapy is started and to determine whether an adverse reaction is occurring. Check the patient for swelling in the feet or ankles. If the patient has diabetes, check the blood glucose level.

**Common Side Effects**
**Alpha-Beta Blockers**

Dizziness, Light-headedness    Weakness    Hypotension

Diarrhea    Hyperglycemia    Impotence

### What To Do *After* Giving Alpha-Beta Blockers

Be sure to review the general nursing responsibilities related to antihypertensive therapy (p. 227) in addition to these specific responsibilities after giving alpha-beta blockers.

For patients with diabetes, check blood glucose levels more frequently because this drug may cause an increase in these levels.

Check intake and output and daily weights and look for any signs of fluid overload (swelling, difficulty breathing, crackles, and weight gain).

### What To *Teach* Patients About Alpha-Beta Blockers

Be sure to teach patients about general issues and precautions related to antihypertensive therapy (p. 227) in addition to these specific teaching points for alpha-beta blockers.

Explain that to suddenly stop taking the drug can lead to life-threatening problems. Tell patients to contact the prescriber for irregular heart rate, heart rate less than 50 beats per minute, or blood pressure changes.

Tell patients not to drive or operate machines because the drug may cause dizziness or drowsiness. Remind them to change positions slowly.

Tell patients taking labetalol (Normodyne) that they may become more sensitive to cold and may need to dress warmly.

Remind patients with diabetes to carefully watch for signs of changes in blood sugar. These drugs may interfere with or mask some of the signs of low blood sugar. Patients may need to check their glucose levels more frequently and adjust the timing of their meals.

### Life Span Considerations for Alpha-Beta Blockers

*Considerations for Pregnancy and Breastfeeding.* Alpha-beta blockers are pregnancy category C drugs. Safe use in pregnancy or breastfeeding has not been researched and established. These drugs cross the placenta and into breast milk. They may cause slowed heart rate, hypotension, hypoglycemia, and respiratory depression in the newborn.

## CENTRAL-ACTING ADRENERGIC AGENTS

### How Central-Acting Adrenergic Agents Work

Central-acting adrenergic drugs stimulate central nervous system receptors to decrease constriction of blood vessels, which leads to dilation (widening) of arteries, and to lower blood pressure. Be sure to consult a drug reference book for information about any specific central-acting adrenergic agent.

### Dosages for Common Central-Acting Adrenergic Agents

| Drug | Dosage |
|------|--------|
| clonidine 100 (Catapres, Dixarit♦, Novo-Clonidine♦) | *Adults:* 0.1 mg (100 mcg) orally twice daily; usual maintenance dosage range is 0.2-0.6 mg daily in 2-3 divided doses<br>*Adults:* Transdermal: 0.1-0.3 mg (100-300 mcg) patch applied every 7 days<br>*Children:* 0.05-0.4 mg (50-400 mcg) orally twice daily |
| methyldopa (Aldomet, Dopamet♦, Nu-Medpa♦) | *Adults:* PO: 250 mg orally 2-3 times daily; may increase up to 3 g daily in divided doses<br>*Adults:* IV: 250-500 mg every 6 hr over 30-60 min; may increase up to 1 g every 6-8 hr<br>*Children:* PO: 10-65 mg/kg orally daily in 2-4 divided doses; do not exceed 3 g daily<br>*Children:* IV: 20-65 mg/kg daily in 4 divided doses |

100 100 Top drugs prescribed.

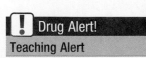

**! Drug Alert!**

**Teaching Alert**

Many blood pressure–lowering drugs can cause drowsiness or dizziness. Teach patients taking these drugs *not* to drive or operate machines.

### Intended Responses
- Vasodilation (widening) of arteries is increased.
- Blood pressure is lowered.
- Heart workload is decreased.

*Side Effects.* Central-acting adrenergic agents have a higher incidence of side effects than other blood pressure–lowering drugs. Common side effects include drowsiness, lethargy, dry mouth, and nasal congestion. Less common side effects include decreased mental status, bradycardia, edema, hypotension, depression, palpitations, constipation, nausea, vomiting, rash, sweating, salt retention, and weight gain.

*Adverse Effects.* Myocarditis associated with allergic type reactions to methyldopa are rare but have been known to cause death.

### What To Do *Before* Giving Central-Acting Adrenergic Agents
Be sure to review the general nursing responsibilities related to antihypertensive therapy (p. 226) in addition to these specific responsibilities before giving central-acting adrenergic drugs.

Obtain a baseline weight on the patient.

When administering a clonidine patch, be aware that it is packaged with two patches. The smaller patch contains the drug, and the larger patch is used to cover the drug patch. If the patch falls off, a new patch should be placed on the patient. Be sure to record the date and time and initial the patch before placing it on the patient.

### What To Do *After* Giving Central-Acting Adrenergic Agents
Be sure to review the general nursing responsibilities related to antihypertensive therapy (p. 227) in addition to these specific responsibilities after giving central-acting adrenergic drugs.

Keep track of the patient's intake and output. Check feet and ankles for swelling. Listen to the patient's lungs for crackles. Watch for signs of mental status changes suggesting that blood pressure may be too low. Look for psychiatric signs of depression such as difficulty concentrating, sleep changes, or a loss of interest in daily activities.

### What To *Teach* Patients About Central-Acting Adrenergic Agents
Be sure to teach patients about general issues and precautions related to antihypertensive therapy (p. 227) in addition to these specific teaching points for central-acting adrenergic drugs.

Teach patients that these drugs should be discontinued gradually. If the drugs are stopped suddenly, blood pressure could become dangerously high.

For dry mouth, encourage patients to perform frequent mouth care with rinses, tooth brushing, and the use of sugarless gum.

If the patient is using transdermal clonidine, teach that the patch can stay on during bathing or swimming. Teach patients that this medication is packaged with two patches. The smaller patch contains the actual drug; and the larger patch, which does not contain medication, is used to cover the drug patch. If the patch falls off, tell the patient to apply a new patch.

### Life Span Considerations for Central-Acting Adrenergic Agents
*Considerations for Pregnancy and Breastfeeding.* Clonidine is a pregnancy category C drug. Safe use of clonidine (Catapres) in pregnancy or breastfeeding has not been researched or established. This drug should be avoided during pregnancy and breastfeeding. Methyldopa (Aldomet) is a pregnancy category B drug when prescribed by mouth and a pregnancy category C drug when prescribed intravenously. Methyldopa has been used safely during both pregnancy and breastfeeding. It is also safely used to treat pregnancy-induced hypertension.

**Common Side Effects**

**Central-Acting Adrenergic Agents**

  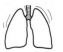

Drowsiness   Dry mouth   Nasal congestion

◄ ⊖-Video 13-1: Administering Topical Medications

**! Drug Alert!**

**Action/Intervention Alert**

Frequent mouth rinses, oral care, and chewing sugarless gum can relieve the dry-mouth side effect of central-acting adrenergic agents.

◄ ⊖-Learning Activity 13-6

*Considerations for Older Adults.* Older adults are very sensitive to the actions of central-acting adrenergic agents and tend to have an increased risk of orthostatic hypotension. Teach older adults to change positions slowly and to ask for help getting up because of the increased risk for dizziness and falling. Lower doses of these drugs are recommended.

## DIRECT VASODILATORS

### How Direct Vasodilators Work

A vasodilator is any drug that relaxes blood vessel walls. Direct vasodilators act directly on the peripheral arteries, causing them to dilate (widen), which leads to lower blood pressure. Be sure to consult a drug reference book for information on any specific direct vasodilator.

### Dosages for Common Direct Vasodilators

| Drug | Dosage |
| --- | --- |
| hydralazine (Apresoline, Novo-Hylazine🍁) | *Adults:* PO: 10 mg orally 4 times daily; may gradually increase up to 300 mg daily |
| | *Adults:* IV: 5-40 mg daily in 4 divided doses; may repeat as needed |
| | *Children:* 0.75 mg/kg orally daily in 2-4 divided doses; may gradually increase to 7.5 mg/kg daily in 2-4 divided doses |
| | *Children:* IM, IV: 1.7 mg/kg daily in 4-6 divided doses |
| minoxidil (Loniten) | *Adults:* 5 mg orally daily may increase gradually up to 100 mg daily; do not exceed 100 mg daily |
| | *Children less than 12 years old:* 0.2 mg/kg orally daily (maximum 5 mg daily); may increase gradually to 0.25-l mg/kg daily (maximum 50 mg daily) |

*Intended Responses*
- Vasodilation (widening) of arteries is increased.
- Blood pressure is lowered.
- Heart workload is decreased.

## Common Side Effects

### Direct Vasodilators

Tachycardia

Hypernatremia

*Side Effects.* Direct vasodilators, along with central-acting adrenergic agents, have a higher incidence of side effects. Common side effects include tachycardia and salt (sodium) retention (hypernatremia). Less common side effects may include dizziness, drowsiness, fatigue, headache, chest pain, edema, dysrhythmias, low blood pressure, diarrhea, nausea, vomiting, rashes, and peripheral neuropathies.

*Adverse Effects.* Stevens-Johnson syndrome may occur with minoxidil. This is a severe inflammatory eruption of the skin and mucous membranes (see Figure 13-4).

### What To Do *Before* Giving Direct Vasodilators

Be sure to review the general nursing responsibilities related to antihypertensive therapy (p. 226) before giving direct vasodilators. Also be sure to obtain a baseline weight for the patient.

### What To Do *After* Giving Direct Vasodilators

Be sure to review the general nursing responsibilities related to antihypertensive therapy (p. 227) in addition to these specific responsibilities after giving direct vasodilators.

These drugs increase the risk for fluid retention and edema formation. Keep track of intake and output. Check the patient's feet and ankles for swelling. Listen to the patient's lungs for crackles.

### What To *Teach* Patients About Direct Vasodilators

Be sure to teach patients about general issues and precautions related to antihypertensive therapy (p. 227) in addition to these specific teaching points for direct vasodilators.

Instruct patients to contact the prescriber if more than two doses are missed. These drugs should be discontinued gradually because blood pressure can become dangerously high if they are stopped suddenly.

Tell patients to report any persistent heart rate increase of more than 20 beats per minute to the prescriber. This may be a sign of heart failure.

Teach patients to weigh themselves and check their feet and ankles for swelling twice a week. Tell them to report a weight gain of more than 3 pounds in 1 week to the prescriber, because this may indicate heart failure.

### Life Span Considerations for Direct Vasodilators

*Pediatric Considerations.* The same side effects that occur with adults may affect children. Doses for children are based on weight.

*Considerations for Pregnancy and Breastfeeding.* Hydralazine (Apresoline) is a pregnancy category C drug and has been used safely during both pregnancy and breastfeeding to decrease high blood pressure in women. Small amounts of this drug pass into breast milk, putting infants at minimal risk for side effects. A woman who plans to breastfeed should discuss this with the prescriber.

> **! Drug Alert!**
> **Action/Intervention Alert**
>
> With vasodilator drugs, a sustained increase in heart rate of more than 20 beats per minute should be reported to the prescriber immediately.

## Get Ready for Practice!

### Key Points

- Hypertension is defined as a systolic blood pressure greater than 140 mm Hg and/or a diastolic blood pressure greater than 90 mm Hg.
- Untreated hypertension can lead to many health problems, including heart attack, stroke, and kidney disease.
- Beta blockers slow the heart rate and decrease the force of the contraction of the heart.
- ACE inhibitors slow the production of angiotensin II, a potent vasoconstrictor, by the body.
- Angiotensin II receptor antagonists block the action of angiotensin II, leading to increased vasodilation (widening) of arteries.
- Angioedema (swelling of the face, eyes, lips, and tongue) is a life-threatening adverse effect of angiotensin II receptor antagonists and ACE inhibitors.
- Calcium channel blockers decrease the force of the contractions of the heart and dilate the arteries.
- Alpha blockers relax blood vessels, leading to arterial widening and lower blood pressure.
- Alpha-beta blockers combine the effects of alpha blockers and beta blockers to lower blood pressure.
- Monitor patients with diabetes carefully when taking alpha-beta blockers because these drugs cause hyperglycemia (high blood sugar).
- Methyldopa, a central-acting adrenergic drug, is the drug of choice for controlling high blood pressure during pregnancy.
- A sustained heart rate increase of more than 20 beats per minute should be reported to the prescriber when a patient is taking a direct vasodilator drug.
- Always check blood pressure, heart rate, and weight and look for swelling of the ankles or feet before and after giving antihypertensive drugs.

- Encourage patients to adopt lifestyle changes that will help to control high blood pressure such as weight loss, regular exercise, and low-salt diets.
- Be sure that patients know how to check their heart rate and blood pressure and understand the importance of follow-up checks.

### Additional Learning Resources

**evolve** Go to your Evolve website (http://evolve.elsevier.com/Workman/pharmacology/) for the following FREE learning resources:

- eLearning Activities
- Animations
- Video Clips
- Interactive Review Questions
- Audio Key Points
- Audio Glossary
- Audio Glossary—Spanish-English
- Drug Dosage Calculators
- Patient Teaching Handouts

**SG** Go to your Study Guide for additional learning activities to help you master this chapter content.

### Review Questions

1. A patient who is taking a beta blocker for hypertension asks how this drug lowers blood pressure. What is your best response?

   A. "It eliminates excess water and salt from the body."
   B. "It blocks the conversion of angiotensin II."
   C. "It reduces the heart rate."
   D. "It dilates the arteries."

2. A patient who is taking captopril (Capoten) 25 mg twice daily develops a cough. What is your priority action?

   A. Ask the physician to prescribe a cold remedy.
   B. Withhold the dose and notify the prescriber.
   C. Provide lozenges as ordered.
   D. Obtain a sputum culture.

3. A patient prescribed losartan (Cozaar) develops swelling of the face, including the eyes, lips, and tongue. What is your best action?

   A. Elevate the head of the patient's bed 180 degrees.
   B. Reassure the patient that this is an expected side effect.
   C. Document these findings as the only action.
   D. Hold the drug and notify the prescriber.

4. Which statement by a patient who is prescribed enalapril (Vasotec) indicates the need for additional teaching?

   A. "I will use a salt substitute instead of table salt."
   B. "I will avoid alcohol while I'm taking this medicine."
   C. "I will wear a sunscreen and hat when I go outdoors."
   D. "I will call my prescriber right away if I notice swelling in my face."

5. A woman who is taking an ACE inhibitor to control hypertension wishes to become pregnant. Why must she discuss this with her prescriber?

   A. ACE inhibitors pass into breast milk.
   B. ACE inhibitors affect women differently than men.
   C. ACE inhibitors have fewer side effects than other hypertension drugs.
   D. ACE inhibitors have caused birth defects in laboratory animal studies.

6. A patient takes losartan (Cozaar) 50 mg once a day to control high blood pressure. For which life-threatening adverse effect do you assess the patient?

   A. Myocarditis
   B. Angioedema
   C. Liver failure
   D. Stevens-Johnson syndrome

7. Which signs/symptoms must you be sure to check before giving a drug to treat high blood pressure? (Select all that apply.)

   A. Swelling in ankles or feet
   B. Oral temperature
   C. Hand grasp strength
   D. Crackles in lungs
   E. Blood pressure
   F. Heart rate
   G. Weight

8. Which points must you be sure to teach the patient who is going home and continuing to take clonidine (Catapres) 0.2 mg twice daily for blood pressure control? (Select all that apply.)

   A. Do not drive or operate machines.
   B. Avoid salt substitutes.
   C. Remember to change positions slowly.
   D. Use frequent mouth rinses for dry mouth.
   E. Take the drug every day at the same time.
   F. Avoid aspirin or aspirin-containing products.

9. A 33-year-old female patient is currently taking HCTZ (Hyzaar) 50 mg and metoprolol (Lopressor) 100 mg daily to control her blood pressure. She tells her prescriber that she plans to become pregnant. What drug will the prescriber most likely prescribe now?

   A. nadolol (Corgard)
   B. clonidine (Catapres)
   C. methyldopa (Aldomet)
   D. lisinopril (Prinivil, Zestril)

10. The prescriber orders hydrochlorothiazide (Hyzaar) 50 mg orally once a day for a patient with high blood pressure. The pharmacy sends HCTZ 25 mg per tablet. How many tablets will you give the patient? _____ tablet(s)

11. The prescriber orders oral prazosin (Minipress) 50 mcg/kg daily for an 8-year-old child in 2 divided doses. The child weighs 30 kg. How much prazosin will you give for each dose? _____ mcg

12. A patient is to receive metoprolol (Lopressor) 5 mg IV to control high blood pressure. Metoprolol comes in a solution of 1 mg/mL. How many milliliters will you give? _____ mL

## Critical Thinking Activities

Mrs. Smith is 62 years old with a new diagnosis of primary hypertension. She states that she is in good health but is 45 pounds overweight, does not exercise, and likes to eat fast food several times a week.

1. What initial type of drug is her prescriber most likely to prescribe?

2. What should you teach Mrs. Smith about taking antihypertensive drugs?

3. What other strategies can you suggest to Mrs. Smith that may help control her high blood pressure?

# Drugs for Heart Failure

## Objectives

*After studying this chapter you should be able to:*

1. List the common names, actions, usual adult dosages, possible side effects, and adverse effects of vasodilators and cardiac glycosides (digoxin).
2. Describe what to do before and after giving vasodilators and cardiac glycosides.
3. Explain what to teach patients taking vasodilators and cardiac glycosides, including what to do, what not to do, and when to call the prescriber.
4. Describe life span considerations for vasodilators and cardiac glycosides.
5. List the common names, actions, usual adult dosages, possible side effects, and adverse effects of human B-type

natriuretic peptides, positive inotropes, potassium, and magnesium.

6. Describe what to do before and after giving human B-type natriuretic peptides, positive inotropes, potassium, and magnesium.
7. Explain what to teach patients taking human B-type natriuretic peptides, positive inotropes, potassium, and magnesium, including what to do, what not to do, and when to call the prescriber.
8. Describe life span considerations for human B-type natriuretic peptides, positive inotropes, potassium, and magnesium.

## Key Terms

**afterload** (ĂF-tŭr-lōd) (p. 249) Total peripheral resistance that the heart must overcome to pump blood out of the heart. It includes mean arterial pressure (MAP).

**angiotensin II** (ăn-jē-ō-TĔN-sĭn) (p. 253) A substance produced by the body that causes blood vessels to narrow (constrict), raising blood pressure.

**cardiac output** (KĂR-dē-ăk ŌWT-pŭt) (p. 253) The amount of blood pumped by the heart in 1 minute.

**contractility** (kŏn-trăk-TĬL-ĭ-tē) (p. 253) The ability of the fibers of living muscle to contract or shorten.

**diastolic left heart failure** (dī-ă-STŎL-ĭk LĔFT HĂRT FĂL-yŭr) (p. 251) Inadequate relaxation or "stiffening" of the ventricle that prevents the heart from filling enough before contraction.

**ejection fraction** (ē-JĔK-shŭn FRĂK-shŭn) (p. 251) The amount (percentage) of blood that is pumped out of the heart to the body with each heartbeat.

**heart failure** (HĂRT FĂL-yŭr) (p. 248) Occurs when the heart cannot pump enough blood to meet the needs of the body. Also called pump failure.

**jugular vein distention** (JŬG-yū-lŭr VĀN dĭs-TĔN-shŭn) (p. 251) Prominent, enlarged, pulsing jugular veins when a patient is sitting up. A sign of heart failure.

**mean arterial pressure (MAP)** (MĒN ăr-TĒR-ē-ŭl PRĔSH-ŭr) (p. 250) Average systolic blood pressure in the large arteries, including the aorta. For the average healthy adult the normal MAP is around 100 mm Hg.

**myocardial hypertrophy** (mī-ō-KĂR-dē-ŭl-hī-PŬR-trō-fē) (p. 253) Enlargement of the myocardial (heart) muscle.

**preload** (PRĒ-lōd) (p. 249) The stretch, tension, or volume of blood present in the ventricles of the heart after passive filling and atrial contraction and before ventricular contraction.

**renin-angiotensin system (RAS)** (RĔN-ĭn ăn-jē-ō-TĔN-sĭn SĬS-tĕm) (p. 253) A body system pathway that causes release of two chemicals, angiotensin II and aldosterone, which act together to increase blood pressure.

**systolic left heart failure** (sĭs-TŎL-ĭk LĔFT HĂRT FĂL-yŭr) (p. 250) Condition in which the heart is unable to contract forcefully enough to pump enough blood to meet the needs of the body.

◀ⓔ-Learning Activity 14-1

## OVERVIEW

**Heart failure** occurs when the heart cannot pump enough blood to meet the needs of the body. As the world population ages, the number of people diagnosed with heart failure is increasing. About 5 million people live with heart failure in the United States, and as many as 500,000 new cases occur each year. Heart failure can occur at any age. However, it is much more common in older people because they often have disorders that damage the heart muscle (for example, high blood pressure), and age-related changes in the heart can make it pump less efficiently.

Most heart failure is caused by hypertension. Many of the drugs used to treat hypertension are also used to treat heart failure. Other causes of heart failure include myocardial infarction, coronary artery disease, cardiomyopathy, substance abuse (alcohol and illicit or prescribed drugs), heart valve disease, congenital defects, cardiac infections and inflammations, and conditions that increase cardiac output and energy demands such as sepsis.

## REVIEW OF RELATED PHYSIOLOGY AND PATHOPHYSIOLOGY

The heart is a muscular organ that is hollow and divided into four chambers: right atrium, right ventricle, left atrium, and left ventricle. The atrial and ventricular chambers are separated by one-way valves that open when the pressure in the first chamber is higher than that in the second chamber (Figure 14-1).

Blood enters the heart from the vena cava into the right atrium. This blood comes from the rest of the body; most of the oxygen has been used. From the right atrium the blood moves through the tricuspid valve into the right ventricle. The muscle of the right ventricle contracts to make the pressure in this chamber higher than the pressure in the blood vessel known as the pulmonary artery. When right ventricular pressure is high enough, the pulmonary valve opens and allows blood to move from the right ventricle into the pulmonary artery. From there blood moves into the lungs, where it picks up oxygen. The oxygenated blood then moves into the left atrium. When the pressure in the left atrium is high enough, the blood moves through the mitral valve (also called the bicuspid valve) into the left ventricle. The muscles of the left ventricle are the strongest ones in the heart. They must

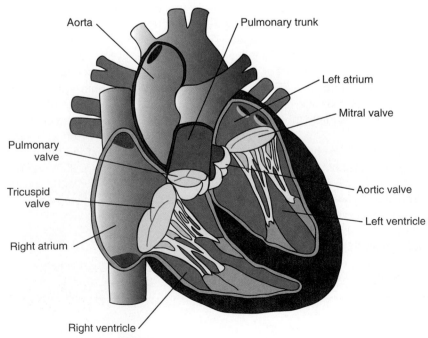

**FIGURE 14-1** Heart chambers and valves.

contract and increase the pressure in the left ventricle to force the blood to leave the left ventricle through the aortic valve and into the aorta. Once oxygenated blood enters the aorta, it circulates throughout the entire body to deliver oxygen to every tissue and organ. So it is important that the muscles of the left ventricle have the best contraction to force blood into the aorta.

The muscles of the left ventricle are similar to other body muscles in that they contract best and strongest after a stretch. Think of a baseball pitcher winding up to throw a fastball. He or she first moves the arm back as far as possible to stretch the throwing muscles. This stretching before throwing allows the muscles to contract harder and faster, resulting in a better throw. When the muscles of the left ventricle are stretched to the best level, the result is a stronger contraction that moves more blood from the left ventricle into the aorta. Usually this stretch occurs naturally when the right amount of blood fills the ventricle (preload). If the muscle is not stretched enough, the resulting contraction is weak and moves only a small amount of blood into the aorta (just as a small windup before a pitch results in a weak and short throw).

One problem that can occur with the muscle of the left ventricle is that it can become *overstretched*. When any muscle is overstretched, its contraction is weaker. Think about a person with a rubber band. Not stretching the rubber band or stretching it only a little results in a weak snap. Stretching it more increases the snap. However, if the rubber band is overstretched, it becomes so flabby that it cannot "snap" back. When the muscles of the left ventricle are overstretched or flabby and the contraction is weak, too much blood remains in the left ventricle, and more blood arriving from the left atrium is added to it. This overstretches the muscle more and continues to weaken contractions, leading to heart failure (Figure 14-2). Blood then backs up into other heart chambers, leading to congestion in the lungs and the peripheral veins (Figure 14-3).

Some of the drugs used to treat heart failure work by actually making the muscles contract better. Others work by reducing the amount of blood in the left ventricle (preventing overstretching). Still others work by lowering the pressure in the aorta (afterload) so muscles of the left ventricle do not have to contract as hard or as strong to move blood out of the ventricle and into the aorta.

Heart function and blood pressure work together for good blood circulation and blood flow to ensure that oxygen is delivered to all body tissues and organs. Heart contractions must be strong enough to move blood into the arteries. Then arterial pressure must be high enough to move blood through the arteries and into the tissues

◄ -Animation 14-1: Structure of the Heart

 Memory Jogger

*Preload* is the "stretching" of the muscle caused by blood filling left ventricle.

 Memory Jogger

*Afterload* is the pressure in the aorta that the left ventricle must overcome before blood can move from it into the aorta.

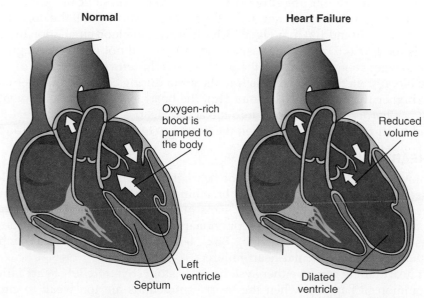

**Normal**  **Heart Failure**

Oxygen-rich blood is pumped to the body

Reduced volume

Left ventricle

Septum

Dilated ventricle

**FIGURE 14-2** Normal heart and heart with heart failure.

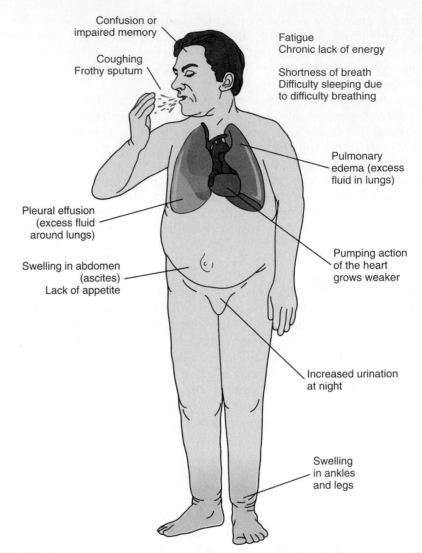

**FIGURE 14-3** Signs and symptoms of heart failure and peripheral and pulmonary congestion.

and organs. **Mean arterial pressure (MAP)** is the average systolic blood pressure in the large arteries, including the aorta. For the average healthy adult the normal MAP range is between 70 and 100 mm Hg, which ensures good blood circulation to tissues. If MAP is too low (<60 mm Hg), tissues and organs will not receive enough blood to ensure oxygenation. MAP also is the pressure that the left ventricle must overcome to move blood from the left ventricle into the aorta during contraction (afterload). If MAP is higher than normal (>110 mm Hg), the heart, especially the left ventricle, has to work harder to move blood into the aorta. Heart attacks (myocardial infarction) and heart failure can occur when the heart has to work too hard for too long.

## LEFT HEART FAILURE

When blood collects in the left side of the heart, it results in congestion in the lungs, decreased lung function, and difficulty breathing. Because the left ventricle pumps blood to the body, symptoms include signs of decreased cardiac output (such as fatigue and weakness) and signs of pulmonary congestion (such as crackles and wheezes detected with a stethoscope). Box 14-1 lists the key signs and symptoms associated with left ventricular heart failure.

Left heart failure can be either systolic or diastolic. **Systolic left heart failure** is more common. It happens when the heart contractions are too weak to circulate enough blood to meet the needs of the body. The decrease in contractility causes a

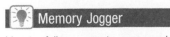

**Memory Jogger**

Heart failure most commonly occurs in the left ventricle.

| Box **14-1** | Signs and Symptoms of Left Heart Failure |
|---|---|

| **DECREASED CARDIAC OUTPUT** | **PULMONARY CONGESTION** |
|---|---|
| • Fatigue | • Hacking cough, worse at night |
| • Weakness | • Dyspnea, breathlessness |
| • Decreased urine output (oliguria) during the day | • Crackles or wheezes in lungs |
| • Angina | • Frothy, pink-tinged sputum |
| • Confusion, restlessness | • Tachypnea |
| • Dizziness | • $S_3$ and $S_4$ summation gallop (abnormal heart sounds) |
| • Tachycardia, palpitations | |
| • Paleness (pallor) | |
| • Weak peripheral pulses | |
| • Cool extremities | |

Adapted from Ignatavicius D, Workman L (2010): *Medical-surgical nursing: patient-centered collaborative care,* 6th edition, Philadelphia: Sanders, p. 768.

| Box **14-2** | Signs and Symptoms of Right Heart Failure |
|---|---|

| **SYSTEMIC CONGESTION** | |
|---|---|
| • Jugular (neck vein) distention | • Increased urine output (polyuria) at night |
| • Enlarged liver and spleen | • Weight gain |
| • Anorexia and nausea | • Increased blood pressure (from excess volume) or decreased blood pressure (from heart failure) |
| • Dependent edema (legs and sacrum) | |
| • Distended abdomen | |
| • Swollen hands and fingers | |

From Ignatavicus D, Workman L (2010): *Medical-surgical nursing: patient-centered collaborative care,* 6th edition, Philadelphia: Sanders, p. 768.

decrease in the amount of blood pumped out with each contraction, leaving more blood in the ventricle and causing an increase in preload. Afterload increases because of increased peripheral resistance usually as a result of high blood pressure. These two changes cause a decrease in ejection fraction (percentage of blood pumped with each contraction) from a normal of 50% to 70% to less than 40%. The lower ejection fraction leads to less blood (cardiac output) for tissue perfusion. Blood collects in the pulmonary blood vessels, causing signs of lung congestion.

Diastolic left heart failure occurs when the left ventricle is not able to relax enough during diastole and causes a decrease in filling of the ventricles (preload) before contraction. A decrease in cardiac output results, and not enough blood is pumped to meet the needs of the body. With diastolic failure the patient's ejection fraction may be very close to normal.

### RIGHT HEART FAILURE

With right heart failure the right ventricle does not empty. This causes increased volume and pressure in the right side of the heart. When the right ventricle contracts poorly, signs and symptoms of peripheral congestion occur (Box 14-2) such as weight gain, swelling in the legs, jugular vein distention (Figure 14-4), and increased blood pressure. The pathophysiology of heart failure is summarized in Figure 14-5.

### COMPENSATORY MECHANISMS FOR HEART FAILURE

The body has several ways to compensate for heart failure. In response to tissue hypoxia (not enough oxygen), the sympathetic nervous system is stimulated, and the hormones epinephrine and norepinephrine (catecholamines) are released. These hormones act on the heart in two ways. First they increase the heart rate. Second they increase the power of the heart muscle fibers to contract or shorten so the heart pumps more forcefully. The ability of the heart fibers to shorten is called

 **Memory Jogger**

Normal ejection fraction is 50% to 70%. With systolic heart failure the ejection fraction is less than 40%.

 **Memory Jogger**

Cardiac output (CO) is the product of heart rate (HR) and stroke volume (SV). The formula for this is $CO = HR \times SV$. An increase in heart rate and/or stroke volume results in an increase in cardiac output.

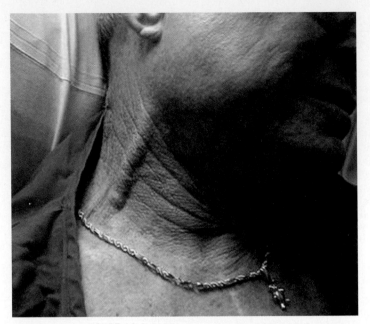

**FIGURE 14-4** Jugular vein distention (JVD).

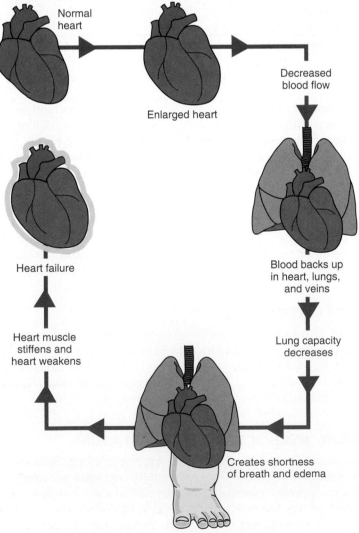

**FIGURE 14-5** Pathophysiology of heart failure.

contractility. These actions increase the amount of blood pumped by the heart in 1 minute, known as the cardiac output.

Sympathetic nervous system stimulation also causes arterial vasoconstriction (narrowing of the arteries). This helps the body to maintain blood pressure and improve blood flow to the tissues. The downside to this compensation is that narrowing of the arteries leads to increased afterload, more work for the heart, and increased oxygen needs. *Increased afterload can lead to worsening heart failure.*

When heart failure causes decreased blood flow to the kidneys, another compensation process called the renin-angiotensin system (RAS) is activated. This pathway causes release of two body chemicals: angiotensin II and aldosterone. Angiotensin II causes blood vessel constriction (increased afterload), whereas aldosterone leads to sodium and water retention (increased preload). Activation of the RAS leads to increased blood pressure.

A third way that the body can compensate for heart failure is by myocardial hypertrophy (enlargement) of the heart muscle. Increase in the heart muscle size can lead to more forceful contractions and increased cardiac output. But when the heart muscle becomes too big, it outgrows its blood supply. The thickened muscle also becomes "stiff," resulting in less effective contractions and diastolic heart failure.

**Memory Jogger**

The renin-angiotensin system causes vasoconstriction and body retention of sodium and water.

◄ ⊖-Learning Activity 14-2

## TREATMENT FOR HEART FAILURE

Continuous heart function is needed for life. Unmanaged heart failure leads to death. Heart failure is usually a chronic disorder. Goals for treatment include (1) making physical activity more comfortable, (2) improving quality of life, and (3) prolonging life. Interventions focus on:
- Treating the cause of heart failure.
- Controlling factors that can cause it to worsen.
- Treating its symptoms.

Lifestyle changes are an important part of a treatment plan. Suggested changes include weight loss, smoking cessation, and a low-salt and low-fat diet. Nurses play an important role in teaching patients the need for these changes and how to accomplish them. Drug therapy only improves heart function; drugs do not cure heart failure. Because the damage to the heart muscle is not reversible, the only real cure for heart failure is a heart transplant.

**Memory Jogger**

The only real cure for heart failure is a heart transplant because the damage to the heart muscle is irreversible.

## GENERAL ISSUES IN HEART FAILURE THERAPY

There are several classes of drugs for heart failure that have both common and different actions and effects. Nursing responsibilities for these common actions and effects are listed in the following discussion. Specific responsibilities are listed with each class of heart failure drugs.

*Before administering any heart failure drug,* obtain a complete list of drugs that the patient is currently taking, including over-the-counter and herbal drugs. Check the patient's blood pressure and heart rate. If the blood pressure is low (less than 90/60 mm Hg) or the heart rate is low (less than 60 beats per minute), check with the prescriber about whether the patient should receive the drug because so many of these drugs lower heart rate further. Check the drug order because some prescribers provide guidelines for when to administer and when to hold these drugs. Obtain a baseline weight for each patient because weight gain is a sign of worsening heart failure. Ask female patients of childbearing years if they are pregnant, breastfeeding, or planning to become pregnant.

*After administering any heart failure drug,* reassess and continue to monitor the patient's blood pressure and heart rate. Notify the prescriber if either measure is low. Ensure that the call light is within easy reach and tell the patient to call for assistance when getting out of bed because of the increased risk for dizziness, light-headedness, and hypotension with these drugs. Check for any signs or symptoms of allergic reactions or infections.

*Teach patients receiving a heart failure drug* to change positions slowly to prevent dizziness and falls. Instruct them to go from a lying position to sitting before standing up. Talk with them about lifestyle changes that will also help to manage hypertension such as weight loss; exercise; smoking cessation; and a low-salt, low-fat diet.

Tell patients to take the drug at the same time every day. Remind them that taking these drugs will help to control but will not cure heart failure; the drugs may be prescribed for life. Talk with patients and their families about the importance of regular blood pressure and heart rate checks, at least once a week. Teach them proper techniques for checking blood pressure and heart rate. Teach the importance of regular follow-up visits to check and maintain control of their heart failure. Remind patients to check with their prescriber before taking any over-the-counter drugs, including cough or allergy remedies or herbal preparations. Tell patients to notify their prescriber for any weight gain or increase in shortness of breath because these are signs of worsening heart failure.

Instruct patients who experience dizziness, drowsiness, or light-headedness not to drive, use machines, or do anything that could be dangerous or require increased alertness until they know how the drug affects them. Encourage patients to get a medical alert bracelet identifying the use of any drug for heart failure.

## TYPES OF DRUGS USED TO TREAT HEART FAILURE

Heart failure is a complex problem in which more than one normal action is disrupted. For this reason usually a combination of drugs is used to manage symptoms and improve heart-pumping function. Some of these drugs have other uses. For example, antihypertensive drugs are commonly used in heart failure therapy for several reasons. First, hypertension is a common cause of heart failure. In addition, by lowering blood pressure these drugs allow the heart to pump more easily. Therefore drugs such as angiotensin-converting enzyme (ACE) inhibitors, angiotensin II receptor blockers (ARBs), and most beta-adrenergic blockers are part of drug therapy for heart failure. Diuretics help in the treatment of heart failure by reducing blood volume, relaxing arteries, and improving heart muscle pumping. Diuretic drugs are discussed in detail in Chapter 12; Chapter 13 discusses antihypertensive drugs. Other drugs used in the treatment of heart failure include anticoagulants (Chapter 17), which may be used to prevent clots from forming in the heart chambers; and antidysrhythmic drugs (Chapter 15), which may be prescribed for abnormal heart rhythms. This chapter focuses primarily on the drugs with intended actions that are specific for the heart.

### ACE INHIBITORS

ACE inhibitors are often among the first drugs prescribed to treat heart failure. Dosages for these drugs are different when used to treat heart failure rather than high blood pressure. The most common ACE inhibitors are listed in the following table. Be sure to consult a drug handbook for information about any specific ACE inhibitor. Refer to Chapter 13 for more general information about ACE inhibitors.

### Dosages for Common ACE Inhibitors for Heart Failure

| Drug | Dosage |
|------|--------|
| captopril (Capoten) | *Adults:* 12.5-100 mg orally 2-3 times daily |
| enalapril 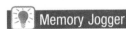 (Vasotec) | *Adults:* 2.5-20 mg orally twice daily |
| fosinopril (Monopril) | *Adults:* 10-40 mg orally once daily |
| lisinopril 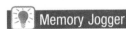 (Zestril, Prinivil) | *Adults:* 2.5-40 mg orally once daily |
| quinapril (Accupril) 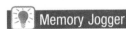 | *Adults:* 5-20 mg orally once or twice daily |
| ramipril (Altace) | *Adults:* 1.25-5 mg orally once or twice daily |
| trandolapril (Mavik) | *Adults:* 1-4 mg orally once daily |

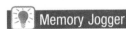 Top 100 drugs prescribed.

**Memory Jogger**

The major classes of drugs to treat heart failure are:
- ACE inhibitors.
- Beta blockers.
- Vasodilators.
- Cardiac glycosides.
- Diuretics.
- Human B-type natriuretic peptides.
- Positive inotropes.

## BETA BLOCKERS

### How Beta Blockers Work

Beta blockers block the effects of epinephrine (adrenaline) on the heart. They decrease the heart rate and the force of heart contractions, which results in a decrease in blood pressure. As a result the heart does not work as hard and requires less oxygen.

◄ ⊖-Animation 14-2: Beta Blockers

These drugs are often used with ACE inhibitors to treat heart failure. They may temporarily worsen heart failure symptoms; but, when taken over a long period, they improve heart function.

Most dosages are the same as when used for high blood pressure. See Chapter 13 for the usual dosages and ranges. Those drugs with specific limits when used for heart failure are listed in the following table. Only the sustained-release form of metoprolol is used to treat heart failure. Be sure to consult a drug handbook for specific information about any specific beta blocker. Refer to Chapter 13 for more general information about beta blockers.

### Dosages for Common Beta Blockers for Heart Failure

| Drug | Dosage |
| --- | --- |
| carvedilol ❶ (Coreg, Coreg CR) | *Adults:* 3.125 mg orally twice daily (do not exceed 25-50 mg twice daily; weight-based dose); CR—10 mg daily (increase every 2 weeks; do not exceed 80 mg daily) |
| metoprolol 🔟❶ (Toprol XL) | *Adults:* 12.5-25 mg orally once daily (do not exceed 200 mg/day) |

🔟 Top 100 drugs prescribed; ❶ High-alert drug.

## VASODILATORS

### How Vasodilators Work

Vasodilators act directly on the peripheral arteries to cause them to dilate (widen). This leads to lowering of blood pressure and decreases the workload of the heart. Vasodilators are often given to patients who cannot take ACE inhibitors or angiotensin II receptor blockers. The vasodilator that is most commonly prescribed for heart failure is hydralazine (Apresoline).

Other vasodilators used for treating chronic heart failure include isosorbide dinitrate (Isordil) and nitroglycerin. Isosorbide dinitrate and nitroglycerin (NTG) produce greater venous vasodilation than arterial vasodilation. Nitroglycerin also increases coronary blood flow by dilating the coronary arteries. With vasodilation the heart is better able to pump blood out to meet the needs of the body. Be sure to consult a drug handbook for information about any specific vasodilator.

### Dosages for Common Vasodilators for Heart Failure

| Drug | Dosage |
| --- | --- |
| hydrALAZINE (Apresoline) | *Adults:* 25-50 mg orally 4 times daily; may increase to 300 mg daily in 3-4 divided doses |
| isosorbide dinitrate 🔟 (Isordil, Imdur, Ismo, Isotrate ER, Monoket) | *Adults:* Ismo and Monoket : 20 mg orally twice daily 7 hours apart<br>*Adults:* Imdur: 30-60 mg orally once daily (up to 240 mg/day) |
| nitroglycerin (many brand names) | *Adults:* Sublingual or buccal: 0.3-0.6 mg; may repeat every 5 minutes 3 times<br>*Adults:* Sublingual or lingual spray: 1-2 sprays; may repeat every 5 minutes 3 times<br>*Adults:* Oral (sustained-release capsules): 2.5-9 mg every 6-8 hr<br>*Adults:* IV: 5 mcg/min; may increase as needed<br>*Adults:* Transdermal ointment: 1-2 inches every 6-8 hours<br>*Adults:* Transdermal patch: 0.1-0.8 mg/hr up to 0.8 mg/hr; patch is worn 12-14 hr/day. |

🔟 Top 100 drugs prescribed.

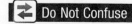

**Do Not Confuse**

**Apresoline** *with* **Priscoline**

An order for Apresoline may be confused with Priscoline. Apresoline is a vasodilator, whereas Priscoline is an alpha-adrenergic antagonist often used for persistent pulmonary hypertension in newborns.

**Do Not Confuse**

**Isordil** *with* **Plendil**

An order for Isordil may be confused with Plendil. Isordil is a vasodilator, whereas Plendil is a calcium channel blocker.

## Common Side Effects
### Vasodilators

Tachycardia

Hypernatremia

Headache

Dizziness

Hypotension

*Intended Responses*
- Vasodilation of arteries (hydralazine) is increased.
- Venous vasodilation (nitroglycerin, isosorbide) is increased.
- Blood flow to coronary arteries (nitroglycerin) is increased.
- Blood pressure is lowered.
- Heart workload is decreased.

*Side Effects.*   Common side effects of hydralazine include tachycardia and salt retention. Less common side effects may include dizziness, palpitations, drowsiness, fatigue, headache, chest pain, edema, dysrhythmias, low blood pressure, diarrhea, nausea, vomiting, rashes, and peripheral neuropathies (numbness and tingling).

Common side effects of nitroglycerin and isosorbide include hypotension, headache, dizziness, and tachycardia. Allergic reactions include skin rash, especially on the face.

*Adverse Effects.*   Adverse effects are very rare with hydralazine. They include neutropenia and shock with overdose. Neutropenia is an acute disease marked by high fever and a sharp drop in circulating white blood cells. Decreased white blood cells can lead to life-threatening infections. Adverse effects of nitroglycerin and isosorbide are also very rare. Circulatory collapse and shock may occur with nitroglycerin overdose.

### What To Do *Before* Giving Vasodilators

Be sure to review the general nursing responsibilities related to heart failure therapy (p. 253) in addition to these specific responsibilities before giving vasodilators.

Wear gloves when administering nitroglycerin ointment. This drug can cause headaches if it is absorbed through the skin. Squeeze the ointment onto the special ruled paper. Choose an unused site on a hairless area of the patient's chest, back, or upper arm. Place the application paper on the skin drug side down. Gently press on the paper to evenly disperse the drug. Be careful not to spread ointment outside the borders of the paper. Put tape over the paper to keep it in place (Figure 14-6).

### What To Do *After* Giving Vasodilators

Be sure to review the general nursing responsibilities related to heart failure therapy (p. 253) in addition to these specific responsibilities after giving vasodilators.

For safe skin care, be sure to apply the drug patch to a different site with each dose when the patient is prescribed nitroglycerin patches or ointment. Remove the previous dose and use a tissue to remove any ointment left on the patient's skin before applying the next dose. Avoid rubbing the skin too much because this can cause more ointment to be absorbed or could tear the skin. Note that leaving the ointment from the previous dose on a patient's skin is like giving a double dose of the drug. Nitroglycerin (ointment or patch) loses its effectiveness when used continuously. This is why it is good to have some "drug-free" time during a 24-hour period. Usually the patches are removed at night when the patient has his or her longest sleeping period because the heart is less stressed during that time.

Monitor intake and output. Check the patient's feet and ankles for swelling. Listen with a stethoscope for crackles in the lungs. Ask the patient about headache or dizziness. A mild headache pain reliever such as acetaminophen (Tylenol) may be required for headaches related to nitroglycerin.

### What To *Teach* Patients About Vasodilators

Be sure to teach patients general care needs and precautions related to drugs for heart failure (p. 254) in addition to these specific points for vasodilators.

---

## !  Drug Alert!
### Administration Alert

Wear gloves to administer nitroglycerin ointment to prevent absorbing the drug through your skin.

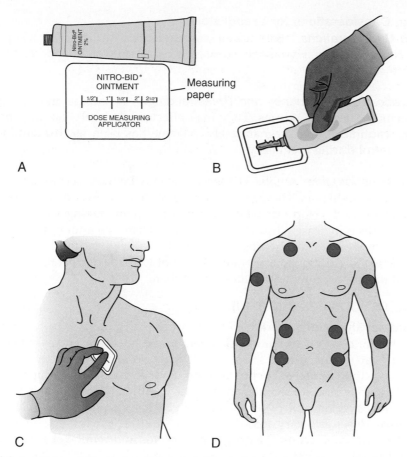

**FIGURE 14-6** Application of nitroglycerin ointment. **A,** Check ointment dose and paper. **B,** Apply dose to the paper. **C,** Apply paper with the drug to the patient. **D,** Appropriate sites for drug application.

Contact the prescriber if more than two doses are missed because these drugs should be discontinued gradually. When the drugs are stopped suddenly, blood vessels constrict too much (known as a rebound response), causing less blood flow to the heart and a rapid rise in blood pressure.

Tell patients to report any heart rate increase of more than 20 beats per minute. An increase in headaches, dizziness, or light-headedness should also be reported to the prescriber.

Remind patients that sublingual and buccal nitroglycerin should be kept in place until dissolved. Nitroglycerin should cause a tingling sensation, which indicates that the drug is potent. Patients should not eat or drink until the tablet is dissolved. Note that, if one tablet does not relieve chest pain, the patient should notify the prescriber.

Teach patients to store nitroglycerin tablets in the drug container distributed by the pharmacy. Remind them that the drug degrades (loses its strength or potency) quickly, especially when exposed to light or moisture. *A nitroglycerin tablet that has lost its potency will not have any helpful effect.* Also remind them to make certain the drug container is labeled so that if another person is helping the patient during an attack of chest pain, the right drug will be given.

Instruct patients about the proper techniques for using nitroglycerin ointment or patches. Remind them to remove these drugs at night.

Teach patients that, while acetaminophen may be needed at first to relieve headaches, most people develop a tolerance for nitroglycerin and isosorbide, and the headaches decrease or disappear.

Tell patients to weigh themselves and check their feet and ankles for swelling at least twice a week. A weight gain of more than 3 pounds in 1 week is a result of water retention, which is an indicator of worsening heart failure.

 **Clinical Pitfall**

Sublingual and buccal nitroglycerin should *not* be swallowed. When swallowed, the liver destroys most of the drug so it is not effective.

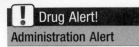
## Life Span Considerations for Vasodilators

***Pediatric Considerations.*** Safe use of isosorbide and nitroglycerin has not been established for children. Hydralazine dosage is based on weight and has been used safely with children.

***Considerations for Pregnancy and Breastfeeding.*** Isosorbide and nitroglycerin are pregnancy category C drugs. They may affect fetal circulation and should be used with caution during pregnancy. Hydralazine has been used safely for blood pressure control during pregnancy.

***Considerations for Older Adults.*** Older adults may be more sensitive to hypotensive effects of vasodilators. They may need to be started on lower doses. Older adults are more likely to develop orthostatic hypotension while taking vasodilators, and their risk of falls is increased. Box 10-3 in Chapter 10 lists precautions to help prevent falls. Stress the need to change positions slowly and use handrails when going up or down steps. In addition, warn older adults not to drive or operate heavy equipment until they know how vasodilators affect them.

⊖-Learning Activity 14-3▶

## CARDIAC GLYCOSIDES (DIGOXIN)

### How Cardiac Glycosides Work

Cardiac glycosides work on the muscle fibers in the heart and increase the force of each heart beat (contractility). They also slow down a heart rate that is too fast, allowing more time for the left ventricle to fill. Both of these actions improve cardiac output. Digoxin is used for maintenance therapy with heart failure. It comes in oral (tablet, capsules, elixir) and IV forms. Prescribed doses are age and weight dependent. Digoxin doses also vary according to whether the dose is a loading or a maintenance dose. Be sure to consult a drug handbook for information about any specific cardiac glycoside.

### Dosages for Common Cardiac Glycosides

| Drug | Dosage |
|---|---|
| digoxin ❶ (Digitek, Lanoxicaps, Lanoxin) | ***Digitalizing Doses***<br>*Adults:* Oral tablets: 0.5-0.75 mg, then 0.125-0.375 mg every 6-8 hr (total of 0.75-1.25 mg in 24 hr)<br>*Adults:* Oral capsules: 0.4-0.6 mg, then 0.1-0.3 mg every 6-8 hr (total of 0.6-1 mg in 24 hr)<br>*Adults:* IV: 0.4-0.6 mg, then 0.1-0.3 mg every 6-8 hr (total of 0.6-1 mg in 24 hr)<br>*Children over 10 years:* 10-15 mcg/kg orally/IV<br>*Children 2-10 years:* 20-40 mcg/kg orally/IV<br>*Children less than 2 years:* 40-60 mcg/kg orally/IV<br>*Term neonate:* 25-35 mcg/kg orally/IV<br>*Preterm neonate:* 20 mcg/kg orally/IV<br>(Children and neonate digitalizing doses are divided into 3 or more doses, with the first dose one half of the total; give the second and third doses at 6- to 8-hour intervals.)<br>***Maintenance Doses***<br>*Adults:* 0.1-0.375 mg/day orally/IV<br>*Children over 10 years:* 3-5 mcg/day orally/IV<br>*Children 5-10 years:* 7.5-10 mcg/kg/day orally/IV<br>*Children 2-5 years:* 10-15 mcg/kg/day orally/IV<br>*Term neonate:* 8-10 mcg/kg/day orally/IV<br>*Premature neonate:* 4-8 mcg/kg/day orally/IV<br>(Dose varies depending on drug form and route ordered) |

❶ High-alert drug.

***Intended Responses***
- Contractility is increased.
- Cardiac output is increased.
- Heart rate is decreased.

*Side Effects.*  The most common side effects of digoxin (Lanoxin) are heart rhythm disturbances that are related to digoxin toxicity. Other common side effects to watch for include fatigue, bradycardia (slow heart rate less than 60 beats per minute), anorexia (loss of appetite), nausea, and vomiting.

Less common side effects include headache, fatigue, drowsiness, confusion, weakness, blurred vision, yellow halos or light around objects, electrocardiogram (ECG) changes, diarrhea, *gynecomastia* (breast enlargement in men) with long-term use, and *thrombocytopenia* (low platelet count).

*Adverse Effects.*  Signs and symptoms of overdose include early signs such as loss of appetite, nausea, vomiting, diarrhea, or vision problems. Other signs include changes in heart rate or rhythm (irregular or slow), palpitations, or fainting. In infants and small children the earliest signs of overdose are changes in heart rate and rhythm. Children may not have the same symptoms as adults.

Dysrhythmias (abnormal and irregular heart rhythms) caused by digoxin can be life threatening.

### What To Do *Before* Giving Cardiac Glycosides

Be sure to review the general nursing responsibilities related to heart failure therapy (p. 253) in addition to these specific responsibilities before giving cardiac glycosides.

Check the apical heart rate with a stethoscope for a full minute because these drugs can decrease heart rate and cause dysrhythmias. Note whether the heart rate is regular or irregular. If it is less than 60 beats per minute, greater than 100 beats per minute, or irregular, notify the prescriber. For a heart rate lower than 60 beats per minute hold the dose; notify the prescriber and ask if the patient should receive this drug.

If the prescriber has ordered a cardiac monitor for the patient, make sure that the monitor is in place and ask the monitor watcher about the patient's baseline rhythm.

Ask female patients of childbearing years if they are pregnant, breastfeeding, or planning to become pregnant because digoxin passes from the mother to the fetus and also passes into breast milk.

Ask patients if they have a history of electrolyte disorders, heart rhythm problems, kidney or liver disease, or thyroid disease.

### What To Do *After* Giving Cardiac Glycosides

Be sure to review the general nursing responsibilities related to heart failure therapy (p. 253) in addition to these specific responsibilities after giving cardiac glycosides.

Check the apical heart rate for a full minute after giving each dose of this drug. If the heart rate is less than 60 beats per minute or irregular, hold the drug and notify the prescriber.

If the patient is on a heart monitor, ask the monitor watcher whether his or her heart rate and rhythm have changed after each dose. Check the patient's current potassium, magnesium, and calcium laboratory values. Abnormal values may affect how this drug works. Monitor the patient for signs and symptoms of digoxin overdose such as loss of appetite, nausea, vomiting, and vision problems.

### What To *Teach* Patients About Cardiac Glycosides

Be sure to teach patients general care needs and precautions related to drugs for heart failure (p. 254) in addition to these specific points for cardiac glycosides.

Explain that the heart rate should be checked every day before taking digoxin. Remind patients to tell the prescriber if their heart rate drops below 60 beats per minute, is greater than 100 beats per minute, or becomes irregular. Describe the signs and symptoms of overdose and instruct patients to report any of these to the prescriber.

---

**Common Side Effects**

**Digoxin**

Dysrhythmias, Bradycardia   Fatigue   Anorexia, Nausea/ Vomiting

---

**Clinical Pitfall**

Report common side effects of digoxin to the prescriber immediately because they are probably signs of digoxin toxicity, which can be life threatening.

---

**Drug Alert!**

**Action/Intervention Alert**

Digoxin has a very narrow therapeutic range (0.8 to 2 ng/mL), and levels above 2 ng/mL are considered toxic. When a patient shows any signs of overdose (digoxin toxicity), a blood level for digoxin is drawn, and the digoxin dose is held.

---

**Drug Alert!**

**Administration Alert**

Always check the apical heart rate for a full minute before giving a cardiac glycoside.

---

 **Did You Know?**

Foxglove is the name of a common garden plant that contains digitalis. Foxglove and its extract digitalis have been used as both a poison and a heart drug for hundreds of years.

---

**Drug Alert!**

**Teaching Alert**

Teach patients taking digoxin to check their pulse before taking the drug. Tell them to notify the prescriber if their heart rate is slower than 60 beats per minute, faster than 100 beats per minute, or irregular.

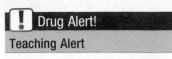
Remind patients to weigh themselves every day and to report a weight gain of greater than 2 pounds per day to the prescriber.

Teach patients to take digoxin exactly as ordered by the prescriber. Digoxin should be taken every day at the same time, and a dose should not be skipped. A missed dose may be taken within 12 hours of its scheduled time. After that time it should be skipped because a double dose can lead to toxicity.

Remind patients to avoid taking antacids within 2 hours of digoxin because antacids can affect the absorption of this drug.

### Life Span Considerations for Cardiac Glycosides

*Pediatric Considerations.*    Doses of digoxin are specific and age related. It has been used in newborns and children of all ages.

*Considerations for Pregnancy and Breastfeeding.*    Digoxin is a pregnancy category C drug. It passes from the mother to the fetus during pregnancy. It also passes to the baby through breast milk. Therefore breastfeeding is not recommended during digoxin therapy.

*Considerations for Older Adults.*    Older adults are more sensitive to the effects of this drug and more likely to develop side effects, including digitalis toxicity. In addition, older adults may be taking diuretics that alter blood potassium levels, increasing the risk for changes in the activity of cardiac glycosides. Encourage older adults to take their medication exactly as prescribed and to keep all appointments for laboratory work to measure potassium and drug levels.

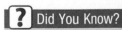-Learning Activity 14-4 ▶

## DIURETICS

Spironolactone (Aldactone), a potassium-sparing diuretic, is used to treat heart failure when systolic dysfunction is present. When prescribed in low doses, this drug blocks the action of aldosterone, which causes the body to hold onto salt and water. When spironolactone is prescribed, usually another diuretic will also be prescribed at its regular dose to decrease the volume of fluid in the blood vessels and reduce the workload of the heart. Used together, these drugs help the body maintain a more normal blood potassium level.

For usual doses of thiazide and loop diuretics, see Chapter 12. The doses of potassium-sparing diuretics when they are used to treat heart failure are listed in the following table. Be sure to consult a drug handbook for information about any specific diuretic.

### Dosages for Common Potassium-Sparing Diuretics for Heart Failure

| Drug | Dosage |
| --- | --- |
| amiloride (Midamor) | *Adults:* 5-10 mg orally daily |
| spironolactone (Aldactone) | *Adults:* 12.5-50 mg orally daily<br>*Children:* 1-3 mg/kg orally daily |
| triamterene (Dyrenium) | *Adults:* 100 mg orally twice daily<br>*Children:* 2-4 mg/kg orally once daily or once every other day |

## HUMAN B-TYPE NATRIURETIC PEPTIDES

### How Natriuretic Peptides Work

Nesiritide (Natrecor) is human B-type natriuretic peptide, a hormone that is produced by the heart ventricles. It is also produced as a drug. The actions of this drug include increased water elimination and blood vessel dilation. Both are helpful when treating a patient with heart failure. This drug is given by the IV route and helps the body get rid of extra salt and water, thus lowering blood pressure. As a result the patient is less short of breath and has less edema.

Dosages for Common Natriuretic Peptides for Heart Failure

| Drug | Dosage |
|------|--------|
| nesiritide ❶ (Natrecor) | *Adults:* 2 mcg/kg IV bolus followed by 0.01 mcg/kg/min continuous infusion |

❶ High-alert drug.

### Common Side Effects
**Natriuretic Peptides**

Hypotension    Dizziness, Light-headedness    Frequent urination

Nausea    Confusion    Palpitations

*Intended Responses*
- Excess sodium and water in the body are decreased.
- Urine output is increased.
- Vasodilation is increased.
- Blood pressure is lowered
- Shortness of breath and swelling are decreased.

*Side Effects.* Side effects of natriuretic peptides include hypotension, dizziness, light-headedness, frequent urination, nausea, vomiting, nervousness, confusion, and palpitations.

*Adverse Effects.* Apnea (absence of breathing) is a life-threatening adverse effect of nesiritide.

### What To Do *Before* Giving Nesiritide
Be sure to review the general nursing responsibilities related to heart failure therapy (p. 253) in addition to these specific responsibilities before giving nesiritide.

Monitor for normal heart rate (60 to 100 beats per minute), blood pressure, and respiratory rate (12 to 20 breaths per minute). Remember that apnea is a life-threatening adverse effect of this drug.

Check the IV site for patency. Look for any signs of infection. This drug is given as an IV bolus followed by a continuous infusion.

### What To Do *After* Giving Nesiritide
Be sure to review the general nursing responsibilities related to heart failure therapy (p. 253) in addition to these specific responsibilities after giving nesiritide.

Continue to monitor blood pressure, heart rate, and respiratory rate during nesiritide infusion. Continue to check the IV line for patency and signs of infection. Tell the patient to report any pain or discomfort at the IV site.

### What To *Teach* Patients About Nesiritide
Be sure to teach patients general care needs and precautions related to drugs for heart failure (p. 254) in addition to these specific points for nesiritide.

Explain to patients why this drug has been prescribed and how it will help them. Tell patients that frequent blood pressure checks are necessary to screen for hypotension and that you will be measuring urine output.

### Life Span Considerations for Nesiritide
Nesiritide is a pregnancy category C drug and has not been tested during pregnancy or in children. Older adults have the same side effects as younger adults but are at greater risk for confusion. Teach family members to assess the level of alertness and thought processes of an older adult who has recently started taking prescribed nesiritide, especially during the first week of drug therapy.

### POSITIVE INOTROPES (HEART PUMP DRUGS)
### How Positive Inotropes Work
Positive inotropes (heart pump drugs) make the heart muscle contract more forcefully. They also relax blood vessels so blood can flow better. These drugs are used for people with severe heart failure symptoms. They are given intravenously to stimulate stronger heart contractions and keep blood circulating. Although some

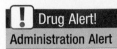

### Do Not Confuse

#### DOPamine with DOBUTamine

An order for DOPamine can be confused with DOBUTamine. Both drugs are positive inotropes that increase the force of heart contractions.

### Drug Alert!

#### Administration Alert

The effects of DOPamine are dose related. Low-dose DOPamine (0.5-3 mcg/kg/min) causes renal vasodilation and increased urine output. Moderate-dose DOPamine (2-20 mcg/kg/min) causes increased force of heart contraction. High-dose DOPamine (more than 10 mcg/kg/min) causes peripheral vasoconstriction to increase blood pressure.

### Common Side Effects

#### Positive Inotropes

Hypertension    Tachycardia, Dysrhythmias

### Drug Alert!

#### Administration Alert

Positive inotropic (heart-pump) drugs are given intravenously. Be sure that the IV line is patent so the drug does not go into the patient's tissues and cause damage.

---

patients with heart failure receive these drugs while in the hospital, many also receive them at home using an infusion pump.

### Dosages for Common Positive Inotropes

| Drug | IV Dosage |
|---|---|
| inamrinone ❗ (Inocor) | *Adults:* 0.75 mg/kg loading dose followed by 5-10 mcg/kg/min continuous infusion<br>*Infants:* 3-4.5 mg/kg in divided doses followed by 5-10 mcg/kg/min infusion<br>*Neonates:* 3-4.5 mg/kg in divided doses followed by 3-5 mcg/kg/min infusion |
| DOBUTamine ❗ (Dobutrex) | *Adults/Children:* Start low (0.5-1 mcg/kg/min) and titrate up as needed (usual range is 2-20 mcg/kg/min) |
| DOPamine ❗ (Intropin) | *Adults:* 2-50 mcg/kg/min<br>*Children:* 2-30 mcg/kg/min |
| milrinone ❗ (Primacor) | *Adults:* Loading dose 50 mcg/kg followed by continuous infusion (0.375-0.75 mcg/kg/min) |

❗ High-alert drug.

### Intended Responses
- Contractility is increased.
- Cardiac output is increased.
- Blood vessel dilation is increased.
- Preload and afterload are decreased.
- Heart function and contractility are improved.
- Blood pressure is lowered.
- Circulation is improved.

**Side Effects.** Common side effects of positive inotrope drugs include hypertension, increased heart rate, premature ventricular contractions, and other dysrhythmias.

Other side effects include headache, palpitations, irregular or rapid heart rate, light-headedness, fainting, and leg muscle cramps.

Inamrinone and milrinone can cause hypotension.

**Adverse Effects.** Ventricular dysrhythmias may occur with milrinone and may be life threatening. Rarely a patient may have allergic reactions to these drugs, including rash, fever, bronchospasm, and chest pain.

### What To Do *Before* Giving Positive Inotropes

Be sure to review the general nursing responsibilities related to heart failure therapy (p. 253) in addition to these specific responsibilities before giving heart-pump drugs.

During infusion of a heart-pump drug, frequently monitor the patient's heart rate and blood pressure (at least every 1 to 2 hours). Make sure that the patient's IV line is patent. Double check the IV rate by asking another nurse to check the calculation. These drugs cause vasoconstriction, so if infiltration occurs, reduced blood flow to the tissues can result in severe tissue damage and even tissue necrosis.

Ask whether the patient has a history of high blood pressure or heart dysrhythmias.

### What To Do *After* Giving Positive Inotropes

Be sure to review the general nursing responsibilities related to heart failure therapy (p. 253) in addition to these specific responsibilities after giving heart-pump drugs.

Watch the IV site for patency and any signs of infection such as pain, redness, swelling, and warmth. Remind the patient to immediately report any pain or discomfort at the IV site.

## What To *Teach* Patients About Positive Inotropes

Be sure to teach patients general care needs and precautions related to drugs for heart failure (p. 254) in addition to these specific points for heart-pump drugs.

Teach patients about the signs and symptoms of IV lines that are no longer patent or that have developed an infection (for example, burning or pain, redness, swelling, warmth). Tell them to report any of these signs immediately.

For patients receiving these drugs at home, demonstrate how to use the infusion pump. Instruct them to report any problems with the pump immediately.

Tell patients why this drug has been ordered and give instructions not to stop the drug unless told to do so by the prescriber. Teach patients to inform the prescriber of any chest pain, dyspnea, numbness, or tingling or burning in the extremities.

## Life Span Considerations for Positive Inotropes

Safe use of these drugs has not been determined during pregnancy or breastfeeding or with children. Positive inotrope drugs are pregnancy category C drugs, except for dobutamine (Dobutrex) which is a pregnancy category B drug.

*Considerations for Older Adults.* Older adults may be more likely to experience adverse effects of these drugs, especially chest pain and hypertension. Monitor the older adult receiving any positive inotropic drug at least every 2 hours for changes in blood pressure, heart rate, and heart rhythm.

## POTASSIUM AND MAGNESIUM

### How Potassium and Magnesium Work

Patients taking diuretic drugs for heart failure can lose some potassium and magnesium in their urine. To keep blood levels of potassium and magnesium within normal ranges, supplements are often prescribed.

### Dosages for Common Potassium and Magnesium Supplements

| Drug | Dosage |
|------|--------|
| potassium 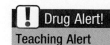 (K-Dur, K-Lor, Kaon CL, K-Lyte, Slow-K, Klotrix, Kaochlor 10%) | *Adults:* PO: 20 mEq orally daily to prevent potassium deficit; 40-100 mEq orally daily to treat potassium deficit<br>*Adults:* IV: Up to 200-400 mEq IV drip daily; do *not* exceed 10 mEq/hr<br>*Children:* PO: 2-5 mEq/kg orally daily<br>*Children:* IV: Up to 3 mEq/kg IV drip daily |
| magnesium ❶ (Max-Oxide, Uro-Mag) | Oral doses are age dependent:<br>*Adults/Children older than 10 years:* 270-400 mg daily<br>*Children:* 3-6 mg/kg daily in 3-4 divided doses. |

🔝 Top 100 drugs prescribed; ❶ High-alert drug.

### *Intended Responses*

- Blood values for potassium and magnesium are normal (Table 14-1).
- Low potassium and magnesium levels are prevented.
- Some abnormal heart rhythms are prevented.

*Side Effects.* Common side effects of potassium and magnesium include nausea, vomiting, diarrhea, gas, and abdominal discomfort.

| Table 14-1 | Normal Electrolyte Values |
|------------|---------------------------|
| **ELECTROLYTE** | **NORMAL RANGE** |
| Sodium | 135 to 145 mEq/L |
| Potassium | 3.5 to 5.0 mEq/L |
| Calcium | 9.0 to 10.5 mg/dL |
| Magnesium | 1.2 to 2.1 mEq/L |

**Drug Alert!**

**Administration Alert**

Monitor the IV site carefully when a patient is receiving IV potassium because this drug can be very irritating to peripheral IV sites. Give it with an infusion pump or controller to ensure safe administration. Do *not* ignore a patient's reports of pain or discomfort at the IV site.

**Memory Jogger**

Signs of increased blood potassium level include slow and irregular heart rhythm, fatigue, muscle weakness, paresthesia (numbness and tingling), confusion, difficulty breathing, and ECG changes.

**Memory Jogger**

Signs of increased blood magnesium level include muscle and generalized weakness, decreased reflexes (neuromuscular depression), hypotension, abnormal cardiac rhythm, drowsiness, decreased alertness and concentration, decreased rate of breathing/respiratory paralysis, CNS depression, and coma.

Less common side effects include flushing, sweating, confusion, restlessness, weakness, ECG changes, and paresthesia (numbness and tingling). When potassium is given intravenously, it can cause irritation at the IV site.

*Adverse Effects.*   High potassium or magnesium levels can cause life-threatening ECG changes and abnormal heart rhythms. *Potassium should never be given via IV push.*

Black, tarry, or bloody stools are signs of stomach bleeding and should be reported to the prescriber immediately.

### What To Do *Before* Giving Potassium or Magnesium

Be sure to review the general nursing responsibilities related to heart failure therapy (p. 253) in addition to these specific responsibilities before giving potassium or magnesium.

Check and recheck the dosage of potassium prescribed and the concentration of the drug in the vial. Concentrations vary considerably. An overdose of intravenous potassium can be lethal.

If the patient is on a heart monitor, check the heart rhythm or ask the monitor watcher about it. Check the patient's current laboratory values for potassium and magnesium. If these values are outside of the normal range, notify the prescriber. (See Table 14-1 for a listing of normal ranges.)

If the potassium level is low (less than 3.5 mEq/L), assess handgrip strength and bowel sounds at least every shift. Also assess respiratory rate and effort and oxygen saturation. Notify the prescriber if oxygen saturation drops below 90%.

### What To Do *After* Giving Potassium or Magnesium

Be sure to review the general nursing responsibilities related to heart failure therapy (p. 253) in addition to these specific responsibilities after giving potassium or magnesium.

Make sure that any follow-up laboratory values are drawn and sent to the laboratory.

If the patient has an IV site, recheck it for signs of irritation every 2 to 4 hours. Instruct the patient to report any pain or discomfort in the IV site immediately.

Watch for signs of potassium overdose *(hyperkalemia)*, including slow and irregular heart rhythm, fatigue, muscle weakness, *paresthesia* (numbness and tingling), confusion, difficulty breathing, and ECG changes.

Also watch for signs of increased magnesium level such as muscle and generalized weakness, decreased reflexes (neuromuscular depression), hypotension, abnormal cardiac rhythm, drowsiness, decreased alertness and concentration, decreased rate of breathing/respiratory paralysis, central nervous system (CNS) depression, and coma.

### What To *Teach* Patients About Potassium and Magnesium

Be sure to teach patients general care needs and precautions related to drugs for heart failure (p. 254) in addition to these specific points for potassium and magnesium.

Tell patients why a potassium or magnesium supplement has been ordered. If they miss a dose, it should be taken within 2 hours. *Patients should not take a double dose of either potassium or magnesium.* Instruct them to take potassium and magnesium supplements with food or right after meals with a full glass of water or fruit juice. Taking potassium on an empty stomach can cause nausea and vomiting.

Remind patients to avoid using salt substitutes that contain potassium. Provide a list of dietary sources of potassium (Box 14-3) and magnesium (Box 14-4).

Teach patients about the signs of too much potassium (such as palpitations, skipped heart beats, muscle twitching or weakness, or numbness and tingling) and tell them to report these signs to the prescriber immediately. Advise patients to have any laboratory values drawn as instructed to monitor responses to these supplements.

Box **14-3**   Dietary Sources of Potassium

- Baked potato
- Bananas
- Beet greens
- Clams
- Halibut, tuna, cod fish
- Molasses
- Prune, carrot, tomato juice
- Soybeans
- Spinach
- Sweet potato
- Tomato paste, sauce, puree
- White, lima beans
- Winter squash
- Yogurt

Box **14-4**   Dietary Sources of Magnesium

- Almonds
- Black beans
- Bran cereal
- Brazil nuts
- Buckwheat flour
- Cashews
- Halibut
- Mixed nuts
- Pumpkin and squash seed kernels
- Sesame seeds
- Soybeans
- Spinach
- Walnuts
- White beans
- Whole grain rice

### Life Span Considerations for Potassium and Magnesium

Potassium is a pregnancy category C drug, and magnesium is pregnancy category A or B.

◄ ⊜-Learning Activity 14-5

### OTHER DRUGS USED TO TREAT HEART FAILURE

Anticoagulants such as heparin and warfarin (Coumadin) prevent clots from forming or getting bigger and may be prescribed to treat heart failure (refer to Chapter 17). The antidysrhythmic drug amiodarone (Cordarone) may be used to prevent or treat irregular heart rhythms that begin in the ventricles such as ventricular tachycardia (refer to Chapter 15). Irregular heart rhythms can be life threatening.

## Get Ready for Practice!

### Key Points

- Most heart failure is caused by high blood pressure.
- Most heart failure begins in the left ventricle and progresses to right heart failure.
- Left heart failure causes symptoms in the lungs, and right heart failure causes peripheral symptoms.
- Drugs for heart failure are prescribed to make physical activity more comfortable, improve quality of life, and prolong life.
- The only cure for heart failure is a heart transplant because the damage to the heart muscle is not reversible.
- Angiotensin-converting enzyme (ACE) inhibitors, angiotensin II receptor blockers (ARBs), vasodilators, and human B-type natriuretic peptides may be prescribed to decrease afterload.
- Diuretics may be prescribed to decrease preload by reducing the circulating blood volume.
- Digoxin and other positive inotropic drugs increase the force of heart contraction.

- Always check the heart rate for a full minute before giving a cardiac glycoside (digoxin).
- Digoxin (Lanoxin) has a narrow therapeutic range (0.8 to 2 ng/mL), and a value above 2 is considered toxic.
- Low-dose spironolactone (Aldactone) is used to block the action of aldosterone, a hormone that causes the body to hold onto salt and water.
- Instruct patients to report weight gain of more than 2 pounds in a day or 5 pounds in a week to the prescriber.
- Nesiritide (Natrecor) (a human B-type natriuretic peptide) causes water elimination and blood vessel dilation.
- Dopamine (Intropin), a positive inotropic drug, has effects that are dose related. At low doses it increases kidney perfusion, at moderate doses it increases contractility of the heart muscle, and at high doses it causes constriction of the blood vessels.
- Rates of IV drugs for heart failure should always be controlled by an infusion controller device.

## Additional Learning Resources

**evolve** Go to your Evolve website (http://evolve.elsevier.com/Workman/pharmacology/) for the following FREE learning resources:

- eLearning Activities
- Animations
- Video Clips
- Interactive Review Questions
- Audio Key Points
- Audio Glossary
- Audio Glossary—Spanish-English
- Drug Dosage Calculators
- Patient Teaching Handouts

**SG** Go to your Study Guide for additional learning activities to help you master this chapter content.

## Review Questions

1. A patient who has just been prescribed hydralazine (Apresoline) for hypertension asks you how the drug will work. What is your best response?

   A. "It will cause your arteries to dilate."
   B. "It will slow your heart rate."
   C. "It will decrease the fluid in your blood vessels."
   D. "It will increase the contraction strength of your heart."

2. Which symptoms will you likely see in a patient with right heart failure? (Select all that apply.)

   A. Ankle edema
   B. Full jugular veins when sitting
   C. Pulmonary congestion
   D. Weight gain
   E. Distended abdomen
   F. Crackles in the lungs

3. A patient who has recently started on isosorbide dinitrate (Isordil) 20 mg twice daily reports having terrible headaches. What is your best action?

   A. Notify the prescriber immediately
   B. Close the door and turn off the television
   C. Suggest that an ice bag be placed on the forehead
   D. Offer the patient a dose of prescribed PRN acetaminophen

4. Which drug can be used safely during pregnancy to control high blood pressure?

   A. digoxin (Lanoxin)
   B. isosorbide (Isordil)
   C. hydralazine (Apresoline)
   D. captopril (Capoten)

5. A patient prescribed potassium (K-Lyte) 20 mEq tells you he has skipped heartbeats. What is your best first action?

   A. Check the most recent blood potassium level.
   B. Hold the drug and notify the prescriber.
   C. Document the finding as the only action.
   D. Assess patient reflexes.

6. A patient is receiving potassium chloride 10 mEq in 100 mL 0.9 saline IV over 1 hour. For which side effects should you monitor? (Select all that apply.)

   A. Pain at the IV site
   B. Abdominal discomfort
   C. Drowsiness
   D. Nausea and vomiting
   E. ECG changes
   F. Hypotension

7. What is the most important teaching point for a patient who will go home taking 0.125 mg of digoxin each day?

   A. Have blood pressure checked every day.
   B. Avoid foods that are high in potassium.
   C. Check pulse for a full minute before taking digoxin.
   D. Do not take digoxin within 1 hour of taking an antacid

8. What should you teach the family of an older adult who has recently been prescribed nesiritide?

   A. Check the blood pressure 3 to 4 times a day.
   B. Avoid grapefruit juice while taking this drug.
   C. Assist with feeding at all meals.
   D. Assess level of alertness and thought processes.

9. A patient has been prescribed potassium bicarbonate (K-Lyte) 40 mEq to be given in 2 divided doses with a full glass of water or fruit juice. How much K-Lyte will you give with each dose? _____ mEq per dose

10. The prescriber has ordered dobutamine (Dobutrex) 2 mcg/kg/min for a patient who weighs 72 kg. What is the correct infusion rate for this patient? _____ mcg/min

11. A patient has been ordered spironolactone (Aldactone) 12.5 mg every morning. Spironolactone comes in 25-mg tablets. How many tablets will you give the patient for each dose? _____ tablet(s)

## Critical Thinking Activities

Ms. Keats is a 68-year-old woman who was diagnosed with heart failure 6 years ago. Her signs and symptoms include reports of being tired and weak, a nagging dry cough, and a weight gain of 5 pounds over the past week. On assessment you find 2+ ankle swelling, enlarged jugular neck veins, weak pedal and radial pulses, and crackles and wheezes when listening to her lungs. Her currently prescribed drugs include lisinopril (Prinivil) 5 mg once a day, spironolactone (Aldactone) 12.5 mg/day, and furosemide (Lasix) 40 mg/day.

1. What type of heart failure does Ms. Keats' assessment indicate?

2. Which assessment finding indicates that Ms. Keats's heart failure may be worsening?

3. Why did the health care provider prescribe two diuretics?

4. What changes in Ms. Keats' current drug prescriptions do you expect?

# Antidysrhythmic Drugs

## Objectives

*After studying this chapter you should be able to:*

1. Explain how different classes of drugs are used to treat abnormal heart rhythms.
2. List the common names, actions, usual adult dosages, possible side effects, and adverse effects of atropine, digoxin, adenosine, and magnesium sulfate.
3. Describe what to do before and after giving atropine, digoxin, adenosine, and magnesium sulfate.
4. Explain what to teach patients taking atropine, digoxin, adenosine, and magnesium sulfate, including what to do, what not to do, and when to call the prescriber.
5. Describe life span considerations for atropine, digoxin, adenosine, and magnesium sulfate.
6. List the common names, actions, usual adult dosages, possible side effects, and adverse effects of class I, II, III,

and IV antidysrhythmic drugs used to treat rapid abnormal heart rhythms.

7. Describe what to do before and after giving class I, II, III, and IV antidysrhythmic drugs used to treat rapid abnormal heart rhythms.
8. Explain what to teach patients taking class I, II, III, and IV antidysrhythmic drugs used to treat rapid abnormal heart rhythms, including what to do, what not to do, and when to call the prescriber.
9. Describe life span considerations for class I, II, III, and IV antidysrhythmic drugs used to treat rapid abnormal heart rhythms.

## Key Terms

**antidysrhythmic drugs** (ăn-tī-dĭs-RĬTH-mĭk DRŬGZ) (p. 272) Drugs used to treat abnormal heart rhythms.

**asystole** (ā-SĬS-tō-lē) (p. 273) An absence of electrical or contraction activity within the heart. Appears on the electrocardiogram (ECG) monitor as a straight line or "flatline."

**atrial fibrillation** (Ā-trē-ŭl fĭb-rĭl-LĀ-shŭn) (p. 271) Quivering of the atria. Atrial fibrillation decreases cardiac output because the atrial portion of the output of the heart is lost when the atria do not contract.

**atrioventricular (AV) node** (ā-trē-ō-věn-TRĬK-yū-lŭr NŌD) (p. 269) Specialized cardiac tissue capable of generating electrical impulses that cause the heart to contract; the secondary pacemaker of the heart.

**automaticity** (ŏ-tō-mă-TĬS-ĭ-tē) (p. 273) Ability of the cardiac muscle cells to fire an impulse on their own.

**bradycardia** (brā-dē-KĂR-dē-ă) (p. 270) Slow heart rate, usually considered to be less than 60 beats per minute.

**bradydysrhythmia** (brā-dē-dĭs-RĬTH-mē-ă) (p. 273) An abnormally slow heart rhythm.

**cardiac output** (KĂR-dē-ăk ŌWT-pŭt) (p. 270) The amount of blood ejected by the heart in 1 minute. A normal adult heart can easily pump 5 quarts (4.7 liters) of blood a minute.

**conductivity** (kŏn-dŭk-TĬV-ĭ-tē) (p. 273) Ability or power of heart muscle cells to transmit electrical impulses.

**dysrhythmia** (dĭs-RĬTH-mē-ă) (p. 270) An abnormal heart rhythm.

**electrical conduction system** (ē-LĔK-trĭ-kŭl kŏn-DŬK-shŭn SĬS-tŭm) (p. 268) The electrical conduction system that controls the heart rate. It causes electrical impulses and conducts them through the muscle of the heart, stimulating the heart to contract and pump blood.

**His-Purkinje system** (HĬZ pŭr-KĬN-jē SĬS-tŭm) (p. 269) Specialized cardiac tissue that normally conducts impulses from the AV node to the ventricles.

**normal sinus rhythm** (NŌR-mŭl SĪ-nŭs RĬTH-ŭm) (p. 269) The normal rhythm of the heart as measured by an electrocardiogram.

**pacemaker** (PĀS-mā-kŭr) (p. 268) A part of the body such as the special cardiac muscle fibers of the sinoatrial node that sets the rate or rhythm of the heart.

**premature contractions** (prē-mă-CHŬR kŏn-TRĂK-shŭnz) (p. 270) Heart contractions that occur earlier than expected.

**refractory period** (rē-FRĂK-tŏr-ē PĒR-ē-ŭd) (p. 273) Time following an action potential during which normal stimulation will not cause another action potential. During the *absolute refractory period* no stimulation will cause an electrical impulse. The *relative refractory period* requires a higher-than-normal stimulus to cause an electrical impulse.

**sinoatrial (SA) node** (sī-nō-Ā-trē-ŭl NŌD) (p. 268) Specialized cardiac tissue capable of generating electrical impulses that cause the heart muscle to contract; the normal pacemaker of the heart located in the upper right atrium.

**syncope** (SĬN-kō-pē) (p. 271) A brief loss of consciousness caused by a temporary deficiency of oxygen in the brain.

**tachycardia** (tăk-ē-KĂR-dē-ă) (p. 270) Rapid heart rate, usually considered to be greater than 100 beats per minute.

**tachydysrhythmia** (tăk-ē-dĭs-RĬTH-mē-ă) (p. 277) An abnormally rapid heart rhythm.

**torsades de pointes** (tōr-SŌDZ dě PWĂNT) (p. 278) A life-threatening ventricular tachycardia. In French it means "twisting of the points." It is primarily caused by a low blood magnesium level and seen in malnourished people.

**ventricular fibrillation** (věn-TRĬK-yū-lŭr fĭb-rĭl-LĀ-shŭn) (p. 271) Quivering of the ventricles. Ventricular fibrillation is life threatening and can lead to death in minutes because there is no cardiac output when the ventricles do not contract.

⊖-Learning Activity 15-1 ▶

## REVIEW OF RELATED PHYSIOLOGY AND PATHOPHYSIOLOGY

The basic function of the heart is to pump blood to the lungs and body. The right side of the heart receives oxygen-poor blood from the body and sends it to the lungs. The left side of the heart receives oxygen-rich blood from the lungs and pumps it out to the body (Figure 15-1). To perform this function well, the heart must be strong and have its own well-oxygenated blood supply. The blood supply to the heart muscle is delivered by the coronary arteries.

### PACEMAKERS AND THE CARDIAC CONDUCTION SYSTEM

The heart has its own system of electrical impulses that travel through the heart muscle, causing the heart to contract and pump blood. It is this process, called the **electrical conduction system**, that controls the heart rate and rhythm. The part of the system that sets the heart rate and rhythm by generating impulses is called the **pacemaker**. Under normal circumstances the **sinoatrial (SA) node** composed of special muscle fibers capable of causing electrical impulses is the pacemaker and

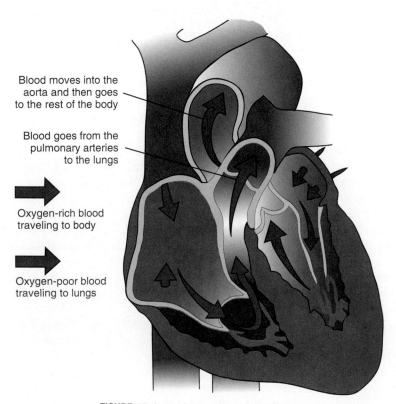

Blood moves into the aorta and then goes to the rest of the body

Blood goes from the pulmonary arteries to the lungs

➡ Oxygen-rich blood traveling to body

➡ Oxygen-poor blood traveling to lungs

**FIGURE 15-1** Blood flow through the heart.

controls the heart rate. The SA node initiates electrical impulses at a rate of 60 to 100 per minute. These impulses travel across pathways to the **atrioventricular (AV) node** and then down through the **His-Purkinje system** to cause the ventricles to contract and pump blood out of the heart (Figure 15-2).

When the SA node does not function, the AV node takes over as the second pacemaker of the heart. This secondary pacemaker usually causes 40 to 60 electrical impulses per minute, which results in a slower heart rate. If both the SA and the AV nodes are not working, the ventricular muscle cells become the third pacemaker of the heart, with a very slow rate of 20 to 40 impulses per minute. This slow rate of heart contractions is not enough to supply the body with the blood and oxygen it needs to function, and the patient may have symptoms such as confusion or a change in level of consciousness.

## HEART RATE

Sometimes it is normal for the heart to beat faster or slower. Heart rate is related to a person's state of health and whether he or she is exercising or resting. For example, a young athlete may have a normal resting heart rate of 50 beats per minute with an exercising heart rate of 100, whereas an older adult may have a resting heart rate of 80 or 90 beats per minute and an exercising heart rate of 120 to 140. Normal heart rate ranges for adults and children are summarized in Table 15-1.

How fast the heart beats depends on how much oxygen-rich blood your body needs. During activity, excitement, fever, or shock, your body needs more oxygen-rich blood, so your heart rate may increase to 100 beats per minute or more. When you are resting or sleeping, your body needs less oxygen-rich blood, so your heart rate decreases sometimes to less than 60 beats per minute.

## Normal Heart Rhythm

When the heart beats normally, each impulse that starts from the SA node causes the atria and ventricles to contract regularly and in sequence at a rate between 60 and 100 beats per minute. This normal rhythm of the heart is called **normal sinus**

**Memory Jogger**

The normal pacemaker of the heart, the SA node, initiates 60 to 100 electrical impulses per minute.

**Memory Jogger**

The electrical impulses that cause normal sinus rhythm begin in the SA node.

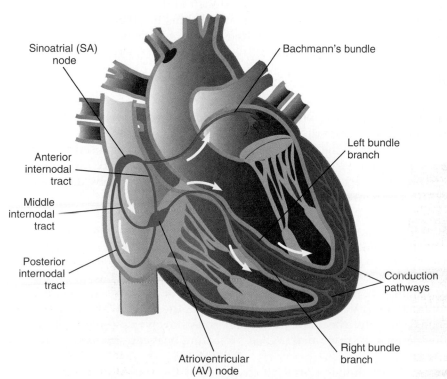

**FIGURE 15-2** Electrical conduction system of the heart.

| Table 15-1 | Normal Heart Rates |
|---|---|
| **AGE-GROUP** | **RANGE (BEATS/MIN)** |
| Adults | 60-100 |
| Children | 70-120 |
| Toddlers | 90-150 |
| Infants | 120-160 |

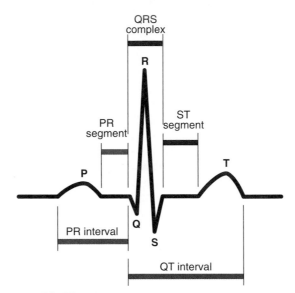

**FIGURE 15-3** Normal sinus rhythm of the heart.

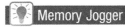

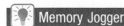

rhythm (Figure 15-3). This means that the impulse begins in the SA node and travels normally to cause the atria to contract and then to the ventricles to contract. A slow heart rhythm started by the SA node is called sinus **bradycardia** (less than 60 beats per minute). A rapid heart rhythm started by the SA node is called sinus **tachycardia** (more than 100 beats per minute).

### Dysrhythmias

**Dysrhythmias** are abnormal heart rhythms (Box 15-1). They often begin with an abnormal unexpected impulse somewhere in the heart muscle tissue (but not from the SA node). Abnormal rhythms are often caused by problems with the electrical conduction system of the heart. Dysrhythmias may also be caused by heart muscle contractions that are irregular or faster or slower than normal. Most dysrhythmias have a negative effect on how well the heart works as a pump by decreasing **cardiac output** (the amount of blood the heart pumps in a minute).

Dysrhythmias can be named according to where they begin. *Atrial dysrhythmias* begin in the atria, whereas *supraventricular dysrhythmias* originate above the ventricles and *ventricular dysrhythmias* begin within the ventricles.

Heartbeats that occur earlier than expected are called **premature contractions.** They can begin in the atria (premature atrial contractions [PACs]), in the AV node region (premature junctional contractions [PJCs]), or ventricles (premature ventricular contractions [PVCs]). A patient may notice the feeling of a skipped beat. An occasional premature beat is usually not serious; however, premature beats may lead to other serious dysrhythmias. When premature beats are frequent, cardiac output is decreased.

Other dysrhythmias cause the chambers of the heart (atria and ventricles) to quiver (*fibrillate*) instead of contracting normally and effectively. This fibrillation

Box **15-1**   List of Common Dysrhythmias

**ATRIAL**
- Atrial fibrillation
- Atrial flutter
- Premature atrial contractions
- Sick sinus syndrome
- Supraventricular tachycardia

**VENTRICULAR**
- Asystole
- Premature ventricular contractions
- Pulseless electrical activity
- Ventricular fibrillation
- Ventricular tachycardia

**JUNCTIONAL**
- Junctional tachycardia
- Premature junctional contractions

**HEART BLOCKS**
- First-degree heart block
- Second-degree heart block
  - Mobitz type I/Wenckebach
  - Mobitz type II
- Third-degree heart block (complete heart block)

Box **15-2**   Common Symptoms of Dysrhythmias

- Chest pain
- Dizziness
- Fainting (syncope)
- Fluttering in the chest
- Light-headedness
- May have *no* symptoms
- Rapid heart rate
- Shortness of breath
- Slow heart rate

results from totally disorganized electrical activity and produces ineffective contraction and pumping of blood. When the atria fibrillate, it is called **atrial fibrillation.** Atrial fibrillation decreases cardiac output, because the atrial portion of cardiac output is lost when the atria do not contract. **Ventricular fibrillation** is the name for the condition in which the ventricles fibrillate. Ventricular fibrillation is life threatening and can lead to death in minutes because no blood is pumped from the heart (cardiac output) when the ventricles quiver and do not contract.

***Dysrhythmia Symptoms.*** Dysrhythmias may or may not cause symptoms in patients (Box 15-2). Often abnormal rhythms cause symptoms such as a fluttery feeling in the chest, racing heartbeats, slow heartbeats, chest pain, shortness of breath, light-headedness, dizziness, and fainting (**syncope**). Having symptoms does not always mean having a serious dysrhythmia. Some people with symptoms do not have a serious dysrhythmia, whereas others with no symptoms may have a life-threatening dysrhythmia.

***Risk Factors for Dysrhythmias.*** Several factors increase the risk of a person developing a heart dysrhythmia (Box 15-3). Older adults with age-related heart changes are more likely to have dysrhythmias. Genetics and family history increase the risk for them. For example, some people are born with an extra electrical impulse pathway and may develop *Wolff-Parkinson-White syndrome,* a type of dysrhythmia. Some disease processes may lead to dysrhythmias. Diabetes increases the risk of developing high blood pressure and coronary artery disease. High blood pressure and obesity increase the risk of developing coronary artery disease, with narrow arteries and heart damage that may cause abnormal heart rhythms. Thyroid problems may cause rapid or slow heart rates. *Obstructive sleep apnea* (a sleep disorder with pauses in breathing during sleep) can cause bradycardia and episodes of atrial fibrillation. Electrolyte imbalances can cause the heart to initiate abnormal electrical impulses. When electrolyte levels (such as potassium, sodium, calcium, and magnesium) are too high or too low, dysrhythmias may occur.

 Clinical Pitfall

Without immediate intervention ventricular fibrillation leads to death within minutes.

 Clinical Pitfall

Some patients *with* symptoms do *not* have serious dysrhythmias, whereas others *without* symptoms may have life-threatening dysrhythmias.

◄ ⊜-Learning Activity 15-2

Box **15-3**    Risk Factors for Developing Dysrhythmias

- Age (older adults)
- Genetics (family history)
- Coronary artery disease
- Thyroid problems
  - Hypothyroidism—bradycardia
  - Hyperthyroidism—tachycardia
- Drugs and supplements
  - Cough/cold remedies with pseudoephedrine
- High blood pressure
- Obesity
- Diabetes
- Low blood sugar (hypoglycemia)
- Obstructive sleep apnea
- Electrolyte imbalance
  - Potassium
  - Sodium
  - Calcium
  - Magnesium
- Alcohol abuse
- Stimulant use
  - Caffeine
  - Nicotine
- Illicit drugs
  - Cocaine
  - Amphetamines

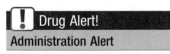

**Drug Alert!**

**Administration Alert**

Over-the-counter cough and cold drugs that contain pseudoephedrine (Sudafed) can cause abnormal rapid heart rhythms.

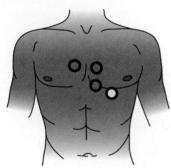

**FIGURE 15-4** Location of the apical pulse.

ⓔ-Learning Activity 15-3 ►

Drugs may also affect heart rhythm. Over-the-counter cold and cough drugs containing pseudoephedrine (for example, Sudafed) can cause tachycardia. Stimulants such as caffeine and nicotine can cause premature heartbeats and rapid (tachycardic) rhythms. Too much alcohol also can change the conduction of electrical impulses and increase the chance of atrial fibrillation. Illegal drugs such as cocaine and amphetamines can cause serious heart rhythm problems, including ventricular fibrillation, which can lead to sudden death.

### Measuring the Heart Rate

The most accurate way to measure a patient's heart rate is to listen with a stethoscope over the apical region of the chest for a full minute. The apical heart rate is measured at the left fifth intercostal space in the midclavicular area (usually two fingers below the left nipple) (Figure 15-4). Listen with a stethoscope for a full minute. Count the number of heartbeats. Note any irregular rhythms.

An important part of teaching for a patient with an abnormal heart rate is how to count the heart rate. Tell the patient to obtain a watch or clock that has a second hand. Instruct him or her to place the index and middle finger of the dominant hand on the inner wrist of the opposite arm just below the base of the thumb (Figure 15-5). In this way the patient should feel the pulsing of the radial artery against the fingers. Have him or her count the number of pulse beats for a full minute. Also tell him or her to note whether the heart rhythm is regular or irregular when measuring the heart rate. A normal heart rhythm is regular.

### GENERAL ISSUES RELATED TO ANTIDYSRHYTHMIC THERAPY

Antidysrhythmic drugs are used to treat abnormal heart rhythms and may be prescribed to increase or decrease the heart rate. The actions of drugs prescribed to treat rapid heart rates may be to decrease spontaneous contraction of myocardial cells, including pacemaker cells (automaticity), slow ability of heart muscle cells to transmit electrical impulses (conductivity), or prolong the refractory period of heart cells. The refractory period is the period of time following an impulse generation during which normal stimulation will not cause another impulse. During the absolute refractory period an impulse *cannot* be conducted. During the relative refractory period an impulse must be stronger than normal to be conducted.

*Before giving any antidysrhythmic drug,* be sure to get a complete list of the drugs that the patient is using, including over-the-counter and herbal drugs. Check the patient's heart rate and blood pressure. Watch for decreased or increased heart rate (less than 60 beats per minute or more than 100 beats per minute) and decreased blood pressure (less than 90/60 mm Hg), which may indicate decreased blood flow to the tissues. *Be sure to check the heart rate by listening to the apical pulse for a full minute.* If a cardiac monitor is being used, ask the monitor watcher, charge nurse, or prescriber about the patient's rhythm. Get a baseline weight for each patient because the dosage of many of these drugs is based on weight.

*After giving any antidysrhythmic drug,* be sure to recheck the patient's heart rate and blood pressure. Ask the monitor watcher about changes in the heart rhythm. Ensure that the call light is within easy reach and instruct the patient to call for help before getting out of bed. Instruct patients to get up and change positions slowly because of the possibility of decreased blood pressure, which can cause dizziness or fainting.

*Teach patients receiving any antidysrhythmic drug* proper techniques for how to check and record their heart rate and blood pressure daily. Remind patients to take these drugs exactly as instructed by the prescriber. Patients should never take a double dose. Tell them to talk with the prescriber before taking any over-the-counter drugs. Stress the importance of follow-up appointments with the prescriber to monitor the progress of dysrhythmia treatment. Advise them to wear a medical identification bracelet stating that an antidysrhythmic drug is being used and the reason for its use.

Warn patients to get up and change positions slowly because of the side effects of dizziness and drowsiness. Teach them to sit on the side of the bed for a few minutes before standing up. Caution them against driving or operating machines that require alertness until responses to the drugs are known.

## TYPES OF ANTIDYSRHYTHMIC DRUGS

### ATROPINE FOR BRADYDYSRHYTHMIAS

#### How Atropine Works on the Heart

Atropine is used to treat abnormally slow heart rhythms known as bradydysrhythmias. Atropine blocks the actions of the vagus nerve on the heart. The vagus nerve slows down the heart rate. By blocking the action of this nerve, atropine causes an increase in electrical impulse conduction and heart rate. This drug is used for a patient who has symptoms of bradycardia. Atropine may also be used in emergency situations when a patient's heart rhythm is in asystole. Asystole is the absence of electrical or contraction activity within the heart. It appears on the electrocardiogram (ECG) monitor as a straight line or "flatline." In emergency settings atropine may also be given through the endotracheal (ET) tube of a patient who has been intubated. Usually twice the normal dose is used, and it is mixed with 5 to 10 mL of normal saline.

Atropine may also be given by the intraosseous (into the bone) route. Specially trained emergency care providers give drugs by endotracheal tube and intraosseous routes. Be sure to consult a drug handbook for specific information about atropine. Other uses for atropine include as a preoperative drug to decrease production of gastrointestinal and respiratory secretions and laryngospasm, bradycardia, and hypotension during anesthesia. This drug is also used topically to dilate pupils before eye examinations.

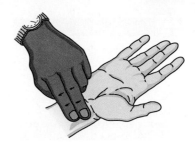

**FIGURE 15-5** Checking the radial pulse.

**! Drug Alert!**

**Administration Alert**

A patient with liver or kidney problems needs smaller doses of most antidysrhythmic drugs to avoid drug overdose and drug toxicity.

**! Drug Alert!**

**Teaching Alert**

Teach patients who have been prescribed antidysrhythmic drugs to check and record their heart rate and blood pressure daily.

**Memory Jogger**

Use the acronym NAVEL to remember drugs that may be given by ET tube: *N*arcan, *a*tropine, *V*alium, *e*pinephrine, and *l*idocaine.

◄⊖-Learning Activity 15-4

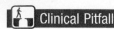

### Clinical Pitfall

Do *not* give large doses of atropine to older adults because they are more sensitive to its effects and may experience confusion.

### Common Side Effects

**Atropine**

Drowsiness    Blurred vision    Tachycardia

Dry mouth    Urinary retention

### Clinical Pitfall

Administering a dose of atropine less than 0.5 mg may make bradycardia worse (paradoxical bradycardia).

### Dosage for Atropine

| Drug | Dosage |
|---|---|
| atropine (Atropine Sulfate) | *Adults:* 0.5-1 mg IV every 5 min up to 3 mg or 0.04 mg/kg<br>*Children:* 0.01-0.03 mg/kg IV every 5 min up to 1 mg in children and 2 mg in adolescents |

### *Intended Responses*
- Heart rate is increased.
- Cardiac output is increased.
- Symptoms such as dizziness and light-headedness are decreased.

***Side Effects.***    Common side effects of atropine include drowsiness, blurred vision, tachycardia, dry mouth, and urinary hesitancy or retention.

Less common side effects include confusion (especially in older adults); dry eyes; palpitations; constipation; and decreased sweating, which can lead to heat emergencies. Other vision side effects include cycloplegia (paralysis of the ciliary muscles of the eye, resulting in the loss of visual accommodation) and mydriasis (dilation of the pupils).

***Adverse Effects.***    A rare but serious and life-threatening effect of atropine is the occurrence of ventricular fibrillation. Because atropine increases heart rate and workload, it can also worsen heart ischemia (decreased blood flow to the heart muscle, causing chest pain) and heart blocks. Atropine can also cause PVCs or ventricular tachycardia.

Doses of atropine smaller than 0.5 mg may make bradycardia worse (paradoxical bradycardia).

### What To Do *Before* Giving Atropine
Be sure to review the general nursing responsibilities related to antidysrhythmic therapy (p. 273) in addition to these specific responsibilities before giving atropine.

Check the patient's heart rate and blood pressure. Look for decreased heart rate and blood pressure, which may indicate decreased blood flow to the tissues.

Assess the intravenous (IV) site for patency and signs of infection and infiltration such as redness, swelling, warmth, or decreased IV flow. Ask the patient if the IV site is causing any discomfort.

Ask patients about eye problems such as glaucoma because atropine can make this problem worse.

### What To Do *After* Giving Atropine
Be sure to review the general nursing responsibilities related to antidysrhythmic therapy (p. 273) in addition to these specific responsibilities after giving atropine.

Recheck the patient's heart rate and blood pressure because these should improve after atropine is given. Continue to monitor the IV site for patency. Check the patient's pulse for regularity and strength.

Monitor urine output because urinary retention can be a side effect of atropine. Ask whether the patient is experiencing any problems with dry mouth, vision, or drowsiness. Report serious side effects to the prescriber. Check for bowel sounds and abdominal tenderness because atropine can also cause constipation.

### What To *Teach* Patients About Atropine
Be sure to teach patients the general care needs and precautions related to antidysrhythmic therapy (p. 273) in addition to these specific points for atropine.

Atropine is not prescribed for long-term use. It is usually given in a patient care setting and should be administered exactly as ordered by the prescriber. It may cause drowsiness, so caution patients about getting up without assistance.

Tell patients that atropine should increase heart rate and blood pressure. Improved blood flow to the tissues should lead to decreased symptoms such as dizziness. Atropine is used for short-term treatment for some patients with bradydys-rhythmias; you will need to instruct them about more permanent solutions such as pacemakers.

Teach patients to use mouth rinses and frequent mouth hygiene to help relieve dry mouth and prevent tooth decay.

Remind patients to notify the prescriber or nurse for any vision problems. Atropine can affect the ability of the body to regulate heat, so caution patients to avoid strenuous activity in a hot setting.

### Life Span Considerations for Atropine
***Considerations for Pregnancy and Breastfeeding.*** Atropine is pregnancy category C. Intravenous atropine may cause tachycardia in the fetus and should be used with caution in pregnant women. However, it may be necessary when the mother's heart rate becomes too slow; otherwise the fetus may not receive enough oxygen and damage may occur.

***Pediatric and Older Adult Considerations.*** Atropine should be used carefully in pediatric patients and older adults because they are more sensitive to its effects and more likely to have side effects. In addition, the risk for drug-induced myocardial infarction is greater in the older adult. Although all patients receiving atropine must be monitored, extra-close monitoring is needed when the drug is used for pediatric patients or older adults.

### DIGOXIN

### How Digoxin Works
Digoxin (Lanoxin) may be used for atrial fibrillation because it helps to slow the heart rate by blocking the number of electrical impulses that pass through the AV node to the heart ventricles. Digoxin also helps to strengthen the contractions in the ventricles so the heart is able to pump more blood with each heartbeat. See Chapter 14 for the usual doses of digoxin and more detailed information about this drug.

### Intended Responses
- Heart rate decreased.
- Contractility is increased.
- Cardiac output is increased.
- Signs and symptoms of cardiac output are reduced.

***Side Effects.*** Watch for these common side effects of digoxin: fatigue, bradycardia (less than 60 beats/minute), anorexia (loss of appetite), nausea, and vomiting.

Less common side effects include headache; fatigue; drowsiness; confusion; weakness; blurred vision; seeing halos around lights; yellow vision; ECG changes and irregular heart rhythms; diarrhea; gynecomastia (breast enlargement in men) with long-term use; and thrombocytopenia (low platelet count), which places the patient at risk for bleeding.

***Adverse Effects.*** Signs and symptoms of overdose (toxicity) include these early signs: loss of appetite, nausea, vomiting, diarrhea, or vision problems. Other signs include changes in heart rate or rhythm (irregular or slow), palpitations, or fainting. In infants and small children the earliest signs of overdose are changes in heart rate and rhythm. Children may not have the same symptoms as adults. Digoxin has a very narrow therapeutic range (0.8 to 2 ng/mL—levels above 2 ng/mL are considered toxic).

Digoxin can also cause life-threatening dysrhythmias.

### What To Do *Before* Giving Digoxin
Be sure to review the general nursing responsibilities related to antidysrhythmic therapy (p. 273) in addition to these specific responsibilities before giving digoxin.

---

**Common Side Effects**

**Digoxin**

Fatigue   Bradycardia   Anorexia, Nausea/Vomiting

---

**Drug Alert!**

**Administration Alert**

Common side effects of digoxin are also signs of drug toxicity and should be reported to the prescriber immediately.

---

**Drug Alert!**

**Action/Intervention Alert**

When a patient shows any signs of overdose (digoxin toxicity), a blood level for digoxin is drawn, and the digoxin dose is held. *Digoxin immune fab* (Digibind, DigiFab) is an antidote for digoxin toxicity. It binds with digoxin to prevent its action.

Check the heart rate (apical pulse) for a full minute. Note whether the heart rate is regular or irregular. If the heart rate is less than 60 beats per minute, hold the dose, notify the prescriber, and ask if the patient should receive the drug. If the heart rate is irregular, notify the prescriber. A 12-lead ECG may be ordered.

Ask whether the patient has a history of electrolyte disorders; heart rhythm problems; and kidney, liver, or thyroid disease. Any of these conditions may alter the effects of digoxin. Low potassium levels place the patient at risk for digoxin toxicity.

### What To Do *After* Giving Digoxin

Be sure to review the general nursing responsibilities related to antidysrhythmic therapy (p. 273) in addition to these specific responsibilities after giving digoxin.

Check the heart rate (apical pulse) for a full minute before giving each dose of this drug. If the heart rate is less than 60 beats per minute or irregular, hold the drug and notify the prescriber immediately.

Check the patient's chart for current levels of potassium, magnesium, and calcium laboratory values. Abnormal values may affect how the drug works. Normal values for these electrolytes are summarized in Table 15-2. Check the patient for signs and symptoms of digoxin overdose such as loss of appetite, nausea, vomiting, and vision problems. If the patient has symptoms of toxicity, a digoxin level should be drawn, and the dose of digoxin held.

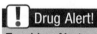
-Learning Activity 15-5 ▶

### What To *Teach* Patients About Digoxin

Be sure to teach patients the general care needs and precautions related to antidysrhythmic therapy (p. 273) in addition to these specific points for digoxin.

Explain that the heart rate must be checked every day before taking digoxin. Remind patients to tell the prescriber if their heart rate drops below 60 beats per minute, is greater than 100 beats per minute, or becomes irregular. Give instructions about the signs and symptoms of overdose (toxicity) and the need to report these to the prescriber. Remind patients about the importance of laboratory tests to monitor electrolytes and blood levels of digoxin.

Instruct patients to weigh themselves every day and to keep a record of their weight. Remind them to report a weight gain of more than 2 pounds per day to the prescriber, because this much weight gain may indicate heart failure.

Digoxin should be taken every day at the same time, and a dose should not be skipped. A missed dose may be taken within 12 hours of its scheduled time, *but double doses should not be taken because this can lead to overdose (toxicity).*

Tell patients to talk with their prescriber before taking any over-the-counter drugs for colds, allergies, upset stomach, or weight loss because these drugs can interact with digoxin. Remind patients to avoid taking antacids within 2 hours of digoxin because they can affect the absorption of the drug.

### Life Span Considerations for Digoxin

*Pediatric Considerations.*  Doses of digoxin are specific and age related (see Chapter 14). It has been used in newborns and children of all ages. When giving digoxin to an infant or child, be sure to check the dose with another nurse or with a pharmacist. The doses are very small, and a mistake could lead to serious problems or death.

| Table **15-2** Normal Blood Electrolyte Levels | |
| --- | --- |
| **ELECTROLYTE** | **NORMAL VALUE** |
| Sodium | 136 to 145 mEq/L |
| Potassium | 3.5 to 5.2 mEq/L |
| Calcium | 8.5 to 10.2 mg/dL |
| Magnesium | 1.8 to 3.0 mg/dL |

***Considerations for Pregnancy and Breastfeeding.***   Digoxin is pregnancy category C and is contraindicated during pregnancy and breastfeeding. It passes from the mother to the fetus during pregnancy and to the baby through breast milk.

***Considerations for Older Adults.***   Older adults are more sensitive to the effects of digoxin and are more likely to develop side effects, including toxicity. In addition, many older adults are prescribed diuretics, which decrease blood potassium levels. When potassium levels are reduced, the heart muscle is more sensitive to the effects of digoxin and toxicity develops more quickly. Teach older adults to take potassium supplements as prescribed and to keep all appointments for blood electrolyte testing.

## DRUGS FOR TACHYDYSRHYTHMIAS

A **tachydysrhythmia** is an abnormally rapid heart rhythm. Drugs used to treat rapid abnormal heart rhythms work in one of three ways. They may reduce automaticity of the heart muscle cells, slow down conduction of electrical impulses through the heart, or prolong the refractory period of heart cells. Several classes of drugs are used to treat these dysrhythmias (Table 15-3). The drugs are classified by the way they work. Some drugs have characteristics of more than one classification.

Goals of treatment with these drugs include preventing and relieving symptoms, prolonging life, and suppressing the abnormal rhythms. Recent trends in the treatment of these heart rhythms include a decrease in the use of class I drugs and an increase in the use of class II and III drugs because there are more side effects with class I drugs.

### *CLASS I: SODIUM CHANNEL BLOCKERS*

There are three subclasses of sodium channel blocker drugs. Different subclasses are used to treat different tachydysrhythmias.

### CLASS IA DRUGS

#### How Class Ia Drugs Work
This group of drugs is used to treat patients who have symptoms associated with PVCs, supraventricular tachycardia (SVT), and ventricular tachycardia. Another use of these drugs is to prevent the occurrence of ventricular fibrillation.

Class Ia drugs decrease the excitability of the heart muscle cells and slow the conduction of electrical impulses through the heart. Together, these actions slow the heart rate and make the rhythm more regular. Procainamide may also decrease

> **Memory Jogger**
>
> The three ways that drugs work to treat rapid abnormal heart rhythms are by:
> - Reducing automaticity of the heart muscle cells.
> - Slowing down conduction of electrical impulses through the heart.
> - Prolonging the refractory period of heart cells.

### Table **15-3**   Classes of Common Antidysrhythmic Drugs for Tachydysrhythmias

| CLASS | PURPOSE |
|---|---|
| Class I: Sodium channel blockers | |
|    Class Ia | Treat symptomatic PVCs, SVT, VT; prevent VF |
|    Class Ib | Treat symptomatic PVCs, VT; prevent VF |
|    Class Ic | Treat life-threatening VT or VF and SVT unresponsive to other drugs |
| Class I: Miscellaneous | Treat life-threatening ventricular dysrhythmias |
| Class II: Beta blockers | Treat SVT |
| Class III: Potassium channel blockers | Treat VT, VF; conversion of A fib and A flutter to sinus rhythm; maintain sinus rhythm |
| Class IV: Calcium channel blockers | Treat SVT |
| Unclassified | |
|    Adenosine | Treat SVT |
|    Magnesium sulfate | Treat torsades de pointes |

*A fib*, atrial fibrillation; *A flutter*, atrial flutter; *PVC*, Premature ventricular contraction; *SVT*, supraventricular tachycardia; *VF*, ventricular fibrillation; *VT*, ventricular tachycardia.

the strength of heart contractions. Common doses of class Ia drugs are listed in the following table. Be sure to consult a drug handbook for information about any specific class Ia antidysrhythmic drug.

**Dosages for Common Class Ia Antidysrhythmic Drugs**

| Drug | Dosage |
|---|---|
| quinidine (Quinidine sulfate, Quinaglute, Quinate♣) | *Adults:* As sulfate—200-400 mg orally every 6-8 hr (immediate release); 300-600 mg every 8-12 hr (extended release)<br>As gluconate (extended release)—324 mg orally every 8-12 hr<br>*Children:* As sulfate, 6 mg/kg orally 5 times daily |
| procainamide (Pronestyl, Procanbid) | *Adults:* Up to 50 mg/kg orally daily in divided doses every 3-6 hr to maintain therapeutic blood levels (every 6-12 hr if extended release)<br>IM—Up to 50 mg/kg daily in divided doses every 3-6 hr<br>IV—1000 mg loading dose over 60 min and then 2-6 mg/min as a continuous infusion<br>*Children:* 15-50 mg/kg orally daily in 3-6 divided doses |
| disopyramide (Norpace, Rythmodan♣) | *Adults:* 300 mg orally loading dose followed by 150 mg every 6 hr (range 400-800 mg in 4 divided doses) |

### Do Not Confuse

**quinidine *with* quinine**

An order for quinidine may be confused with quinine. Quinidine is a class Ia antidysrhythmic drug, whereas quinine is an antimalarial drug.

### Common Side Effects

**Class Ia Antidysrhythmic Drugs**

Hypotension | Anorexia, Abdominal cramping, Diarrhea, Nausea

### Intended Responses
- Heart rate is decreased.
- Abnormal supraventricular and ventricular rhythms are decreased.
- Heart rhythm is normal and regular.
- Cardiac output is increased.

**Side Effects.**   Common side effects include hypotension, loss of appetite, abdominal cramping, diarrhea, and nausea. As many as 30% to 50% of patients develop gastrointestinal side effects while taking these drugs. Disopyramide also commonly causes constipation, dry mouth, urinary retention, and urinary hesitation.

Less common side effects of class Ia drugs may include dizziness, confusion, headache, fainting, blurred vision, tachycardia, rash, decreased platelet count with increased risk for bleeding *(thrombocytopenia)*, bitter taste in the mouth, gas (flatulence), and dry eyes or throat.

**Adverse Effects.**   Life-threatening adverse effects vary with the drug prescribed. Patients taking quinidine may become hypotensive or develop an abnormal life-threatening ventricular rhythm called torsades de pointes. The life-threatening effects of procainamide include seizures, heart block, asystole, and decreased white blood cell count with increased risk for infection. Disopyramide has been known to cause heart failure.

Allergic reactions to class Ia antidysrhythmic drugs are rare but serious. Signs of allergic reaction include fever, neutropenia, Raynaud's syndrome (ice-cold hands), muscle aches, skin rashes, and blood vessel inflammation in the fingers.

### What To Do *Before* Giving Class Ia Drugs
Be sure to review the general nursing responsibilities related to antidysrhythmic therapy (p. 273) in addition to these specific responsibilities before giving class Ia drugs.

Although these drugs are best absorbed on an empty stomach with a full glass of water, if the patient develops gastrointestinal problems, you may need to give them with food.

If the patient being started on disopyramide has been taking quinidine, wait 6 to 12 hours after the last dose of quinidine to begin disopyramide. If immediate-release procainamide was being used, wait 6 hours after the last dose of procainamide to begin disopyramide.

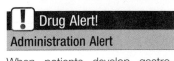

### Drug Alert!

**Administration Alert**

When patients develop gastrointestinal symptoms, give class Ia drugs with food to help reduce the symptoms.

**1+ Trace**
A barely perceptible pit (2 mm)

**2+ Mild**
A deeper pit, with fairly normal contours, that rebounds in 10 to 15 seconds (4 mm)

**3+ Moderate**
A deep pit; may last for 30 seconds to more than 1 minute (6 mm)

**4+ Severe**
An even deeper pit, with severe edema that may last as long as 2 to 5 minutes before rebounding (8 mm)

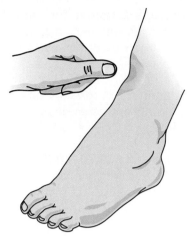

**FIGURE 15-6** Pitting edema scale.

## What To Do *After* Giving Class Ia Drugs

Be sure to review the general nursing responsibilities related to antidysrhythmic therapy (p. 273) in addition to these specific responsibilities after giving class Ia drugs.

Keep a record of intake and output because these drugs may affect urine retention. Also monitor daily weights. For the patient taking disopyramide, watch for signs of heart failure such as swelling (Figure 15-6), shortness of breath, and crackles when you listen to the lungs with a stethoscope.

Ask the patient about stomach upset or diarrhea. Remind the patient taking quinidine to call for help before getting up and to change positions slowly because of the potential for hypotension (low blood pressure).

If he or she is also taking digoxin, watch for signs of digoxin toxicity because these drugs may lead to increased blood level of digoxin by as much as 50%. Indications of early digoxin toxicity include loss of appetite, nausea, vomiting, diarrhea, or vision problems. Other signs include changes in heart rate or rhythm (irregular or slow), palpitations, or fainting.

## What To *Teach* Patients About Class Ia Drugs

Be sure to teach patients the general care needs and precautions related to antidysrhythmic therapy (p. 273) in addition to these specific points for class Ia drugs.

Remind patients to monitor urine output and to check and record daily weights. Instruct patients to report weight gain of more than 2 pounds a day to their prescriber. Demonstrate how to check ankles for swelling and tell patients to report any swelling or shortness of breath to their prescriber. Increased weight gain, ankle swelling, or shortness of breath are signs of worsening heart failure.

Remind patients that the blood level of these drugs must be maintained to achieve the expected actions. This is best achieved by taking the drug at the same time every day and exactly as prescribed.

Disopyramide can cause increased sun sensitivity (photosensitivity). Instruct patients to avoid exposure to sunlight and to wear protective sun block and clothing.

Teach patients taking quinidine to avoid high-alkaline ash foods (such as citrus fruits; milk; and vegetables such as broccoli, cabbage, and carrots). Although rare, these foods affect the excretion of quinidine and may lead to toxic levels of this drug.

Teach patients to avoid the herb St. John's wort while taking quinidine because it can cause a decreased blood level of this drug.

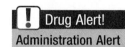

**Drug Alert!**
**Administration Alert**

Monitor patient weight and intake and output because class Ia antidysrhythmic drugs can cause urinary retention.

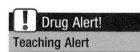

**Drug Alert!**
**Teaching Alert**

Teach patients taking quinidine to *avoid* large amounts of high-alkaline ash foods because they affect excretion of the drug and can lead to drug toxicity.

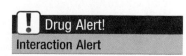

**Drug Alert!**
**Interaction Alert**

The herb St. John's wort can cause a decreased blood level of quinidine.

### Life Span Considerations for Class Ia Drugs

*Pediatric Considerations.*   Although some class Ia drugs (quinidine and procainamide) have been used for children with dysrhythmias, their safety has not been studied or established.

*Considerations for Pregnancy and Breastfeeding.*   Class Ia drugs are pregnancy category C and are generally not considered safe for use during pregnancy or breastfeeding.

*Considerations for Older Adults.*   Older adults may eliminate class Ia drugs more slowly and are at higher risk for side effects and toxicity. Emphasize to older adults the importance of monitoring urine output and checking and recording daily weights. Instruct patients to report a weight gain of more than 2 pounds a day to their prescriber. Also demonstrate how to check ankles for swelling, and tell patients to report any swelling or shortness of breath to their prescriber because these are signs of heart failure.

### CLASS IB DRUGS

### How Class Ib Drugs Work

Class Ib antidysrhythmic drugs are used to treat ventricular tachycardia and PVCs that cause patient symptoms. They are also used to prevent ventricular fibrillation, a life-threatening dysrhythmia.

Most of these drugs inhibit the ability of the ventricles to contract prematurely. This decreases the number of PVCs and episodes of ventricular tachycardia. In an emergency setting amiodarone is the first-line drug prescribed for ventricular tachycardia followed by lidocaine (Xylocaine).

Lidocaine is only given intravenously or by airway inhalation (ET tube—remember "NAVEL") because, when given by mouth, the liver destroys most of the drug, making it ineffective. Lidocaine may be given intramuscularly in an emergency situation if an IV line is not available.

Common doses of class Ib drugs are listed in the following table. Be sure to consult a drug handbook for information about a specific class Ib antidysrhythmic drug.

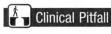 **Clinical Pitfall**

Lidocaine (Xylocaine) should *never* be used for patients with severe heart block dysrhythmias. Because the normal heart pacemaker is not functioning, this can lead to cardiac arrest.

### Dosages for Common Class Ib Antidysrhythmic Drugs

| Drug | Dosage |
|---|---|
| lidocaine ❶ (Betacaine🍁, Xylocaine) | *Adults:* 50-100 mg IV bolus (may repeat once) followed by continuous infusion of 1-4 mg/min<br>*Children:* 1 mg/kg IV bolus (up to 100 mg) followed by 20 mcg/kg/min continuous infusion (range 20-50 mcg/kg/min)<br>*Adults/Children >50 kg:* 300 mg IM (4.5 mg/kg); may repeat in 60-90 min |
| mexiletine (Mexitil) | *Adults:* 200-300 mg orally every 8 hr (maximum 1200 mg daily)<br>*Children:* 1.4-5 mg/kg orally every 8 hr |
| tocainide (Tonocard) | *Adults:* 400-600 mg orally every 8 hr (maximum 2400 mg daily) |
| phenytoin (Dilantin) | *Adults:* 50-100 mg IV every 10-15 min until dysrhythmia is gone (up to 15 mg/kg) |

❶ High-alert drug.

### Intended Responses
- Number of PVCs is decreased.
- Risk for ventricular tachycardia is decreased.
- Heart rhythm is regular and normal.
- Cardiac output is increased.

*Side Effects.*   Common side effects include confusion and drowsiness. IV lidocaine may cause stinging at the IV site. Common side effects of mexiletine and tocainide include dizziness, tremors, nervousness, nausea, vomiting, and heartburn. A patient may also have visual disturbances, vertigo, or ringing in the ears (tinnitus). Dizziness and falls are more likely with older adults.

Less common side effects include slurred speech, respiratory depression, psychosis, and seizures. Additional side effects for lidocaine include numbness and tingling, decreased blood pressure and heart rate, a sense of anxiousness, and rarely coma.

***Adverse Effects.*** A life-threatening adverse effect of lidocaine is cardiac arrest. Dysrhythmias may worsen with mexiletine and tocainide. A patient may develop pneumonitis, pulmonary fibrosis, or pulmonary edema while taking tocainide. Decreased white blood cell count with increased risk for infection (*neutropenia*) is an adverse effect of both tocainide and phenytoin. Two additional adverse effects of phenytoin are aplastic anemia and Stevens-Johnson syndrome, a skin disorder resulting from an allergic reaction to drugs, infections, or illness. See Chapter 13 for more information about this syndrome.

### What To Do *Before* Giving Class Ib Drugs

Be sure to review the general nursing responsibilities related to antidysrhythmic therapy (p. 273) in addition to these specific responsibilities before giving class Ib drugs.

Ask specifically about herbal preparation use. St. John's wort may decrease the blood level of lidocaine in the blood.

To monitor for drug side effects, ask patients if they have ever had any problems with tremors, dizziness, light-headedness, visual problems, or ringing in the ears.

For IV drugs be sure to check the IV site for patency and signs of infection. Ask the patient about stinging at the IV site.

### What To Do *After* Giving Class Ib Drugs

Be sure to review the general nursing responsibilities related to antidysrhythmic therapy (p. 273) in addition to these specific responsibilities after giving class Ib drugs.

Tell the patient to report any chest pain or shortness of breath immediately. Watch for side effects, including confusion, tremors, dizziness, light-headedness, visual difficulties, and tinnitus (ringing in the ears).

Ask about any shortness of breath and listen to the patient's lungs with a stethoscope for crackles, a sign of heart failure. Watch the IV site for patency and any signs of infection. Ask whether the patient feels any stinging or burning at the IV site. Also ask him or her about numbness, which can be caused by lidocaine and may mask the signs of IV infiltration.

With older adults, check for signs of confusion and other side effects because they are more sensitive to the effects of these drugs. Confusion may be a sign of lidocaine toxicity in these patients. Heart rate changes include decreased heart rate and asystole with hypotension and shock.

### What To *Teach* Patients About Class Ib Drugs

Be sure to teach patients the general care needs and precautions related to antidysrhythmic therapy (p. 273) in addition to these specific points for class Ib drugs.

Tell patients to report any of the following symptoms to the prescriber immediately:
- Irregular rhythms
- Heart rates less than 60 beats per minute or more than 100 beats per minute
- Chest pain
- Shortness of breath
- Wheezing

**⚠ Drug Alert!**

**Administration Alert**

Sudden changes in level of consciousness, confusion, and heart rate may be signs of lidocaine toxicity in older adults.

## Life Span Considerations for Class Ib Drugs

*Considerations for Pregnancy and Breastfeeding.* Class Ib drugs should not be used during pregnancy or breastfeeding because they cross the placenta and enter breast milk. All Class 1b drugs are pregnancy category C except phenytoin (Dilantin), which is class D.

*Considerations for Older Adults.* Older adults are more likely to experience dizziness and falls while taking these class Ib drugs. Instruct them to change positions slowly and to hold the handrails when using stairs to reduce the risk of falling. In addition, older adults are more likely to become confused. Instruct family members to assess them for confusion or any changes in level of cognition.

⊖-Learning Activity 15-6 ▶

## CLASS IC DRUGS

### How Class Ic Drugs Work

Class Ic antidysrhythmic drugs are used to treat life-threatening ventricular tachycardia or fibrillation and supraventricular tachycardia that does not go away when other drugs are used.

Flecainide (Tambocor) and propafenone (Rythmol) are oral drugs given to adults to slow the electrical impulse conduction of the heart. Common doses of class Ic drugs are listed in the following table. Be sure to consult a drug handbook for information about any specific class Ic antidysrhythmic drug.

### Dosages of Common Class Ic Antidysrhythmic Drugs

| Drug | Dosage |
| --- | --- |
| flecainide (Tambocor) | *Adults:* 100-200 mg orally every 12 hr |
| propafenone (Rythmol) | *Adults:* 150-300 mg orally every 8 hr; sustained-release (SR)—225-425 mg every 12 hr |

### Common Side Effects
**Class Ic Antidysrhythmic Drugs**

| Light-headedness | Altered taste, Constipation, Nausea/ Vomiting | Blurred vision |

### ⚠ Drug Alert!
**Administration Alert**

Side effects of class Ic antidysrhythmic drugs are more likely to occur as the dosage increases.

*Intended Responses*
- Episodes of ventricular and supraventricular dysrhythmias are decreased.
- Cardiac output is increased.
- Symptoms are decreased.
- Heart rhythm is normal and regular.

*Side Effects.* Common side effects of class Ic antidysrhythmic drugs include dizziness, conduction system abnormalities leading to heart blocks, altered sense of taste, constipation, nausea, and vomiting. Patients taking flecainide may also have blurred vision and difficulty focusing. Side effects are more likely to occur with higher doses of these drugs.

Less common side effects of these drugs include shaking, weakness, chest pain, bradycardia, hypotension, diarrhea, dry mouth, rash, and joint pain.

*Adverse Effects.* Adverse life-threatening effects of class Ic drugs include supraventricular and ventricular dysrhythmias such as heart blocks and ventricular tachycardia.

### What To Do *Before* Giving Class Ic Drugs

Be sure to review the general nursing responsibilities related to antidysrhythmic therapy (p. 273) in addition to these specific responsibilities before giving class Ic drugs.

Check whether the patient has a history of bronchospasm because patients with this condition should not take propafenone.

### What To Do *After* Giving Class Ic Drugs

Be sure to review the general nursing responsibilities related to antidysrhythmic therapy (p. 273) in addition to these specific responsibilities after giving class Ic drugs.

Ask the patient about dizziness, altered taste sensation, constipation, nausea, vomiting, and vision changes, which are indications of drug toxicity. Report any of these symptoms to the prescriber immediately.

### What To *Teach* Patients About Class Ic Drugs

Be sure to teach patients the general care needs and precautions related to antidysrhythmic therapy (p. 273) in addition to these specific points for class Ic drugs.

Tell patients to report any visual disturbances or other symptoms, including fever, sore throat, chills, unusual bleeding or bruising, chest pain, shortness of breath, excessive sweating (diaphoresis), or palpitations, to the prescriber at once. These symptoms may indicate toxicity or life-threatening dysrhythmias.

### Life Span Considerations for Class Ic Drugs

*Pediatric Considerations.* Class Ic antidysrhythmic drug use is not recommended for children since safety and effectiveness have not been established.

*Considerations for Pregnancy and Breastfeeding.* Class Ic drugs are pregnancy category C and should be used during pregnancy only when the potential benefit outweighs the risk to the fetus. It is not known whether class Ic drugs are excreted in breast milk. Because of possible serious adverse reactions in nursing infants, a different method of infant feeding should be considered.

*Considerations for Older Adults.* A slight increase in the incidence of dizziness has been seen in older adults. Instruct them to change positions slowly and to hold handrails when using stairs to reduce the risk for falls. Because of the possible increased risk of liver and kidney problems in older adults, class Ic drugs should be used with caution in this group. The effective dose may be lower in these patients.

## CLASS II: BETA BLOCKERS

### How Beta Blockers Work

Beta blockers are used to treat supraventricular tachycardia. These drugs block the effects of epinephrine (adrenaline) on the heart (see Figure 13-2). They decrease the heart rate and the force of heart contractions, which results in a decrease in blood pressure. Beta blockers are often used to slow the rate of ventricular contractions with supraventricular tachycardia, including rapid atrial fibrillation or flutter. As a result the heart does not work as hard and requires less oxygen. Cardioselective beta blockers work only on the cardiovascular system. Noncardioselective beta blockers have systemic effects. See Chapter 13 for more information on beta blockers.

When a beta blocker is prescribed for a patient with kidney damage, a lower dose of the drug is ordered, or the time between doses is increased. An older adult patient may also be started on a lower drug dose.

Common doses of class II beta blockers approved for use with dysrhythmias are listed in the following table. Be sure to consult a drug handbook for information about a specific class II beta blocker antidysrhythmic drug.

 **Memory Jogger**

Beta blockers may work on the cardiovascular system (cardioselective) or have systemic effects (noncardioselective).

**Dosages for Common Class II Beta Blocker Antidysrhythmic Drugs**

| Drug | Dosage |
|---|---|
| acebutolol ❶ (Monitan✤, Sectral) | *Adults:* 200 mg orally twice daily (usual therapeutic range 600-1200 mg daily) |
| esmolol ❶ (Brevibloc) | *Adults:* 500 mcg/kg/min IV as loading dose, followed by maintenance dose of 50 mcg/kg/min; may repeat loading and maintenance dose every 5-10 min until dysrhythmia is gone |

*Continued*

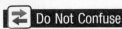
**Common Side Effects**

**Beta Blockers**

Erectile dysfunction | Dizziness | Drowsiness, Insomnia

Weakness, fatigue

### Dosages for Common Class II Beta Blocker Antidysrhythmic Drugs—cont'd

| Drug | Dosage |
|---|---|
| propranolol ❶ (Detensol✦, Inderal, NovoPranol✦) | *Adults:* 1-3 mg IV at a rate of 1 mg/min; 10-20 mg orally 3-4 times daily |
| sotalol ❶ (Betapace, Sotacar✦) | *Adults:* 80 mg orally every 12 hr; may increase (average dosage 150-320 mg/day) |

❶ High-alert drug.

### *Intended Responses*

* Heart rate is decreased.
* Force of heart contraction is decreased.
* Workload of heart is decreased.
* Blood pressure is lowered.
* There are fewer episodes of supraventricular tachycardia.

**Side Effects.** Fairly common side effects of beta blockers include decreased sexual ability, dizziness or light-headedness, drowsiness, trouble sleeping (insomnia), and fatigue or weakness. In patients with diabetes, beta blockers can mask the symptoms of low blood glucose levels (hypoglycemia), increasing the risk of severe hypoglycemia.

Less common side effects that must be reported to the prescriber include difficulty breathing or wheezing; cold hands or feet; mental depression; shortness of breath; slow heart rate (less than 60 beats per minute); and swelling in the ankles, feet, or lower legs.

Rare side effects include back or joint pain, chest pain, dark urine, dizziness or fainting when getting up (orthostatic hypotension), fever or sore throat, hallucinations, irregular heart rate, skin rash, unusual bleeding or bruising, and yellow eyes or skin. These drugs can affect the blood glucose level of a patient and may cause hypoglycemia or hyperglycemia.

Depression is another side effect that has been associated with taking beta blockers. A patient with a history of depression may notice that this gets worse while taking these drugs. Beta blockers may also cause depression for the first time.

**Adverse Effects.** Signs of drug overdose include very slow heart rate, severe dizziness or fainting, fast or irregular heart rate, difficulty breathing, bluish-colored fingernails and palms, and seizures. Report any of these signs and symptoms to the prescriber at once.

Adverse effects also include "passing out" (syncope) or falling when changing positions.

### What To Do *Before* Giving Beta Blockers

Be sure to review the general nursing responsibilities related to antidysrhythmic therapy (p. 273) in addition to these specific responsibilities before giving beta blockers.

For patients with diabetes, check their blood sugar regularly. Beta blockers can decrease or increase blood sugar levels. They can also mask signs of hypoglycemia such as rapid heart rate, making it difficult to recognize and treat.

### What To Do *After* Giving Beta Blockers

Be sure to review the general nursing responsibilities related to antidysrhythmic therapy (p. 273) in addition to these specific responsibilities after giving beta blockers.

Be sure to measure the patient's fluid intake and urine output. Check for any signs of heart failure, including weight gain, dependent swelling, and crackles in the lungs when listening with a stethoscope. Ask whether the patient is experiencing any dizziness, drowsiness, or light-headedness.

**❗ Drug Alert!**

**Administration Alert**

Be sure to regularly check the blood sugar of a patient with diabetes who is taking beta blockers.

## What To *Teach* Patients About Beta Blockers

Be sure to teach patients the general care needs and precautions related to antidysrhythmic therapy (p. 273) in addition to these specific points for beta blockers.

Tell patients that it's important not to miss any doses of the drug, especially if they are receiving only one dose per day. If a dose is missed, instruct the patient to take it as soon as possible; but, if it is within 4 hours of the next dose, teach them to skip the missed dose and get back on the regular dosing schedule. Remind the patient not to stop taking these drugs suddenly but rather to check with the prescriber. It may be necessary to gradually decrease the daily amount of drug before stopping it. Suddenly stopping the drug can increase the danger of a heart attack (myocardial infarction), tachycardia, and hypertensive crisis.

Ensure that patients have an adequate supply of the drug to "cover" weekends, holidays, and travel.

Instruct patients to notify their prescriber of a weight gain of 2 pounds per day or 5 pounds per week or any increase in shortness of breath. These are signs of heart failure.

Tell patients to always notify their prescribers or dentists of beta blocker use before any form of surgery or emergency treatment. They should also tell their prescriber about beta blocker use before any medical tests or allergy shots. These drugs can affect test results and cause a serious reaction to allergy shots because they narrow the air passages and may lead to a life-threatening asthma attack.

If a patient has or develops chest pain during activity, it should be reported to the prescriber immediately. Patients should discuss safe activity levels with their prescriber.

Beta blockers can cause increased sensitivity to sunlight and cold. Tell patients to stay out of direct sunlight, use a sun block skin protector, and wear protective clothing. Patients should dress warmly during cold weather because decreased blood flow to the hands increases the risk for conditions such as frostbite.

> **Drug Alert!**
> **Teaching Alert**
> Teach patients that stopping beta blockers suddenly increases the danger of a heart attack, tachycardia, or hypertensive crisis.

> **Drug Alert!**
> **Teaching Alert**
> Teach patients taking beta blockers to use sunscreens, wear protective clothes when exposed to sunlight, and dress warmly during cold weather.

### Life Span Considerations for Beta Blockers

*Pediatric Considerations.*   Beta blockers can worsen asthma. They should be used cautiously with infants and children because changing the heart rate is how blood pressure is controlled in pediatric patients.

*Considerations for Pregnancy and Breastfeeding.*   Beta blockers are pregnancy category B (acebutolol, sotalol) and C (propranolol, esmolol). Use of some beta blockers during pregnancy has been associated with low blood sugar, breathing problems, a lower heart rate, and low blood pressure in the newborn infant. Before taking any of these drugs, a woman should notify her prescriber if she is pregnant or thinking of becoming pregnant. All beta blockers pass into breast milk. Problems such as low blood sugar, slow heartbeat, low blood pressure, and trouble in breathing have been reported in nursing babies. These drugs should not be used during breastfeeding.

*Considerations for Older Adults.*   Side effects are more likely to occur in older adults because they are usually more sensitive to the effects of beta blockers. Beta blockers may also reduce tolerance to cold temperatures in these patients. In addition, older adults are more likely to be taking oral antidiabetic drugs for type 2 diabetes. Beta blockers can mask the symptoms of hypoglycemia. Teach older adults to check their blood glucose levels more often when taking a beta blocker, especially if 4 hours or more have passed since the last meal. Urge them to carry a quick source of glucose with them at all times (for example, hard sugar candy or glucose tablets) and to wear a medical alert bracelet indicating diabetes.

◄ ⊖-Learning Activity 15-7

## CLASS III: POTASSIUM CHANNEL BLOCKERS

### How Potassium Channel Blockers Work

Class III antidysrhythmic drugs are potassium channel blockers. They are used to treat ventricular tachycardia and ventricular fibrillation, convert atrial fibrillation or flutter to normal sinus rhythm, and maintain normal sinus rhythm (amiodarone). Amiodarone (Cordarone) given intravenously is used to slow conduction through the AV node with atrial fibrillation and control ventricular tachycardia and fibrillation. Oral amiodarone is used to prevent recurrence of ventricular tachycardia and fibrillation and to maintain a normal sinus rhythm after conversion from atrial fibrillation or flutter. Dofetilide (Tikosyn) is given orally to keep a patient in normal sinus rhythm after conversion from atrial fibrillation. Ibutilide (Corvert) is given intravenously and makes cardioversion of a patient with atrial fibrillation or flutter to normal sinus rhythm more likely to be successful.

**-Animation 15-1: ►**
**Amiodarone**

Common dosages of class III potassium channel blockers approved for use with dysrhythmias are listed in the following table. Be sure to consult a drug handbook for information about any specific class III potassium channel blocker antidysrhythmic drug.

### Dosages of Common Class III Potassium Channel Blockers

| Drug | Dosage |
|------|--------|
| amiodarone ❶ (Cordarone) | *Adults:*<br>IV loading dosage: 150 mg over 10 min, then 360 mg over the next 6 hr, then 540 mg over the next 18 hr<br>IV maintenance dosage: 720 mg over 24 hr<br>Oral loading dosage: 800-1600 mg daily for 1-3 wk<br>Oral maintenance dosage: 200-400 mg daily |
| dofetilide ❶ (Tikosyn) | *Adults:* 125-500 mcg orally twice daily |
| ibutilide ❶ (Corvert) | *Adults:* IV weight based:<br>More than 60 kg: 1 mg IV over 10 min<br>Less than 60 kg: 0.01 mg/kg IV over 10 min<br>Dose can be repeated once after 10 min if necessary |
| sotalol ❶ (Betapace, Sotacar🍁)* | *Adults:* 80 mg orally every 12 hr; may increase (average dosage 150-320 mg daily) |

❶ High-alert drug.
*Sotalol is a beta blocker but is considered a class III antidysrhythmic drug.

### Common Side Effects

**Class III Potassium Channel Blockers**

Dizziness    Fatigue    Hypotension

Nausea, Anorexia

### Intended Responses
- Blood vessel constriction is decreased.
- Blood flow to coronary arteries and heart muscle is increased.
- Electrical impulse conduction in all heart muscle tissues is slowed.
- Heart rate is decreased.
- Strength of contractions in the left ventricle is decreased.
- Success of cardioversion to normal sinus rhythm (ibutilide) is increased.
- Normal heart rhythm and rate (oral amiodarone and dofetilide) are maintained.

**Side Effects.**   Common side effects of class III potassium channel blockers include dizziness, fatigue, malaise, bradycardia, hypotension, loss of appetite, constipation, nausea, vomiting, unsteady gait (ataxia), involuntary movement, numbness and tingling, poor coordination, and tremor. Side effects unique to amiodarone include photosensitivity, hypothyroidism, peripheral neuropathy, and microdeposits on the corneas

Less common side effects include headache, difficulty sleeping, abnormal sense of smell and taste, dry eyes, increased light sensitivity, abdominal pain, and decreased sex drive. Hyperthyroidism may occur with amiodarone. Thyroid problems are more likely to occur during the first few weeks of treatment. A patient who is taking amiodarone for a long period may develop blue discoloration of the face, neck, and arms.

*Adverse Effects.* Several potential life-threatening effects are associated with amiodarone, including adult respiratory distress syndrome (ARDS), pulmonary fibrosis, heart failure, worsening of heart dysrhythmias, decreased liver function, and toxic epidermal necrolysis. Toxic epidermal necrolysis is a rare but life-threatening skin disorder that is caused by an allergic reaction.

With dofetilide, patients also may experience chest pain or life-threatening ventricular dysrhythmias. It may also cause heart dysrhythmias.

### What To Do *Before* Giving Potassium Channel Blockers

Be sure to review the general nursing responsibilities related to antidysrhythmic therapy (p. 273) in addition to these specific responsibilities before giving potassium channel blockers.

If the patient is to receive an IV drug, check the IV site for patency and signs of infection.

### What To Do *After* Giving Potassium Channel Blockers

Be sure to review the general nursing responsibilities related to antidysrhythmic therapy (p. 273) in addition to these specific responsibilities after giving potassium channel blockers.

For IV drugs, continue to watch the IV line for patency and signs of infection.

Watch for signs of pulmonary problems such as ARDS (including crackles when you listen to the lungs with a stethoscope), difficulty breathing, fatigue, cough, and fever.

Look for signs of thyroid problems, including weight gain; lethargy; and swelling in the hands, feet, or around the eyes. Report any of these signs to the prescriber immediately.

Make sure that any follow-up laboratory tests (for example, liver and thyroid function tests) and ECGs are completed.

### What To *Teach* Patients About Potassium Channel Blockers

Be sure to teach patients the general care needs and precautions related to antidysrhythmic therapy (p. 273) in addition to these specific points for potassium channel blockers.

Tell patients taking amiodarone that they may need to wear dark glasses when going outside because of the potential for increased sensitivity to light. Also teach them to wear protective clothing and a sunscreen barrier for increased sun sensitivity (photosensitivity) while taking these drugs.

Remind patients that side effects may not appear for several days or weeks. Explain that long-term use of amiodarone may cause the development of a bluish discoloration of the face, neck, and arms. This side effect is reversible and will disappear over several months.

Tell patients that they will need eye examinations every 6 to 12 months to determine if corneal microdeposits or other eye changes have occurred. These changes would not necessarily be apparent to the patient during the early stages.

Be sure to advise male patients to tell the prescriber immediately about any pain or swelling in the scrotum. The prescriber may need to decrease the dosage of amiodarone.

### Life Span Considerations for Potassium Channel Blockers

*Considerations for Pregnancy and Breastfeeding.* Potassium channel blockers are pregnancy category C (dofetilide, ibutilide) and D (amiodarone). Pregnant women should not take amiodarone because it can harm the fetus. Women who are breastfeeding should not use these drugs; if the treatment is necessary, breastfeeding should be discontinued.

*Pediatric and Older Adult Considerations.* Potassium channel blockers should be used cautiously in pediatric patients and older adults.

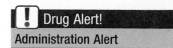

**Drug Alert!**

**Administration Alert**

Be sure to monitor the respiratory status of patients taking amiodarone.

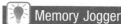

**Memory Jogger**

Signs of IV patency include blood return and easy flushing. Signs of infection include swelling, redness, warmth, fever, and pain.

**Drug Alert!**

**Administration Alert**

Monitor for signs of thyroid problems such as changes in heart rate, which are more likely to occur during the first few weeks of treatment with amiodarone (Cordarone).

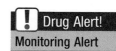

**Drug Alert!**

**Monitoring Alert**

Male patients may experience pain or swelling in the scrotum while taking amiodarone (Cordarone), which should be reported to the prescriber immediately.

◄ ℮-Learning Activity 15-8

## CLASS IV: CALCIUM CHANNEL BLOCKERS

### How Calcium Channel Blockers Work

Class IV antidysrhythmic drugs include the calcium channel blockers diltiazem (Cardizem) and verapamil (Calan, Isoptin). They are used primarily for the treatment of supraventricular tachycardia. As antidysrhythmic drugs, they act by slowing conduction through the SA and AV nodes of the conduction system of the heart, leading to a decreased heart rate. When these drugs are prescribed for older adults or patients with hepatic (liver) or renal (kidney) impairment, lower initial dosages are used.

Common dosages of class IV calcium channel blockers approved for use with dysrhythmias are listed in the following table. Be sure to consult a drug handbook for information about any specific class IV calcium channel blocker antidysrhythmic drug. For more generalized information on calcium channel blockers, see Chapter 13.

### Dosages of Common Class IV Calcium Channel Blockers

| Drug | Dosage |
|---|---|
| diltiazem (Apo-Diltiaz🍁, Cardizem, Syn-Diltiazem🍁) 🔝 | *Adults:*<br>Oral: 30-120 mg 3-4 times daily; slow-release capsules 60-120 mg twice daily; extended-release capsules 240-360 mg once daily<br>IV: 0.25 mg/kg over 2 min; second dose 0.35 mg/kg may be given after 15 min if needed; then follow with continuous infusion 5-15 mg/hr for up to 24 hr |
| verapamil (Calan, Isoptin, Novo-Verapamil🍁, Nu-Verap🍁) 🔝 | *Adults:*<br>Oral: 40-120 mg every 6-8 hr<br>IV: 5-10 mg; may give 10 mg after 30 min if needed<br>*Children less than 1 year:* 0.1-0.2 mg/kg IV over 2 min<br>*Children 1 to 15 years:* 0.1-0.3 mg/kg IV (maximum 5 mg) over 2 min; may repeat in 30 min if needed |

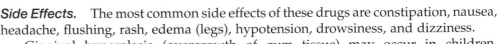 Top 100 drugs prescribed.

### Intended Responses
- Heart contraction is decreased.
- Artery dilation (widening) is increased.
- Heart workload is decreased.
- Blood pressure is lowered.
- Blood flow and oxygen to the heart is increased.
- There are fewer episodes of supraventricular tachycardia.

**Side Effects.** The most common side effects of these drugs are constipation, nausea, headache, flushing, rash, edema (legs), hypotension, drowsiness, and dizziness.

Gingival hyperplasia (overgrowth of gum tissue) may occur in children. Gynecomastia (development of the enlarged male breasts) may also occur with rare unusual secretion of milk when taking verapamil.

**Adverse Effects.** Rare but serious adverse effects include difficulty breathing; irregular, rapid, or pounding heart rhythm; slow heart rate (less than 50 beats per minute); bleeding; chest pain; and vision problems.

Heart failure symptoms may worsen with verapamil and diltiazem because of their increased ability to reduce the strength and rate of heart contractions.

Stevens-Johnson syndrome (erythema multiforme) is a skin disorder resulting from an allergic reaction to drugs, infections, or illness. It causes damage to blood vessels of the skin. Symptoms include many different types of skin lesions, itching, fever, joint aches, and generally feeling ill. This syndrome has the potential to be fatal.

---

### Common Side Effects
### Calcium Channel Blockers

Hypotension | Constipation, Nausea | Headache

Dizziness

---

### ⚠ Drug Alert!
### Administration Alert

Always check the patient for skin lesions, itching, fever, and achy joints. Report these signs of Stevens-Johnson syndrome immediately to the prescriber.

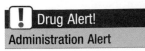

## What To Do *Before* Giving Calcium Channel Blockers

Be sure to review the general nursing responsibilities related to antidysrhythmic therapy (p. 273) in addition to these specific responsibilities before giving calcium channel blockers.

Check whether the patient has any health problems that may be affected by these drugs such as heart failure, blood vessel disease, and liver or kidney disease.

## What To Do *After* Giving Calcium Channel Blockers

Be sure to review the general nursing responsibilities related to antidysrhythmic therapy (p. 273) in addition to these specific responsibilities after giving calcium channel blockers.

Check for any signs of heart failure, including weight gain, swelling, and crackles in the lungs, when you listen with a stethoscope. Report any chest pain immediately to the prescriber.

## What To *Teach* Patients About Calcium Channel Blockers

Be sure to teach patients the general care needs and precautions related to antidysrhythmic therapy (p. 273).

## Life Span Considerations for Calcium Channel Blockers

*Considerations for Pregnancy and Breastfeeding.*   Calcium channel blockers are pregnancy category C and should not be used during pregnancy or breastfeeding. Calcium channel blockers may cause birth defects, longer-than-usual pregnancy, poor bone development in children, and stillbirth. Diltiazem and verapamil pass into breast milk.

*Considerations for Older Adults.*   Older adults may be especially sensitive to the effects of calcium channel blocking agents. This may increase the chance of side effects during treatment. A lower starting dose may be required.

◄ ⊜-Learning Activity 15-9

# UNCLASSIFIED ANTIDYSRHYTHMIC DRUGS

## ADENOSINE

### How Adenosine Works

Adenosine (Adenocard) is used to treat supraventricular tachycardia. Its action is similar to that of calcium channel blockers. It slows electrical impulse conduction through the AV node to help restore a patient to a normal sinus rhythm. Adenosine is an IV drug given as a rapid IV bolus injection. When given slowly, adenosine is eliminated from the body before it can reach the heart and act to slow the rhythm. After giving adenosine there will be a very brief period of asystole; then the heart will resume a normal rhythm. Be sure to consult a drug handbook for specific information about adenosine.

### Dosages for Adenosine

| Drug | Dosage |
| --- | --- |
| adenosine (Adenocard) | *Adults/Children over 50 kg:* 6 mg IV given rapidly over 1-2 seconds; flush with normal saline and elevate arm after giving drug IV push; second and third doses of 12 mg can be given if necessary<br>*Children under 50 kg:* 0.05-0.1 mg/kg IV over 1-2 seconds; may repeat in 1-2 min if necessary |

### Intended Responses

- Impulse conduction through the AV node is slower.
- Heart rate is decreased.

---

**[!] Drug Alert!**
**Monitoring Alert**

Monitor patients who have been prescribed calcium channel blockers for chest pain, and report any chest pain to the prescriber.

---

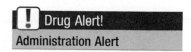

**[!] Drug Alert!**
**Administration Alert**

Always give IV adenosine (Adenocard) *rapidly over 1 to 2 seconds.*

- Supraventricular tachycardia is eliminated.
- Heart rhythm is normal and regular.

*Side Effects.*    Common side effects of adenosine include facial flushing, shortness of breath, and transient dysrhythmias such as atrial fibrillation and atrial flutter.

Less common side effects include apprehension, dizziness, headache, head pressure, light-headedness, blurred vision, throat tightness, chest pressure or pain, hyperventilation, hypotension, palpitations, metallic taste, nausea, burning sensation, sweating, neck and back pain, numbness and tingling, and a heavy feeling in the arms or groin.

*Adverse Effects.*    Allergic reactions are rare. Adenosine should not be used with heart block unless the patient has an artificial pacemaker in place because it may lead to asystole.

Fatal cardiac arrest, sustained ventricular tachycardia, and nonfatal myocardial infarction have been reported after giving injections of adenosine. Patients with unstable angina may be at greater risk. Emergency equipment must be available before this drug is given.

### What To Do *Before* Giving Adenosine

Be sure to review the general nursing responsibilities related to antidysrhythmic therapy (p. 273) in addition to these specific responsibilities before giving adenosine.

Tell the patient that there will be a brief period of asystole that may feel like a "mule kick" to the chest before the heart goes back into a normal rhythm.

Bring emergency equipment to the bedside before giving this drug. Check the IV line for patency and any signs of infection. Draw the bolus up into a syringe and remember that it must be given by IV push *rapidly* over 1 to 2 seconds.

### What To Do *After* Giving Adenosine

Be sure to review the general nursing responsibilities related to antidysrhythmic therapy (p. 273) in addition to these specific responsibilities after giving adenosine.

Check blood pressure every 15 to 30 minutes immediately after adenosine has been given. Be sure to check the heart monitor for changes in heart rhythm.

### What To *Teach* Patients About Adenosine

Be sure to teach patients the general care needs and precautions related to antidysrhythmic therapy (p. 273) in addition to these specific points for adenosine.

Explain the purpose of giving adenosine. Warn patients that facial flushing may occur with this drug. Tell patients to call for help when getting up and to change positions slowly because doses of 12 mg or more can cause hypotension.

Instruct patients to report any facial flushing, shortness of breath, or dizziness immediately.

### Life Span Considerations for Adenosine

*Considerations for Pregnancy and Breastfeeding.*    Adenosine is pregnancy category C and should not be used during pregnancy because its safe use has not been studied or established.

*Considerations for Older Adults.*    Older adults may be more sensitive to the effects of adenosine; however, these effects have not been studied.

### MAGNESIUM SULFATE

### How Magnesium Sulfate Works

Magnesium sulfate is used intravenously to prevent the ventricular dysrhythmia *torsades de pointes* from returning after a patient has been defibrillated (given an

---

**Common Side Effects**

**Adenosine**

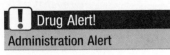

| Facial flushing | Shortness of breath | Dysrhythmias |

---

**(!) Drug Alert!**

**Administration Alert**

Always have emergency equipment, including the crash cart and defibrillator, at the bedside before giving an IV dose of adenosine.

electric shock) to return into a normal rhythm. An IV magnesium sulfate bolus can sometimes eliminate torsades de pointes in a patient who is not symptomatic. A normal level of magnesium in the blood keeps the heart muscle from becoming overexcited and reduces the risk for this life-threatening dysrhythmia. The common dose of magnesium sulfate used is listed in the following table. For more generalized information about magnesium sulfate, see Chapter 14. Be sure to consult a drug handbook for specific information about magnesium sulfate.

### Dosages for Magnesium Sulfate

| Drug | Dosage |
|---|---|
| magnesium sulfate ❶ | *Adults:* 1-2 g IV diluted with 10 mL of D₅W solution; give over 30 seconds (patient should be on cardiac monitor when receiving this drug)<br>*Children:* Dosage not established |

❶ High-alert drug.

### Intended Responses
- Heart muscle excitability is decreased.
- There are no further episodes of torsades de pointes.

**Side Effects.**   The only common side effect of IV magnesium sulfate is diarrhea. Less common side effects include drowsiness, decreased respiratory rate, bradycardia, hypotension, flushing, and sweating.

**Adverse Effects.**   Adverse effects are rare and include complete heart block and respiratory arrest. With higher doses, muscle weakness and a loss of deep tendon reflexes can occur.

### What To Do *Before* Giving Magnesium Sulfate
Be sure to review the general nursing responsibilities related to antidysrhythmic therapy (p. 273) in addition to these specific responsibilities before giving magnesium sulfate.

Check the IV site for patency and signs of infection. Check the patient's current blood magnesium level.

### What To Do *After* Giving Magnesium Sulfate
Be sure to review the general nursing responsibilities related to antidysrhythmic therapy (p. 273) in addition to these specific responsibilities after giving magnesium sulfate.

Ask the monitor watcher or charge nurse whether the heart rhythm has changed. Make sure that any follow-up magnesium levels are drawn and sent to the laboratory. Monitor blood levels of magnesium and monitor patients for signs and symptoms of excessive blood levels of magnesium (hypermagnesemia). The most common problems that occur when magnesium levels exceed 4 mg/dL are seen in the cardiac, central nervous, and neuromuscular systems.

Cardiac changes include bradycardia, peripheral vasodilation, and hypotension. ECG changes show a prolonged PR interval and a widened QRS complex. Bradycardia can be severe and cardiac arrest is possible. Hypotension is also severe with a diastolic pressure lower than normal. *Patients with severe hypermagnesemia are in grave danger of cardiac arrest.*

Central nervous system changes result from depressed nerve impulse transmission. Patients may become drowsy or lethargic. Coma may occur if the imbalance is prolonged or severe.

Deep tendon reflexes are reduced or absent. Skeletal muscle contractions become progressively weaker and finally stop. When the respiratory muscles are weak, respiratory insufficiency can lead to respiratory failure and death.

**Common Side Effects**

**Magnesium Sulfate**

Diarrhea

### What To *Teach* Patients About Magnesium Sulfate

Be sure to teach patients the general care needs and precautions related to antidysrhythmic therapy (p. 273) in addition to these specific points for magnesium sulfate.

Explain the purpose of giving IV magnesium sulfate. Teach the patient about food sources of magnesium because low magnesium levels are the main cause of torsades de pointes. See Box 14-4 for dietary sources of magnesium.

### Life Span Considerations for Magnesium Sulfate

*Considerations for Pregnancy and Breastfeeding.* Magnesium sulfate is pregnancy category A and is safe to give during pregnancy. It is used during labor to lower the risk of seizures for patients with eclampsia. The infant may have decreased reflexes for the first 24 hours after birth when magnesium is used during labor.

### OTHER DRUGS USED TO TREAT DYSRHYTHMIAS

Anticoagulants such as heparin and warfarin (Coumadin) are prescribed for rhythms when the patient is at increased risk for blood clots such as atrial fibrillation. For more information on these drugs, see Chapter 17.

## Get Ready for Practice!

### Key Points

- The normal pacemaker of the heart is the SA node, which initiates 60 to 100 electrical impulses to the heart.
- Dysrhythmias are abnormal heart rhythms.
- Some patients with symptoms do *not* have serious dysrhythmias, whereas others with *no* symptoms may have life-threatening dysrhythmias.
- Ventricular fibrillation causes death within minutes if not treated.
- A watch or clock with a second hand is needed to check heart rate.
- Always check a patient's blood pressure, heart rate, and heart rhythm before and after giving an antidysrhythmic drug.
- Always check IV sites for patency and signs of infection before and after a patient is given an IV antidysrhythmic drug.
- Teach patients taking antidysrhythmic drugs to check and record their heart rate and rhythm every day and to report any abnormal findings to their prescriber.
- Check patients for signs of heart failure after receiving antidysrhythmic drugs. Check daily weights, listen for crackles in the lungs, and look for swelling.
- An older adult patient may need decreased doses of antidysrhythmic drugs because of increased sensitivity and age-related body changes.
- Adenosine must always be given by IV push rapidly over 1 to 2 seconds to be effective.
- Always have emergency equipment brought to the bedside before giving IV adenosine because of the risk of dysrhythmias and cardiac arrest.
- Magnesium sulfate is given to prevent the ventricular dysrhythmia torsades de pointes from returning after the patient's rhythm has been returned to a normal sinus rhythm.
- Anticoagulants are prescribed for abnormal heart rhythms with increased risk for clot formation such as atrial fibrillation or atrial flutter.

### Additional Learning Resources

evolve Go to your Evolve website (http://evolve.elsevier.com/Workman/pharmacology/) for the following FREE learning resources:

- eLearning Activities
- Animations
- Video Clips
- Interactive Review Questions
- Audio Key Points
- Audio Glossary
- Audio Glossary—Spanish-English
- Drug Dosage Calculators
- Patient Teaching Handouts

SG Go to your Study Guide for additional learning activities to help you master this chapter content.

### Review Questions

1. A patient with an abnormally slow heart rate is dizzy, light-headed, and short of breath. How will administration of IV atropine treat his bradydysrhythmia?
   - A. Atropine stimulates the heart to beat faster.
   - B. Atropine blocks the actions of the vagus nerve on the heart.
   - C. Atropine increases the strength of heart contractions.
   - D. Atropine decreases the demand for blood supply to the heart.

2. What is the maximum dose of atropine (Atropine Sulfate) for an adult patient?

   A. 1 mg
   B. 2 mg
   C. 3 mg
   D. 4 mg

3. What action must you take for a patient who is prescribed digoxin (Lanoxin) 0.25 mg once daily and whose heart rate is 54 beats per minute?

   A. Give the drug as prescribed.
   B. Give half the prescribed dosage.
   C. Hold the dose and notify the prescriber.
   D. Document the heart rate.

4. A patient asks you why digoxin (Lanoxin) has been prescribed for atrial fibrillation. What is your best response?

   A. "It will increase your heart rate."
   B. "It will slow your heart rate."
   C. "It will increase your urinary output."
   D. "It will increase the force of contraction in your heart."

5. What priority action do you take before giving a dose of digoxin to an infant or child?

   A. Monitor for signs of low blood potassium.
   B. Count the apical heart rate for 2 full minutes.
   C. Place the infant or child on a heart monitor.
   D. Check the dosage with another nurse or pharmacist.

6. Which symptom is developed by as many as 50% of patients taking a class Ia antidysrhythmic drug?

   A. Gastrointestinal upset
   B. Hypotension
   C. Dizziness
   D. Confusion

7. What laboratory value must you be sure to check before giving a beta blocker to a patient with diabetes?

   A. Serum potassium level
   B. Serum sodium level
   C. Serum magnesium level
   D. Serum glucose level

8. What important point do you include in your teaching plan for the female patient going home with the class III antidysrhythmic drug amiodarone (Cordarone)?

   A. "Women need lower doses initially when taking this drug than men."
   B. "Be sure to use a sunscreen before you spend time outside."
   C. "The blue discoloration on your face will not go away."
   D. "This drug is safe for use during pregnancy."

9. Which side effect after giving the class Ib antidysrhythmic drug lidocaine (Xylocaine) indicates drug toxicity in an older adult?

   A. Hypotension
   B. Confusion
   C. Tremors
   D. Nausea

10. A patient is to receive propafenone (Rythmol) 450 mg per day in 3 divided doses. How many milligrams will you give per dose? _____ mg

11. A child who weighs 21 kg is to be given an IV dose of adenosine (Adenocard) 0.1 mg/kg. How many milligrams will you give? _____ mg

12. The prescriber has ordered amiodarone (Cordarone) 800 mg per day in 2 divided doses. The pharmacy sent amiodarone 200 mg per tablet. How many tablets will you give per dose? _____ tablet(s)

## Critical Thinking Activities

Mr. Jonas is 79 years old and has been diagnosed with new-onset atrial fibrillation. He has an irregular heart rate that ranges between 110 and 150 beats per minute. On admission to the cardiac step-down unit, his symptoms include dizziness, feeling weak, and fainting. The prescriber orders sotalol (Betapace) 80 mg orally every 12 hours.

1. When you assess Mr. Jonas's heart rate and rhythm, what would you expect to find?

2. What is the expected action of sotalol in treating this dysrhythmia?

3. After a dose of sotalol, Mr. Jonas's heart rate is 56 beats per minute and irregular. What is your next action?

4. Mr. Jonas wants to get up and use the bathroom. What would you tell him to do?

# Drugs for High Blood Lipids

evolve

http://evolve.elsevier.com/Workman/pharmacology/

## Objectives

*After studying this chapter you should be able to:*

1. Explain how antihyperlipidemic drugs work to lower blood lipid levels.
2. List the common names, actions, usual adult dosages, possible side effects, and adverse effects of statins, bile acid sequestrants, cholesterol absorption inhibitors, and fibrate drugs.
3. Describe what to do before and after giving drugs to lower blood lipid levels.
4. Explain what to teach patients taking drugs to lower blood lipid levels, including what to do, what not to do, and when to call the prescriber.
5. Describe life span considerations for drugs to lower blood lipid levels.
6. List the common names, actions, usual adult dosages, possible side effects, and adverse effects of nicotinic acid.
7. Describe what to do before and after giving nicotinic acid.
8. Explain what to teach patients taking nicotinic acid, including what to do, what not to do, and when to call the prescriber.
9. Describe life span considerations for nicotinic acid.

## Key Terms

**antihyperlipidemics** (ăn-tī-hī-pŭr-lĭp-ĭ-DĒ-mĭks) (p. 294) Drugs that work against high levels of lipids (fats) in the blood.

**bile acid sequestrants** (BĪ-ŭl ĂS-ĭd sĕ-KWĔS-trĕnts) (p. 300) Cholesterol-lowering drugs that bind with cholesterol-containing bile acids in the intestines and remove them via bowel movements.

**cholesterol** (kō-LĔS-tŭr-ŏl) (p. 295) A fatty, waxy material that our bodies need to function. It is present in cell membranes everywhere in the body.

**cholesterol absorption inhibitors** (kō-LĔS-tŭr-ŏl ăb-SŌRP-shŭn ĭn-HĬB-ĭ-tŭrz) (p. 302) Cholesterol-lowering drugs that prevent the uptake of cholesterol from the small intestine into the circulatory system.

**familial hyperlipidemia** (fă-MĬL-ē-ŭl hī-pŭr-lĭp-ĭ-DĒ-mē-ă) (p. 295) High blood fat levels that are related to genetic or inherited factors.

**fibrates** (FĪ-brāts) (p. 303) Lipid-lowering drugs that are used primarily to lower triglycerides and, to a lesser extent, LDL ("bad") cholesterol.

**high-density lipoprotein (HDL)** (HĪ DĔN-sĭ-tē lī-pō-PRŌ-tēn) (p. 297) The "good" cholesterol that exists in the body.

**hyperlipidemia** (hī-pŭr-lĭp-ĭ-DĒ-mē-ă) (p. 295) High levels of blood fats (plasma lipoproteins).

**hypertriglyceridemia** (hī-pŭr-trī-GLĬS-ŭr-ĭ-DĒ-mē-ă) (p. 295) High levels of triglycerides in the blood.

**low-density lipoprotein (LDL)** (LŌ DĔN-sĭ-tē lī-pō-PRŌ-tēn) (p. 295) The "bad" cholesterol that exists in the body.

**nicotinic acid** (nĭ-kō-TĬN-ĭk ĂS-ĭd) (p. 305) Special type of vitamin B that helps to decrease blood cholesterol levels.

**rhabdomyolysis** (răb-dō-mī-Ŏ-lĭ-sĭs) (p. 299) A condition in which skeletal muscle cells break down, releasing myoglobin. Risks with this condition include muscle breakdown and kidney failure because myoglobin is toxic to the kidneys.

**statins** (STĂ-tĭnz) (p. 298) A class of drugs used to lower LDL ("bad") cholesterol and triglycerides by inhibiting their production by the body.

**triglyceride** (trī-GLĬS-ŭr-īd) (p. 295) The chemical form of most fats in foods and the human body.

🌐-Learning Activity 16-1 ►

🌐-Animation 16-1: ►
Cholesterol-Lowering Medications

## OVERVIEW

Lipid-lowering drugs are those that decrease the amount of lipids (fats) or cholesterol in a person's blood. These drugs are also called antihyperlipidemics because they work against high levels of lipids in the blood. Lipid-lowering drugs are used with diet changes (for example, decreased intake of fat) to reduce the amount of certain fats and cholesterol in the blood. Some lipid-lowering drugs work to decrease the production of cholesterol in the body and increase the ability of the liver to remove the "bad" cholesterol (**low-density lipoprotein** or **LDL**). Others reduce the amount of fat from food that the body absorbs. Still others bind with cholesterol-containing bile acids in the intestines and promote cholesterol loss in the stool.

## REVIEW OF RELATED PHYSIOLOGY AND PATHOPHYSIOLOGY

**Cholesterol** is a fatty, waxy material that the body needs to function. It is present in cell membranes everywhere in the body. It is used to produce hormones, vitamin D, and bile acids that help digest fat. A person needs some cholesterol for important body functions. Cholesterol is produced by the liver, and it is in the foods that you eat (Figure 16-1). However, your body needs only a small amount of cholesterol; too much in the bloodstream contributes to the development of narrowed arteries such as atherosclerosis and coronary artery disease. The chemical form of most fats in foods and the human body is **triglycerides.** Both cholesterol and triglycerides are present in the blood, making up the plasma lipids.

A high level of blood fats (plasma lipoproteins) is called **hyperlipidemia.** Table 16-1 lists the normal values for a patient's lipid profile. A high level of triglycerides in the blood is called **hypertriglyceridemia.** Chronic hyperlipidemia can lead to many health problems, including:

- Atherosclerosis.
- Coronary artery disease (angina, heart attack).
- Hypertension.
- Pancreatitis.
- Peripheral vascular disease, which leads to organ damage or impairment.
- Stroke.
- Xanthomas (skin atheromas—abnormal fat deposits).

## CORONARY ARTERY DISEASE

The coronary arteries supply blood, oxygen, and nutrients to the heart muscle (myocardium). Atherosclerosis, a major contributor to development of coronary artery disease, begins by forming a fatty streak on an arterial wall, leading to fat buildup (plaques). Fat buildup in the walls of coronary arteries can result in partial or complete blockage of blood flow to the heart muscle (Figure 16-2). The main lipids involved are cholesterol and triglycerides. Partial blockage in the coronary arteries can result in chest pain (*angina*); complete blockage can result in heart attack (*myocardial infarction*). Table 16-2 summarizes lipid levels related to the risk of developing coronary artery disease (CAD).

## FAMILIAL HYPERLIPIDEMIA

Some people develop high blood fat levels that are related to genetic or inherited factors. This is called **familial hyperlipidemia** or sometimes *familial hypercholesterolemia.* The liver makes too much cholesterol and other fats, which lead to increased

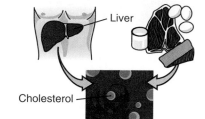

**FIGURE 16-1** Cholesterol is produced by the liver, but it is also consumed in meat and dairy products.

| Table **16-1**   Lipid Profile Normal Values | |
|---|---|
| **TYPE OF LIPID** | **NORMAL VALUE** |
| Total cholesterol | <200 mg/dL |
| Low-density lipoprotein (LDL) | 60-180 mg/dL |
| Very low–density lipoprotein (VLDL) | 25%-50% |
| High-density lipoprotein (HDL) | Male: >45 mg/dL<br>Female: >55 mg/dL |
| Triglycerides | Male: 40-160 mg/dL<br>Female: 35-135 mg/dL |

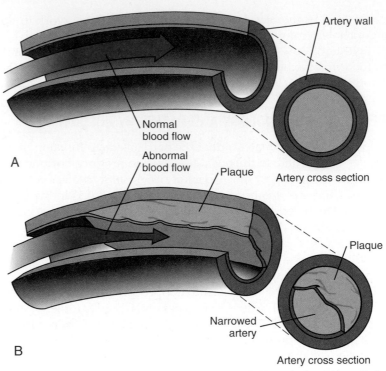

**FIGURE 16-2** Cholesterol can form plaques that narrow arteries. **A,** Normal, clean artery. **B,** Artery with plaque formation.

| Table 16-2 | Lipid Values and Risk for Coronary Artery Disease | |
| --- | --- | --- |
| **LIPID** | **VALUE (mg/dL)** | **RISK FOR CORONARY ARTERY DISEASE** |
| Total cholesterol | <200 | Low |
| | 200-239 | Borderline high |
| | >239 | High |
| HDL ("good" cholesterol) | >35 | Low |
| | <35 | High |
| LDL ("bad" cholesterol) | <129 | Low |
| | 130-159 | Borderline high |
| | >159 | High |
| Triglycerides | <200 | Low |
| | 201-399 | Borderline high |
| | 400-1000 | High |
| | >1000 | Very high |

*HDL,* High-density lipoprotein; *LDL,* low-density lipoprotein.

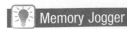 **Memory Jogger**

High blood lipid levels may result from genetic factors (familial hyperlipidemia).

⊜-Learning Activity 16-2 ▶

levels of fats in the blood and the development of atherosclerosis. The reason for this condition is not completely clear; however, it tends to occur in families. For people who have a genetic factor leading to hyperlipidemia, simply reducing fatty foods does not help lower blood lipid levels. Antilipidemic drugs are prescribed to lower them.

## GENERAL ISSUES FOR ANTIHYPERLIPIDEMIC THERAPY

Lipid-lowering drugs are used most often to treat high blood lipid levels that fail to decrease with lifestyle changes such as reduced-fat diets, increased exercise, smoking cessation, and weight loss. When such changes do not result in lower blood lipid levels, the patient remains at risk for development of heart disease, especially in the

**Table 16-3** Normal Liver Function Values

| LIVER FUNCTION TEST | NORMAL VALUE |
|---|---|
| Aspartate aminotransferase (AST) | 10-34 international units/L |
| Alanine aminotransferase (ALT) | 5-35 international units/L |
| Alkaline phosphatase (ALP) | 20-140 international units/L |
| Gamma-glutamyltransferase (GGT) | 0-51 international units/L |
| Bilirubin | Direct bilirubin: 0-0.3 mg/dL<br>Total bilirubin: 0.3-1.9 mg/dL |
| Albumin | 3.4-5.4 g/dL |
| Total protein | 6.0-8.3 g/dL |

presence of other risk factors such as high blood pressure (hypertension) and diabetes.

Lipid-lowering drugs may be prescribed for high total cholesterol or triglyceride levels, high levels of low-density lipoproteins (LDLs, or "bad" cholesterol), or low levels of **high-density lipoproteins** (**HDLs**, or "good" cholesterol). Some health problems for which these drugs are used include:

- Coronary artery disease (heart disease).
- Hypertension.
- Stroke.

Several classes of drugs affect blood lipid levels. Each class has both common and different actions and effects. Nursing responsibilities for the common actions and effects are listed in the following paragraphs. Specific nursing responsibilities are listed with each individual drug class.

*Before giving any antihyperlipidemic drug,* obtain a complete list of drugs that the patient is currently taking, including herbal and over-the-counter drugs. Ask women of childbearing age if they are pregnant, planning to become pregnant, or breastfeeding. Check patient histories for liver or muscle problems.

Before giving the first dose, be sure that the patient has baseline blood lipid and liver function tests drawn. Check his or her lipid blood tests (*lipid profile*) (see Table 16-1) and liver function tests (Table 16-3). Notify the prescriber about any abnormal results.

*After giving any antihyperlipidemic drug,* be sure to notify the prescriber if liver function laboratory tests are elevated. Ask patients about symptoms of muscle damage such as soreness, pain, or weakness. Assess patients for signs of liver damage, including jaundice, dark urine, or light-colored stools.

*Teach patients receiving any antihyperlipidemic drug* to continue lifestyle changes that help lower cholesterol such as a low-fat diet, exercise, and weight control. Remind them to check with their prescriber before using any over-the-counter drugs.

Instruct patients not to eat or drink for 8 hours before having follow-up laboratory tests drawn (lipid profile, liver function tests) because these test results can be changed by substances in some foods and fluids. Remind them that these blood tests must be repeated every 3 to 6 months to monitor the effectiveness of lipid-lowering drugs.

Advise female patients to tell their prescriber if they plan to become pregnant or are at risk of becoming pregnant.

Teach that all lipid-lowering drugs reduce high blood lipid levels but that they do not cure the problem. Treatment is long term, and these drugs must be taken even after blood fat levels are normal. Remind patients to take the drug exactly as prescribed because this ensures the best result.

Tell patients to report signs and symptoms of decreased liver function, muscle problems, or changes in urine output to their prescriber.

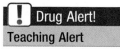

**Drug Alert!**

**Teaching Alert**

Instruct patients to fast (no eating or drinking) for at least 8 hours before a lipid profile blood test is abtained.

Memory Jogger

All lipid-lowering drugs reduce high blood lipid levels, but they do not cure the problem; treatment is long term, and these drugs must be taken even after blood fat levels are normal.

## TYPES OF LIPID-LOWERING DRUGS

There are five main types of lipid-lowering drugs. The group most commonly used is the "statins" (HMG CoA reductase inhibitors). They control the rate of cholesterol produced by the liver. The other drug types include bile acid sequestrants, cholesterol absorption inhibitors, fibrates, and nicotinic acid.

### STATINS

#### How Statins Work

**Statins** inhibit HMG CoA reductase, an enzyme that controls cholesterol production in the body. They lower blood lipid levels by slowing the production of cholesterol and increasing the ability of the liver to remove LDL cholesterol from the blood (Figure 16-3). Be sure to consult a drug reference book for information on any specific statin.

#### Dosages for Common Statins

| Drug | Dosage |
|---|---|
| atorvastatin (Lipitor) **TOP 100** | *Adults:* 10-80 mg orally once daily |
| fluvastatin (Lescol) | *Adults:* 20-40 mg orally once daily at bedtime or twice daily; extended-release (XL)—80 mg once daily |
| lovastatin (Mevacor, Altocor) | *Adults:* 20-80 mg orally once daily with evening meal |
| pravastatin (Pravachol) | *Adults:* 10-40 mg orally once daily |
| rosuvastatin (Crestor) | *Adults:* 5-40 mg orally once daily |
| simvastatin (Zocor) **TOP 100** | *Adults:* 5-80 mg orally once daily in the evening |

**TOP 100** Top 100 drugs prescribed.

#### Intended Responses
- Total cholesterol is decreased.
- Triglycerides are decreased.
- LDL is decreased.

***Side Effects.***   Side effects of statins are rare. Upset stomach, gas, constipation, abdominal pain, and cramps may occur. These symptoms are usually mild and disappear as the body adjusts to the drug.

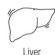

**Memory Jogger**

The generic names of HMG CoA reductase inhibitors ("statins") all end in "*-statin*" (for example, simvastatin).

**Do Not Confuse**

**Zocor** *with* **Cozaar**

An order for Zocor may be confused with Cozaar. Zocor is a lipid-lowering statin, whereas Cozaar is a blood pressure–lowering angiotensin II receptor antagonist.

*-Learning Activity 16-3 ▶

**Common Side Effects**

**Statins**

Musculoskeletal discomfort   GI discomfort   Liver problems

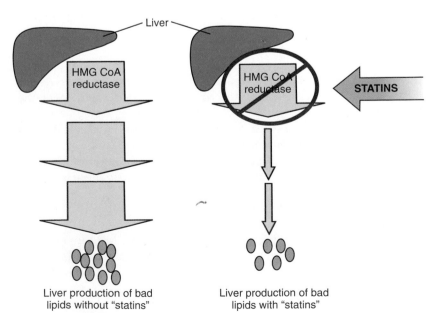

FIGURE 16-3 The action of statins to lower blood lipid levels.

***Adverse Effects.*** Patients may develop rhabdomyolysis (muscle breakdown). Signs and symptoms of rhabdomyolysis include general muscle soreness, muscle pain and weakness, vomiting, stomach pain, and brown urine. The urine turns brown because small reddish-brown pieces of broken-down muscle are removed from the body through the urine.

Statins may cause decreased liver function. Because of this danger, the prescriber should monitor liver function tests regularly (every 3 to 6 months). These tests are important because early, mild liver problems do not cause symptoms. Late symptoms of liver disease include yellowing (*jaundice*) of the skin, whites of the eyes, and roof of the mouth; pain over the liver on the right side just below the ribs; darkened urine; and pale gray-colored stools. The bile and bilirubin made by the liver normally leave the body in the stool, giving stool a medium-to–dark brown color. When the liver isn't working well, these products do not reach the stool, so the stool becomes a light gray or green instead of brown. Bilirubin enters the urine, turning it dark, and gets into skin and mucous membranes, turning them yellow.

◄ⓔ-Learning Activity 16-4

◄ⓔ-Learning Activity 16-5

### What To Do *Before* Giving Statins

Be sure to review the general nursing responsibilities related to antihyperlipidemic therapy (p. 297) in addition to these specific responsibilities before giving statins.

Ask about the patient's baseline kidney function tests (blood urea nitrogen [BUN] and creatinine) because kidney failure can be a side effect of rhabdomyolysis. Normal values are listed in Table 1-5 in Chapter 1.

Ask patients about their alcohol consumption. Statins should not be given to patients who consume more than two alcoholic drinks per day because drinking alcohol puts even more stress on the liver.

### What To Do *After* Giving Statins

Be sure to review the general nursing responsibilities related to antihyperlipidemic therapy (p. 297) in addition to these specific responsibilities after giving statins.

Regularly assess the patient for signs and symptoms of decreased liver function or muscle breakdown, including constant fatigue, itchy skin, general weakness, and jaundice (yellowish color of the skin and sclera). Report these signs and symptoms to the prescriber immediately.

Be sure to monitor the patient's urine output. Renal failure can occur if rhabdomyolysis develops because protein released from broken-down muscle can block urine flow through the kidneys. Continue to check the patient's BUN and creatinine levels.

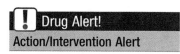

**Drug Alert!**
**Action/Intervention Alert**

After a patient begins taking a statin drug, be sure to monitor for signs of rhabdomyolysis.

### What To *Teach* Patients About Statins

Be sure to teach patients the general care needs and precautions related to antihyperlipidemic therapy (p. 297) in addition to these specific points for statins.

Remind patients that some statins should be taken in the evening and some may be taken twice a day.

### Life Span Considerations for Statins
***Pediatric Considerations.*** Safe use of statin drugs in children under 8 years of age has not been established. Statin use in older children is rare but may be prescribed for children with familial hypercholesterolemia.

***Considerations for Pregnancy and Breastfeeding.*** Statins are pregnancy category X and should not be given to women who are pregnant, plan to become pregnant, or are breastfeeding. Statins decrease the amount of fat in the body. Fat is essential to brain development in the fetus and infant. When there is not enough fat in the body during pregnancy and infancy, the fetus can suffer poor brain development and mental retardation.

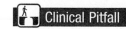

**Clinical Pitfall**

Women who are pregnant or breastfeeding should *not* take statin drugs.

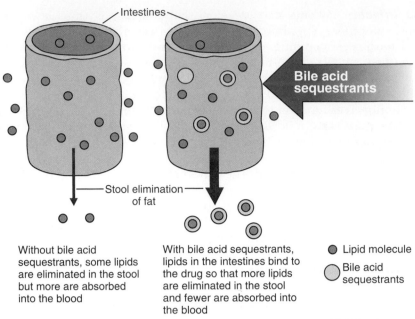

FIGURE 16-4 The action of bile acid sequestrants to lower blood lipid levels.

***Considerations for Older Adults.*** Statin drugs are safe for use in older adults if there is no history of muscle problems *(myopathy)* or liver disease. Remind older adults to contact their prescriber if they notice any new muscle weakness, muscle aches, or joint aches. Patients may think any muscle ache or weakness is related to aging, but this could be an indication of the adverse reaction rhabdomyolysis.

## BILE ACID SEQUESTRANTS

### How Bile Acid Sequestrants Work

The class of lipid-lowering drugs called **bile acid sequestrants** helps the body lose cholesterol. The drugs are taken by mouth and work directly on dietary fats in the intestine. They bind with cholesterol in the intestine, preventing the fats from being absorbed into the blood. This action then eliminates the cholesterol from the body through the stool (Figure 16-4). Be sure to check a drug reference book for information on any specific bile acid sequestrant drug.

### Dosages for Common Bile Acid Sequestrants

| Drug | Dosage |
|------|--------|
| cholestyramine (LoCHOLEST, Prevalite, Questran, Questran Light) | *Adults:* 4-24 g orally 1-6 times daily<br>*Children:* 240 mg/kg orally daily in 3 divided doses (do not exceed 8 g/day) |
| colesevelam (Welchol) | *Adults:* 3 oral tablets (625 mg each) twice daily or 6 tablets once daily; may increase to 7 tablets daily |
| colestipol (Colestid) | *Adults:*<br>Granules: 5 g orally 1-2 times daily; may be increased monthly up to 30 g/day in 1-2 doses<br>Tablets: 2 g orally 1-2 times daily; may be increased monthly up to 16 g/day in 1-2 doses |

**Common Side Effects**

**Bile Acid Sequestrants**

GI discomfort, Nausea/Vomiting, Constipation, Gas

***Intended Responses***
- LDL cholesterol level is decreased.
- HDL cholesterol level is increased.

***Side Effects.*** Side effects of bile acid sequestrants are rarely serious. The most common side effects are gastrointestinal symptoms, including constipation, bloating, nausea, vomiting, and gas.

***Adverse Effects.***   Bile acid sequestrants decrease the ability of the body to absorb oral drugs. They also inhibit fat-soluble vitamins (A, D, E, and K), so patients may need to take a daily vitamin supplement. Bile acid sequestrants may change the action of the anticoagulant warfarin (Coumadin) in two ways. They can decrease the absorption of vitamin K, which would intensify the effects of warfarin and increase the risk of bleeding. Bile acid sequestrants can also directly bind warfarin in the intestinal tract and cause its rapid elimination. This action inactivates the activity of warfarin and increases the risk of clot formation. Therefore it is always important to monitor the international normalized ratio (INR) of a patient taking both warfarin and bile acid sequestrants.

### What To Do *Before* Giving Bile Acid Sequestrants

Be sure to review the general nursing responsibilities related to antihyperlipidemic therapy (p. 297) in addition to these specific responsibilities before giving bile acid sequestrants.

Do not give any bile acid sequestrants within 2 hours after giving any other oral drug because they can inhibit the absorption of other drugs.

Ask patients whether they are experiencing constipation. This is a very common side effect of the drug and can make the patient uncomfortable.

### What To Do *After* Giving Bile Acid Sequestrants

Be sure to review the general nursing responsibilities related to antihyperlipidemic therapy (p. 297) in addition to these specific responsibilities after giving bile acid sequestrants.

After giving a bile acid sequestrant, assess the patient for gastrointestinal symptoms such as constipation, bloating, gas, nausea, or vomiting.

If the patient is taking warfarin, monitor for signs of bleeding such as easy bruising, clammy skin, pale skin, dizziness, increased heart rate, decreased blood pressure, shortness of breath, or confusion. Monitor INRs for changes that are higher or lower than the patient's prescribed therapeutic range. Give vitamin supplements if ordered.

Continue to monitor the patient for constipation.

### What To *Teach* Patients About Bile Acid Sequestrants

Be sure to teach patients the general care needs and precautions related to antihyperlipidemic therapy (p. 297) in addition to these specific points for bile acid sequestrants.

Teach patients to take bile acid sequestrants with meals because they bind with cholesterol in the intestine. Remind them not to take other drugs at least 2 hours before or 4 to 6 hours after bile acid sequestrants because bile acid sequestrants may interfere with absorption of other drugs. Tell patients to mix the powder forms of bile acid sequestrants with 4 to 6 ounces of fruit juice or water.

Tablet forms should be taken with large amounts of water (at least 12 to 16 ounces) to prevent stomach and intestinal problems such as bowel obstruction. Teach patients about the signs of bowel obstruction, including abdominal pain, bloating, vomiting, and diarrhea or constipation.

Tell patients that these drugs may be prescribed along with a statin drug to reduce cholesterol level further.

### Life Span Considerations for Bile Acid Sequestrants

***Pediatric Considerations.***   Cholestyramine (Questran) and colestipol (Colestid) should be avoided in children because they can cause intestinal obstructions. Safe use of colesevelam (Welchol) has not been established in children.

***Considerations for Pregnancy and Breastfeeding.***   Bile acid sequestrants are pregnancy category C (cholestyramine, colesevelam) and B (colestipol). Safe use of colesevelam (Welchol) has not been established for pregnancy or breastfeeding.

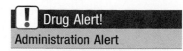

**Drug Alert!**

**Administration Alert**

If administering a bile acid sequestrant to a patient taking warfarin (Coumadin), be prepared to administer vitamin K, the antidote for warfarin.

**Drug Alert!**

**Action/Intervention Alert**

Always ask patients about constipation before administering bile acid sequestrants because these drugs can cause constipation.

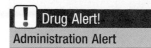

**Drug Alert!**

**Administration Alert**

Bile acid sequestrants should be taken 2 hours before or 2 hours after antacids.

◄ⓔ-Learning Activity 16-6

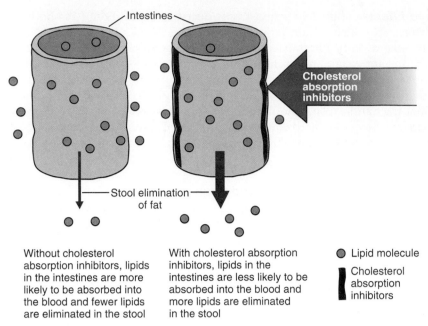

**FIGURE 16-5** The action of cholesterol absorption inhibitors to lower blood lipid levels.

The value of lowering cholesterol levels during pregnancy is controversial because the fetus needs a constant level of cholesterol for brain development.

## CHOLESTEROL ABSORPTION INHIBITORS

### How Cholesterol Absorption Inhibitors Work

Cholesterol absorption inhibitors are used when a low-fat, low-cholesterol diet does not control blood cholesterol levels. These drugs work to reduce the amount of cholesterol absorbed by the body (Figure 16-5). They are useful for patients who cannot take statin drugs because of side effects. They may also be used with statin drugs to increase the cholesterol-lowering effects. Be sure to consult a drug reference book for information on a specific cholesterol absorption inhibitor.

#### Dosage for Common Cholesterol Absorption Inhibitor

| Drug | Dosage |
| --- | --- |
| ezetimibe (Zetia, Ezetrol🍁) 🔲 | 10 mg orally once daily |

🔲 Top 100 drugs prescribed.

### *Intended Responses*
- Level of LDL cholesterol is decreased.
- Level of total cholesterol is decreased.

*Side Effects.*  Common side effects of cholesterol absorption inhibitors include gastrointestinal discomforts such as stomach pain and diarrhea. Other common side effects include fatigue, back pain, joint pain, rash, and sinusitis.

Less common side effects include cough, sore throat, and viral infections. When combined with a statin drug, side effects may include chest pain, dizziness, headache, muscle pain, and upper respiratory infections.

Fenofibrate (Tricor), gemfibrozil (Lopid), and cyclosporine increase blood levels of ezetimibe (Zetia). Rare side effects include muscle problems such as pain, aches, tenderness, or weakness.

*Adverse Effects.*  Angioedema is a rare adverse effect of ezetimibe. Angioedema is swelling beneath the skin, usually around the eyes, nose, and lips, caused

**Common Side Effects**

**Cholesterol Absorption Inhibitors**

GI discomfort,    Joint pain,    Rash
Diarrhea         Fatigue

by blood vessel dilation. Swelling may be life threatening when it affects the airways.

Rare adverse effects include allergic reactions, liver problems, pancreas inflammation, nausea, gallbladder inflammation, and gallstones.

### What To Do *Before* Giving Cholesterol Absorption Inhibitors

Be sure to review the general nursing responsibilities related to antihyperlipidemic therapy (p. 297) in addition to these specific responsibilities before giving cholesterol absorption inhibitors.

Ask if the patient has a history of liver disease or muscle disorders. Also check his or her liver function tests because the use of this drug may worsen liver disease when prescribed with a statin drug.

### What To Do *After* Giving Cholesterol Absorption Inhibitors

Be sure to review the general nursing responsibilities related to antihyperlipidemic therapy (p. 297) in addition to these specific responsibilities after giving cholesterol absorption inhibitors.

Check the patient for signs of decreased liver function such as decreased appetite, fatigue, jaundice, weakness, or muscle problems, including aches and pains. Monitor for fatigue or abdominal pain.

Monitor the patient for facial swelling, which may be an indicator of the adverse effect of angioedema. If this problem develops, hold the next dose and notify the prescriber immediately.

### What To *Teach* Patients About Cholesterol Absorption Inhibitors

Be sure to teach patients the general care needs and precautions related to antihyperlipidemic therapy (p. 297) in addition to these specific points for cholesterol absorption inhibitors.

Tell patients to be sure to report any muscle pain, tenderness, or weakness to their prescriber. Teach them to take the drug once a day at the same time every day. Not only does this habit help the patient remember to take the drug, but it also can help make the timing of any intestinal symptoms from the drug more predictable. It can be taken at the same time as a statin drug but should be given at least 2 hours before or 4 hours after bile acid sequestrants.

Stress to patients that they should go to the nearest emergency department if they develop swelling of the face or tongue or start to have difficulty breathing or swallowing. These are signs of angioedema, a serious adverse reaction.

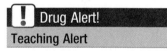

**Drug Alert!**

**Teaching Alert**

Teach patients to go to the nearest emergency department if swelling of the face or tongue occurs.

### Life Span Considerations for Cholesterol Absorption Inhibitors

*Pediatric Considerations.*   Safe use of these drugs in children under the age of 10 years has not been established.

*Considerations for Pregnancy and Breastfeeding.*   Ezetimibe is pregnancy category C, and safe use of this drug during pregnancy has not been established. During breastfeeding, this drug should only be used if the benefits outweigh possible risks to the infant because it is not known if ezetimibe passes into breast milk.

◄ ⊜-Learning Activity 16-7

## FIBRATES

### How Fibrates Work

Fibrates activate cell lipid receptors that bind to and collect cholesterol and other lipids from the blood and break them down for elimination. The main effects of fibrates are to decrease blood triglyceride levels and cause a mild increase in HDL (or "good" cholesterol). These drugs decrease liver production of triglycerides and increase the use of triglycerides by the fat tissues for metabolism. Fibrates also increase cholesterol excretion in bile. Be sure to consult a drug reference book for information on a specific fibrate drug.

**Dosages for Common Fibrates**

| Drug | Dosage |
|------|--------|
| fenofibrate (Tricor) | *Adults:* 67 mg orally daily<br>*Special Considerations:* May increase to maximum of 3 capsules (201 mg) daily |
| gemfibrozil (Lopid) | *Adults:* 600 mg orally twice daily<br>*Special Considerations:* Give 30 min before morning and evening meal; may increase up to 1500 mg daily |

### Common Side Effects

**Fibrates**

GI discomfort, Diarrhea    Musculoskeletal discomfort    Headache

Rash

---

!  **Drug Alert!**

**Interaction Alert**

Fibrates can increase the effectiveness of warfarin (Coumadin) by causing a prolonged prothrombin time, which can lead to excessive bleeding.

---

*Intended Responses*
- Triglycerides are decreased.
- HDL cholesterol is mildly increased.

*Side Effects.*  The side effects of fibrates are usually mild. The most common side effects are stomach upset and diarrhea. Other common side effects include gastrointestinal discomfort such as indigestion or heartburn (dyspepsia) and nausea. Patients may also experience muscle weakness, headache, pruritus, and rash.

*Adverse Effects.*  In the patient with kidney disease, fibrates may cause increased creatinine levels. Fibrates increase cholesterol loss in bile, which may lead to the development of cholesterol-based gallstones. Bleeding can also occur in the patient taking fibrates.

Gemfibrozil (Lopid) interferes with the breakdown of statin drugs, causing higher levels of statins in the blood. This can lead to statin side effects such as muscle damage, muscle weakness, rhabdomyolysis, or liver damage.

### What To Do *Before* Giving Fibrates

Be sure to review the general nursing responsibilities related to antihyperlipidemic therapy (p. 297) in addition to these specific responsibilities before giving fibrates.

Ask patients about a history of kidney, liver, or gallbladder disease.

### What To Do *After* Giving Fibrates

Be sure to review the general nursing responsibilities related to antihyperlipidemic therapy (p. 297) in addition to these specific responsibilities after giving fibrates.

Monitor the patient for indications of kidney, liver, or gallbladder disease such as changes in urine output, decreased appetite, fatigue, weakness, nausea, and vomiting.

If the patient is also taking warfarin (Coumadin), monitor for signs of bleeding such as easy bruising, clammy skin, paleness, dizziness, increased heart rate, decreased blood pressure, shortness of breath, and confusion.

Remind the patient that his or her prescriber will check liver and kidney function laboratory tests periodically.

### What To *Teach* Patients About Fibrates

Be sure to teach patients the general care needs and precautions related to antihyperlipidemic therapy (p. 297) in addition to these specific points for fibrates.

Teach patients to take fibrates 30 minutes before meals. Remind them that these drugs are usually given before the morning and evening meals. Instruct patients to avoid heavy alcohol use (more than 2 drinks per day). Tell patients *not* to drink grapefruit juice with fibrates.

Teach patients who are also taking warfarin to report any sign or symptom of bleeding such as easy bruising, clammy skin, pale skin, dizziness, increased heart rate, decreased blood pressure, shortness of breath, or confusion.

---

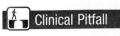 **Clinical Pitfall**

Patients should *not* drink grapefruit juice while taking fibrates because it interferes with the metabolism (breakdown) of fibrates in the body, making them less effective.

**Life Span Considerations for Fibrates**

*Considerations for Pregnancy and Breastfeeding.*   Fibrates are pregnancy category C. Safe use of these drugs during pregnancy or breastfeeding has not been established. Fibrates can cross the placenta and affect fetal brain development.

*Considerations for Older Adults.*   Older adults are more likely to be taking the drug warfarin (Coumadin) and are at greater risk for bleeding problems. In addition to assessing themselves for signs and symptoms of bleeding, it is important that the INR be tested weekly. Remind the older adult to keep all appointments for INR testing.

## NICOTINIC ACID AGENTS

### How Nicotinic Acid Agents Work

Nicotinic acid (niacin) is a special type of vitamin B that helps to decrease triglyceride, total cholesterol, and LDL cholesterol levels. It also helps to increase HDL cholesterol. Nicotinic acid is given in doses much higher than the normal daily requirement. Although the effects of niacin are well known, the drug action leading to the lipid-lowering effect is not known. Be sure to consult a drug reference book for information about a specific form of niacin.

### Dosages for Common Nicotinic Acid Agents

| Drug | Dosage |
|---|---|
| niacin (immediate-release) (Niacor, Novo-Niacin❤) | *Adults:* 1-2 g orally 2-3 times daily<br>*Special Considerations:*<br>Do not exceed 6 g daily<br>Supplied in 500-mg tablets<br>Start at low dose (500 mg) and increase slowly over several weeks |
| niacin (extended-release) (Niaspan; Slo-Niacin) | *Adults:* One 500-mg tablet (usual starting dose)<br>*Special Considerations:*<br>Every 4 weeks the prescriber may increase dosage by 500 mg up to maximum of 2000 mg taken once daily, depending on response to drug; maximum dose is 2000 mg daily |

*Intended Responses*
- Total cholesterol level is decreased.
- Total triglyceride level is decreased.
- LDL cholesterol level is decreased.
- HDL cholesterol level is increased.

*Side Effects.*   Nicotinic acid agents may cause many side effects. The most common are itching and nasal inflammation because the drug makes blood vessels dilate.

   Other common side effects include gastrointestinal symptoms such as nausea, indigestion, gas, vomiting, diarrhea, and abdominal pain. The patient may also experience flushing (redness) and hot flashes, chills, dizziness, fainting, headaches, rapid heart rate (tachycardia), shortness of breath (dyspnea), sweating (diaphoresis), and swelling caused by fluid retention.

*Adverse Effects.*   Liver problems, including toxicity, can occur, although liver failure is rare. Gout (painful swelling and redness of the toes, feet, or ankles) can occur because of a buildup of excess uric acid and calcium. Other adverse effects can include high blood sugar (hyperglycemia) and stomach ulcer flare-up. Nicotinic acid preparations are contraindicated for people who have hypertension, peptic ulcer disease, or any other active bleeding.

**Common Side Effects**

**Nicotinic Acid Agents**

Itching    GI discomfort    Headache

Tachycardia    Dizziness

### What To Do *Before* Giving Nicotinic Acid Agents

Be sure to review the general nursing responsibilities related to antihyperlipidemic therapy (p. 297) in addition to these specific responsibilities before giving nicotinic acid agents.

Obtain baseline vital signs, including blood pressure and heart rate. Also check a baseline blood sugar level for patients with diabetes.

Find out if patients have a history of liver disease or diabetes. Ask them about their usual alcohol intake. Also ask if they have ever had gout.

### What To Do *After* Giving Nicotinic Acid Agents

Be sure to review the general nursing responsibilities related to antihyperlipidemic therapy (p. 297) in addition to these specific responsibilities after giving nicotinic acid agents.

Notify the prescriber if liver function laboratory tests are elevated or if elevations of these tests are associated with nausea, vomiting, or weakness. Liver function tests that are three times the upper limits of normal indicate that the drug may need to be discontinued. (See Table 16-3 for normal liver function ranges.)

Check the patient's heart rate and blood pressure and notify the prescriber about any changes. Flushing or hot flashes can be reduced by the use of aspirin or nonsteroidal anti-inflammatory drugs (NSAIDs) 30 minutes before taking nicotinic acid or by taking nicotinic acid during or after meals.

Monitor blood glucose levels regularly for patients with diabetes because nicotinic acid can increase serum glucose levels.

### What To *Teach* Patients About Nicotinic Acid Agents

Be sure to teach patients the general care needs and precautions related to antihyperlipidemic therapy (p. 297) in addition to these specific points for nicotinic acid agents.

Tell patients that nicotinic acid dosage is usually started low and gradually increased. Teach patients about side effects of nicotinic acid and the importance of notifying their prescriber for any side effects or adverse effects of these drugs. Instruct patients who are also taking a statin drug to notify their prescriber about any muscle pain, tenderness, or weakness.

To decrease gastrointestinal side effects, teach patients to take nicotinic acid agents with meals or snacks. Remind them to take bile acid sequestrants and nicotinic acid agents 4 to 6 hours apart.

Do not substitute a sustained-release form of the drug for an immediate-release form. Extended-release forms of the drug should be swallowed whole and never crushed or chewed.

Be sure to teach patients with diabetes that nicotinic acid may increase blood glucose levels. Doses of drugs used to control blood glucose may need to be increased.

Before any surgery or dental work, the surgeon or dentist should be notified that the patient is taking a nicotinic acid agent because this drug can slow the clotting process and excessive bleeding can occur. These problems are made worse if the patient also takes aspirin or an NSAID daily along with a nicotinic acid agent.

### Life Span Considerations for Nicotinic Acid Agents

*Considerations for Pregnancy and Breastfeeding.* Nicotinic acid is pregnancy category C. It is secreted in breast milk. If a woman plans to breastfeed, she should avoid breastfeeding or discontinue the nicotinic acid agent to prevent the newborn from receiving large amounts of nicotinic acid.

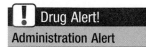

**Drug Alert!**

**Administration Alert**

Gastrointestinal symptoms can be decreased by giving nicotinic acid with food.

**Clinical Pitfall**

Extended-release forms of these drugs should *never* be crushed or mixed with water because crushing the drug causes immediate release of the entire drug dose and could lead to an overdose.

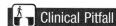

-Learning Activity 16-8 ▶

# Get Ready for Practice!

## Key Points

- Low-density lipoproteins (LDLs) are the "bad" lipids.
- High-density lipoproteins (HDLs) are the "good" protective lipids.
- Hyperlipidemia (high level of fats in the blood) can lead to cardiovascular disease.
- Familial hyperlipidemia is a form of high blood fat that is related to genetic or inherited factors.
- Lipid-lowering drugs decrease the amount of fat in a patient's blood.
- The major types of lipid-lowering drugs include statins, bile acid sequestrants, cholesterol absorption inhibitors, nicotinic acid agents, and fibrates.
- Lipid-lowering drugs should not be given if a woman is pregnant or plans to become pregnant.
- Muscle breakdown (rhabdomyolysis) is a rare but serious adverse effect of statin drugs that can lead to kidney failure.
- Bile acid sequestrants can increase the action of warfarin (Coumadin) and cause excessive bleeding.
- Extended-release forms of lipid-lowering drugs (for example, niacin) should not be crushed or given by feeding tube.
- Immediate-release forms of lipid-lowering drugs (for example, niacin) should not be substituted for extended-release drugs.
- Fibrates increase cholesterol excretion in bile, predisposing patients to gallstone formation.

## Additional Learning Resources

**evolve** Go to your Evolve website (http://evolve.elsevier.com/Workman/pharmacology/) for the following FREE learning resources:
- eLearning Activities
- Animations
- Video Clips
- Interactive Review Questions
- Audio Key Points
- Audio Glossary
- Audio Glossary—Spanish-English
- Drug Dosage Calculators
- Patient Teaching Handouts

**SG** Go to your Study Guide for additional learning activities to help you master this chapter content.

## Review Questions

1. A patient asks you how statin drugs lower blood lipid levels. What is your best response?
   - A. "They eliminate cholesterol in the stool."
   - B. "They decrease production of cholesterol by the liver."
   - C. "They bind with cholesterol bile acids."
   - D. "They decrease the absorption of cholesterol by the body."

2. A patient recently started on a statin drug reports muscle ache in the calf. What is your best first action?
   - A. Ask the patient to exercise the calf to resolve the leg cramp.
   - B. Massage the patient's calf to eliminate the pain.
   - C. Administer a dose of acetaminophen 650 mg by mouth.
   - D. Hold the drug and notify the prescriber immediately.

3. Before giving a statin drug, what information must you be sure to obtain? (Select all that apply.)
   - A. A complete list of drugs that the patient is currently taking
   - B. The possibility of pregnancy
   - C. A history of diabetes
   - D. Any history of muscle problems
   - E. How much alcohol the patient consumes each day

4. A patient's triglyceride level is very high. Which drug and drug dosage do you teach the patient might correct this level?
   - A. simvastatin (Zocor) 5 mg by mouth every evening
   - B. ezetimibe (Zetia) 10 mg by mouth every day
   - C. gemfibrozil (Lopid) 600 mg twice a day
   - D. nicotinic acid (Niacor) 1 g 3 times a day

5. A 28-year-old female patient who has been prescribed atorvastatin (Lipitor) to control familial hyperlipidemia tells you that she and her husband plan to have a child in the next 1 to 2 years. What is your best action?
   - A. Discuss the importance of continuing a low-fat diet during pregnancy.
   - B. Instruct her to discuss becoming pregnant with her prescriber.
   - C. Suggest that she begin a regular exercise program.
   - D. Refer her to a smoking cessation program.

6. The patient prescribed niacin 1 gram 3 times a day experiences nausea and vomiting when taking this drug. What is your best action?
   - A. Hold the drug.
   - B. Ask the prescriber to order an antiemetic drug.
   - C. Give the drug with food.
   - D. Reassure the patient that this is an expected side effect.

7. What action should you take for a diabetic patient prescribed niacin (Niacor)?
   - A. Give insulin only when the patient's meal tray is at the bedside.
   - B. Instruct the patient to ambulate in the halls at least 4 times daily.
   - C. Check the patient's blood potassium level before giving the drug.
   - D. Monitor the patient's blood glucose before each meal and at bedtime.

8. You are providing teaching to a patient who has been prescribed nicotinic acid (Niacor). What information should you be sure to include in the teaching plan?

   A. "Take Niacor with meals or a low-fat snack."
   B. "Drink lots of water with Niacor to prevent upset stomach."
   C. "Avoid taking Niacor for at least 1 hour after antacids."
   D. "Mix Niacor with juice or water before taking your dose."

9. What do you teach a woman prescribed niacin (Niacor) who is planning to become pregnant and breastfeed her baby?

   A. This drug is safe for use during pregnancy.
   B. This drug is safe for use during breastfeeding.
   C. This drug is secreted in breast milk.
   D. This drug is pregnancy category X.

10. A child who weighs 35 kg is to receive cholestyramine (Questran) 240 mg/kg/day in 3 equally divided doses. What is the correct dose to administer to this child? _____ mg per dose

11. A patient is to be given Niacor 1 g orally. Niacor is supplied in 500-mg tablets. How many tablets will you administer? _____ tablet(s)

12. A patient is prescribed colestipol (Colestid) tablets 8 g per day in 2 divided doses. Tablets come in 1-g tablets. How many tablets will you give for each dose? _____ tablet(s) per dose

## Critical Thinking Activities

Mrs. Lowe is a 60-year-old woman who goes to her prescriber for an annual check-up. Routine laboratory tests reveal elevated total cholesterol, LDL, and triglyceride levels. The physician places Mrs. Lowe on a low-fat diet and moderate exercise program with a follow-up appointment and laboratory tests in 3 months.

Mrs. Lowe complies with the dietary and activity changes suggested by her physician. However, her follow-up laboratory tests show even higher levels of blood lipids.

1. What is the most likely cause of the findings from the follow-up laboratory values?

2. Which class of lipid-lowering drugs is the physician most likely to prescribe at this time?

3. About what two major side effects of the prescribed drug should you be sure to tell the patient?

# Drugs That Affect Blood Clotting

## Objectives

*After studying this chapter you should be able to:*

1. Explain how different classes of drugs affect blood clotting.
2. List the common names, actions, usual adult dosages, possible side effects, and adverse effects of thrombin inhibitors, clotting factor synthesis inhibitors, antiplatelet drugs, and thrombolytic (fibrinolytic) drugs.
3. Describe what to do before and after giving thrombin inhibitors, clotting factor synthesis inhibitors, antiplatelet drugs, and thrombolytic drugs.
4. Explain what to teach patients taking thrombin inhibitors, clotting factor synthesis inhibitors, antiplatelet drugs, and thrombolytic drugs, including what to do, what not to do, and when to call the prescriber.
5. Describe life span considerations for thrombin inhibitors, clotting factor synthesis inhibitors, antiplatelet drugs, and thrombolytic drugs.
6. List the common names, actions, usual adult dosages, possible side effects, and adverse effects of drugs that improve clotting.
7. Describe what to do before and after giving drugs that improve clotting.
8. Explain what to teach patients taking drugs that improve clotting, including what to do, what not to do, and when to call the prescriber.
9. Describe life span considerations for drugs that improve clotting.

## Key Terms

**activated partial thromboplastin time (aPTT)** (ĂK-tĭ-vā-tĭd PĂR-shŭl thrŏm-bō-PLĂS-tĭn TĪM) (p. 313) Plasma coagulation test developed for monitoring the effects of unfractionated heparin, in which plasma coagulation is activated in two steps.

**anticoagulant** (ăn-tē-kō-ĂG-yū-lĕnt) (p. 310) A drug used to prevent clot formation or to prevent a clot that has already formed from getting bigger.

**antiplatelet drug** (ăn-tē-PLĂT-lĕt) (p. 319) A drug that prevents platelets from forming plugs that lead to clots.

**blood clot** (BLŬD KLŎT) (p. 310) Blood that has been converted from a liquid to a solid state. It is also called a thrombus when occurring in a blood vessel or the heart.

**clotting cascade** (KLŎT-tĭng kăs-KĀD) (p. 310) The series of blood protein reactions among clotting factors that cause blood to clot; also called the coagulation cascade.

**clotting factor synthesis inhibitors** (KLŎT-tĭng FĂK-tŭr SĬN-thĕ-sĭs ĭn-HĬB-ĭ-tŭrz) (p. 316) Drugs that decrease the production of clotting factors in the liver.

**coagulation** (kō-ăg-yū-LĀ-shŭn) (p. 310) The process by which a blood clot forms.

**embolus** (ĔM-bō-lŭs) (p. 310) Something that travels through the bloodstream, lodges in a blood vessel, and blocks its blood flow (for example, detached blood clot, a clump of bacteria, or foreign material such as air).

**fibrin** (FĪ-brĭn) (p. 310) The protein formed during normal blood clotting that is the essence of the clot.

**hemorrhage** (HĔM-ŏr-ĕj) (p. 310) Excessive loss of blood from the blood vessels; profuse bleeding.

**international normalized ratio (INR)** (ĭn-tŭr-NĂ-shŭn-ăl NŌR-mŭl-īzd RĂ-shē-ō) (p. 316) A system established by the World Health Organization (WHO) and the International Committee on Thrombosis and Hemostasis for reporting the results of warfarin anticoagulation.

**platelets** (PLĂT-lĕts) (p. 310) Irregular, disk-shaped elements in the blood that help with blood clotting.

**pulmonary embolism** (PŬL-mŭn-ār-ē ĔM-bō-lĭz-ŭm) (p. 311) An embolus that travels to the lungs and can be life threatening.

**thrombin inhibitors** (THRŎM-bĭn ĭn-HĬB-ĭ-tŭrz) (p. 313) Drugs that interfere with blood clotting by blocking the action of thrombin, which converts fibrinogen to fibrin to form clots.

**thrombolytic** (thrŏm-bō-LĬT-ĭk) (p. 321) A drug that breaks down a clot that has already formed. Fibrinolytic drugs are a class of thrombolytics.

**thrombolytic event** (thrŏm-bō-LĬT-ĭk ē-VĔNT) (p. 310) Any dangerous blood clot such as a thrombus or an embolus.

**thrombosis** (thrŏm-BŌ-sĭs) (p. 310) Forming of a blood clot in the cardiovascular system.

**thrombus** (THRŎM-bŭs) (p. 310) A blood clot in a blood vessel or within the heart.

**venous thromboembolism (VTE)** (VĒ-nŭs thrŏm-bō-ĔM-bō-lĭz-ŭm) (p. 310) A condition in which there is a clot in a vein. It may be referred to as deep vein thrombosis.

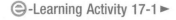 -Learning Activity 17-1 ►

## OVERVIEW

The body of a normal, healthy person is able to prevent continuous bleeding by forming clots. A blood clot is blood that has been converted from a liquid to a solid state. Dangerous clots are called thrombolytic events. One type of thrombolytic event is a clot that forms in the heart or blood vessels known as a thrombus. Another is an embolus, which occurs when something like a clot, air bubble, or fat travels through the bloodstream until it lodges in a blood vessel and blocks the blood flow. A healthy body knows how to protect itself from dangerous clots. People who have an increased risk for a thrombolytic event include patients who have had surgery or dialysis or who are bedridden.

To prevent these life- and limb-threatening events, prescribers often use drugs called anticoagulants. Anticoagulant drugs are used to reduce clot formation or to prevent an already-existing clot from becoming bigger. When a clot already exists, a thrombolytic drug may be prescribed to dissolve it. Drug dosage and therapy with these drugs is guided by coagulation laboratory values (Table 17-1).

## REVIEW OF RELATED PHYSIOLOGY AND PATHOPHYSIOLOGY

### CLOT FORMATION

When a person is injured or wounded, the body protects itself from excessive bleeding or hemorrhage by allowing the part of the blood called *platelets* and other proteins in the plasma to stick together and form a clot. Forming a clot is a normal body defense. This process begins with an enzyme called *thrombin* that acts on the protein fibrinogen, converting it into fibrin. Fibrin creates threads that make the plasma sticky and able to form a clot. Platelets clump together to create the initial plug that helps to stop bleeding. This process of cellular reactions is called the clotting cascade (Figure 17-1) or, simply, coagulation. Ideally clot formation occurs only where it is needed to prevent hemorrhage.

### THROMBOSIS

Thrombosis occurs when a clot (thrombus) forms in the cardiovascular system (Figure 17-2). This process is often triggered by atherosclerotic damage to blood vessels. Atherosclerosis refers to deposits of fatty plaque in the arteries. These fatty deposits narrow the arteries. When a thrombus develops in a coronary artery and blocks the blood supply to a part of the heart muscle, a heart attack (*myocardial infarction*) occurs. If a clot forms in an artery in the brain, a stroke can be the result. A clot in a deep vein such as a leg vein is a venous thromboembolism, or VTE (formerly called *deep vein thrombosis [DVT]*). VTEs mostly affect the larger veins in the lower legs, blocking blood flow. A clot that forms a VTE may also break off, forming an

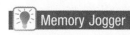 Memory Jogger

DVT (deep vein thrombosis) is now called a VTE (venous thromboembolism.

### Table **17-1**   Normal and Therapeutic Coagulation Values

| TEST | NORMAL RANGE | THERAPEUTIC RANGE |
|---|---|---|
| Activated partial thromboplastin time (aPTT) | Mean normal range in seconds established by laboratory | 1.5-2.5 times mean normal range in seconds established by laboratory |
| International normalized ratio (INR) | 0.8-1.2 | 2.0-3.0 |

embolus that travels through the bloodstream to another part of the body such as the brain or lungs.

## EMBOLUS

An embolus travels through the bloodstream until it lodges in a blood vessel and blocks it (see Figure 17-2). It can be a clump of bacteria, fat, or air; but it is often a blood clot or portion of a clot. An embolus that travels to the brain can cause a stroke. An embolus in the lung is called a **pulmonary embolism** (Figure 17-3). Pulmonary embolism is a life-threatening condition that causes severe problems in the respiratory system with symptoms of shortness of breath, chest pain, and rapid heart and respiratory rates. When a patient does not respond well to anticoagulant drugs and is at continued risk for pulmonary emboli, a metal filter may be placed in the vena cava to trap clots.

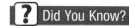
**Did You Know?**

An embolus can be a clump of baeteria or fat or an air bubble. Most often it is a clot or part of a clot.

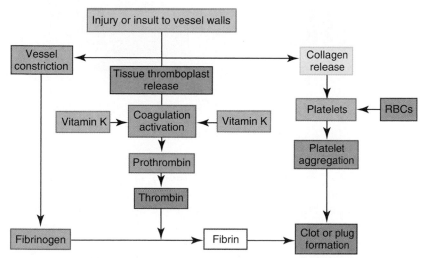

**FIGURE 17-1** The clotting cascade. *RBC*, Red blood cell.

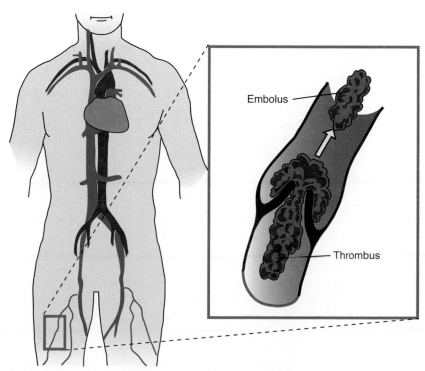

**FIGURE 17-2** Thrombus and embolus.

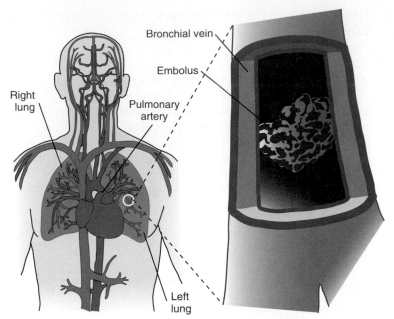

FIGURE 17-3 Pulmonary embolism.

> **Memory Jogger**
>
> Anticoagulant drugs do *not* "thin" the blood or dissolve existing clots but will prevent new clots from forming and existing clots from becoming larger.

⊖-Learning Activity 17-2 ▶

> **Memory Jogger**
>
> Thrombolytic drugs are used to dissolve clots that already exist in the body.

## GENERAL ISSUES FOR ANTICOAGULANT THERAPY

Anticoagulant drugs are prescribed to decrease the ability of the blood to form clots or to prevent an already-formed clot from becoming larger. These drugs are sometimes called *blood thinners,* but they do not actually thin the blood. They also do not dissolve clots that already exist. Drugs that dissolve existing clots are called *thrombolytics* or sometimes *clot busters.*

Anticoagulant drugs may be prescribed to prevent clots from forming after a heart valve replacement, reduce the risk of stroke or heart attack, or prevent VTEs. They are also used during open heart surgery to prevent clots from forming. These drugs may also be prescribed to prevent clots in patients who are on bed rest for a long period and for patients with heart dysrhythmias such as atrial fibrillation. Atrial fibrillation is an abnormal heart rhythm in which the atria do not contract effectively and there is a high risk of clots forming in the atrial chambers of the heart. The clots may break off and travel to other areas of the body as emboli.

When a clot already exists, thrombolytic drugs may be prescribed. Thrombolytic drugs break down clots that have already formed. They help to prevent death and additional tissue damage for patients with heart attack, stroke, pulmonary embolism, and other clot-related problems.

Several classes of drugs affect blood clotting. Each class has both different and common actions and effects. Nursing responsibilities for these common actions and effects are listed in the following paragraphs. Specific nursing responsibilities are listed with each individual class.

*Before giving any drug that affects blood clotting,* obtain a complete list of current drugs that the patient is taking, including over-the-counter and herbal preparations. Check the heart rate and blood pressure. Also check the patient's baseline coagulation laboratory results.

Ask female patients of childbearing age if they are pregnant, breastfeeding, or planning to become pregnant. Also determine whether the patient has had a baby, a miscarriage, or an abortion within the past 24 hours. These bleeding conditions are made worse by drugs that disrupt blood clotting and can lead to serious hemorrhage.

Ask if the patient has a history of bleeding problems. Check the patient for any bruising and ask whether he or she bruises easily. Ask if he or she is currently taking any drugs by injection.

Teach about the side effects and signs of bleeding. These include bleeding from the gums while brushing teeth, bleeding or oozing from cuts or wounds, bruising, and nosebleeds that are excessive and hard to control. Signs of more serious bleeding include paleness around the mouth and nailbeds, rapid heart and respiratory rates, sensation of light-headedness or dizziness, and thirst.

*After giving any drug that affects blood clotting,* check patients frequently for signs of bleeding or allergic reaction. Recheck the patient's blood pressure and heart rate. Watch for changes that may indicate bleeding such as a decrease in blood pressure (less than 90/60 mm Hg) or an increase in heart rate (more than 100 beats per minute). Notify the prescriber immediately if the patient develops any signs or symptoms of bleeding.

Avoid giving intramuscular (IM) or intravenous (IV) injections. If you must give an IM or IV drug, hold pressure over the site for at least 5 minutes. Use the smallest needle possible if you must give an IM injection.

Make sure that follow-up coagulation laboratory values are drawn and be sure to check these values because they determine the drug dose that is prescribed.

*Teach patients receiving any drug that affects blood clotting* about the importance of regular follow-up and blood tests that measure blood-clotting time. If a dose is missed, the patient should take it as soon as possible but should *never take a double dose because this could cause bleeding.* Teach patients to keep a record of each dose to prevent mistakes.

Teach patients to use a soft toothbrush and electric shaver. Tell them to inform other prescribers, including dentists, about the use of these drugs before any surgery or dental work. Remind them to take the drug exactly as prescribed. Patients should also be reminded to report any signs of bleeding or allergic reaction to the prescriber.

Tell patients to avoid contact sports and activities that may cause injuries because they can cause internal bleeding. Some activities that can cause internal bleeding (especially in the kidneys) and bleeding into the joints include running, jogging, jumping for any reason, and high-impact exercise. Encourage patients to make their home safe from falls or injuries that may cause bleeding.

Suggest that patients get and wear a medical alert bracelet that states they are taking an anticoagulant drug.

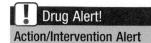

Hold pressure over an IM or IV site for at least 5 minutes when a patient is taking drugs that slow clotting.

◀ 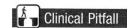-Learning Activity 17-3

## TYPES OF DRUGS THAT AFFECT BLOOD CLOTTING

### *ANTICOAGULANT DRUGS*

Anticoagulant drugs come in three categories: thrombin inhibitors (for example, heparin), clotting factor synthesis inhibitors (for example, warfarin [Coumadin]), and antiplatelet drugs (for example, aspirin). These drugs prevent or slow the formation of clots. For this reason their use is prohibited in people who have bleeding ulcers and those who have had surgery or delivered a baby within the previous 24 hours.

**Clinical Pitfall**

Anticoagulant drugs are generally *not* used in patients who are at risk for bleeding.

### THROMBIN INHIBITORS

#### How Thrombin Inhibitors Work

Thrombin inhibitors indirectly or directly interfere with blood clotting by blocking the action of thrombin, which converts fibrinogen into fibrin to form clots. Indirect thrombin inhibitors work by blocking a substance in the blood first and then blocking thrombin. This class of drugs includes heparin, low-molecular weight heparin, and fondaparinux (Arixtra). Direct thrombin inhibitors such as lepirudin (Refludan), argatroban, and bivalirudin (Angiomax) block thrombin directly.

Heparin may be given by IV or subcutaneous routes. IV heparin is usually given in the form of an IV push bolus followed by a continuous infusion. The bolus dose is usually based on the patient's weight; the infusion rate is based on and adjusted according to the patient's activated partial thromboplastin time (aPTT) laboratory results. Activated partial thromboplastin time (aPTT) is a plasma coagulation test

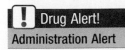

**Drug Alert!**

**Action/Intervention Alert**

Always get a current and accurate weight for a patient who is to be placed on continuous-infusion heparin because the initial IV bolus dose is based on the patient's weight.

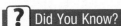

**Drug Alert!**

**Administration Alert**

For continuous heparin infusion the rate is based on the patient's aPTT laboratory results.

**? Did You Know?**

A major advantage of using LMW heparin is that patients do not need to have laboratory work drawn to guide their therapy.

developed for monitoring the effects of unfractionated heparin, lepirudin, argatroban, and bivalirudin.

The goal of this therapy is to keep the aPTT within a therapeutic range to prevent clots from forming. The therapeutic range for heparin is based on establishing a mean normal reference by the laboratory processing the tests. The therapeutic range should yield an aPTT that is 1.5 to 2.5 times greater than the mean normal range, also called the *control value*. For example, if a laboratory establishes a mean normal range of 28 seconds, the therapeutic range should be 1.5 to 2.5 times 28 seconds or 42 to 70 seconds. For heparin, blood may be drawn for the aPTT 4 to 6 hours after the initial bolus and repeated every 6 hours until a therapeutic dose is achieved. Once two consecutive aPTT results are within the therapeutic range, the serum aPTT is drawn only once every 24 hours. Although the usual therapeutic range is 1.5 to 2.5 times the control, it may be extended to as high as 3.5 depending on why the patient's blood clotting is being controlled. Always check with the prescriber to determine the exact range the patient requires, and ensure this information is recorded in the patient's record.

Subcutaneous heparin may be prescribed for therapeutic anticoagulation or prevention of clots and emboli. Subcutaneous injections are usually given every 8 to 12 hours.

Low-molecular-weight (LMW) heparin and fondaparinux are given by the subcutaneous route. Most commonly they are used to prevent VTE and pulmonary embolism. They are often given after surgeries that pose an increased risk of thrombolytic events such as knee or hip replacement and abdominal surgeries.

The direct thrombin inhibitors are given intravenously to prevent clot formation or embolic complications. These drugs are used to treat patients who have developed a reaction to heparin *(heparin-induced thrombocytopenia [HIT])*. They may also be given with antiplatelet drugs to treat chest pain and some heart attacks. Be sure to consult a drug reference book for information about a specific thrombin inhibitor.

### Dosages for Common Thrombin Inhibitors

| Drug | Dosage |
|---|---|
| heparin ❶ (Calcilean✤, Hepalean✤, heparin sodium) | *Adults:* IV bolus: weight-based (usual range 5000-10,000 units) followed by continuous infusion<br>Subcutaneous: 5000 units every 8-12 hr<br>*Children:* IV bolus of 50 units/kg followed by continuous infusion of 100 units/kg/4 hr |
| low-molecular-weight heparins ❶<br>dalteparin (Fragmin)<br>enoxaparin (Lovenox)<br>tinzaparin (Innohep) | *Adults:* Subcutaneous<br>2500-5000 units per day<br>30-40 mg twice daily<br>175 units/kg once daily |
| argatroban ❶ (Argatroban) | *Adults:* IV infusion of 2 mcg/kg/min |
| bivalirudin ❶ (Angiomax) | *Adults:* IV bolus of 0.75 mg/kg followed by IV infusion of 1.75 mg/kg/hr (angioplasty) |
| fondaparinux ❶ (Arixtra) | *Adults:* 2.5-10 mg daily |
| lepirudin ❶ (Refludan) | *Adults:* IV bolus of 0.4 mg/kg followed by continuous infusion of 0.15 mg/kg/hr |

❶ High-alert drug.

**⇄ Do Not Confuse**

**heparin** *with* **Hespan**

An order for heparin may be confused with Hespan. Heparin is an anticoagulant drug, whereas Hespan is a trade name for hetastarch, a plasma volume expander.

### *Intended Responses*
- Clotting time is increased.
- Clot formation is decreased.
- Existing clots do not become larger.

- Thrombolytic events are prevented.
- Blood flow is maintained.

*Side Effects.*   A patient who is receiving anticoagulant therapy is always at increased risk for bleeding. Bleeding from the gums while brushing teeth, bleeding or oozing from cuts and wounds, bruising, and nosebleeds may occur. Female patients may develop heavy menstrual bleeding.

Other side effects include increased blood potassium (hyperkalemia), thinning of the bones (osteoporosis), decreased number of platelets (thrombocytopenia), decreased aldosterone, blood clots in the spinal cord, and hair loss (alopecia) with prolonged use.

*Adverse Effects.*   Some patients develop allergic reactions (hypersensitivity) to these drugs. Signs of allergic reaction include changes in skin color of the face, fast or irregular breathing, puffiness or swelling around the eyes, shortness of breath or difficulty breathing, chest tightness, wheezing, skin rash, hives, and itching. Allergic reactions to heparin may be severe and life threatening because of respiratory complications and airway swelling.

Hemorrhage (excessive bleeding) is a risk of all anticoagulant drugs and may be life threatening. Many factors increase the risk of bleeding (Box 17-1). Signs of bleeding include abdominal swelling or pain, back pain, bloody urine, bloody stools (black and tarry), constipation, coughing up blood, dizziness, headaches, joint pain, and vomiting emesis that looks like coffee grounds.

HIT is a low blood platelet count as a result of heparin use. It can lead to blood clots that can be mild or serious and fatal.

Heparin-induced skin necrosis is a rare but serious complication caused by subcutaneous heparin, most commonly seen on the abdomen where injection sites are located. Management is to stop the heparin and begin warfarin. In severe cases surgery may be needed to remove necrotic skin.

### What To Do *Before* Giving Thrombin Inhibitors

Be sure to review the general nursing responsibilities related to anticoagulant therapy (p. 312) in addition to these specific responsibilities before giving thrombin inhibitors.

Check the current aPTT result. Ask the patient if he or she has ever had an allergic reaction of any kind to foods, preservatives, or dyes. Be sure to ask him or her about taking aspirin-containing products.

Ensure that the antidote to heparin, protamine sulfate, is readily available whenever a patient is receiving heparin therapy.

LMW heparin should be given by deep subcutaneous injection with the patient lying down. To avoid losing any of the drug, do not expel the air bubble before injection. The needle should be inserted into a skinfold held between the thumb and forefinger (Figure 17-4). *Remember to not aspirate before injection to avoid tissue damage.* The skinfold should be held until the injection is completed. To avoid bruising, do not rub the injection site.

---

| Common Side Effects |
| --- |

**Thrombin Inhibitors**

Bleeding       Dizziness       Hyperkalemia

---

💡 **Memory Jogger**

Signs of allergic reaction to thrombin inhibitors include:
- Changes in skin color of the face.
- Chest tightness.
- Fast or irregular breathing.
- Puffiness or swelling around the eyes.
- Shortness of breath, difficulty breathing, or wheezing.
- Skin rash, hives, itching.

---

⚠ **Drug Alert!**
**Action/Intervention Alert**

The antidote to heparin is IV protamine sulfate.

---

◀ⓔ**Video 17-1:** Administering a Subcutaneous Injection

---

| Box **17-1** | Factors That Increase Bleeding Risk with Anticoagulant Therapy |
| --- | --- |

| | |
| --- | --- |
| • Bleeding disorders such as hemophilia | • Recent major surgery or injury |
| • Blood vessel or organ abnormalities | • Recent stroke |
| • History of bleeding in the brain | • Severe diabetes |
| • History of brain tumor | • Severe kidney disease |
| • History of cerebral aneurysm | • Severe liver disease |
| • Low platelet count | • Uncontrolled high blood pressure |
| • Recent internal bleeding (for example, peptic ulcer) | |

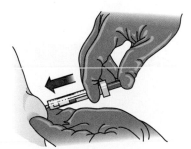

**FIGURE 17-4** Injection technique for low-molecular-weight heparin.

### What To Do *After* Giving Thrombin Inhibitors

Be sure to review the general nursing responsibilities related to anticoagulant therapy (p. 313) in addition to these specific responsibilities after giving thrombin inhibitors.

For patients receiving continuous IV heparin, adjust the flow rate based on the prescriber's orders and the results of follow-up aPTT tests. Monitor the IV site for patency and signs of infection or phlebitis.

Avoid giving IM or IV injections. If you must give an IM or IV drug, hold pressure over the injection site for at least 5 minutes. Use the smallest needle possible if you must give an IM injection.

### What To *Teach* Patients About Thrombin Inhibitors

Be sure to teach patients the general care needs and precautions related to anticoagulant therapy (p. 313) in addition to these specific points for thrombin inhibitors.

While taking heparin, patients should avoid contact sports and other activities that may result in injury. Any falls, blows to the body or head, headaches that won't go away (described as "the worst headache in my life"), or other injuries should be reported to their prescriber right away. Instruct the patient to go to the nearest emergency department if bleeding or bruising occurs and does not stop when ice is applied to the area.

Instruct patients not to take aspirin or aspirin-containing products while taking these drugs and to read the labels on both over-the-counter and prescription drugs to see if they contain aspirin. Patients should be taught not to take ibuprofen without asking their prescriber. Taking aspirin or ibuprofen while taking heparin increases the risk for bleeding.

### Life Span Considerations for Thrombin Inhibitors

*Considerations for Pregnancy and Breastfeeding.*    Although heparin is pregnancy category C, it has not been shown to cause birth defects with pregnancy. It does not pass into breast milk, so it is safe while a mother is breastfeeding. Heparin is the *drug of choice* when anticoagulation therapy is needed during pregnancy and breastfeeding. It may cause bleeding problems in the mother during the last trimester of pregnancy and delivery of the baby.

*Considerations for Older Adults.*    Older adults are more sensitive to the effects of thrombin inhibitors and therefore more likely to experience side effects such as bleeding. This is especially true for older women. Because of this, older adults may require lower drug doses. Bruising in general and at the injection site can be quite severe. Teach older adults to immediately apply cold compresses or ice packs to the injured area to reduce bruising and bleeding. Remind them to keep all appointments for blood-clotting tests.

## CLOTTING FACTOR SYNTHESIS INHIBITORS

### How Clotting Factor Synthesis Inhibitors Work

Clotting factor synthesis inhibitors decrease the production of clotting factors in the liver. The drug that fits this category is warfarin (Coumadin). Warfarin interferes with liver synthesis of vitamin K–dependent clotting factors (II, VII, IX, and X). It is most often given as an oral drug and is prescribed for adults and children to prevent forming of clots and emboli. Most patients are started on warfarin before being taken off of heparin. Patients may be prescribed heparin and warfarin together for a few days until the international normalized ratio (INR) is within the therapeutic range. Then the heparin is discontinued.

The international normalized ratio (INR) is a blood test used to monitor the effects of warfarin. The dosage of warfarin is based on the results of the INR laboratory test. Some patients may require higher or lower doses, depending on other medical conditions. The normal range for the INR is 0.8 to 1.2; a therapeutic range is generally considered to be 2.0 to 3.0. If a patient has a mechanical heart valve, the

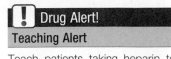

**Drug Alert!**

**Teaching Alert**

Teach patients taking heparin to avoid contact sports and any other activities that may lead to injury.

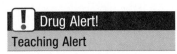

**Drug Alert!**

**Teaching Alert**

Teach patients to read labels of all over-the-counter and prescription drugs to see if they contain aspirin.

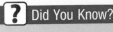-Learning Activity 17-4 ►

**?  Did You Know?**

Warfarin was originally developed as a rat poison and is still used for that purpose today.

therapeutic range is 2.5 to 3.5 because of the increased risk for clots forming on the valve.

◄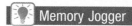-Learning Activity 17-5

Initially the INR is performed once a day, and the dose of warfarin is prescribed on the basis of the test results. Once a therapeutic range is established, the prescriber will monitor the test results periodically and adjust the dosage as needed. Lower doses of warfarin are needed for older patients, patients with liver impairment, and those with other bleeding risk factors such as dialysis.

 **Memory Jogger**

The normal INR range is 0.8 to 1.2; the therapeutic range is from 2.0 to 3.0.

### Dosages for Common Clotting Factor Synthesis Inhibitors

| Drug | Dose |
| --- | --- |
| warfarin ❗ (Coumadin, Warfilone🍁) 🔳 | *Adults:* Oral/IV—2.0-10 mg once daily for 2-4 days, then adjusted based on INR laboratory test results<br>*Children:* Oral/IV—0.2 mg/kg once daily; maximum dosage is 10 mg; adjust based on INR laboratory test results |

🔳 Top 100 drugs prescribed; ❗ High-alert drug.

### Intended Responses
- Clotting time is increased.
- Clot formation is decreased.
- Existing clots do not become larger.
- Thrombolytic events are prevented.
- Blood flow is maintained.

*Side Effects.*   Side effects of warfarin are uncommon but include bleeding, blood in urine or stool, headache, upset stomach, diarrhea, fever, and skin rash.

*Adverse Effects.*   Hemorrhage (excessive bleeding), although rare, can be life threatening. Symptoms include unusual bleeding or bruising, black or bloody stools, blood in the urine, fatigue, unexplained fever, chills, sore throat, stomach pain, or headaches that won't go away (described as "the worst headache of my life"). Patients may also vomit emesis that resembles coffee grounds, indicating bleeding in the gastrointestinal system.

Warfarin-induced skin necrosis (Figure 17-5) is a rare but serious complication that typically happens in women who are obese and going through menopause. It is associated with large doses of warfarin and usually occurs within 1 to 10 days of starting the drug. In women the breast, buttocks, and thighs are the most common

**Common Side Effects**

**Clotting Factor Synthesis Inhibitors**

Bleeding

Headache

Upset stomach, Diarrhea

Fever

Rash

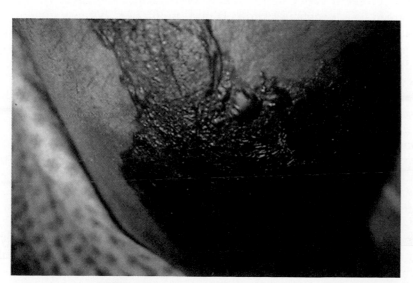

**FIGURE 17-5**   Warfarin-induced skin necrosis.

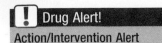

**Action/Intervention Alert**

The antidote for warfarin is IM or IV vitamin K.

sites. In men the abdomen, buttocks, thighs, and the skin of the penis may be affected. Management involves using high doses of IM or IV vitamin K as an antidote for warfarin and heparin for anticoagulation. Vitamin K should be readily available when a patient in taking warfarin.

### What To Do *Before* Giving Clotting Factor Synthesis Inhibitors

Be sure to review the general nursing responsibilities related to anticoagulant therapy (p. 312) in addition to these specific responsibilities before giving clotting factor synthesis inhibitors.

Check the patient's INR laboratory results. Ensure that vitamin K, the antidote for warfarin, is readily available. A common brand of this antidote is phytonadione (AquaMEPHYTON).

Find out if the patient is following a vegetarian diet because some vegetables are rich in vitamin K (for example, green leafy vegetables), which can decrease the action of warfarin. (Remember that vitamin K is the antidote for warfarin.)

Ask female patients of childbearing age if they are pregnant or planning to become pregnant because warfarin can cause birth defects and bleeding in an unborn baby.

Because many drugs and herbal supplements interfere with warfarin, be sure to check the patient's current drug list for interactions.

### What To Do *After* Giving Clotting Factor Synthesis Inhibitors

Be sure to review the general nursing responsibilities related to anticoagulant therapy (p. 313) in addition to these specific responsibilities after giving clotting factor synthesis inhibitors.

Tell the patient that an INR will be performed regularly to help adjust the dose of this drug.

Remind him or her to avoid intermittent large amounts of foods rich in vitamin K (especially leafy green vegetables) because they interfere with the action of warfarin.

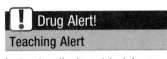

**Teaching Alert**

Instruct patients not to take over-the-counter drugs (especially aspirin or aspirin-containing drugs) or herbal supplements without asking their prescriber first.

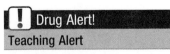

**Teaching Alert**

Be sure to teach patients taking warfarin to make their homes safe from falls.

### What To *Teach* Patients About Clotting Factor Synthesis Inhibitors

Be sure to teach patients the general care needs and precautions related to anticoagulant therapy (p. 313) in addition to these specific points for clotting factor synthesis inhibitors.

Teach patients to maintain their current diet and to not attempt a "fad" diet such as an all-vegetarian or Atkins diet. Abrupt changes in a person's diet can alter the INR results. It is important for patients to tell their prescriber if they have recently eaten or are presently eating large amounts of foods that are rich in vitamin K (such as liver, green leafy vegetables, broccoli, and cauliflower) because vitamin K interferes with the action of warfarin. These foods should be avoided. Teach patients to also inform their prescriber if they are not presently eating vegetables (for example, Atkins diet). Warn that alcohol can interfere with the action of warfarin and advise patients to talk to their prescriber before drinking alcohol.

Remind patients that it takes several days after stopping warfarin for the body to recover its normal clotting ability.

### Life Span Considerations for Clotting Factor Synthesis Inhibitors

*Pediatric Considerations.* Although warfarin is rarely used in children, there are cases in which it is needed. Side effects and risks are the same as for adults. Parents should be taught that their child should not receive IM injections, take aspirin-containing drugs, or participate in contact sports while taking this drug.

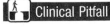

**Clinical Pitfall**

Warfarin should *not* be given during pregnancy.

*Considerations for Pregnancy and Breastfeeding.* Warfarin is pregnancy category X, and women who are of childbearing age should use birth control while taking this drug. It causes birth defects and bleeding in an unborn child.

***Considerations for Older Adults.*** Older adults may require lower doses of warfarin because they are more sensitive to its effects and more likely to develop side effects such as bleeding and bruising. In addition, older adults are more likely to be taking drugs that change the activity of warfarin. Many drugs increase the action of warfarin (for example, aspirin, acetaminophen, statin drugs, oral contraceptives, and some antibiotics), and some decrease its action (for example, cholestyramine [Questran], sucralfate [Carafate], and barbiturate drugs). Older patients may need more frequent monitoring of the INR. Remind older patients to take the drug exactly as prescribed and to keep all appointments for blood-clotting tests. In addition, warfarin tablets are usually very light colored, and distinguishing between dosage strengths can be difficult for an older adult with vision problems. Teach the older adult who may have more than one dosage strength on hand to ensure that drug label dosages are clearly marked and to read the labels carefully when taking the drug.

## ANTIPLATELET DRUGS

### How Antiplatelet Drugs Work

Antiplatelet drugs block platelets from clumping together (*aggregating*) to form harmful clots. They work well in the arterial circulation where other anticoagulant drugs are not effective. They are given by the oral or IV route. Aspirin is the most common antiplatelet drug. Antiplatelet drugs are prescribed for primary and secondary prevention of clots in the brain and cardiovascular system. They are used to treat patients with coronary artery disease, heart attack, angina, stroke, transient ischemic attacks (TIAs), and peripheral artery disease. These drugs may also be prescribed following percutaneous transluminal coronary angioplasty (PTCA) with stent placement, after heart bypass surgery, and to prevent clot formation in patients with the heart dysrhythmia atrial fibrillation. Be sure to consult a drug reference book for information about a specific antiplatelet drug.

### Dosages for Common Antiplatelet Drugs

| Drug | Dose |
| --- | --- |
| aspirin (Acuprin, Arthrinol✿, Ecotrin, Entrophen✿, many trade names) | *Adults:* 81-325 mg orally once daily |
| clopidogrel ❶ (Plavix) 🔲 | *Adults:* 75 mg orally once daily |
| eptifibatide ❶ (Integrilin) | *Adults:* 180 mcg/kg IV bolus followed by continuous IV infusion of 2 mcg/kg/min |
| ticlopidine ❶ (Ticlid) | *Adults:* 250 mg orally twice daily with food |
| tirofiban ❶ (Aggrastat) | *Adults:* 0.4 mcg/kg/min IV for 30 min, then 0.1 mcg/kg/min |

🔲 Top 100 drugs prescribed; ❶ High-alert drug.

### Intended Responses
- Clotting time is increased.
- Platelet aggregation and clot formation are decreased.
- Existing clots do not become larger.
- Thrombolytic events are prevented.
- Blood flow is maintained.

***Side Effects.*** Common side effects of antiplatelet drugs include bleeding, nausea, vomiting, upset stomach, gas, stomach pain, loss of appetite, diarrhea, headache, rash, and itching.

***Adverse Effects.*** Hemorrhage can be life threatening. Signs of bleeding include dizziness, weakness, severe headache, blood in urine or stools, unexpected nosebleeds, unusual bleeding or bruising (especially in the joints), heavy bleeding

**? Did You Know?**

Aspirin, the most commonly prescribed antiplatelet drug, comes in tablet, capsule, gum, and suppository forms.

**Do Not Confuse**

**Aggrastat** *with* **Argatroban**

An order for Aggrastat may be confused with Argatroban. Aggrastat is a platelet inhibitor, whereas argatroban is a thrombin inhibitor used for patients who develop heparin-induced thrombocytopenia (HIT).

**Do Not Confuse**

**Ticlid** *with* **Tequin**

An order for Ticlid may be confused with Tequin. Ticlid is a platelet inhibitor, whereas Tequin is a quinolone antibiotic used to treat infections.

**Common Side Effects**

**Antiplatelet Drugs**

| Bleeding | Nausea, Upset stomach | Itching, Rash |

from cuts or injuries, black and tarry-appearing stools, coughing up blood, or vomiting coffee-ground emesis. Women may experience heavy menstrual or vaginal bleeding.

Allergic reactions to these drugs are not common. Signs of an allergic reaction include hives, rash, and itching; difficulty breathing or swallowing; wheezing; chest tightness or pain; and swelling of face, tongue, lips, eyes, and extremities. The patient may also show fever, sore throat, chills, and other signs of infection. A side effect of aspirin-containing drugs is ringing in the ears (tinnitus).

Salicylate poisoning can cause vomiting, tinnitus, confusion, hyperthermia, respiratory alkalosis, metabolic acidosis, and multiple organ failure. Ingestion of more than 150 mg/kg can cause severe toxicity. Muscle breakdown (*rhabdomyolysis*), kidney failure, or respiratory failure may occur.

Children who take aspirin or aspirin-containing products are at risk for Reye's syndrome, a rare but serious illness that affects brain and liver function.

### What To Do *Before* Giving Antiplatelet Drugs

Be sure to review the general nursing responsibilities related to anticoagulant therapy (p. 312) in addition to these specific responsibilities before giving antiplatelet drugs.

Ask the patient if he or she is allergic to aspirin or nonsteroidal anti-inflammatory drugs (NSAIDs). Be sure to check his or her platelet count.

Antacids interfere with the absorption of antiplatelet drugs. Give antiplatelet drugs 2 hours after or 1 hour before giving antacids.

### What To Do *After* Giving Antiplatelet Drugs

Be sure to review the general nursing responsibilities related to anticoagulant therapy (p. 313) in addition to these specific responsibilities after giving antiplatelet drugs.

Give antiplatelet drugs with meals or just after eating to decrease side effects such as nausea and upset stomach. Continue to monitor blood platelet count levels.

### What To *Teach* Patients About Antiplatelet Drugs

Be sure to teach patients the general care needs and precautions related to anticoagulant therapy (p. 313) in addition to these specific points for antiplatelet drugs.

To decrease the side effect of nausea, teach patients to take antiplatelet drugs with food.

Remind them that they may need to take these drugs for the rest of their lives to prevent clots from forming. Instruct them to continue taking antiplatelet drugs unless their prescriber stops the therapy.

Instruct patients to read the labels of over-the-counter drugs to ensure that they are aspirin free. Aspirin and NSAIDs may cause bleeding when taken at the same time as an antiplatelet drug.

Although a moderate amount of alcohol is sometimes recommended for patients with heart disease, remind patients taking aspirin not to drink alcohol because it affects the action of aspirin. Drinking alcohol while taking aspirin increases patients' risk of bleeding problems, especially stomach bleeding.

### Life Span Considerations for Antiplatelet Drugs

*Pediatric Considerations.*  Children should not take aspirin because of the risk of developing Reye's syndrome, a rare but dangerous illness that can cause brain damage, liver failure, and even death.

*Considerations for Pregnancy and Breastfeeding.*  Taking antiplatelet drugs during the last 2 weeks of pregnancy can cause bleeding problems in the baby before and after delivery. Antiplatelet drugs can be passed through breast milk to the baby. Aspirin should not be taken during the last 3 months of pregnancy or while breastfeeding. Other NSAIDs need to be avoided during pregnancy because they can cause premature closure of the foramen ovale, an important opening for blood flow through the fetal heart.

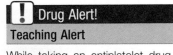

**Drug Alert!**
**Teaching Alert**

While taking an antiplatelet drug, teach patients to read labels of over-the-counter drugs to make sure that they are aspirin free and NSAID free.

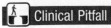

**Clinical Pitfall**

Children should *not* take aspirin-containing products because of the risk for Reye's syndrome.

**⊖-Learning Activity 17-6 ►**

# THROMBOLYTIC DRUGS

## How Thrombolytic Drugs Work

Thrombolytic drugs are drugs that dissolve clots that have already formed. This is why these drugs have the nickname "clot busters." They are prescribed for patients who have had a heart attack, stroke, pulmonary embolism, or some other clot-related problem. All thrombolytic drugs activate plasminogen, an inactive form of plasmin found in body fluids and blood plasma. Plasminogen forms plasmin, an enzyme that dissolves the fibrin in blood clots. All thrombolytics are able to initiate the process of breaking down clots and can prevent new clots from forming.

Clot busters are IV drugs given in a setting with specially trained nurses (e.g., emergency department, cardiac catheterization lab, or intensive care unit). They may be given by a peripheral IV line or through a long catheter that is guided to the clot. If started within 12 hours after the onset of symptoms for heart attack or 3 hours for stroke symptoms, thrombolytics can dissolve the clot that is blocking the artery and restore blood flow. This action may prevent or minimize tissue damage to the heart or brain. The sooner these drugs are begun, the more likely it is that they will achieve a positive result. When thrombolytics are begun within 90 minutes, they have the best success for stroke patients. In as many as 25% of patients, thrombolytic drugs are unable to dissolve clots. About 12% of patients will have clots that form again, especially if the underlying problem that caused the clot has not been treated. In some situations (for example, a heart attack), thrombolytics are not used if more than 6 hours have passed since the symptoms began because tissue damage has already occurred, and at this point the drugs can cause more problems than they prevent.

The most commonly prescribed thrombolytic drugs are alteplase (Activase [t-PA]) tenecteplase (TNKase), and reteplase (Retavase). Some thrombolytic drugs are used to clear long term–use vascular catheters that have been blocked by clots.

**Did You Know?**

The body makes its own naturally occurring clot busters such as tissue-type plasminogen activator.

**Drug Alert!**
**Administration Alert**

The sooner thrombolytic drugs are started, the more likely it is that they will successfully dissolve a clot.

### Dosages for Common Thrombolytic Drugs

| Drug | Dosage |
|---|---|
| alteplase ❶ (Activase [t-PA], Activase rt-PA🍁) | *Myocardial Infarction:*<br>  *Adults:* weight more than 67 kg: 15 mg IV bolus, followed by 50 mg IV over 30 min, then 35 mg IV over 60 min; follow with heparin therapy<br>*Pulmonary Embolism:*<br>  *Adults:* 100 mg IV over 2 hr followed by heparin therapy<br>*Stroke:*<br>  *Adults:* 0.9 mg/kg (no more than 90 mg) IV over 1 hr (10% of dose given as bolus during first min) |
| reteplase ❶ (Retavase) | *Adults:* 10 units IV followed by additional 10 units in 30 min |
| tenecteplase ❶ (TNKase) | *Adults:* IV: weight-based (30-50 mg IV push) |

❶ High-alert drug.

**Do Not Confuse**

**Activase (t-PA)** *with* **tenecteplase (TNKase)**

An order for t-PA can be confused with TNKase. Both are thrombolytic drugs. t-PA is given by IV infusion, whereas TNKase is given by IV push.

◄ⓔ-Learning Activity 17-7

### Intended Responses
- Clotting time is increased.
- Existing clot is dissolved.
- Blood flow is restored in a blocked artery.
- Tissue damage is prevented or minimized.

***Side Effects.*** The most common side effects of thrombolytic drugs include bleeding or oozing from cuts, gums, and wounds and around injection sites. Other common side effects include fever and low blood pressure.

***Adverse Effects.*** Patients who experience allergic reactions may have shortness of breath, fever, chills, chest tightness, swelling, wheezing, skin rash, hives, or itching.

Hemorrhage is a major risk when patients receive thrombolytic therapy because the action of these drugs is to break down clots. They increase the risk of hemorrhagic

**Common Side Effects**
**Thrombolytic Drugs**

Bleeding     Fever     Hypotension

stroke because of the increased risk for bleeding, which includes bleeding into the brain.

### What To Do *Before* Giving Thrombolytic Drugs

Be sure to review the general nursing responsibilities related to anticoagulant therapy (p. 312) in addition to these specific responsibilities before giving thrombolytic drugs.

Find out whether the patient has experienced any of the following events because they increase the risk of serious bleeding:

- Falls or blows to the head or body
- Any injections into a blood vessel
- Placement of any tubes within the body
- Surgery, including dental surgery
- Delivery of a baby within the past 72 hours

Obtain the patient's health history because there are absolute and relative contraindications for thrombolytic therapy (Box 17-2). With absolute contraindications the therapy should *not* be given. With relative contraindications the prescriber weighs the pros and cons of the treatment before making a decision.

Check the patient's coagulation laboratory study results. Make sure that all ordered laboratory tests have been completed and that the patient has IV lines in place.

### What To Do *After* Giving Thrombolytic Drugs

Be sure to review the general nursing responsibilities related to anticoagulant therapy (p. 313) in addition to these specific responsibilities after giving thrombolytic drugs.

Check the patient for any signs of bleeding at least every 2 hours and report these immediately. Ask the patient about headaches and monitor for changes in level of consciousness. Initially check the patient every 15 to 30 minutes, then every 1 to 2 hours, every 4 hours, every shift, and as needed.

Because of the risk for bleeding, do not give any injectable (intramuscular or subcutaneous) drugs to the patient. Do not start or remove IV lines. If a line must be removed, you will need to apply pressure to the site for at least 30 minutes.

At first (during the first 4 to 6 hours), patients are kept in bed while they recover from thrombolytic therapy. They receive IV fluids, including anticoagulation with continuous heparin to prevent additional clots from forming. Make sure that these IV fluids are infusing at the correct rate and that the IV line is patent. Ensure that the call light is within easy reach and tell the patient to call for help before getting out of bed.

Make sure that follow-up laboratory tests for coagulation are completed.

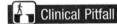

**Clinical Pitfall**

Thrombolytic drugs should *not* be given if there are absolute contraindications (see Box 17-2).

**Clinical Pitfall**

After a patient has received a thrombolytic drug, do *not* start or remove IV lines and do *not* give IM injections.

---

| Box 17-2 | Contraindications for Thrombolytic Drugs |
| --- | --- |

| **ABSOLUTE CONTRAINDICATIONS** | **RELATIVE CONTRAINDICATIONS** |
| --- | --- |
| • Active internal bleeding | • Active peptic ulcer disease |
| • Cerebrovascular processes: | • Current use of oral anticoagulants |
|   • Cranial neoplasm | • Endocarditis or pericarditis |
|   • Recent spinal or cerebral surgery | • Hemostatic defects |
|   • Recent stroke (within 2 months) | • Severe uncontrolled hypertension |
| • Increased blood pressure greater than 200/120 mm Hg | • Surgery within the last 10 days |
| • Known allergy to streptokinase products | • Trauma within the last 10 days |
| • Known bleeding disorders | |
| • Pregnancy or recent delivery (24 hours) | |
| • Prolonged cardiopulmonary resuscitation | |
| • Recent head trauma | |
| • Suspected aortic dissection | |

## What To *Teach* Patients About Thrombolytic Drugs

Be sure to teach patients the general care needs and precautions related to anti-coagulant therapy (p. 313) in addition to these specific points for thrombolytic drugs.

Thrombolytic drugs are given in the hospital setting, so most patient teaching is done there. Instruct patients to report any problems with their IV access sites such as bleeding, swelling, pain, or numbness.

Instruct patients to report any unusual symptoms at once. Also tell them to report any arm or leg pain that seems to be getting worse.

Once discharged, patients should notify their prescribers if any of these conditions develop:

- Fever
- Shortness of breath
- Changes in the arms or legs such as blueness, swelling, or feeling cold
- Signs of bleeding such as light-headedness or dizziness, nausea, and back pain

Remind patients to avoid heavy lifting for a week to 10 days and to drink lots of fluids to help rid the body of dyes that may have been used during procedures. Patients may take a shower, but they should avoid baths to protect the catheter insertion site for a few days until this is allowed by their prescriber.

### Life Span Considerations for Thrombolytic Drugs

*Pediatric Considerations.*   The risk of bleeding is increased in children because they are more sensitive to the effects of thrombolytic drugs.

*Considerations for Pregnancy and Breastfeeding.*   Thrombolytic drugs are pregnancy category C. There is a slight chance that some thrombolytic drugs used during the first 5 months of pregnancy may cause a miscarriage. Delivery of a baby within the past 24 hours is a contraindication to giving these drugs.

*Considerations for Older Adults.*   The risk of bleeding is increased in older adults because they are more sensitive to the effects of thrombolytic drugs.

## *DRUGS THAT IMPROVE BLOOD CLOTTING*

### COLONY-STIMULATING FACTORS

### How Colony-Stimulating Factors Work

Sometimes drugs are needed to *improve* the ability of the blood to clot rather than to decrease clotting. These drugs increase the number of red blood cells (RBCs) and platelets available to improve blood clotting and are known as *colony-stimulating factors (CSFs)*. The bone marrow normally makes these blood components in response to naturally occurring hormones. For example, when a person is *anemic* (has too few RBCs), the ability of the blood to carry oxygen is reduced, and tissues do not receive the normal amount of oxygen. When the kidney receives less oxygen, it secretes erythropoietin into the blood. This substance goes to the bone marrow and stimulates it to increase production of RBCs. Drugs that increase RBC levels are known as erythropoiesis-stimulating agents (ESAs), and those that increase platelet levels are known as thrombopoiesis-stimulating agents (TSAs). ESAs and TSAs are similar to the naturally occurring hormones that trigger the bone marrow to produce more cells. ESAs make the bone marrow increase production of RBCs to the greatest extent, although they do increase all blood cell production to some degree. TSAs are more specific for stimulating the bone marrow to increase production of platelets, although the production of other cells also increases.

ESAs are most often used for patients who have chronic kidney disease, are anemic from cancer chemotherapy, or need to increase RBC counts before surgery. TSAs are most often used for patients who have low platelet counts from cancer chemotherapy. Both types of drugs reduce the need for transfusion of blood and blood products.

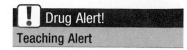

**Drug Alert!**
**Teaching Alert**

Instruct patients to report any problems with IV access sites such as bleeding, swelling, pain, or numbness.

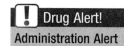

**Drug Alert!**
**Administration Alert**

Bleeding is more likely to occur in children and older adults because they are more sensitive to the effects of thrombolytic drugs.

**Memory Jogger**

ESAs (erythropoiesis-stimulating agents) increase red blood cell (RBC) levels. TSAs (thrombopoiesis-stimulating agents) increase platelet levels.

**Dosages for Common Colony-Stimulating Factors**

| Drug | Dosage |
|------|--------|
| *Erythropoiesis-Stimulating Agents* | |
| darbepoetin alfa (Aranesp) | *Adults/Children:* 0.45 mcg/kg IV or subcutaneously each week (can be given in divided doses 2 to 3 times per week until the hemoglobin level approaches 12 g/dL) |
| epoetin alfa (Epogen, Eprex✦, Procrit) | *Adults/Children:* 50-100 units/kg IV or subcutaneously 3 times per week to maintain hemoglobin levels within the individualized target range |
| *Thrombopoiesis-Stimulating Agents* | |
| oprelvekin (Neumega) | *Adults/Children:* 50 mcg/kg subcutaneously once daily until the platelet count is greater than 50,000/mm³ |

**Common Side Effects**

**Colony-Stimulating Factors**

Hypertension    Headache    Fever, flushing

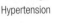

Pain at injection site

## Intended Responses

- Blood cell levels are approaching normal.
- There is a reduced need for transfusion therapy.

**Side Effects.** Because these drugs increase blood cell production, the blood becomes more viscous (thicker). This effect raises blood pressure, increases clot formation, and slows blood movement through small vessels. Other side effects include headaches, general body aches, flushing, fever, chills, and pain at the injection site.

**Adverse Effects.** Because colony-stimulating factors increase blood viscosity and fluid retention, the patient is at risk for hypertension, blood clots, strokes, and heart attacks. In addition, certain types of cancer cells grow faster in the presence of these factors such as head and neck cancer cells, leukemias, and lymphomas. The basis of dosing for these drugs is to monitor individual patient hemoglobin or platelet levels to ensure that just enough cells are produced to avoid the need for transfusion.

### What To Do *Before* Giving Colony-Stimulating Factors

If the patient is receiving a repeat dose of the drug, ask him or her if any allergic reactions or difficulty breathing occurred with a previous dose. If the patient has had such a response, notify the prescriber before giving the drug.

Check the patient's blood counts before therapy. If the platelet count is greater than 50,000/mm³ or if the hemoglobin level is at 12 g/dL (or higher), notify the prescriber before giving the drug.

Check the patient's blood pressure and use this value to monitor for drug-induced hypertension.

Follow the package directions for mixing and preparing the drug.

Ensure that oprelvekin (Neumega) is administered only by deep subcutaneous injection and not intravenously or intradermally.

### What To Do *After* Giving Colony-Stimulating Factors

When giving the first IV dose of a colony-stimulating factor, check the patient every 15 minutes for any signs or symptoms of an allergic reaction (hives at the IV site, low blood pressure, rapid irregular pulse, swelling of the lips or lower face, the patient feeling a "lump in the throat"). If you suspect an allergic reaction, call the rapid response team and notify the prescriber.

Check the patient's blood pressure and complete blood count to determine the effectiveness of the drug and whether increased viscosity is occurring.

### What To *Teach* Patients About Colony-Stimulating Factors

Teach patients to weigh themselves daily and report a weight gain of more than 2 lbs in a 24-hour period or 4 lbs in a week to their prescriber.

Teach them to report any sign of a clot (swelling in one extremity, difference in skin color or temperature in one extremity, pain in one extremity) immediately to their prescriber. Remind them to be sure to have blood tests done as often as prescribed.

Instruct them to go immediately to the emergency department for chest pain, shortness of breath, change in level of consciousness, difficulty speaking, numbness or drooping of one side of the face, or blurred vision. These are signs of a heart attack or stroke.

For patients who are self-administering the drug, teach them the proper technique for subcutaneous injection and how to monitor the site for problems.

### Life Span Considerations for Colony-Stimulating Factors

*Pediatric Considerations.*   Oprelvekin has been known to cause an increase in intracranial pressure (rare). This drug should not be used in children who have brain tumors or any other problem that increases intracranial pressure.

*Considerations for Pregnancy and Breastfeeding.*   Colony-stimulating factors are pregnancy category C drugs. They should be avoided during pregnancy unless the benefits outweigh the possible risks. These drugs should not be used during breastfeeding.

*Considerations for Older Adults.*   The increased viscosity of the blood is more likely to result in hypertension and increase the risk for congestive heart failure, pulmonary edema, heart attacks, and strokes. Older adults should be monitored more closely for blood cell responses, and the therapy should be stopped or decreased when hemoglobin levels approach 11 g/dL or if hypertension develops.

◄ⓔ-Learning Activity 17-8

> **Drug Alert!**
> **Teaching Alert**
>
> Teach patients to report signs of clot formation immediately (e.g., swelling in one extremity, pain in one extremity, a difference in temperature or color in one extremity).

## Get Ready for Practice!

### Key Points

- Clot formation is a normal bodily protective process that prevents blood loss.
- Dangerous forms of clots include thrombi and emboli.
- Anticoagulant drugs prevent clots from forming or already-existing clots from getting bigger.
- An initial IV bolus of heparin is based on the patient's weight; the rate of the continuous infusion is based on the aPTT laboratory results.
- A therapeutic range for the aPTT is 1.5 to 2.5 times the mean normal range, which is established by the laboratory processing the test.
- LMW heparins such as enoxaparin (Lovenox) do not require laboratory tests to guide therapy.
- Protamine sulfate, the antidote to heparin, should be readily available when a patient is receiving heparin.
- Dose prescription for warfarin is guided by the INR laboratory test. A therapeutic INR is 2.0 to 3.0 (normal INR is 0.8 to 1.2).
- Vitamin K, the antidote for warfarin, should be available when a patient is receiving this drug.
- Antiplatelet drugs prevent platelets from clumping together (aggregating) to form clots.
- A patient taking anticoagulant drugs should not take aspirin-containing drugs or NSAIDs at the same time because of the increased risk for bleeding.
- Thrombolytic drugs dissolve existing clots. They are also called *clot busters*.
- Clot busters should be started as soon as possible after symptoms because the sooner they are started, the more likely it is that they will dissolve the clot.
- A complete patient health history is very important before giving thrombolytic drugs because there are reasons why the drugs may not be given (contraindications).
- Colony-stimulating factors are used to improve blood clotting.

### Additional Learning Resources

ⓔvolve Go to your Evolve website (http://evolve.elsevier.com/Workman/pharmacology/) for the following FREE learning resources:
- eLearning Activities
- Animations
- Video Clips
- Interactive Review Questions
- Audio Key Points
- Audio Glossary
- Audio Glossary—Spanish-English
- Drug Dosage Calculators
- Patient Teaching Handouts

**SG** Go to your Study Guide for additional learning activities to help you master this chapter content.

## Review Questions

1. Which drug will dissolve an already existing clot?

   A. heparin
   B. warfarin (Coumadin)
   C. aspirin
   D. alteplase (Activase)

2. For which adverse effect must you monitor in a woman taking a platelet inhibitor?

   A. Vaginal bleeding
   B. Gastrointestinal bleeding
   C. Severe bruising
   D. Nosebleeds

3. Which action is essential before beginning continuous IV heparin therapy?

   A. Have the laboratory draw an INR blood test
   B. Get an accurate baseline patient weight
   C. Make a sign that states, "no IM or subcutaneous injections"
   D. Instruct the patient to remain on bed rest and use the call light

4. A patient asks you why only one aspirin a day has been prescribed. What is your best response?

   A. "To help prevent any pain"
   B. "To keep your platelets from forming a clot"
   C. "To dissolve any small clots that may form"
   D. "To keep any clots in your body from growing"

5. Which anticoagulant drug is relatively safe to use during pregnancy?

   A. ticlopidine (Ticlid)
   B. warfarin (Coumadin)
   C. enoxaparin (Lovenox)
   D. clopidogrel (Plavix)

6. What is an intended response when a patient is prescribed epoetin alfa (Epogen)?

   A. Blood cell levels normalize.
   B. New blood clots do not form.
   C. Clotting time is increased.
   D. Thrombolytic events are prevented.

7. The patient is prescribed the first dose of a colony-stimulating factor drug. What action must you perform after giving this drug?

   A. Check the patient's aPTT.
   B. Teach the patient to use a soft toothbrush.
   C. Assess the patient for edema in the legs.
   D. Check the patient every 15 minutes for an allergic reaction.

8. Which teaching point do you include in a care plan for a patient being discharged on a prescribed colony-stimulating factor drug?

   A. Take this drug with food to prevent GI discomfort.
   B. Blood tests will need to be performed to monitor the effects of this drug.
   C. This drug works by preventing new clots from forming.
   D. Report a weight gain of 1 pound in a week to your prescriber.

9. What is the danger for an older adult who is taking a colony-stimulating drug?

   A. Development of type 2 diabetes
   B. Confusion
   C. Hypertension
   D. Increased risk for falls

10. A patient is to receive 4000 units of subcutaneous heparin. Heparin comes as 5000 units in 1 mL. How many milliliters will you give? _____ mL

11. The prescriber orders clopidogrel (Plavix) 150 mg orally. Clopidogrel comes in 75-mg tablets. How many tablets will you give? _____ tablet(s)

12. A child has been ordered warfarin 0.2 mg/kg. The child weighs 21 kg. How many mg will you give? _____ mg

## Critical Thinking Activities

Mr. Jones is a 68-year-old man admitted to the acute care medical floor with pain, swelling, and redness in his left lower leg. The prescriber wrote an order for enoxaparin (Lovenox) 30 mg subcutaneously twice a day.

1. What type of drug is enoxaparin?

2. What is the major side effect of this drug?

3. List three common signs/symptoms of this side effect.

4. List two strategies that you would teach Mr. Jones to avoid injury while taking this drug.

# Drugs for Asthma and Other Respiratory Problems

## Objectives

*After studying this chapter you should be able to:*

1. Describe the names, actions, usual adult dosages, possible side effects, and adverse effects of bronchodilator drugs for respiratory problems.
2. Describe what to do before and after giving bronchodilator drugs.
3. Explain what to teach patients taking bronchodilator drugs, including what to do, what not to do, and when to call the prescriber.
4. Describe life span considerations for bronchodilator drugs.
5. List the names, actions, usual adult dosages, possible side effects, and adverse effects of anti-inflammatory drugs and mucolytics for respiratory problems.
6. Describe what to do before and after giving anti-inflammatory drugs and mucolytics for respiratory problems.
7. Explain what to teach patients taking anti-inflammatory drugs and mucolytics for respiratory problems.

## Key Terms

**alveoli** (ăl-VĒ-ō-lī) (p. 327) Air sacs in the lungs where oxygen moves into the blood.

**asthma** (ĂZ mă) (p. 328) An intermittent disease of airway obstruction caused by constriction of the bronchial smooth muscles that surround the airways and by inflammation in the airways.

**bronchoconstriction** (brŏn-kō-kŏn-STRĬK-shŭn) (p. 328) The tightening of pulmonary smooth muscle, resulting in narrowed airways.

**bronchodilator** (brŏn-kō-DĪ-lā-tŭr) (p. 330) A drug that relaxes the smooth muscle around airways, causing the center openings to enlarge.

**chronic bronchitis** (KRŎ-nĭk brŏn-KĪ-tĭs) (p. 330) A persistent inflammation of the airways.

**chronic obstructive pulmonary disease (COPD)** (KRŎ-nĭk ŏb-STRŬK-tĭv PŬL-mŭn-ār-ē dĭz-ĒZ) (p. 327)

A respiratory disorder that is a combination of chronic bronchitis and emphysema.

**emphysema** (ĕm-fĭ-SĒ-mă) (p. 330) A disease in which the elasticity of air sacs (alveoli) is greatly reduced.

**lumen** (LŪ-mĕn) (p. 328) The open center of a hollow airway.

**mucolytic** (myū-kō-LĬ-tĭk) (p. 338) A drug that reduces the thickness of mucus, making it easier to move out of the airways.

**peak expiratory rate flow (PERF)** (PĒK ĕks-PĬR-ă-tōr-ē RĀT FLŌ) (p. 328) The fastest airflow rate reached at any time during exhalation that measures how well a patient can exhale or blow out his or her breath. Also known as peak expiratory flow.

**wheeze** (WĒZ) (p. 329) A squeaky or snorelike sound present when air moves through narrowed airways.

◄ ⊖ -Learning Activity 18-1

## OVERVIEW

All cells need oxygen ($O_2$) to live, grow, and perform their specific jobs. This oxygen comes from the air you breathe. Air with oxygen enters the nose and mouth and moves through the airways (trachea, bronchi, bronchioles) into air sacs located in the lungs. These air sacs are called **alveoli** and are the sites where oxygen from the air moves into the blood so it can be carried to all tissues and organs. The waste gas created in the tissues, *carbon dioxide ($CO_2$)*, moves from the blood into the alveoli so it can be exhaled. The major health problems of the respiratory system are those that narrow the airways such as asthma or chronic bronchitis and diseases that destroy the alveoli such as emphysema. **Chronic obstructive pulmonary disease (COPD)** is a respiratory disorder that is a combination of chronic bronchitis and emphysema. This chapter is focused on drug therapy for asthma and COPD because they are the most common noninfectious lung disorders. Although any part of the lungs can

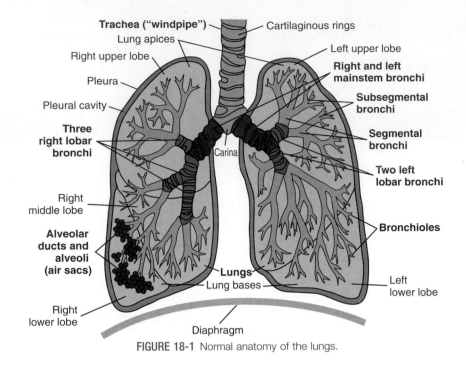

FIGURE 18-1 Normal anatomy of the lungs.

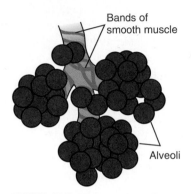

FIGURE 18-2 Close-up view of one small airway with attached alveoli.

**Memory Jogger**

Keeping airways open is critical for air inhalation and ensuring that oxygen reaches the lungs.

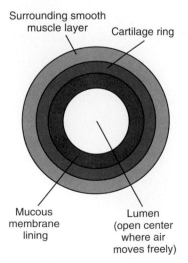

FIGURE 18-3 Cross section of a small airway showing the tissue layers.

become infected, these infections are not respiratory-related causes of disease. Drugs for respiratory infections are discussed in Chapters 9 through 11.

## REVIEW OF RELATED PHYSIOLOGY AND PATHOPHYSIOLOGY

Figure 18-1 shows the normal anatomy of the lungs, including the larger airways and the smaller airways leading to the alveoli. Figure 18-2 shows a close-up of one small airway with the alveoli attached. It is important for the airways to remain open for good airflow to and from the alveoli where oxygen and carbon dioxide are exchanged. As shown in Figure 18-3, the airways have several layers around a hollow middle section.

The open center of the hollow part of the airway is called the lumen. Different health problems can affect the lumen in various ways, making it smaller or even closing it completely. The middle can be blocked by thick mucus and other substances. In addition, the mucous membrane lining of the tube can swell when it is inflamed and block off the open area. One of the layers around the tubes is made up of smooth muscle. If this smooth muscle constricts tightly, the center of the tube can be narrowed or even closed. This is called bronchoconstriction. Table 18-1 shows test values used to measure breathing effectiveness and airway function.

A common method to measure airway function is peak expiratory rate flow (PERF). It is the fastest airflow rate reached at any time during exhalation and measures how well the patient can exhale or blow out his or her breath. PERF is measured by blowing into a handheld meter during exhalation. It can indicate whether the airways are functioning properly or are narrowed. The normal range for PERF is established by age, size, and gender. A decrease in PERF of 15% to 20% below the expected value for a person may occur when the airways are narrowed. *When the PERF value drops below 50%, the patient has dangerously low airflow into and out of the airways.*

### ASTHMA

Asthma is a problem of airway obstruction caused by constriction of the bronchial smooth muscles that surround the airways and by inflammation in the airways. It

| Table 18-1 | Tests Used to Measure Breathing Effectiveness | |
|---|---|---|
| **TEST** | **NORMAL OR EXPECTED VALUES** | **COMMON CHANGES DURING AN ASTHMA ATTACK** |
| Oxygen saturation (Spo₂) by pulse oximetry | 95% to 100% | Decreased |
| Peak expiratory rate flow (PERF), the fastest airflow reached at any time during exhalation | At least 95% of the expected value for size, gender, and age | Less than 80% of expected value for size, gender, and age |
| Arterial blood gases: | | |
| PaO₂ | 95-100 mm Hg | Decreased |
| PaCO₂ | Less than 45 mm Hg | Increased |
| HCO₃⁻ | 22-24 mEq/L | Normal |
| pH | 7.35-7.45 | Increased (early) Decreased (late) |

*HCO₃⁻*, bicarbonate concentration; *PaO₂*, arterial oxygen concentration (partial pressure); *PaCO₂*, arterial carbon dioxide concentration (partial pressure); *pH*, hydrogen ion concentration.

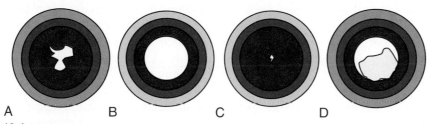

**FIGURE 18-4** Different causes of narrowed airways. **A,** Mucosal swelling. **B,** Constriction of smooth muscle. **C,** Mucosal swelling and constriction of smooth muscle. **D,** Mucus plug.

occurs in episodes or attacks. Between attacks the airways are open. Thus the problem is intermittent and reversible. Only the airways are affected, not the alveoli. Two problems can narrow the airways: bronchoconstriction (smooth muscle tightening) and inflammation, as shown in Figure 18-4. Bronchoconstriction blocks the airways from the outside of the airway, and inflammation causes swelling of the mucous membranes and obstructs the lumen, or the inside, of airways. This problem is worse when mucus plugs also form. Airway inflammation also can trigger bronchoconstriction so the airways are blocked by two processes at the same time.

Inflammation of the mucous membranes lining the airways is a key event in triggering an asthma attack. It occurs in response to the presence of allergens; irritants such as cold air, dry air, or fine particles in the air; microorganisms; and aspirin. As described in Chapter 8, histamine and leukotrienes are released into the mucous membranes. When this happens, blood vessels dilate, the tissue swells, and mucus increases. These same factors also may cause the smooth muscles around the airways to tighten (constrict).

A patient with mild-to-moderate asthma has no symptoms between asthma attacks. Symptoms of an acute asthma attack are increased respiratory rate and a "wheeze." A wheeze is a squeaky or snorelike sound made when air moves through narrowed airways. At first the wheeze is heard only when the patient exhales. As airways continue to narrow, wheezes also are heard when the patient inhales. With inflammation the patient also has increased coughing. As breathing becomes less effective, blood oxygen levels decrease, and blood carbon dioxide levels increase. If the asthma attack is so severe that oxygen levels become too low, the patient can die. Refer to Table 18-1 for changes in test values that can occur during an asthma attack.

 **Memory Jogger**

The two causes of airway obstruction with asthma are bronchoconstriction and inflammation.

 **Memory Jogger**

A severe asthma attack can lead to death.

◀ ⊖-Animation 18-1: Asthma

## CHRONIC OBSTRUCTIVE PULMONARY DISEASE

Chronic obstructive pulmonary disease (COPD) is a combination of chronic bronchitis and emphysema. **Chronic bronchitis** is a *persistent* inflammation of the airways. The mucous membranes of the airways are swollen, and the mucus-producing cells enlarge. This creates large amounts of thick, sticky mucus that narrow the airways. As a result, moving air into and out of the lungs is more difficult (see Figure 18-4). **Emphysema** is a problem in which the normal elastic tissue in the alveoli becomes loose and flabby. Because exhalation depends on recoil of the alveoli (just as the "stretch" of a full balloon helps it to deflate quickly), a loss of good elastic tissue makes moving air out of the lungs more difficult. Both chronic bronchitis and emphysema are progressive and become worse with time. No cure currently exists for either problem; the most common cause is cigarette smoking.

COPD is similar to asthma in terms of airway blockage. However, the symptoms of COPD *never* go away completely, even with drug therapy. The alveoli are damaged in COPD but not in asthma. Thick, sticky mucus is continuously produced in the patient with COPD.

💬-Learning Activity 18-2 ▶

## TYPES OF DRUGS FOR ASTHMA AND COPD

When asthma is well controlled, the airway narrowing is temporary and reversible. With poor control attacks become worse, happen more often, and can become so severe that the person dies during an attack from lack of oxygen. The goals of drug therapy for asthma are to improve airflow, reduce symptoms, and prevent asthma attacks. The drugs used to help prevent airway closure from asthma come from several categories, depending on the exact problem that is triggering the airways to narrow.

Drug therapy for asthma in adults and children is based on disease severity. Some patients may need drug therapy with a *rescue drug* only during an asthma episode. Others need daily drugs as *prevention* to keep asthma attacks from happening. Total therapy involves the use of drugs that make the smooth muscle around the airways relax (**bronchodilators**) and anti-inflammatory drugs. Thus some drugs reduce the attack severity or stop the attack (*rescue* drugs), and other drugs actually prevent the attack (*prevention* or *controller* drugs).

Although COPD cannot be reversed, its progression can be slowed, and the symptoms reduced with proper drug therapy. Drug therapy for COPD is based on disease severity and the patient's responses to the drugs. Because the chronic bronchitis airway problems of COPD are essentially the same as the airway changes occurring during an asthma attack, most of the drugs used to treat COPD are the same as those used to treat asthma. Sometimes the drug dosage or frequency differs, with the person who has COPD taking higher or more frequent doses.

The patient with asthma or chronic bronchitis can help manage his or her disease by assessing symptom severity at least twice daily with a peak flowmeter and adjusting prescribed drugs for inflammation and bronchospasms to prevent or relieve symptoms. The patient should first establish a baseline or "personal best" peak expiratory rate flow (PERF) by measuring his or her PERF twice daily for 2 to 3 weeks when asthma is well controlled or COPD symptoms are minimal, and recording the results. This way the patient will be able to know when his or her peak flow is reduced to the point that more drugs or emergency assistance is needed. When the patient has established a "personal best," all other readings are compared to this value in terms of percent of personal best. Some meters are color coded to help the patient interpret the results (Figure 18-5), and other meters just show numbers. Green zone readings are at least 80% of the "personal best." This is the ideal range for breathing control and indicates that no increases in drug therapy are needed. Yellow is a range between 50% and 80% of personal best. When a patient has a reading in this range, he or she needs to use the "rescue drug" as prescribed. Red is a range below 50% of the patient's personal best and indicates serious respiratory obstruction. The patient needs to seek emergency assistance immediately.

**Memory Jogger**

Rescue drugs stop an asthma attack or reduce its severity; prevention (controller) drugs prevent an attack from starting.

**Memory Jogger**

Teach patients who have a reading in the red zone or less than 50% of their personal best to use the rescue drugs immediately and seek emergency help.

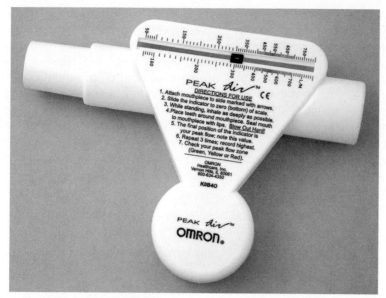

**FIGURE 18-5** A peak flow meter. This model will show faster exhalation rates in green, reduced exhalation rates in yellow, and seriously reduced exhalation rates in red.

Because the airway narrowing associated with asthma and COPD have more than one cause, drug management usually requires the use of more than one drug type. The types of drugs usually prescribed for asthma and COPD are the bronchodilators, anti-inflammatories, and mucolytics. All of these drugs are used to manage asthma and COPD, although the doses, routes, and timing of the drugs may differ between the two disorders.

## BRONCHODILATORS

Bronchodilators relax smooth muscle. They have no effect on inflammation. So when a patient's asthma or chronic bronchitis is caused by both bronchoconstriction and inflammation, at least two types of drug therapy are needed. These drugs types include beta$_2$-adrenergic agonists, cholinergic antagonists, and methylxanthines.

### How Bronchodilators Work

*Beta$_2$-adrenergic agonists* bind to the beta$_2$-adrenergic receptors and cause an increase in the production of a substance that triggers pulmonary smooth muscle relaxation. The name of this substance is *cyclic adenosine monophosphate*, known as *cAMP*.

Short-acting beta$_2$-adrenergic agonists (SABAs) provide rapid but short-term relief. They are *rescue drugs* because they are most useful when an asthma attack begins and when the patient is about to start an activity that is likely to induce an asthma attack. These drugs are used for COPD when the patient feels more breathless than usual. When inhaled, the drug is delivered directly to the lungs, and systemic effects are minimal (unless the agent is overused or abused).

Long-acting beta$_2$-adrenergic agonists (LABAs) work in the same way as SABAs but need time to build up an effect. *Therefore LABAs are used to prevent an asthma attack because their effects last longer but have no value during an acute attack.* For COPD these drugs are taken daily to maintain open airways. The patient with COPD may use a nebulizer and mask for some of these drugs rather than a hand-held inhaler.

*Cholinergic antagonists (anticholinergic drugs)* block the parasympathetic nervous system. This blockade allows a person's natural epinephrine and norepinephrine to bind to smooth muscle receptors; bronchodilation results. These inhaled drugs also bind to mucous membrane receptors and decrease airway secretions. Like LABAs, they are *prevention* drugs and must be taken on a daily basis to prevent asthma attacks and reduce airway blockage in COPD. The patient with COPD is more likely to be prescribed a longer-acting cholinergic antagonist. *These drugs are used to prevent an asthma attack but have no value during an acute attack.*

**Memory Jogger**

Types of drugs for asthma treatment and prevention and COPD maintenance include:
- Bronchodilators.
- Anti-inflammatories.
- Mucolytics.

**Memory Jogger**

Drugs for prevention must be taken daily and exactly as prescribed, even on days when no symptoms are present.

*Methylxanthines* are powerful but have many side effects. They are given systemically rather than by inhaler and increase the amount of cAMP in cells. When the amount of cAMP is increased in respiratory smooth muscle cells, they relax, causing bronchodilation. Methylxanthines are used only when other types of management are ineffective. Blood levels of these drugs must be monitored closely because the drug level that causes dangerous side effects is not much higher than the level needed to dilate the bronchioles. The most dangerous side effects result from cardiac and central nervous system overstimulation. The patient with a severe acute asthma attack may be prescribed these drugs intravenously. Daily oral therapy with these drugs is used only for the patient with severe asthma and the patient with COPD.

**Dosages for Common Bronchodilators**

| Drug Category | Drug Name | Dosage |
|---|---|---|
| Short-acting beta$_2$-agonists (SABAs) | albuterol 🔝 (Apo-Salvent🍁, PMS-Salbutamol🍁, Proventil HFA, Ventolin HFA, VoSpire ER) | 1-2 inhalations every 4 to 6 hr |
| | pirbuterol (Maxair) | 1-2 puffs every 4 to 6 hr |
| | terbutaline (Brethine, Bricanyl🍁) | *Adults:* 2.5-5 mg orally every 6 hr<br>*Children:* 2.5 mg orally every 6 hr while awake |
| Long-acting beta$_2$-agonists (LABAs) | arformoterol (Brovana) | 15 mcg (contents of one 2-mL vial) every 12 hr via nebulization |
| | formoterol (Foradil, Oxeze🍁, Perforomist) | 1 puff every 12 hr |
| | salmeterol (Serevent) | 1 puff every 12 hr |
| Cholinergic antagonists | ipratropium (Apo-Ipravent🍁, Atrovent 🔝, Novo-Ipramide🍁, Nu-Ipratropium🍁) | 2-4 puffs 3-4 times daily |
| | tiotropium (Spiriva) | 1 puff (18 mcg) daily (DPI) |
| Methylxanthines | aminophylline (Truphylline) | 5-7 mg/kg IV as a loading dose; 0.4-0.7 mg/kg/hr IV for maintenance |
| | theophylline (Bronkodyl, Theo-Dur, Theolair, Uniphyl) | Immediate-release:<br>  *Adults:* 100-300 mg orally every 8 hr<br>  *Children:* 3-5 mg/kg every 6 hr<br>Sustained-release:<br>  *Adults/Children:* 10-12 mg/kg (up to 800 mg) orally once daily or in 2-3 divided doses |

*DPI,* Dry-powder inhaler; 🔝 Top 100 drugs prescribed.

### Intended Responses
- Pulmonary smooth muscles relax.
- Airways widen, allowing air to move more freely into and out of the alveoli.
- Wheezing decreases or disappears.
- PERF increases compared with readings taken right before drug therapy.

***Side Effects.*** Bronchodilators that are inhaled have few side effects unless the inhaler is heavily used. Using an inhaler too often allows the drug to be absorbed through the mucous membranes of the mouth, throat, or respiratory linings and enter the bloodstream. Once a drug has entered the bloodstream, it can have systemic effects. Some of the systemic effects of bronchodilators include rapid heart rate, increased blood pressure, a feeling of nervousness, and difficulty sleeping. The inhaled drugs can dry the mouth and throat and also may leave a bad taste in the mouth.

Anticholinergic agents can cause some specific side effects if they reach the bloodstream. These effects include urinary retention, blurred vision, eye pain, nausea, and headache.

*Adverse Effects.*   Some brands of inhaled bronchodilators contain preservatives that can cause minor-to-severe allergic reactions. Warn patients to check with their prescriber if a rash, chest pain, or light-headedness occurs within a few minutes after using the inhaler. In addition, if a patient uses the inhaler more frequently than prescribed, enough drug can reach the blood to cause the blood vessels in the heart to constrict, leading to angina or a heart attack (*myocardial infarction*).

The methylxanthines are systemic drugs, and their side effects can be severe. In addition to increased heart rate and blood pressure, these drugs can cause seizures and life-threatening heart rhythm problems (*dysrhythmias*). Adverse effects are most likely to occur when they are given intravenously but can occur when taken orally.

### What To Do *Before* Giving Bronchodilators

Many patients have never used an oral inhaler or a spacer (Figure 18-6) and may not know the correct technique. Ask whether the patient has ever used an inhaler. If the answer is yes, ask him or her to demonstrate or describe the technique used. If the patient has not used an inhaler or a spacer, teach the correct technique. Box 18-1 describes teaching tips for using an aerosol inhaler (also called a metered-dose inhaler) with a spacer; Box 18-2 describes teaching tips for using an aerosol inhaler without a spacer.

The powder used in a dry-powder inhaler may already be loaded in the inhaler or may have to be placed in the inhaler each time it is used. The technique used with dry-powder inhalers differs from that of standard aerosol inhalers because the powder must remain dry to be active. Box 18-3 describes teaching tips for how to use a dry-powder inhaler.

Use a stethoscope to listen to the lungs of the patient before administering an inhaled bronchodilator. This information can be used to determine drug effectiveness by comparing it with the patient's breath sounds after therapy.

Take the vital signs of a patient who is to receive parenteral or oral methylxanthines. These drugs always increase heart rate and blood pressure. Also, because an adverse effect of methylxanthines is increased central nervous system activity with possible seizures, assess the temperature and mental status of the patient and document the findings. Check the patient's hands for tremors. Use a pump or controller to deliver the IV drug to prevent accidental rapid infusion and overdose. Have suction and oxygen equipment in the room with the patient during IV methylxanthine therapy in case seizures occur.

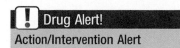
**Drug Alert!**
**Action/Intervention Alert**

Assess for chest pain in the patient taking a bronchodilator.

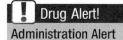
◀ -Video 18-1: Using a Metered-Dose Inhaler

**Drug Alert!**
**Administration Alert**

Always use an IV pump or controller when giving methylxanthines intravenously.

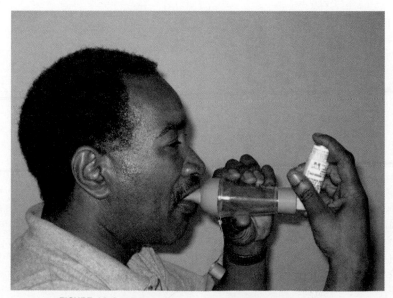

**FIGURE 18-6** Patient using an aerosol inhaler with a spacer.

---

**Box 18-1** Teaching Tips for Using an Aerosol Inhaler with a Spacer

- Before each use remove the caps from the inhaler and the spacer.
- Insert the mouthpiece of the inhaler into the nonmouthpiece end of the spacer.
- Shake the whole unit 3 or 4 times vigorously to mix the drug in the inhaler.
- Hold the inhaler canister between your thumb and index finger.
- Place the mouthpiece of the spacer into your mouth, over your tongue. Seal your lips around the mouthpiece.
- Squeeze the canister firmly between your thumb and index finger to release one dose of the drug into the spacer.
- Breathe in slowly and deeply. If the spacer makes a whistling sound, you are breathing in too fast.
- Remove the mouthpiece from your mouth, closing your lips immediately.
- Keep your lips closed and hold your breath for at least 10 seconds, then slowly breathe out.
- If you are prescribed to take two puffs, wait at least 1 minute before taking the second puff.
- Use the same technique for the second puff as you did for the first.
- When finished, remove the inhaler canister from the spacer.
- Replace the caps on the inhaler and the spacer.
- At least once each day clean the plastic mouthpiece and the cap of the inhaler by thoroughly rinsing them in warm, running tap water.
- Clean the spacer and its mouthpiece at least weekly by thoroughly rinsing them in warm, running tap water.

---

**Box 18-2** Teaching Tips for Using an Aerosol Inhaler Without a Spacer*

**PREFERRED TECHNIQUE**
1. Before each use remove the cap and shake the inhaler according to the instructions in the package insert.
2. Tilt your head back slightly and breathe out fully.
3. Open your mouth and place the mouthpiece 1 to 2 inches away.
4. As you begin to breathe in deeply through your mouth, press down firmly on the canister of the inhaler to release one dose of the medication.
5. Continue to breathe in slowly and deeply (usually over 3 to 5 seconds).
6. Hold your breath for at least 10 seconds to allow the medication to reach deep into the lungs; then breathe out slowly.
7. Wait at least 1 minute between puffs.
8. Replace the cap on the inhaler.
9. At least once a day remove the canister and clean the plastic case and cap of the inhaler by thoroughly rinsing in warm, running tap water.

**ALTERNATIVE METHOD**
1. Follow steps 1 and 2 for the Preferred Technique.
2. Place the mouthpiece into your mouth, over your tongue, and seal your lips tightly around it.
3. Follow steps 4 to 9 for the Preferred Technique.

*Avoid spraying in the direction of the eyes.

---

### What To Do *After* Giving Bronchodilators

Check the patient's breathing status after giving short-acting inhaler drugs to determine whether the drugs are effective. Breathing improvement as measured by a slower respiratory rate, decreased or absent wheezes, and pulse oximetry values of 95% or higher usually occurs within 5 minutes of inhalation of short-acting bronchodilators. If a peak expiratory flowmeter is used to check breathing improvement, the peak flow should increase by at least 15% after using the drug.

Compare the patient's heart rate and blood pressure within 15 minutes after giving the drug to determine whether any systemic effects are present. Ask about any chest pain. Report severe tachycardia, a rapid rise in blood pressure, or chest

### Box 18-3   Teaching Tips for Using a Dry-Powder Inhaler

For inhalers requiring loading:
- First load the drug by:
  - Turning the device to the next dose of drug, *or*
  - Inserting the capsule into the device, *or*
  - Inserting the disk or compartment into the device.

After loading the drug and for inhalers that do not require drug loading:
- Read your health care provider's instructions for how fast you should breathe for your particular inhaler.
- Place your lips over the mouthpiece and breathe in forcefully (there is no propellant in the inhaler; only your breath pulls the drug in).
- Remove the inhaler from your mouth as soon as you have inhaled (breathed in).
- Never exhale (breathe out) into your inhaler. Your breath will moisten the powder, causing it to clump and not be delivered accurately.
- Never wash or place the inhaler in water.
- Never shake your inhaler.
- Keep your inhaler in a dry place at room temperature.
- If the inhaler is preloaded, discard the inhaler after it is empty.
- Because the drug is a dry powder and there is no propellant, you may not feel, smell, or taste it as you inhale.

pain immediately to the prescriber. If the patient receiving a methylxanthine begins to have tremors or has an increase in restlessness, slow the infusion rate and report this finding immediately.

If a patient is to receive two or more drugs by inhaler for breathing problems, give the bronchodilator first and wait at least 5 minutes before giving the next drug. This action allows time for the bronchodilator to widen the airways so the next drug can be inhaled more deeply into the respiratory tract and be more effective.

### What To *Teach* Patients About Bronchodilators

Inhaled bronchodilators can be very effective in controlling or preventing an asthma attack if used correctly. Teach patients to carry a short-acting beta agonist (SABA) inhaler with them at all times and to ensure that it contains enough drug to be effective. Demonstrate how to check aerosol inhaler drug levels by placing the inhaler in water (Figure 18-7). Full inhalers sink to the bottom. An empty inhaler floats on its side. Teach patients that, if the short-acting inhaler is needed increasingly more often as a "rescue" from asthma attacks, the prescriber should be notified, and other therapy options discussed.

Long-acting beta-adrenergic agonists (LABAs) should be taken as prescribed even when symptoms of asthma are not present because these drugs are used to *prevent* an attack, not stop an attack that has already started. *Therefore teach patients not to use LABAs to rescue them during an attack or when wheezing is getting worse but to use a SABA. Relying on LABAs during an attack can lead to worsening of symptoms and death.*

### Life Span Considerations for Bronchodilators

***Considerations for Older Adults.***   Older adults may be more sensitive to the cardiac and nervous system side effects of bronchodilators. Teach older patients to check their pulse rates before and after taking a bronchodilator. Tell them to report any new development of tremors or sleep difficulties to their prescriber. Instruct them to call the life squad or go to the nearest emergency department if chest pain occurs.

Dry-powder inhalers that must be loaded by the patient can be difficult for older patients who have trouble with fine motor movements. Assess the older patient's ability to load and handle the inhaler. If he or she has difficulty, ask the prescriber to consider an inhaler type that does not require the patient to load the drug.

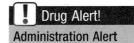

**Drug Alert!**

**Administration Alert**

When giving two or more inhalation drugs for asthma at the same time, give the bronchodilator first and wait at least 5 minutes before giving the second and third drugs.

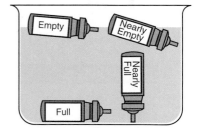

**FIGURE 18-7** Checking the drug level in an aerosol inhaler.

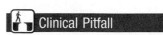

**Clinical Pitfall**

Do not use long-acting adrenergic inhalers for immediate relief of symptoms during an asthma attack.

◄ ⊖-Learning Activity 18-3

## ANTI-INFLAMMATORY DRUGS

There are many anti-inflammatory drugs for inflammation, but the drug types used as therapy for asthma and COPD are the corticosteroids, mast cell stabilizers, and leukotriene inhibitors.

### How Anti-Inflammatory Drugs for Respiratory Problems Work

*Corticosteroids* decrease the production of body chemicals that trigger inflammation. Inhaled corticosteroids can prevent inflammation in the respiratory tract and reduce inflammation that has already started. Although inhaled corticosteroids do not cause relaxation of pulmonary smooth muscle, their presence enhances the effects of some bronchodilators.

*Mast cell stabilizers* prevent the release of histamine (and other chemicals that cause inflammation) when allergens bind to mast cell receptors. The exact way the mast cell membranes are inhibited from opening *(degranulating)* is not known.

*Leukotriene inhibitors* work in several ways to prevent an asthma episode and reduce the inflammation of chronic bronchitis. Zileuton (Zyflo) prevents leukotriene production within white blood cells. Montelukast (Singulair) and zafirlukast (Accolate) block the leukotriene receptors on inflammatory cells. With these drugs a person develops less inflammation in respiratory tissues.

None of the anti-inflammatory drugs induce bronchodilation. See Chapter 8 for a more detailed discussion of how anti-inflammatory drugs work.

### Dosages for Common Anti-inflammatory Drugs for Asthma and COPD

| Drugs | Dosage |
|---|---|
| *Inhaled Corticosteroids* | |
| beclomethasone (QVAR) | *Adults:* 1-2 puffs twice daily |
| | *Children:* 1-2 puffs twice daily |
| budesonide (Pulmicort) | *Adults/Children:* 1-2 puffs 1-2 times daily |
| flunisolide (AeroBid) | *Adults/Children:* 2 puffs twice daily |
| fluticasone (Flovent, Flovent Diskus) | *Adults:* 2 puffs twice daily |
| | *Children:* 1 puff twice daily |
| triamcinolone (Azmacort) | *Adults/Children:* 1-2 puffs 3-4 times daily |
| *Mast Cell Stabilizers* | |
| cromolyn sodium (Intal Inhaler) | *Adults/Children:* 2 puffs 4 times daily |
| nedocromil sodium (Tilade) | *Adults/Children:* 2 puffs 4 times daily |
| *Leukotriene Inhibitors* | |
| montelukast sodium (Singulair) 🔟⁰ | *Adults:* 10 mg orally daily |
| | *Children:* 4-5 mg orally daily |
| zafirlukast (Accolate) | *Adults:* 20 mg orally twice daily |
| | *Children:* 10 mg orally twice daily |
| zileuton (Zyflo CR) | *Adults:* 1200 mg orally twice daily |

🔟⁰ Top 100 drugs prescribed.

### Intended Responses

- Swelling of pulmonary mucous membranes is reduced.
- Pulmonary secretions are reduced.
- Airway lumens open, allowing air to move more freely into and out of the alveoli.
- Wheezing decreases or disappears.
- PERF remains within the patient's "personal best" range.

**Side Effects.** Side effects of inhaled anti-inflammatories are local and include bad taste, mouth dryness, and an increased risk for oral infection. Side effects of oral leukotriene inhibitors include headache and abdominal pain.

---

💡 **Memory Jogger**

Anti-inflammatory drugs reduce inflammation but do not cause bronchodilation.

---

🔁 **Do Not Confuse**

**Zyflo** *with* **Zyrtec or Zyban**

An order for Zyflo may be confused with Zyrtec or Zyban. Zyflo is a leukotriene inhibitor, whereas Zyrtec is another type of anti-inflammatory drug, and Zyban is a drug used to decrease symptoms of withdrawal during smoking cessation.

---

**Common Side Effects**

**Inhaled Anti-inflammatory Drugs**

Dry mouth    Tearing    Headache

*Adverse Effects.*   The propellant and preservatives in inhaled drug mixtures can irritate tissues, causing the patient to cough severely or have bronchospasms.

When inhaled corticosteroids are used as prescribed, they have a low risk for any adverse effect. However, when heavily used, they can be absorbed into the bloodstream and cause adrenal gland suppression just as systemic corticosteroids do. Although this is possible, it rarely occurs. In addition, when used excessively, inhaled corticosteroids reduce the local immune response, which allows oral infections to occur.

Leukotriene inhibitors may cause liver impairment and allergic reactions, including hives and anaphylaxis. Both of these responses are rare.

### What To Do *Before* Giving Anti-Inflammatory Drugs for Respiratory Problems

Inspect the patient's mouth and throat to determine whether an infection is present. The most common oral infection associated with inhaled corticosteroids is a fungal infection known as *thrush*. It appears as white or cream-colored patches of a cheesy coating on the mucous membranes, roof of the mouth, and tongue.

Many patients have never used an oral inhaler or a spacer (see Figure 18-6) and may not know the correct technique. If the patient has not used an inhaler or a spacer, teach the correct technique (see Boxes 18-1 and 18-2).

If the patient also is receiving an inhaled bronchodilator, give the bronchodilator first and wait at least 5 minutes before giving the inhaled anti-inflammatory. Giving the bronchodilator first allows the greatest widening effect on the airways so the anti-inflammatory can be inhaled more deeply into the respiratory tract and be more effective.

When a new canister of nedocromil (Tilade) is being used for the first time, prime it by pressing the actuation valve three times before giving the dose to the patient.

### What To Do *After* Giving Anti-Inflammatory Drugs for Respiratory Problems

For inhaled drugs, assist the patient to rinse with water or mouthwash to remove the drug from the mouth. This practice helps reduce the bad taste and mouth dryness.

Regularly assess the patient taking a leukotriene inhibitor for signs and symptoms of decreased liver function, including constant fatigue, itchy skin, and jaundice of the skin or sclera.

### What To *Teach* Patients About Anti-Inflammatory Drugs for Respiratory Problems

Anti-inflammatory drugs can be very effective in controlling or preventing an asthma attack and reducing the inflammation of chronic bronchitis in COPD if used correctly. They carry a warning that the risk for death from asthma is increased when using these drugs. This is because the anti-inflammatory drugs for respiratory problems may help prevent inflammation but do not cause bronchodilation.

Remind patients to use anti-inflammatory inhalers at least 5 minutes after using an inhaled bronchodilator.

Teach patients to take the drug as prescribed even when symptoms of asthma are not present because these drugs are used to *prevent* an attack, not stop an attack that has already started. However, when acute asthma is present, patients should continue to take these prevention drugs as prescribed in addition to the rescue drugs. Teach patients with COPD the importance of taking the drug daily to prevent worsening of chronic bronchitis. Tell patients to be careful about how the inhaler is used because the risk for oral and respiratory infection increases with increased use. In addition, more systemic side effects are likely to occur.

Tell patients using an inhaled drug that rinsing the mouth after using the drug can reduce the bad taste and mouth dryness.

Teach patients to check the gums, mouth, and throat daily in the mirror for increased redness or the presence of white/cream-colored patches that may indicate

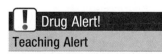

**Drug Alert!**
**Teaching Alert**

Teach patients not to rely on anti-inflammatory drugs alone to stop or reduce bronchoconstriction.

◄ⓔ-Learning Activity 18-4

an infection. Also tell patients to use good oral hygiene at least 3 times a day to prevent oral infections.

### COMBINATION BRONCHODILATOR AND ANTI-INFLAMMATORY DRUGS

A newer option for people with asthma and COPD is the use of inhalers that contain both a bronchodilator and a corticosteroid for prevention therapy. One such drug is Advair, which is a combination of the corticosteroid fluticasone and the long-acting bronchodilator salmeterol. It comes in different combinations of dosages. Another drug is Symbicort, which is a combination of the corticosteroid budesonide and the long-acting bronchodilator formoterol. The therapeutic effects, side effects, adverse effects, precautions, and patient education are the same as for each drug individually.

### MUCOLYTICS

> **Memory Jogger**
>
> Mucolytics improve airflow by reducing the thickness of mucus in the airways.

Most people with COPD take a drug daily to reduce the thickness of mucus, allowing the mucus to more easily move out of the airways. This type of drug is called a mucolytic. Patients with asthma may use mucolytics when increased secretions are a problem.

Guaifenesin (Mucinex, Naldecon Senior EX, Organidin) is a systemic mucolytic that is taken orally. The major mucolytic drug prescribed for a person with COPD is acetylcysteine (Mucomyst). Mucus contains protein molecules and mucus molecules held tightly together. This drug works by breaking the connections that hold the protein and mucus molecules. This results in thinner, less sticky mucus that is easier to cough up and spit out.

Acetylcysteine is most commonly delivered with a nebulizer face mask and is also available as an oral drug. Typically 1 to 10 mL of a 20% solution is placed in the medication nebulizer every 6 hours. The patient places the nebulizer mask over the face and breathes in the mist containing the drug. It is also possible to administer small amounts of the drug directly into the tracheal tube of a patient who has a tracheostomy or down the endotracheal tube of a patient who is intubated.

The drug has few side effects but does have a very unpleasant odor. Some patients experience nausea and even vomiting from the smell. It is also possible for the drug to irritate the airways and cause bronchospasms, although this does not occur often. If the secretions are excessive and the patient cannot cough them up completely, aspiration and pneumonia are possible.

Another major use of acetylcysteine is not related to respiratory mucus. This drug is given intravenously as an antidote for acetaminophen (Tylenol) overdose. If given soon enough, acetylcysteine can protect the kidneys and liver from permanent damage as a result of acetaminophen toxicity.

e-Learning Activity 18-5 ►

## Get Ready for Practice!

### Key Points

- Teach patients with asthma to take drugs exactly as prescribed, even when asthma symptoms have not been present for days.
- Teach patients with asthma to carry a short-acting adrenergic inhaler (used for "rescue") at all times.
- When giving two or more inhalation drugs for asthma at the same time, administer the bronchodilator first and wait at least 5 minutes before giving the second and third drugs.
- Teach patients using dry-powder inhalers not to wash the inhaler or exhale into it.

- Always use a pump or controller when giving any of the methylxanthine type of bronchodilators intravenously.
- Remind the patient who is taking more than one inhaled drug for asthma to take the bronchodilator first and wait at least 5 minutes before taking any other inhaled drug.

### Additional Learning Resources

evolve Go to your Evolve website (http://evolve.elsevier.com/Workman/pharmacology/) for the following FREE learning resources:
- eLearning Activities
- Animations

- Video Clips
- Interactive Review Questions
- Audio Key Points
- Audio Glossary
- Audio Glossary—Spanish-English
- Drug Dosage Calculators
- Patient Teaching Handouts

**SG** Go to your Study Guide for additional learning activities to help you master this chapter content.

## Review Questions

1. A patient is using an albuterol inhaler for a rescue treatment of asthma. You monitor the patient's heart rate and find an increase from 70 beats per minute to 86 beats per minute within 5 minutes of using the inhaler. What is your best action?
   A. Notify the prescriber.
   B. Apply the PRN oxygen by mask.
   C. Raise the head of the bed to 45 degrees.
   D. Document the change as the only action.

2. A patient who received a bronchodilator 20 minutes ago now has all of the following responses. For which one do you notify the prescriber immediately?
   A. Change in oxygen saturation from 89% to 95%
   B. Bad taste in the mouth
   C. Chest pain on exertion
   D. Dryness of the mouth and throat

3. A patient with asthma has been prescribed a dry-powder inhaler. Which statement made by the patient indicates a need for further teaching about the drug regimen?
   A. "I will not exhale into the inhaler."
   B. "I will keep the inhaler in the drawer of my bedroom dresser."
   C. "I will wash the inhaler mouthpiece daily with soap and water."
   D. "I will inhale twice as hard through this inhaler as I do with my aerosol inhaler."

4. What precaution is most important to teach an older patient taking a methylxanthine bronchodilator on a daily basis?
   A. "Avoid coffee and other caffeinated beverages."
   B. "Avoid beer and other alcohol-containing beverages."
   C. "Be sure to take this drug 1 hour before or 2 hours after meals."
   D. "Use sunscreen and protective clothing whenever you go out in the sun."

5. A patient is prescribed a leukotriene inhibitor for respiratory problems. Which health problem is a possible adverse effect of the therapy?
   A. Moon face
   B. Hypertension
   C. Jaundice of the skin
   D. Bad taste in the mouth

6. When a patient is prescribed an inhaled bronchodilator and a mast cell stabilizer at the same time, why must he or she wait 5 minutes after using the bronchodilator before using the mast cell stabilizer?
   A. When the two drugs are taken one right after the other, the effects of both are reduced.
   B. When the two drugs are taken one right after the other, the side effects are more severe.
   C. Giving the bronchodilator first allows the mast cell stabilizer to be more effective.
   D. Giving the bronchodilator first reduces the risk for an allergic reaction to the mast cell stabilizer.

7. What is the most important issue to teach patients about anti-inflammatory drugs for respiratory problems?
   A. To keep the drug with them at all times to use for sudden narrowing of the airways
   B. To take the drug daily, even when symptoms of airway obstruction are not present
   C. To avoid crowds and people who are ill because of the increased risk for infection
   D. To brush their teeth at least 4 times daily to remove the drug from the mouth and improve taste

8. A patient who weighs 198 pounds is prescribed 7 mg of aminophylline per kilogram of body weight intravenously as a loading dose.
   How many kilograms is 198 lbs? _____ kg
   How much drug should this patient receive? _____ mg

9. A child is prescribed 10 mg of zafirlukast (Accolate). You have on hand 20-mg tablets. How many tablets will you give? _____ tablet(s)

## Critical Thinking Activities

It is March in Minnesota, and a 22-year-old female college athlete comes to the health clinic with loud wheezes on exhalation. She explains between breaths that she was running her normal 5 miles on the outdoor track when she started wheezing. She does have asthma and usually carries an albuterol inhaler with her when she runs. Today she forgot her "rescue" inhaler but did take Advair one puff by DPI 2 hours ago. Her vital signs are: pulse 68 beats/min, respirations 34/min, BP 132/92 mm Hg.

1. What additional assessment data should you obtain? Provide a rationale for your choices.

2. Should the patient take another dose of Advair? Why or why not?

3. What should you teach her to help her avoid another episode?

## Objectives

*After studying this chapter you should be able to:*

1. List the common names, actions, usual adult dosages, possible side effects, and adverse effects of antinausea drugs and antiemetic drugs.
2. Describe what to do before and after giving antinausea drugs and antiemetic drugs.
3. Explain what to teach patients taking antinausea drugs and antiemetic drugs, including what to do, what not to do, and when to call the prescriber.
4. Describe life span considerations for antinausea drugs and antiemetic drugs.

5. List the common names, actions, usual adult dosages, possible side effects, and adverse effects of drugs for diarrhea and drugs for constipation.
6. Describe what to do before and after giving drugs for diarrhea and drugs for constipation.
7. Explain what to teach patients taking drugs for diarrhea and drugs for constipation, including what to do, what not to do, and when to call the prescriber.
8. Describe life span considerations for drugs for diarrhea and drugs for constipation.

## Key Terms

**antidiarrheal drugs** (ăn-tē-dī-ŭ-RĒ-ŭl DRŬGZ) (p. 351) Drugs that relieve or control diarrhea or some of the symptoms that go along with diarrhea.

**antiemetic drugs** (ăn-tē-ĕ-MĔT-ĭk DRŬGZ) (p. 342) Drugs that prevent or control nausea and vomiting.

**chemoreceptors** (kē-mō-rē-SĔP-tŭrz) (p. 341) Sensory nerve cells or sense organs such as smell or taste that respond to chemical stimuli and poisonous substances in the intestines.

**constipation** (kŏn-stĭ-PĀ-shŭn) (p. 346) A condition in which bowel movements happen less frequently than is normal for an individual or the stool is small, hard, and difficult or painful to pass.

**diarrhea** (dī-ŭ-RĒ-ă) (p. 351) Frequent watery bowel movements.

**mechanoreceptors** (mĕ-kăn-ō-rē-SĔP-tŭrz) (p. 341) Tension receptors that initiate vomiting because of distention and contraction such as with a bowel obstruction.

**nausea** (NŎ-zē-ă) (p. 341) The state that precedes vomiting; the urge to vomit brought on by many causes such as influenza, medications, pain, and inner ear disease.

**peristalsis** (pĕr-ĭ-STĂL-sĭs) (p. 341) The rippling motion of muscles in the intestines or other tubular organs characterized by alternate contraction and relaxation of the muscles that propel contents forward.

**retching** (RĔCH-ĭng) (p. 341) Labored respiratory movements against a closed throat with contraction of the abdominal muscles, chest wall muscles, and diaphragm but without any expulsion of stomach contents.

**vestibular apparatus** (vĕs-TĬB-yū-lŭr ăp-pŭr-Ă-tŭs) (p. 341) The inner ear structures associated with balance and position sensing.

**vomiting** (VŎM-ĭ-tĭng) (p. 341) The forcing of stomach contents up through the esophagus and out through the mouth.

---

⊖-Learning Activity 19-1 ▶

 **Memory Jogger**

Nausea and vomiting are GI system defenses often used to remove harmful substances from the body.

## OVERVIEW

The gastrointestinal (GI) system begins at the mouth and ends at the anus. It is a hollow tube that is about 25 feet long in an adult (Figure 19-1) and is also called the *digestive system* or the *alimentary canal*. GI system functions include taking in fluids and nutrients (food), breaking down food into forms that the body can use, absorbing useful fluid and nutrients, and eliminating waste products.

The bowel is the lower part of the GI system (see Figure 19-1). Its roles include digesting the food we eat, absorbing the nutrients from digested foods, processing waste products, and expelling the waste products that the body can't use.

The small bowel is where parts of digested food that the body can use are absorbed. It sends waste products to the large bowel *(colon)*. The colon is the waste processing part of the bowel. Waste products have a consistency similar to that of pea soup when entering the colon. The large bowel absorbs fluids from waste products as they move through the colon and form stool *(feces)* (Figure 19-2). Depending on how long stool remains in the colon and how much water is absorbed, the consistency of stool may vary from soft and loose (watery diarrhea) to very hard lumps (constipation).

The rectum and left side of the colon are where stool is stored before a bowel movement occurs. Mass movements (peristalsis) cause stool to enter the rectum (Figure 19-3). These movements can be triggered by food arriving in the stomach or by physical activity such as getting out of bed in the morning, resulting in the sensation that the bowel needs to be emptied. When a person sits on the toilet to move the bowels, first the internal anal sphincter relaxes; then the external sphincter relaxes, and the bowel empties. Bowel movements are complex processes involving several different muscles and nerves located in the pelvic floor. Normal bowel function is different for every person. Bowel movements may occur anywhere between several times per day to several times a week. Consistency of bowel movements is more important than frequency. A person's stool should be soft enough to pass easily out of the bowel but should not be liquid.

## NAUSEA AND VOMITING

### REVIEW OF RELATED PHYSIOLOGY AND PATHOPHYSIOLOGY

Nausea and vomiting are defenses of the GI system and are signs of altered body function. Nausea is the unpleasant sensation of the need to vomit. Vomiting *(emesis)* is the forcing of stomach contents up through the esophagus and out the mouth. The process of vomiting consists of three phases: nausea, retching, and vomiting.

Nausea usually occurs before vomiting. It can be accompanied by cold sweats, pallor, salivation, loss of gastric tone, duodenal contractions, and reflux of intestinal contents into the stomach. It is often followed by retching.

Retching involves labored respiratory movements against a closed throat, with contractions of the abdominal muscles, chest wall muscles, and diaphragm without vomiting. Vomiting does not always follow retching, but retching usually causes enough pressure buildup to lead to vomiting.

Vomiting results from powerful contractions of the abdominal and chest wall muscles, accompanied by lowering of the diaphragm and opening of the sphincter between the stomach and esophagus *(cardiac sphincter)*. It is a reflex, not a voluntary action that involves interactions among the nervous system, vestibular system, vomiting center of the brain, and receptors within the GI tract. The vestibular apparatus is the inner ear structures associated with balance and position sense. When balance or sense of position is upset, vomiting can occur. Tension receptors (mechanoreceptors) initiate vomiting because of distention and contraction such as with a bowel obstruction. Chemoreceptors are sensory nerve cells that respond to chemical stimuli such as poisonous substances (toxins) in the intestines. The mechanoreceptor and chemoreceptor stimuli are sent to the vomiting center in the brain, which controls the act of vomiting (Figure 19-4).

The vomiting center located in the medulla is responsible for initiating the vomiting reflex. It combines the input from the GI tract, vestibular apparatus, and higher brain pressure centers for activation. Once activated, the vomiting center causes vomiting by stimulating the salivary and respiratory centers and the throat (pharyngeal), GI, and abdominal muscles.

There are many causes of nausea and vomiting (Table 19-1). When a person vomits, the body is often trying to remove harmful substances that were ingested. Other possible triggers include disgusting sights, smells, or memories. People often learn to avoid the stimuli that lead to nausea and vomiting because these responses are so unpleasant. Nausea and vomiting are common, severe side effects of chemotherapy.

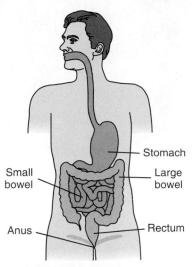

FIGURE 19-1 The GI system.

**? Did You Know?**

Food usually takes 1 to 3 days to be processed by the bowel; about 90% of that time it is spent in the colon.

**💡 Memory Jogger**

The three phases in the process of vomiting are nausea, retching, and vomiting.

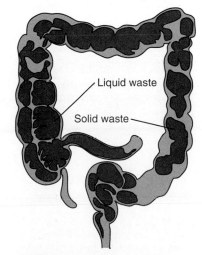

FIGURE 19-2 Fluid is absorbed from the stool by the large bowel as it moves through the colon.

◄⊖-Learning Activity 19-2

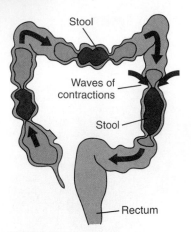

FIGURE 19-3 Peristalsis; mass movements in the colon.

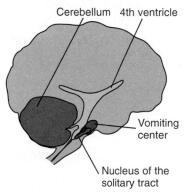

FIGURE 19-4 The vomiting center.

**? Did You Know?**

As many as 25% of patients who could benefit from chemotherapy refuse treatment because the side effects of nausea and vomiting are so unpleasant.

**! Drug Alert!**

**Action/Intervention Alert**

When a patient has nausea and vomiting, be alert for electrolyte, fluid, and nutritional imbalances that must be corrected.

### Table 19-1    Causes of Nausea and Vomiting

| CAUSE | AGENTS |
|---|---|
| Drug- or treatment-induced | Antibiotics<br>Cancer chemotherapy<br>Opiate drugs<br>Radiation therapy |
| Labyrinth disorders | Ménière's disease<br>Motion |
| Endocrine system | Pregnancy |
| Infection | Gastroenteritis<br>Viral labyrinthitis |
| Increased intracranial pressure | Hemorrhage<br>Meningitis |
| Postoperative | Analgesics<br>Anesthetics<br>Procedural |
| Central nervous system | Anticipatory<br>Bulimia nervosa<br>Migraine |

Nausea and vomiting are not only stressful to a person having these experiences; they can also create complications such as bleeding, aspiration pneumonia, dehydration, and reopening of surgical wounds, which can lead to longer hospital stays.

## TYPES OF DRUGS FOR NAUSEA AND VOMITING

### ANTIEMETIC DRUGS

#### How Antiemetic Drugs Work

**Antiemetic drugs** control nausea and prevent vomiting. Nausea and vomiting often occur together, and the same drugs are used for both problems. In addition to drugs, management of a patient with nausea and vomiting includes identifying and treating or eliminating the cause, controlling the symptoms, and correcting imbalances (electrolyte, fluid, and nutritional).

Antiemetic drugs include the phenothiazines, anticholinergics, antihistamines, 5HT$_3$-receptor antagonists, and dopamine receptor antagonists. Each drug affects different receptors, and some drugs affect several sites. For example, 5HT$_3$-receptor antagonists work against nausea and vomiting caused by chemotherapy treatments, whereas antihistamines work against nausea and vomiting caused by opiate drugs or motion. Multiple drugs may be used for nausea and vomiting because different drugs affect different parts of the vomiting reflex pathways.

The phenothiazines block dopamine receptors in the chemotrigger zone of the brain. This action inhibits one or more of the vomiting reflex pathways. The sedating effects help control the sensation of nausea.

Anticholinergic drugs inhibit other pathways of the vomiting reflex. They stop intestinal cramping and inhibit vestibular input (balance and position) into the central nervous system (CNS).

Antihistamines block the action of histamine (a compound released in allergic inflammatory reactions) at the H$_1$ receptor sites. They inhibit the same pathways as anticholinergic drugs and depress inner ear excitability, reducing vestibular stimulation. These different actions work together to control nausea and prevent vomiting.

The 5HT$_3$-receptor antagonists bind to and block serotonin receptors in the intestinal tract and the chemotrigger zone of the brain. By blocking the receptors in both of these sites, at least two pathways of the vomiting reflex are interrupted. These drugs are commonly used to manage the nausea and vomiting resulting from cancer chemotherapy.

Dopamine antagonists directly block dopamine from binding to receptors in the chemotrigger zone and the intestinal tract. Food in the intestinal tract moves along more quickly and is less likely to stimulate responses that trigger the vomiting reflex.

Common names and doses of antiemetic drugs are listed in the following table. Be sure to consult a drug reference for information on specific antiemetic drugs.

## Dosages for Common Antiemetic Drugs

| Drug Class and Name | Dosage |
| --- | --- |
| **Phenothiazines** | |
| promethazine (Histanil✛, Phenergan) | *Adults:* Oral—25 mg at bedtime, or 10-12.5 mg 4 times daily; IM, IV, rectal—25 mg, may repeat in 2 hr<br>*Children:* Oral—5-12.5 mg 3 times daily or 25 mg at bedtime; Rectal (children over 2 years)—0.125 mg/kg every 4-6 hr or 0.5 mg/kg at bedtime |
| prochlorperazine (Compazine, Provazin✛, Stemetil✛) | *Adults/Children over 12 years:* Oral—5-10 mg 3-4 times daily; IM—5-10 mg every 3-4 hr as needed; IV—2.5-10 mg (do not exceed 40 mg/day); Rectal—25 mg twice daily; Elixir—5-10 mg 3-4 times daily<br>*Children less than 12 years* (weight-based): Oral—2.5 mg 1-3 times daily; IM—132 mcg/kg; Rectal (weight-based)—2.5 mg 1-3 times daily |
| **Anticholinergics** | |
| scopolamine (L-hyoscine) | *Adults:* IM, IV, subcutaneous—0.3-0.6 mg; transdermal—1.5 mg<br>*Children:* IM, IV, subcutaneous—6 mcg/kg |
| **Antihistamines** | |
| cyclizine (Marezine) | *Adults:* Oral—50 mg 30 min before travel; IM—50 mg every 4-6 hr as needed<br>*Children:* Oral—25 mg every 4-6 hr as needed; IM—1 mg/kg 3 times daily as needed |
| meclizine (Antivert, Bonamine✛, Dramamine) | *Adults:* Oral—25-50 mg 1 hr before travel for motion sickness, 25-100 mg/day for vertigo |
| **5HT3 Receptor Antagonists** | |
| granisetron (Kytril) | *Adults:* Oral—1 mg twice daily, begin 1 hr before chemotherapy; IV—10 mcg/kg over 30 min, begin 30 min before chemotherapy<br>*Children 2-16 years:* Same as adults |
| ondansetron (Zofran) | *Adults:* Oral—8 mg 30 min before chemotherapy, then every 8 hr and 16 hr after the initial dose; IV—150 mcg/kg infused over 15 min, begin 30 min before chemotherapy<br>*Children over 4 years:* Oral—4 mg 30 min before chemotherapy, then every 8 hr and 16 hr after the initial dose; IV—same dose as adults |
| **Dopamine Antagonists** | |
| metoclopramide (Emex✛, Maxeran✛, Reglan) | *Adults/Children over 14 years:* Oral—10 mg 30 min before symptoms are likely to occur (for example, meals and at bedtime); IV—10 mg<br>*Children 5-14 years:* Dose determined by prescriber |
| trimethobenzamide (Tigan) | *Adults:* Oral—300 mg 3-4 times daily as needed; IM/rectal—200 mg 3-4 times daily as needed |

Top 100 drugs prescribed.

**Drug Alert!**
**Administration Alert**

To *prevent* nausea and vomiting associated with a specific trigger such as cancer chemotherapy or motion, give antiemetics *before* the triggering events and during the time the person usually has these responses.

**Clinical Pitfall**

Ask patients about a history of depression. Metoclopramide (Reglan) can cause mild-to-severe depression and should *not* be prescribed for patients with a history of depression.

**Do Not Confuse**
**Antivert with Axert**

An order for Antivert may be confused with Axert. Antivert is an antihistamine used for nausea, vomiting, and dizziness from motion sickness and for vertigo associated with diseases affecting the inner ear vestibular apparatus. Axert is a vascular headache suppressant used to treat migraine headaches.

*Intended Responses*
- Vomiting reflex is inhibited.
- Vomiting reflex pathways are interrupted or disrupted.
- Patient is sedated.
- Nausea is relieved.
- Vomiting is prevented.

*Side Effects.* Common side effects of antiemetic drugs vary with the prescribed drug. The most common side effects are listed in the following table. Be sure to consult a drug reference for additional information on any specific antiemetic drug.

**Common Side Effects of Antiemetic Drugs**

| Drug | Common Side Effects |
|------|---------------------|
| cyclizine (Marezine) | Drowsiness, dry mouth, hypotension |
| meclizine (Antivert) | Drowsiness |
| metoclopramide (Reglan) | Drowsiness, fatigue, increased depression, restlessness |
| prochlorperazine (Compazine) | Blurred vision, constipation dizziness, dry eyes, dry mouth, involuntary muscle spasms, jitteriness, mouth puckering |
| promethazine (Phenergan) | Confusion, disorientation, dizziness, dry mouth, nausea, vomiting, rash, sedation |
| ondansetron (Zofran) | Abdominal pain, constipation, fatigue, headache |
| granisetron (Kytril) | Headache, constipation, loss of energy |
| scopolamine (L-hyoscine) | Blurred vision, constipation, dilated pupils, dizziness, drowsiness, dry mouth, light-headedness, rash, urinary retention |
| trimethobenzamide (Tigan) | Blurred vision, diarrhea, drowsiness, cramps, headache, hypotension, rectal irritation with suppositories |

Less common side effects include insomnia; diplopia (double vision); tinnitus (ringing in the ears); hypertension; photosensitivity; electrocardiogram (ECG) changes such as tachycardia, bradycardia, and supraventricular tachycardia; pink or reddish-brown urine; urinary retention; anxiety; and depression.

*Adverse Effects.* Adverse effects of antiemetic drugs also vary with the prescribed drug. Promethazine (Phenergan), prochlorperazine (Compazine), and metoclopramide (Reglan) can cause neuroleptic malignant syndrome, a rare and life-threatening side effect in which dangerously high body temperatures can occur. Without prompt and expert treatment, this condition can be fatal in as many as 20% of those who develop it. Signs and symptoms include fever, respiratory distress, tachycardia, seizures, diaphoresis, blood pressure changes, pallor, fatigue, severe muscle stiffness, and loss of bladder control.

Trimethobenzamide (Tigan) may cause coma and seizures. Promethazine (Phenergan) and metoclopramide (Reglan) can cause *tardive dyskinesia*, a chronic disorder of the nervous system. Signs and symptoms include uncontrolled rhythmic movement of the mouth, face, or extremities; lip smacking or puckering; puffing of cheeks; uncontrolled chewing; and rapid or wormlike movements of the tongue. This adverse effect usually occurs after a year or more of continued use of these drugs and is often irreversible. If diagnosed early, tardive dyskinesia may be reversed by stopping the drug.

Promethazine (Phenergan) and prochlorperazine (Compazine) may cause *neutropenia*, a decrease in the number of neutrophils (white blood cells), putting the patient at higher risk for infections. When given by IV push, undiluted promethazine has been associated with severe tissue necrosis.

**Common Side Effects**

**Antiemetic Drugs**

Dizziness   Fatigue   Headache

Blurred vision   Constipation   Drowsiness

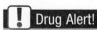 **Drug Alert!**

**Action/Intervention Alert**

Prochlorperazine (Compazine) can cause a decrease in sweating, increasing the risk of overheating of the patient's body. Check body temperature every 4 to 8 hours while a patient is taking this drug.

**Drug Alert!**

**Action/Intervention Alert**

Neuroleptic malignant syndrome is a rare, life-threatening side effect of antiemetic drugs in which dangerously high body temperatures can occur. Be sure to monitor a patient's body temperature every 4 to 8 hours.

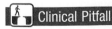 **Clinical Pitfall**

Tardive dyskinesia is an adverse effect of antiemetic drugs that occurs after a year or more of continuous use of these drugs. If it is not diagnosed early, it is *not* reversible.

Respiratory depression (decreased drive for breathing) is a life-threatening effect that can occur with cyclizine (Marezine), promethazine (Phenergan), and scopolamine (L-hyoscine).

## What To Do *Before* Giving Antiemetic Drugs

Check the patient's body temperature, blood pressure, and heart rate and rhythm. Also check his or her baseline respiratory rate and level of consciousness. Obtain a baseline weight and check electrolyte laboratory values. Ask the patient about nausea and vomiting. Ask about any possible causes, allergies, or reactions such as motion sickness.

Use your stethoscope to listen for active bowel sounds in the patient's abdomen. Look for abdominal distention. Ask about the patient's usual diet and fluid intake, bowel movements, constipation, or difficulty swallowing.

Obtain a complete list of drugs the patient is currently taking, including over-the-counter and herbal drugs. Ask whether the patient who is prescribed metoclopramide (Reglan) has experienced depression in the past. If so, notify the prescriber before giving the drug.

If a drug is to be given intravenously, be sure to dilute it first to decrease the risk of tissue necrosis.

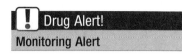

**Drug Alert!**

**Monitoring Alert**

Before giving an antiemetic drug, always observe the abdomen for distention and listen for active bowel sounds.

## What To Do *After* Giving Antiemetic Drugs

Keep track of any episodes of nausea or vomiting to determine the effectiveness of these drugs.

Recheck the patient's body temperature, blood pressure, heart rate and rhythm, and respiratory rate. Obtain daily weights using the same scale and the same amount of clothing at the same time each day. Ask the patient about nausea and vomiting at least every shift. Continue to listen for active bowel sounds and assess for abdominal distention.

Immediately report any signs of respiratory depression to the prescriber. Instruct the patient to call for help getting out of bed and ensure that the call light is within easy reach. Watch for signs of side effects or adverse effects, especially malignant neuroleptic syndrome and tardive dyskinesia. Report any signs immediately to the prescriber.

Check the patient's level of consciousness and watch for sedation effects, especially with older adults.

Some drugs may cause hypotension. Instruct the patient to change positions slowly and call for help when getting out of bed. Be sure that the call light is within easy reach.

Keep track of intake and output (both food and fluid). Ask about GI upset. If these drugs cause GI symptoms, give them with food, milk, or a full glass of water.

Watch for signs of depression in patients taking metoclopramide (Reglan) because this drug may cause mild-to-severe depression. Notify the prescriber immediately because a different drug may be needed to treat the nausea and vomiting.

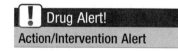

**Drug Alert!**

**Action/Intervention Alert**

Carefully monitor respiratory status and rate while patients are taking antiemetic drugs.

## What To *Teach* Patients About Antiemetic Drugs

Because these drugs may cause drowsiness, caution patients about driving or operating machines. Teach them to use frequent mouth hygiene and mouth rinses to decrease problems associated with dry mouth. Because of sun sensitivity, instruct patients to use sunscreen, wear protective clothing, and avoid tanning beds.

Teach patients about the signs and symptoms of malignant neuroleptic syndrome and tardive dyskinesia. Instruct them to check their body temperature every day and report abnormal signs and symptoms to their prescriber.

Warn patients that prochlorperazine (Compazine) may cause urine to change color to pink or reddish-brown. This condition is temporary and disappears within days after the drug is discontinued.

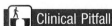
-Learning Activity 19-3 ▶

Tell patients about eating foods with increased bulk and about the importance of drinking enough fluids to prevent constipation. Explain that moderate exercise may also help prevent the side effect of constipation.

Remind patients that for best control of nausea or vomiting, antiemetic drugs should be taken before events that usually cause nausea.

Remind patients to get approval from their prescriber before taking over-the-counter drugs. Advise against using CNS depressants such as alcohol, antihistamines, sedatives, tranquilizers, or sleeping drugs while taking antiemetic drugs.

Suggest the use of a mild analgesic such as acetaminophen for relief from headaches. Teach patients to use frequent mouth rinses and oral care to manage dry mouth. If long-term use of these drugs is planned, remind them to see a dentist regularly to prevent dental disorders.

Remind patients to take a missed dose of the drug as soon as possible but not to take double doses.

### Life Span Considerations for Antiemetic Drugs

*Pediatric Considerations.* Unintentional overdoses of metoclopramide (Reglan) have occurred with infants and children. Teach parents how to read the drug label and correctly give this drug to a child.

Children may have muscle spasms of the jaw, neck, and back, along with jerky movements of the head and face while taking metoclopramide. Balance disturbance is more likely to occur in children with high doses of antiemetic drugs used for cancer chemotherapy.

*Considerations for Pregnancy and Breastfeeding.* Most of these drugs are pregnancy category C, and a woman should check with her prescriber before taking these drugs if she is pregnant or breastfeeding. Some of these drugs, such as metoclopramide (pregnancy category B), pass into breast milk and should be avoided while breastfeeding.

*Considerations for Older Adults.* Older adults are more likely to experience side effects such as acute confusion and dizziness. They may develop a shuffling walk, trembling, and shaking of the hands after taking metoclopramide over a long period of time. They are more likely to develop CNS effects of scopolamine (L-hyoscine) such as confusion, memory loss, unusual excitement, and heat-related disorders. Older adults are also more likely to experience symptoms of balance disturbance with high doses of antiemetic drugs used for cancer chemotherapy and may need lower doses of these drugs.

## CONSTIPATION

### REVIEW OF RELATED PHYSIOLOGY AND PATHOPHYSIOLOGY

Constipation occurs when a person has fewer than three bowel movements a week. Stools become very hard, dry, and difficult to eliminate. Having a bowel movement can be uncomfortable, even painful because of straining, bloating, and having a full bowel. Constipation may also include straining or pushing for longer than 10 minutes when trying to have a bowel movement. Figure 19-5 summarizes how constipation occurs.

Constipation is a symptom, not a disease, usually indicating some other health problem. Just about everyone experiences constipation at some time in his or her life, often because of poor diet. Most episodes of constipation are temporary and are not serious.

The most common causes of constipation are low-fiber diet, lack of physical activity, not taking in enough fluid, and delaying going to the bathroom when the urge to have a bowel movement is felt (Box 19-1). Stress, travel, and other changes

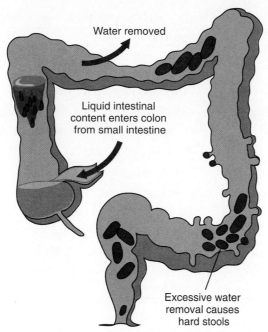

Water removed

Liquid intestinal
content enters colon
from small intestine

Excessive water
removal causes
hard stools

FIGURE 19-5 How constipation occurs.

---

| Box 19-1 | Common Causes of Constipation |

- Abuse of laxatives
- Bowel diseases (for example, irritable bowel syndrome, cancer)
- Changes in life (for example, pregnancy, aging, travel)
- Dehydration
- Drugs
- Ignoring the urge to have a bowel movement
- Lack of physical activity
- Medical problems (for example, hypothyroidism, cystic fibrosis, stroke)
- Mental problems such as depression
- Milk
- Not enough fiber in the diet
- Problems with the colon or rectum
- Problems with intestinal function

---

in bowel habits can lead to constipation. Misuse of laxatives can cause constipation because the body becomes dependent on these drugs, needing higher and higher doses until the bowel no longer works. Bowel diseases, pregnancy, medical illnesses, mental health problems, neurologic problems, and many drugs may also cause constipation (Table 19-2). Drugs may cause constipation by affecting nerve and muscle activity of the colon or binding intestinal fluids. Children often develop constipation when holding back having a bowel movement if they are not yet ready or are afraid of toilet training.

Mild constipation is usually not serious. But, if symptoms are severe, last more than 3 weeks, or complications such as bleeding occur, a health care provider should be informed. Constipation that does not respond to self-treatment, constipation that occurs with rectal bleeding, abnormal pain and cramps, nausea and vomiting, and weight loss should be reported. Patients with severe constipation should be referred to their health care provider to rule out colon cancer. A health care provider should be consulted whenever constipation occurs during pregnancy or breastfeeding.

◄ⓔ-Learning Activity 19-4

### Table 19-2 | Drug Categories That Cause Constipation

| CATEGORY | EXAMPLES |
| --- | --- |
| Antacids | Drugs containing magnesium |
| Anticholinergics | amitriptyline, carbidopa-levodopa, dicyclomine, levodopa, nortriptyline, propantheline |
| Anticonvulsants | phenytoin, valproic acid |
| Antidepressants | amitriptyline, imipramine, phenelzine |
| Antihypertensives | clonidine, methyldopa |
| Antipsychotics | haloperidol, risperidone |
| Bile acid sequestrants | cholestyramine, colestipol |
| Calcium channel blockers | diltiazem, nifedipine, verapamil |
| Calcium supplements | calcium carbonate, PhosCal |
| Iron supplements | Iron-aid (vitamin C, B-12, folic acid), chelated iron |
| Opiates | oxycodone/acetaminophen, propoxyphene napsylate and acetaminophen, drugs containing morphine or codeine |

## TYPES OF DRUGS FOR CONSTIPATION

### LAXATIVES, LUBRICANTS, AND STOOL SOFTENERS

#### How Drugs for Constipation Work

Many people buy over-the-counter drugs to self-treat constipation. The purpose of drugs for constipation is to help the body eliminate hard stools. Products that are available include bulk-forming laxatives, stool softeners, lubricants, saline laxatives, and stimulant laxatives. It is important to remember that laxatives are not meant for long-term use and should not be used for longer than 1 week unless prescribed for longer. Long-term use of laxatives can cause other health problems. The exception is bulk-forming laxatives such as psyllium (Metamucil) that may be taken once a day to help avoid constipation. This drug is not absorbed from the intestines into the body and is safe for long-term use.

Bulk-forming drugs for constipation add bulk to the stool, which increases stool mass that stimulates peristalsis. This helps stool move through the bowel. These drugs may work in as soon as 12 hours but can take as long as 3 days to be effective.

Emollient or softener drugs soften stool, allowing the stool to mix with fatty substances, making it easier to eliminate. Some drugs combine the softening effect with a stimulant to both soften the stool and increase peristalsis to eliminate stool.

Osmotic laxatives cause retention of fluid in the bowel, increasing the water content in stool. Drugs such as lubricants coat the surface of stool and help it hold water so the body can more easily expel it.

Common names and doses of drugs for constipation are listed in the following table. Be sure to consult a drug reference for information on any specific constipation drugs.

> **Clinical Pitfall**
>
> Most laxatives should *not* be used for longer than 1 week, unless a patient is instructed to do so by the prescriber.

#### Dosages for Common Drugs for Constipation

| Drug | Dosage |
| --- | --- |
| *Bulk-Forming Drugs*<br>methylcellulose (Citrucel)<br>psyllium (Fiberall, Karacil✤, Metamucil) | *Adults:* 1 tsp orally 1-3 times daily with 8 oz of fluid<br>*Children:* Give half the adult oral dose with 8 oz of fluid |
| *Emollients/Stool Softeners*<br>docusate (Colace, Regulex✤, Surfak) | *Adults:* 100 mg orally 1-2 times daily<br>*Children:* 10-150 mg orally daily in divided doses; age-based |

### Dosages for Common Drugs for Constipation—cont'd

| Drug | Dosage |
| --- | --- |
| **Emollients Combined with Stimulants** | |
| docusate sodium and casanthranol (Peri-Colace, Diocto C, Silace-C) | *Adults:* 1-4 capsules orally per day<br>*Children:* Not recommended for children <6 years |
| **Stimulants** | |
| bisacodyl (Bisacolax✦, Dulcolax) | *Adults/Children (>12 years):* 5-15 mg single oral dose; 10 mg rectally<br>*Children (<12 years):* 5-10 mg single oral dose; 5-10 mg rectally |
| **Osmotic Laxatives** | |
| lactulose (Cephulac, Cholac, Constilac, Lactulax✦) | *Adults:* 15-30 mL orally 1-2 times daily<br>*Children:* 2.5-10 mL orally twice daily; age-based |
| lubiprostone (Amitiza) | *Adults:* 24 mcg orally twice daily with food |
| magnesium hydroxide (Phillips' Milk of Magnesia) | *Adults:* 5-15 mL orally every 6 hr as needed<br>*Children:* 2.5-5 mL orally 4 times daily as needed |
| polyethylene glycol (GoLYTELY, Klean-Prep✦, MiraLax, Peglyte✦) | *Adults:* Dissolve 17 g in 8 oz and take orally once daily for up to 2 weeks |
| sodium phosphate (Fleet Enema) | *Adults:* One 4.5-oz enema given rectally<br>*Children:* One 2.25-oz enema given rectally |
| **Lubricants** | |
| castor oil (Purge, Emulsoil) | *Adults:* 5-30 mL orally at bedtime<br>*Children:* 5-15 mL orally; 4-oz enema given rectally |
| glycerin suppository (Sani-Supp) | 1 suppository given rectally; hold in rectum 15 min |

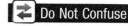

**Do Not Confuse**

**Colace** *with* **Cozaar**

An order for Colace may be confused with Cozaar. Colace is a stool softener, whereas Cozaar is an angiotensin II receptor antagonist used to manage high blood pressure.

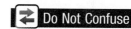

**Do Not Confuse**

**MiraLax** *with* **Mirapex**

An order for MiraLax may be confused with Mirapex. MiraLax is an osmotic diuretic used to treat constipation, whereas Mirapex is a drug used to manage Parkinson's disease.

## Intended Responses
- Stool is softened.
- Stool is passed.
- Constipation is relieved and prevented.

**Side Effects.**   Common side effects of drugs for constipation vary with the prescribed drug. The most common side effects are listed in the following table. Be sure to consult a drug handbook for additional information on any specific constipation drug.

### Common Side Effects of Drugs for Constipation

| Drug | Common Side Effects |
| --- | --- |
| bisacodyl (Dulcolax) | Abdominal cramps, diarrhea, hypokalemia (low potassium), muscle weakness, nausea, rectal burning |
| castor oil (Purge, Emulsoil) | Belching, cramping, diarrhea, nausea |
| docusate (Colace, Surfak) | Mild GI cramps, throat irritation, rashes |
| docusate sodium and casanthranol (Peri-Colace) | Diarrhea, skin rash, stomach cramps, throat irritation |
| glycerin suppository (Sani-Supp) | Abdominal cramps, hyperemia (increased blood flow) of rectal mucosa, rectal discomfort |
| lactulose (Cephulac, Cholac, Constilac) | Abdominal distention, belching, diarrhea, flatulence, GI cramps, hypoglycemia in patient with diabetes |
| lubiprostone (Amitiza) | Abdominal pain and distention, diarrhea, dizziness, dry mouth, gas, headache, nausea, peripheral swelling, reflux |

*Continued*

### Common Side Effects of Drugs for Constipation—cont'd

| Drug | Common Side Effects |
|---|---|
| magnesium hydroxide (Phillips' Milk of Magnesia) | Diarrhea, flushing, sweating |
| polyethylene glycol (MiraLax) | Abdominal bloating, cramping, flatulence (gas), nausea |
| psyllium (Metamucil) | Bronchospasm, GI cramps, intestinal or esophageal obstruction, nausea, vomiting |
| sodium phosphate (Fleet Enema) | Abdominal bloating, abdominal pain, dizziness, electrolyte imbalances (hyperphosphatemia, hypocalcemia, hypokalemia, sodium retention), GI cramping, headache, nausea, vomiting |

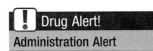

**Common Side Effects**

**Drugs for Constipation**

Diarrhea, Abdominal cramps, Abdominal distention, Nausea

*Adverse Effects.*   Severe life-threatening adverse effects are rare with drugs for constipation. Psyllium (Metamucil) and docusate (Colace) may cause allergic reactions that include difficulty breathing, swelling and closing of the throat, swelling of lips and tongue, or hives.

Side effects of castor oil (Purge) that require medical attention include confusion, irregular heartbeat, muscle cramps, skin rash, and unusual tiredness or weakness.

Lactulose (Cephulac) and bulk-forming drugs containing sugar may cause hyperglycemia (high blood sugar) in patients with diabetes.

Bisacodyl (Dulcolax) may cause hypokalemia, which can lead to life-threatening dysrhythmias.

Fleet Enemas are meant to be used occasionally and can cause electrolyte imbalances when used often.

### What To Do *Before* Giving Drugs for Constipation

Obtain a complete list of drugs that the patient is currently using, including over-the-counter and herbal drugs. Ask the patient about current bowel habits and the nature of his or her normal stools. Check the abdomen for distention and bowel sounds. Obtain baseline vital signs and the patient's weight. If the patient has diabetes, obtain a baseline blood sugar using a fingerstick test.

Ask the patient about abdominal pain. Drugs for constipation should not be given to a patient experiencing undiagnosed abdominal pain or acute abdomen, because these drugs increase peristalsis and the risk of bowel perforation.

Prepare a full glass (8 ounces) of fluid to give with oral drugs. If the patient is also taking antacids, give these drugs at least 1 hour before or after taking them. Be sure to lubricate suppositories before placing them in the rectum.

### What To Do *After* Giving Drugs for Constipation

Recheck the patient's abdomen for distention and bowel sounds. Monitor for bowel movements and assess his or her quality of stools.

Instruct the patient to report bowel movements and any drug side effects to the nursing staff. Be sure to remind patients to drink at least 1500 to 2000 mL of fluid every day to prevent constipation.

### What To *Teach* Patients About Drugs for Constipation

Instruct patients to take oral drugs for constipation with 8 ounces of fluid to be sure the drugs are safe and effective. Advise them to keep a daily record of bowel movements, including the nature of their stools. Tell them that normal bowel patterns vary from person to person and help them determine their normal pattern.

Remind patients that most laxatives should be used only short term (except for bulk-forming drugs such as psyllium, which are safe to take every day). Instruct them to call the prescriber if constipation is not relieved or if rectal bleeding or signs of electrolyte imbalance such as muscle cramps or pain, weakness, or dizziness occur.

Teach patients not to take oral forms of these drugs within 1 hour of taking an antacid drug because antacids decrease absorption.

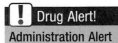

**Drug Alert!**

**Administration Alert**

Do not give constipation drugs if a patient has undiagnosed abdominal pain or acute abdomen because of the increased risk for bowel perforation.

**Drug Alert!**

**Administration Alert**

Give oral drugs for constipation with 8 ounces of fluid at least 1 hour before or after antacids.

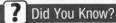

**Did You Know?**

Normal bowel patterns vary widely from several times a day to several times a week. Patients may need your help to determine their normal pattern.

## Life Span Considerations for Drugs for Constipation

*Pediatric Considerations.*   Doses of drugs for constipation given to children 6 to 12 years of age are generally half of the adult dose but should still be given with 8 ounces of fluid. Laxatives or enemas should not be given to children without specific instructions from the prescriber.

*Considerations for Pregnancy and Breastfeeding.*   Most drugs for constipation are considered safe for pregnancy, but the benefits must be assessed by the prescriber before ordering these drugs. Sodium phosphate (Fleet enema) and lubiprostone (Amitiza) are pregnancy category C and should not be used.

*Considerations for Older Adults.*   Constipation is common in older adults, and most constipation drugs are safe for them to use. Psyllium is safe for older adults to use on a daily basis to prevent constipation. Older patients often use laxatives for a longer period and at higher dosages than recommended, which places them at risk for diarrhea and fluid imbalance. Remind older adults to follow package directions for laxative use. Reinforce that increasing fluid intake often relieves constipation without the need for laxatives.

◄ ⊖-Learning Activity 19-5

# DIARRHEA

## REVIEW OF RELATED PHYSIOLOGY AND PATHOPHYSIOLOGY

Diarrhea is an increase in the amount of water in bowel movements and in their volume and frequency. It is not a disease but is a symptom of another health problem. Diarrhea may occur suddenly and usually disappears in a few days even without treatment. It is a fairly common occurrence for all age-groups, and most cases of diarrhea are not serious. However, in children and infants diarrhea can cause dehydration fairly rapidly. It may be an acute, self-limiting occurrence; or it may be a severe, life-threatening illness because of fluid and electrolyte imbalances.

An imbalance between the absorption and secretion functions of the intestines can lead to diarrhea. Absorption is decreased, and secretion is increased (Figure 19-6). Acute diarrhea is three or more loose stools within a 24-hour period, continuing for less than 2 weeks. Most often acute diarrhea goes away within 72 hours. Diarrhea that lasts longer than 2 weeks is considered chronic; however, it may not always include frequent daily passing of loose, watery stools.

There are many causes of diarrhea (Box 19-2), but the most common cause is inflammation of the small bowel *(enteritis)*. Most cases of infectious diarrhea are caused by viruses or bacteria taken in with contaminated food or water or with undercooked meat, poultry, fish, or eggs. Many drugs, including antibiotics, cardiac drugs, GI drugs, and neuropsychiatric drugs can cause diarrhea (Box 19-3). Other causes of diarrhea are radiation therapy, medical problems, gastrectomy, and nerve disorders. The four major types of diarrhea are osmotic, secretory, exudative, and motility disorder (Table 19-3).

## TYPES OF DRUGS FOR DIARRHEA

### ANTIMOTILITY, ADSORBENT/ABSORBENT, AND ANTISECRETORY DRUGS

#### How Antidiarrheal Drugs Work

Drugs for diarrhea (antidiarrheal drugs) are given to control diarrhea and some of the symptoms that occur with this condition. The three types of antidiarrheal drugs are antimotility drugs, adsorbent/absorbent drugs, and antisecretory drugs. The purpose of drugs prescribed for diarrhea is to correct the underlying problem and help the body control diarrhea and its uncomfortable symptoms. Goals of treatment include keeping the patient hydrated, treating the underlying cause, and relieving diarrhea. Be sure to watch for signs and symptoms of electrolyte imbalances that may be caused by diarrhea such as low potassium level *(hypokalemia)*.

**Memory Jogger**

Signs and symptoms of diarrhea are:
- Frequent need to have a bowel movement.
- Abdominal pain and cramping.
- Fever, chills, and generally feeling ill.
- Weight loss.

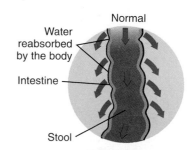

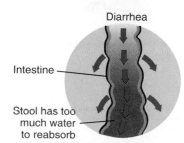

**FIGURE 19-6** Pathophysiology of diarrhea.

**Memory Jogger**

The three types of antidiarrheal drugs are:
- Antimotility drugs.
- Adsorbent/absorbent drugs.
- Antisecretory drugs.

**Memory Jogger**

Signs and symptoms of hypokalemia include cardiac dysrhythmias, muscle pain, general discomfort or irritability, weakness, and paralysis.

---

### Box 19-2  Common Causes of Diarrhea

- Drugs (for example, antibiotics, laxatives, chemotherapy)
- Food poisoning/traveler's diarrhea
- Gastrectomy (partial removal of the stomach)
- High-dose radiation therapy
- Medical conditions (for example, malabsorption, inflammatory bowel diseases such as Crohn's disease or ulcerative colitis, irritable bowel syndrome, celiac disease)
- Nerve disorders (autonomic neuropathy, diabetic neuropathy)
- Other infections (bacterial, parasites)
- Viral gastroenteritis (most common cause)
- Zollinger-Ellison syndrome

---

### Box 19-3  Drugs That Can Cause Diarrhea

**ANTIBIOTICS**
- Ampicillin
- Broad-spectrum antibiotics
- Cephalosporins
- Clindamycin
- Erythromycin
- Sulfonamides
- Tetracycline

**ANTIHYPERTENSIVE DRUGS**
- Guanabenz
- Guanadrel
- Guanethidine
- Methyldopa
- Reserpine

**CARDIAC DRUGS**
- Angiotensin-converting enzyme inhibitors
- Beta blockers
- Digitalis/digoxin
- Diuretics
- Hydralazine
- Procainamide
- Quinidine

**CHOLINERGICS**
- Bethanechol
- Metoclopramide
- Neostigmine

**GASTROINTESTINAL DRUGS**
- Antacids
- Laxatives
- Misoprostol
- Olsalazine

**HYPOLIPIDEMIC DRUGS**
- Clofibrate
- Gemfibrozil
- Statin drugs

**NEUROPSYCHIATRIC DRUGS**
- Alprazolam
- Ethosuximide
- Fluoxetine
- L-Dopa
- Lithium
- Valproic acid

**MISCELLANEOUS**
- Chemotherapy drugs
- Colchicine
- Nonsteroidal anti-inflammatory drugs
- Theophylline
- Thyroid hormones

---

### Table 19-3  Classifications of Diarrhea

| CLASSIFICATION | MECHANISM | CAUSES |
| --- | --- | --- |
| Osmotic | Unabsorbed solutes | Lactose deficiency, magnesium antacid excess |
| Secretory | Increased secretion of electrolytes | *E. coli* infections, ileal resection, thyroid cancer |
| Exudative | Defective colonic absorption, outpouring of mucus and/or blood | Ulcerative colitis, Crohn's disease, shigellosis, leukemia |
| Motility disorder | Decreased contact time | Irritable bowel syndrome, diabetic neuropathy |

Drugs for diarrhea act in several ways. Antimotility drugs slow the movement of stool through the bowel, allowing more time for water and essential salts to be absorbed by the body. Adsorbent/absorbent drugs remove substances that cause diarrhea from the body. Antisecretory drugs decrease secretion of intestinal fluids and slow bacterial activity.

Common names and doses of drugs for diarrhea are listed in the following table. Be sure to consult a drug reference for information on specific antidiarrheal drugs.

### Dosages for Common Antidiarrheal Drugs

| Drug | Dosage |
|---|---|
| *Antimotility Drugs* | |
| difenoxin with atropine (Motofen) | *Adults:* 2 tablets orally followed by 1 tablet after each unformed stool; do not exceed 8 tablets per day |
| diphenoxylate with atropine (Lomotil) | *Adults:* 5 mg orally 4 times daily<br>*Children:* 0.3-0.4 mg/kg orally daily in 4 divided doses (oral solution only; do not use tablets) |
| loperamide (Imodium) | *Adults:* 4 mg orally followed by 2 mg after each unformed stool; do not exceed 16 mg/day<br>*Children:* 1-2 mg orally 3 times daily |
| paregoric (Camphorated Opium Tincture) | *Adults:* 5-10 mL orally after unformed stool; may be given every 2 hr up to 4 times daily<br>*Children:* 0.25-0.5 mL/kg orally 1-4 times daily |
| *Adsorbent/Absorbent Drugs* | |
| attapulgite (Kaopectate❧)<br>bismuth subsalicylate (Kaopectate) | *Adults:* 1200 mg orally after each unformed stool; up to 7 doses per day<br>*Children:* 300-600 mg orally after each unformed stool; up to 7 doses per day |
| calcium polycarbophil (FiberCon) | *Adults:* 1 g orally 1-4 times daily as needed; do not exceed 6 g/day<br>*Children:* 500 mg orally 1-3 times daily as needed; do not exceed 1.5-3 g/day |
| *Antisecretory Drugs* | |
| bismuth subsalicylate (Pepto-Bismol) | *Adults:* 2 tablets or 30 mL orally every 30 min to 1 hr as needed; up to 8 doses per day<br>*Children:* Not recommended for children because it contains subsalicylate |

### Intended Responses
- GI motility is decreased.
- Diarrhea is decreased.
- Fluid from bowel is reabsorbed.
- Secretion of fluids into the bowel is decreased.
- Activity of bacteria is decreased.

***Side Effects.***    Side effects of antidiarrheal drugs are uncommon in healthy adults and vary with the prescribed drug. The most common side effects are listed in the following table. Be sure to consult a drug reference for additional information on any specific antidiarrheal drug.

### Common Side Effects of Antidiarrheal Drugs

| Drug | Common Side Effects |
|---|---|
| attapulgite (Kaopectate) | Constipation, bloating, feeling of fullness |
| bismuth subsalicylate (Pepto-Bismol) | Constipation, gray-black stools, impaction in infants and debilitated patients, tinnitus (ringing in the ears) |

*Continued*

**Common Side Effects**

**Antidiarrheal Drugs**

Constipation, Abdominal discomfort

Dizziness

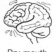

Dry mouth

**Common Side Effects of Antidiarrheal Drugs—cont'd**

| Drug | Common Side Effects |
|------|---------------------|
| calcium polycarbophil (FiberCon) | Abdominal fullness, flatulence (gas), laxative dependence with long-term use |
| difenoxin with atropine (Motofen) | Blurred vision, constipation, confusion, dizziness, drowsiness, dry eyes, dry mouth, flushing, GI distress, headache, insomnia, nausea, nervousness, tachycardia, urinary retention, vomiting |
| diphenoxylate with atropine (Lomotil) | Blurred vision, constipation, confusion, dizziness, drowsiness, dry eyes, dry mouth, flushing, GI distress, headache, insomnia, nervousness, tachycardia, nausea, urinary retention, vomiting |
| loperamide (Imodium) | Abdominal pain/discomfort, allergic reactions, constipation, distention, dizziness, drowsiness, dry mouth, nausea, vomiting |
| paregoric (Camphorated Opium Tincture) | Abdominal pain, constipation, loss of appetite, nausea, vomiting |

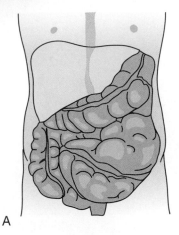

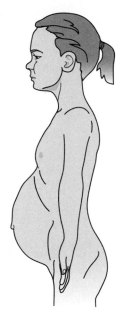

**FIGURE 19-7** Toxic megacolon. **A,** Note the enlarged intestines. **B,** Side view.

---

**! Drug Alert!**

**Action/Intervention Alert**

After giving an antimotility drug, be sure to check the patient for abdominal distention, a sign of toxic megacolon.

---

**! Drug Alert!**

**Action/Intervention Alert**

Bismuth subsalicylate (Pepto-Bismol) contains aspirin. Watch for bleeding because this drug can also increase the effects of the anticoagulant warfarin (Coumadin).

---

***Adverse Effects.*** Adverse effects are rare with antidiarrheal drugs. Calcium polycarbophil (FiberCon) may cause intestinal obstruction.

A potential life-threatening adverse effect of antimotility drugs is *toxic megacolon*, which is a very inflated colon with abdominal distention (Figure 19-7). Other signs and symptoms of this condition include fever, abdominal pain, rapid heart rate, and dehydration. A patient with toxic megacolon may go into shock. When this condition is not recognized and treated early, there is a risk for death.

### What To Do *Before* Giving Antidiarrheal Drugs

Obtain a complete list of drugs that the patient is currently using, including over-the-counter and herbal drugs. Check the patient's baseline weight and set of vital signs. Listen to the abdomen with your stethoscope for active bowel sounds and check for abdominal distention. Observe the patient's skin turgor for signs of dehydration. When a patient is dehydrated, gently pinching and lifting the skin over the sternum, back of the hand, or arm will form a "tent." Use the sternum to test for tenting in the older adult because the skin on the back of hand may tent due to aging. The worse the dehydration, the longer the skin will take to return to its normal position.

Ask patients about allergies or unusual reactions to aspirin or other drugs containing aspirin because bismuth subsalicylate (Pepto-Bismol) contains aspirin. This drug may interact with and increase the effects of anticoagulant drugs such as warfarin (Coumadin).

### What To Do *After* Giving Antidiarrheal Drugs

Reassess the abdomen for bowel sounds and distention. Watch for signs of toxic megacolon if the patient is taking an antimotility drug. If symptoms occur, notify the prescriber immediately.

Recheck and continue to monitor vital signs every 4 to 8 hours. Keep a record of how often the patient has diarrhea stools. Be sure to document the consistency, odor, and appearance of stools. Continue to monitor the skin turgor and encourage the patient to drink plenty of fluids to avoid dehydration.

### What To *Teach* Patients About Antidiarrheal Drugs

Instruct patients to take the drug exactly as ordered by their prescriber. Remind them not to take double doses of these drugs because constipation may result.

Because some of these drugs may cause dizziness or drowsiness, advise patients to avoid driving or performing any activities that require alertness. Tell them that frequent mouth rinses, mouth care, and sugarless gum or candy may be useful to relieve dry mouth. If the drug is a liquid, remind patients to shake well before measuring and taking it.

Remind patients to notify their prescriber if the diarrhea is not relieved in 2 days while taking antidiarrheal drugs or if they develop a fever, abdominal pain, or abdominal distention. Patients should also notify their prescriber if any blood or mucus appears in stools.

Advise patients to avoid the use of alcohol and other CNS depressants while taking these drugs.

Remind patients taking bismuth subsalicylate (Pepto-Bismol) that this drug contains aspirin and that additional aspirin should not be taken because it may cause ringing in the ears (tinnitus). Also tell them that this drug may turn stool and the tongue gray-black.

### Life Span Considerations for Antidiarrheal Drugs

*Pediatric Considerations.*   Children should not be given bismuth subsalicylate because it contains an aspirin-like drug and may cause Reye's syndrome. This is a life-threatening condition that affects the liver and CNS and causes vomiting and confusion. It occurs soon after the onset of a viral illness in which a child was treated with aspirin. Children are more sensitive to the drowsiness and dizziness caused by loperamide (Imodium). Bismuth subsalicylate (Kaopectate) and calcium polycarbophil (Fibercon) are not recommended for preschool children. Infants and children are at increased risk for dehydration with diarrhea.

*Considerations for Pregnancy and Breastfeeding.*   Women who are pregnant or breastfeeding should check with their prescriber before using any antidiarrheal drugs. They should also ask about replacing lost fluids because dehydration can cause a woman to go into early labor.

*Considerations for Older Adults.*   Older adults are at higher risk for dehydration from diarrhea. Be sure that they receive adequate fluid replacement to prevent dehydration. Older adults (over 60) should not use bismuth subsalicylate (Kaopectate) because they are more likely to experience side effects such as constipation.

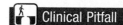

**Clinical Pitfall**

Antidiarrheal drugs should *not* be taken for more than 2 days unless instructed to do so by the prescriber.

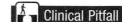

**Clinical Pitfall**

To be safe and prevent Reye's syndrome, children younger than 16 years should *never* be given bismuth subsalicylate (Pepto-Bismol).

◄ ⊖-Learning Activity 19-6

## Get Ready for Practice!

### Key Points

- Nausea and vomiting are distressing for patients and can cause significant clinical complications and extended hospital stays.
- There are many causes of nausea and vomiting involving several central and peripheral neurotransmitter pathways.
- Nausea and vomiting are GI defense mechanisms.
- Drugs for nausea and vomiting are prescribed to manage these symptoms, eliminate the causes, and correct electrolyte and nutritional imbalances.
- Always check a patient's respiratory status before and after giving drugs for nausea and vomiting because respiratory depression can be an adverse effect of some of these drugs.
- Teach patients taking antinausea drugs for motion sickness to take the drug 30 to 60 minutes before expected travel.
- Normal bowel patterns vary widely from several times a day to several times a week.
- Constipation and diarrhea are symptoms, not diseases.
- The most common causes of constipation are poor diet and lack of exercise.

- Always give drugs for constipation with 8 ounces of fluid.
- A person with diarrhea is at high risk for dehydration because of fluid lost in the stool.
- After giving an antimotility drug for diarrhea such as loperamide (Imodium), be sure to check for signs of the life-threatening adverse effect toxic megacolon.
- Teach patients that antidiarrheal drugs should not be taken for more than 2 days unless instructed to do so by their prescriber.

### Additional Learning Resources

ⓔvolve Go to your Evolve website (http://evolve.elsevier.com/Workman/pharmacology/) for the following FREE learning resources:

- eLearning Activities
- Animations
- Video Clips
- Interactive Review Questions
- Audio Key Points
- Audio Glossary
- Audio Glossary—Spanish-English
- Drug Dosage Calculators
- Patient Teaching Handouts

**SG** Go to your Study Guide for additional learning activities to help you master this chapter content.

## Review Questions

1. Which action of metoclopramide (Reglan) helps prevent nausea and vomiting?

    A. Suppressing the vomiting reflex
    B. Helping food move more rapidly through the GI system
    C. Preventing cancer chemotherapy–induced vomiting
    D. Providing a protective coating to the stomach and esophagus

2. Which actions should you take before giving an antinausea drug? (Select all that apply.)

    A. Listen for active bowel sounds.
    B. Look for abdominal distention.
    C. Ask about patient electrolyte values.
    D. Check the respiratory rate.
    E. Ask about patient coagulation tests.
    F. Ask the patient about usual diet intake.

3. What do you teach a patient who is undergoing chemotherapy and is taking an antiemetic drug?

    A. Take this drug with food.
    B. Take the drug 30 minutes before meals.
    C. Take the drug 30 minutes after meals.
    D. Take the drug at bedtime.

4. An older adult taking chemotherapy drugs for cancer is prescribed an antiemetic drug for nausea and vomiting. For which side effects do you monitor?

    A. Muscle spasms of the jaw
    B. Jerky movements of the head
    C. Dizziness
    D. Insomnia

5. Which drug do you expect to be prescribed for a patient who has persistent diarrhea?

    A. meclizine (Antivert)
    B. lactulose (Cephulac)
    C. loperamide (Imodium)
    D. trimethobenzamide (Tigan)

6. What actions must you be sure to take before giving any drug for diarrhea? (Select all that apply.)

    A. Listen for active bowel sounds.
    B. Check for abdominal distention.
    C. Assess skin turgor.
    D. Prepare a full glass of fluid.
    E. Ask about the patient's normal bowel habits.

7. After giving a drug for constipation, how many milliliters of fluid do you instruct the patient to drink every day?

    A. 1000-1200
    B. 1200-1500
    C. 1500-2000
    D. 2000-2400

8. What is the major risk for prescribing bismuth subsalicylate (Pepto-Bismol) to children under 16 years of age?

    A. Hand tremors
    B. Unbalanced gait
    C. Flu-like symptoms
    D. Reye's syndrome

9. A preoperative patient has been ordered scopolamine (L-hyoscine) 0.6 mg intramuscularly. Scopolamine is available in vials with a concentration of 0.3 mg/mL. How many milliliters will you give? _____ mL

10. A patient on chemotherapy is to receive oral metoclopramide (Reglan) 2 mg/kg 30 minutes before each meal. The patient weighs 51 kg. How many milligrams will you give for each dose? _____ mg

11. A patient with dehydration from diarrhea is prescribed IV fluids 1000 mL over 8 hours. How many milliliters per hour will the patient receive? _____ mL/hr

## Critical Thinking Activities

Miss White, who is 80 years old, is admitted to your medical unit with severe diarrhea over the past 3 days. She has been having 8 to 10 watery stools per day and reports abdominal cramps and passing gas (flatulence) frequently. She tells you that she has been unable to eat or drink much during the past 3 days. The prescriber has ordered loperamide (Imodium) 4 mg as an initial dose, followed by 2 mg after each diarrhea stool.

1. What assessments should you make before giving an antidiarrheal drug?

2. Miss White is at risk for what side effect of diarrhea?

3. For what life-threatening adverse effect would you monitor?

4. What should you teach Miss White about this drug?

# Drugs for Gastric Ulcers and Reflux

## Objectives

*After studying this chapter you should be able to:*

1. Explain how different classes of drugs are used to treat peptic ulcer disease (PUD) and gastroesophageal reflux disease (GERD).
2. List the common names, actions, usual adult dosages, possible side effects, and adverse effects of drugs for PUD and GERD.
3. Describe what to do before and after giving drugs for PUD and GERD.
4. Explain what to teach patients taking drugs for PUD and GERD, including what to do, what not to do, and when to call the prescriber.
5. Describe life span considerations for drugs for PUD and GERD.

## Key Terms

**antacids** (ănt-ĂS-ĭdz) (p. 367) Drugs that neutralize the acids produced by the stomach.

**Barrett's esophagus** (BĂR-ĕts ē-SŎF-ŭ-gŭs) (p. 363) A complication of severe chronic GERD involving changes in the cells of the tissue that line the bottom of the esophagus.

**cytoprotective drugs** (sī-tō-prō-TĔK-tĭv DRŬGZ) (p. 369) Drugs that decrease the acid content of the stomach by coating the stomach mucosa and reducing the risk of developing ulcers.

**duodenal ulcer** (dū-ō-DĒ-nŭl ŬL-sŭr) (p. 358) An open sore (ulcer) in the lining of the first part of the small intestine (duodenum).

**dyspepsia** (dĭs-PĔP-sē-ă) (p. 361) Upset stomach; indigestion.

**esophageal ulcer** (ē-sŏf-ŭ-JĒ-ŭl ŬL-sŭr) (p. 358) An open sore (ulcer) in the lining of the esophagus corroded by the acidic digestive juices secreted by the stomach.

**esophagogastroduodenoscopy (EGD)** (ē-SŎF-ŭ-gō-GĂS-trō-DŪ-ŏd-ĕ-NŎS-kō-pē) (p. 359) An upper endoscopy used to evaluate or treat problems of the esophagus, stomach, and part of the small intestine (duodenum).

**gastroesophageal reflux disease (GERD)** (GĂS trō-ē-sŏf-ŭ-JĒ-ŭl RĒ-flŭks dĭz-ÊZ) (p. 357) Esophageal irritation or inflammation often caused by stomach acid that backs up into the esophagus.

**gastric ulcer** (GĂS-trĭk ŬL-sŭr) (p. 358) An open sore (ulcer) in the stomach lining.

***Helicobacter pylori (H. pylori)*** (hĕl-ĭ-kō-BĂK-tŭr pī-LŌR-ē) (p. 359) Bacteria that cause inflammation and ulcers in the stomach.

**histamine H₂ blockers** (HĬS-tă-mēn BLŎ-kŭrz) (p. 363) Drugs that treat the gastric effects of histamine in cases of peptic ulcers, gastritis, and GERD by blocking the effects of histamine on the receptor site known as H₂.

**lower esophageal sphincter (LES)** (LŌ-ŭr ē-sŏf-ŭ-JĒ-ŭl SFĬNK-tŭr) (p. 361) A strong muscular ring located where the esophagus joins the stomach.

**peptic ulcer disease (PUD)** (PĔP-tĭk ŬL-sŭr dĭz-ÊZ) (p. 357) An open sore in the lining of the stomach or duodenum.

**peritonitis** (pĕr-ĭ-tŏn-Ī-tĭs) (p. 360) An inflammation of the abdominal cavity (peritoneum).

**proton pump inhibitor (PPI)** (PRŌ-tŏn PŬMP ĭn-HĬB-ĭ-tŭr) (p. 363) A drug that blocks acid secretion in the stomach.

**regurgitation** (rē-gŭr-jĭ-TĀ-shŭn) (p. 361) Backward flow (reflux) of stomach contents.

**water brash** (WĂ-tŭr BRĂSH) (p. 361) Regurgitation of watery acid from the stomach; a symptom of GERD.

◄ ⊖-Learning Activity 20-1

## OVERVIEW

Peptic ulcer disease (PUD) and gastroesophageal reflux disease (GERD) affect the upper GI system, which consists of the mouth, esophagus, stomach, and upper part of the small intestine (duodenum). PUD may occur in the esophagus, stomach, or upper part of the duodenum. GERD occurs when stomach contents leak backward into the esophagus.

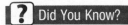
## REVIEW OF RELATED PHYSIOLOGY AND PATHOPHYSIOLOGY

Food is digested and converted into a form that the body can use. The upper GI system is responsible for taking in and moving food to the stomach. Digestion begins in the mouth, where chewing changes the food to a fine texture; saliva moistens it and begins the conversion of starch into simple sugars. The food is then swallowed, passing through the pharynx and down the esophagus to the stomach. Specialized cells in the stomach *(gastric glands)* secrete digestive enzymes and gastric juices, which act on the partially digested food. The stomach also physically churns and mixes the food. Stomach secretions include the enzyme pepsin, which acts on proteins; hydrochloric acid, needed for the action of pepsin; and an enzyme, gastric lipase, which begins the breakdown of fats. These acid substances that digest food also have the potential to damage or break down normal GI tissues.

The stomach secretes thick gel-like mucus to coat and protect it from contact with stomach acids. In most people acid production is balanced by mucus secretion, and ulcers do not form. Whenever acid production exceeds mucus production, the risk for ulcers and tissue damage increases. Health problems, genetic influences, lifestyle influences, and certain drugs can decrease mucus production or increase acid secretion and upset the protective balance. The intestinal tract, unlike the stomach, does not secrete large amounts of the protective mucus. Instead it relies on buffers such as bicarbonate to neutralize stomach acids before they reach the intestines.

### GASTROINTESTINAL ULCERS

GI ulcers are fairly common. About 10% of people in the United States develop an ulcer during their lifetime. A GI ulcer is an open sore found in the mucosal lining of the stomach or duodenum where hydrochloric acid and pepsin are located. These ulcers are also commonly referred to as *peptic ulcer disease (PUD)*. When a peptic ulcer occurs in the stomach, it is called a **gastric ulcer,** and when an ulcer is formed in the duodenum it is called a **duodenal ulcer** (Figure 20-1).

Esophageal ulcers usually occur in the lower part of the esophagus near the stomach. An **esophageal ulcer** is a hole in the lining of the esophagus that has been

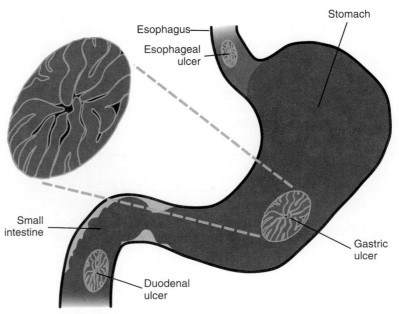

**FIGURE 20-1** Locations of gastric, duodenal, and esophageal ulcers.

damaged by the acidic digestive juices secreted by the stomach cells. This type of ulcer is often associated with chronic GERD when acidic stomach contents back up (reflux) into the esophagus.

In the past the causes of peptic ulcers were believed to be excess acids and lifestyle factors such as stress and too many spicy foods. However, research has shown that 80% to 90% of gastric ulcers are caused by infection with the *Helicobacter pylori (H. pylori)* bacteria. *H. pylori* infection is present in 20% to 30% of people in the United States. Some people experience no signs or symptoms, whereas others develop ulcers. Today it is believed that lifestyle (for example, stress and diet), along with excess acids and *H. pylori* infection, have roles in the development of ulcers; but *H. pylori* is the primary cause. Box 20-1 summarizes the factors that are suspected to have a role in the development of peptic ulcers.

Gastric mucosa resists damage; but, when there is an increase in gastric acidity or a decrease in prostaglandins, which increase the production of bicarbonate and also produce the protective mucus, there is danger of developing an ulcer (Figure 20-2). The mucosa breaks down and an open sore or raw area develops in the stomach or upper part of the intestine (duodenum).

The most common symptom of a peptic ulcer is burning, gnawing pain caused by stomach acid coming into contact with the open wound (ulcer). The pain usually occurs somewhere between the navel (*umbilicus*) and the breastbone (*sternum*) and may last from a few minutes to many hours. It often occurs when the stomach is empty and can be relieved by eating foods that buffer stomach acids or taking a drug that reduces stomach acid such as an antacid. The pain may flare up at night or come and go for a few days to several weeks. Other symptoms of a gastric ulcer include vomiting blood (bright red or black), dark blood in the stool, nausea or vomiting, belching, unexplained weight loss, and chest pain.

A gastric ulcer is diagnosed by either a barium swallow test followed by an upper GI x-ray series or by an upper endoscopy called an **esophagogastroduodenoscopy (EGD)**. An EGD is more accurate but requires that the patient be sedated for the insertion of a flexible tube to inspect the esophagus, stomach, and duodenum for ulcers. The instrument used to perform this procedure is also capable of removing small tissue samples (biopsy) to test for the presence of *H. pylori* infection.

 **Memory Jogger**

The primary cause of 80% to 90% of GI ulcers is infection with the *H. pylori* bacteria.

 **Memory Jogger**

The most common symptom of a peptic ulcer is burning, gnawing pain that occurs between the umbilicus and sternum.

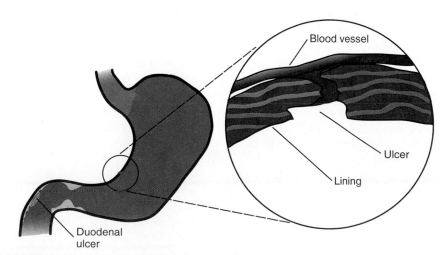

**FIGURE 20-2** Gastric ulcer pathophysiology: The mucosa breaks down and an open sore develops.

| Box 20-1 Factors in the Development of Peptic Ulcers |
| --- |

- Acid and pepsin
- Alcohol
- Caffeine
- *H. pylori* bacteria infection
- Nonsteroidal anti-inflammatory drugs
- Smoking
- Stress

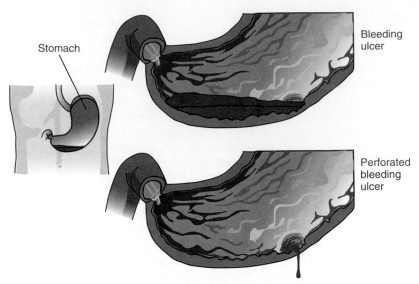

**FIGURE 20-3** A peptic ulcer may lead to bleeding, perforation, or other emergencies.

| Box **20-2** | Signs That Indicate an Ulcer Is Getting Worse |
| --- | --- |

- Blood in stools
- Continuing nausea or repeated vomiting
- Feeling cold or clammy
- Feeling weak or dizzy
- Losing weight
- Pain that doesn't go away after taking drugs
- Pain that radiates to the back
- Sudden severe pain
- Vomiting blood
- Vomiting food eaten hours or days ago

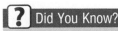 **Did You Know?**

No special diet is recommended for the prevention or treatment of ulcers. A bland diet has not been shown to be effective.

Treatment of ulcers involves not only drugs but also lifestyle changes. Recommended lifestyle changes include avoiding irritating foods, caffeine, and excessive alcohol. Smoking cessation is highly recommended because smoking slows ulcer healing and is related to the return of ulcers. Smoking increases acid secretion; reduces prostaglandin, mucus, and bicarbonate production; and decreases mucosal blood flow. Patients with a gastric ulcer are instructed to avoid excess stress and nonsteroidal anti-inflammatory drugs (NSAIDs). NSAIDs are associated with the development of gastric upset and ulcers because they inhibit prostaglandins. As many as 15% of patients on long-term NSAID treatment may develop ulcers of the stomach or duodenum.

Although most ulcers heal within a few weeks with drug treatment, some serious complications may occur. When an ulcer damages GI tissues, blood vessels may also be damaged, resulting in a bleeding ulcer (Figure 20-3). Sometimes an ulcer causes a hole in the wall of the stomach or duodenum, allowing partly digested food and bacteria to enter the sterile abdominal cavity (*peritoneum*) and causing an inflammation and infection of the abdominal cavity (**peritonitis**). Signs that tell you that an ulcer is getting worse are listed in Box 20-2.

### GASTROESOPHAGEAL REFLUX DISEASE

Most people suffer from occasional heartburn, but when heartburn occurs daily, exposure of the mucosa of the esophagus to stomach acids can cause irritation and inflammation. *Gastroesophageal reflux disease (GERD)* is a condition in which the liquid contents of the stomach back up (*regurgitate* or *reflux*) into the esophagus. At the end of the esophagus where it connects to the stomach is a strong muscle ring called the

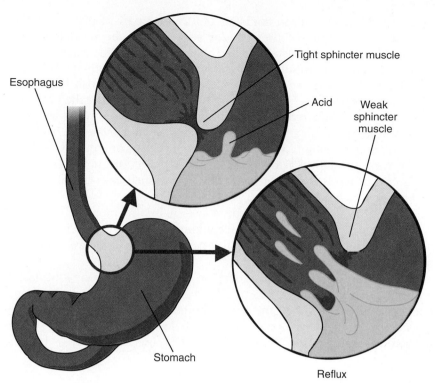

**FIGURE 20-4** Acid reflux in the lower esophageal sphincter.

| Box 20-3 | Risk Factors for GERD |

- Being overweight
- Being pregnant
- Certain diseases (for example, diabetes, asthma, peptic ulcers)
- Certain drugs (for example, nonsteroidal anti-inflammatory drugs)
- Drinking alcohol and caffeinated beverages
- Eating foods with high acid content (for example, tomatoes, orange juice)
- Eating fatty and spicy foods
- Lying down too soon after meals
- Smoking

**lower esophageal sphincter (LES).** The LES stays tightly shut except when food or liquids pass into the stomach. When closed it prevents stomach contents from backing up into the esophagus. Reflux or **regurgitation** happens when the LES is not working correctly (Figure 20-4). The LES may relax during periods of the day or night, or it may become too weak and constantly allow stomach contents to flow upward into the esophagus. When the LES is very weak and GERD is severe, a patient may need surgery to strengthen the LES.

Most people experience reflux occasionally; a person with GERD has reflux more often, and the stomach contents stay in the esophagus for longer periods of time. The regurgitated stomach contents contain stomach acids and pepsin and may also contain bile. These substances can injure the esophagus, causing inflammation and tissue damage, including ulcers. Risk factors for developing GERD are listed in Box 20-3.

The most common symptom of GERD is **dyspepsia** (heartburn). Other common symptoms include sour or bitter taste; bitter stomach fluid going into the mouth, especially during sleep; hoarseness; **water brash** (regurgitation of watery acid from the stomach); a repeated need to clear the throat; difficulty swallowing food or liquid; wheezing or coughing at night; and worsening of symptoms after eating or when bending over or lying down.

 Memory Jogger

The cause of GERD is an LES that is not working correctly and allows stomach contents to back up (reflux) and damage the esophagus.

 Memory Jogger

The most common symptom of GERD is dyspepsia (heartburn).

◄ ⊖-Learning Activity 20-2

GERD is best diagnosed on the basis of a careful patient history by the health care provider. An endoscopy done under sedation can be used to examine the esophagus and stomach for tissue damage and determine the severity of the disease.

GERD is a chronic condition; treatment is lifelong. Treatment of GERD is divided into five stages (Box 20-4) and involves not only drugs but also lifestyle changes (Table 20-1) such as smoking cessation (because nicotine weakens the LES), decreased dietary fat intake, weight reduction, and avoidance of large meals and foods that cause regurgitation. A patient with GERD is instructed to elevate the head of the bed at least 6 to 10 inches using blocks under the top bed legs or a pillow wedge (Figure 20-5). After meals the patient with GERD should remain upright for 3 hours. Patients should also avoid foods that cause increased reflux such as chocolate, peppermint, alcohol, and caffeinated drinks.

Chewing gum after meals may be a useful treatment for GERD because it increases the production of saliva, which contains bicarbonate, and increases the rate of swallowing. The bicarbonate in saliva neutralizes acid in the esophagus and decreases the irritation of refluxed stomach contents.

Complications of GERD occur when the disease is severe or long lasting. The constant irritation of the esophagus by stomach contents can lead to inflammation, ulcers, and bleeding. Bleeding can cause anemia. Over time scarring of the esophagus can cause it to narrow, making it difficult to swallow. Narrowing of the esophagus is called an *esophageal stricture*. Chronic GERD can cause changes in the cells of

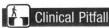
**Clinical Pitfall**

Patients with GERD should *avoid* chocolate, peppermint, alcohol, and caffeinated drinks because they lower the pressure of the LES and promote reflux.

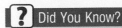
**Did You Know?**

Chewing gum after meals may prevent irritation of the esophagus associated with GERD.

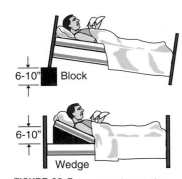

**FIGURE 20-5** How to elevate the head of the bed.

**Box 20-4**   Stages of Treatment for GERD

Stage I: Lifestyle modifications
Stage II: As-needed drug therapy
- Antacid and/or antacid-containing alginic acid
- Over-the-counter histamine H$_2$ blocker
Stage III: Scheduled pharmacologic therapy
- Histamine H$_2$ blocker for 8 to 12 weeks
- For persistent symptoms: high-dose H$_2$ blocker or proton pump inhibitor for additional 8 to 12 weeks
- Proton pump inhibitors as first choice for documented erosive esophagitis
Stage IV: Maintenance therapy
- For patients with symptoms of relapse or complicated disease
- Lowest effective dosage of histamine H$_2$ blocker or proton pump inhibitor
Stage V: Surgery
- For patients with severe symptoms, erosive esophagitis, or disease complications
- Fundoplication procedure to strengthen lower esophageal sphincter

**Table 20-1**   Lifestyle Changes for Treatment of GERD

| LIFESTYLE CHANGE | RATIONALE |
|---|---|
| Avoid eating within 3 hours of bedtime | Decreases risk of nighttime reflux |
| Stop smoking | Nicotine weakens the LES |
| Avoid alcohol (especially red wine), caffeine, chocolate, citrus fruits and juices, fatty foods, milk, peppermint, pepper seasoning, spearmint, and tomato products | These foods cause increased reflux |
| Decrease portions at mealtimes | Decreases reflux |
| Avoid tight-fitting clothes and bending after meals | Decreases reflux |
| Elevate the head of the bed or mattress 6 to 10 inches | Helps keep acid in stomach by gravity while sleeping |
| Lose weight if overweight | Relieves pressure on the stomach and LES |

*LES,* Lower esophageal sphincter.

the esophagus, leading to precancerous cells and cancer. This condition is called **Barrett's esophagus** and occurs in about 10% of patients with GERD. Barrett's esophagus increases the risk of developing esophageal cancer.

## GENERAL ISSUES FOR DRUGS FOR PUD AND GERD

There are several classes of drugs used to treat PUD and GERD that have both different and common actions and effects. Nursing responsibilities for these common actions and effects are listed in the following paragraphs. Specific nursing responsibilities are listed with each individual class of drugs.

*Before giving drugs for PUD or GERD*, be sure to obtain a complete list of drugs currently being used by the patient, including over-the-counter and herbal drugs. Not only can some drugs increase the risk for PUD or GERD, but the drugs used to treat these problems may interfere with the absorption of other drugs.

Obtain a baseline set of vital signs, including body temperature, and obtain a baseline weight. Ask patients about normal bowel habits, appearance of stools, bleeding, vomiting, and reflux (location, duration, character, and factors that cause it to occur).

◄ⓔ-Learning Activity 20-3

Listen to the abdomen with your stethoscope for bowel sounds, check for distention, and ask about abdominal pain. Instruct the patient to report any episodes of heartburn or reflux.

*After giving drugs for PUD or GERD*, be sure to recheck vital signs every shift and weigh patients every morning. Also watch for abnormal heart rhythms (too fast, too slow, irregular). Keep track of bowel movement frequency and consistency. Check the abdomen for active bowel sounds and distention every shift. Remind the patient about the potential for altered bowel functions, including constipation and diarrhea. Ask patients about bowel movements every day. Record any episodes of reflux, heartburn, or indigestion.

*Teach patients taking a drug for PUD or GERD* to take the drug exactly as prescribed for the period of time prescribed, even when they are feeling better. Remind them to take a missed dose as soon as possible but not to take a double dose.

Tell patients to notify their prescriber for difficulty swallowing; persistent abdominal pain; vomiting blood (bright red or coffee grounds–appearing emesis); or black, tarry stools. Remind them that increased fluid intake, fiber-containing foods, and exercise can help prevent constipation.

Advise patients to avoid alcohol, aspirin-containing products, NSAIDs, and foods that cause increased GI irritation. All of these substances increase the risk for ulcer development.

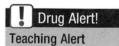

**Drug Alert!**

**Teaching Alert**

Teach patients with PUD or GERD to avoid substances that cause increased GI irritation, such as alcohol, NSAIDs, and aspirin.

## TYPES OF DRUGS FOR PUD AND GERD

Anti-ulcer drugs are used to treat ulcers of the stomach and duodenum. **Histamine H₂ blockers** decrease the secretion of gastric acid, and **proton pump inhibitors (PPIs)** block the secretion of gastric acid. *Cytoprotective drugs* such as sucralfate (Carafate) are used to form a thick coating that covers an ulcer to protect the open sore from further damage and allows healing to occur. Antibiotics are used to treat *H. pylori* infections that are the major cause of ulcers.

Several groups of drugs are used to treat GERD. Drugs used to treat PUD such as histamine H₂ blockers and PPIs are also used to treat GERD. Antacids can neutralize stomach acid and decrease the ability of acid to irritate and inflame the esophagus. Metoclopramide (Reglan), a promotility drug, increases LES tone and helps to empty the stomach.

◄ⓔ-Learning Activity 20-4

### HISTAMINE H₂ BLOCKERS

#### How Histamine H₂ Blockers Work
Histamine H₂ blockers (*antagonists*) cause decreased stimulation of H₂ receptors in gastric cells that secrete hydrochloric acid (*parietal cells*), leading to a decrease in

gastric acid secretion. When histamine binds to receptors in the stomach lining, acid pumps are activated, releasing acid into the stomach. $H_2$ blockers prevent histamine from stimulating the pumps in the stomach that produce hydrochloric acid.

Histamine $H_2$ blockers are used to heal ulcers or relieve the symptoms and pain that occur with GERD. These drugs are available over the counter and by prescription. Over-the-counter $H_2$ blockers are lower dose and are useful for prevention and relief of mild heartburn, indigestion, or sour stomach. Prescription-strength $H_2$ blockers come in higher doses and are used for moderate-to-severe forms of GERD.

Common names and doses of drugs for histamine $H_2$ blockers are listed in the following table. Be sure to consult a drug handbook for information on specific histamine $H_2$ blockers.

### Dosages for Common Histamine $H_2$ Blockers

| Drug | Dosage |
|---|---|
| nizatidine (Axid) | *Adults:* 75-150 mg orally twice daily 30-60 min before meals or 300 mg once daily at bedtime |
| famotidine (Pepcid, Pepcid RPD🍁) | *Adults:* 10-20 mg orally twice daily or 40 mg once daily at bedtime (do not exceed 40 mg/day) |
| ranitidine (Gen-Ranitidine🍁, Zantac, Zantac-C🍁) **TOP 100** | *Adults:* Oral—150 mg twice daily or 300 mg once daily at bedtime (do not exceed 300 mg/day); IV, IM—50 mg every 6 to 8 hr<br>*Children over 12 years:* Oral—l75-150 mg every 12 hr or once daily (do not exceed 300 mg/day); IV, IM—3-6 mg/kg/day divided in doses every 6 hr (do not exceed 200 mg/day) |
| cimetidine (Novo-Cimetine🍁, Peptol🍁, Tagamet) | *Adults:* Oral—300 mg 4 times daily or 400 mg twice daily; IM, IV—300 mg every 6 to 8 hr<br>*Children:* Oral, IM, IV—20-40 mg/kg/day in 4 divided doses |

**TOP 100** Top 100 drugs prescribed.

### *Intended Responses*
- Secretion of gastric acid is decreased.
- Symptoms of GERD are decreased.
- Ulcers are healed and prevented.

***Side Effects.*** The most common side effect of histamine $H_2$ blockers is confusion. Other common side effects include dizziness, drowsiness, headaches, altered sense of taste, constipation, diarrhea, nausea, impotence and decreased sperm count, anemia, neutropenia (decreased number of neutrophil white blood cells), and thrombocytopenia (low platelet count).

Ranitidine (Zantac) may also cause a blackened tongue and dark stools. Nizatidine (Axid) and cimetidine (Tagamet) may cause drug-induced hepatitis.

***Adverse Effects.*** Adverse life-threatening effects of $H_2$ blockers include abnormal heart rhythms (dysrhythmias), decreased white blood cell count (*agranulocytosis*), and anemia caused by deficient red blood cell production by the bone marrow (*aplastic anemia*).

### What To Do *Before* Giving Histamine $H_2$ Blockers
Be sure to review the general nursing responsibilities related to drugs for PUD and GERD (p. 363) in addition to these specific responsibilities before giving histamine $H_2$ blockers.

Check the patient's baseline level of consciousness because drowsiness is a common side effect of these drugs. Use this information to determine patient responses to the drug.

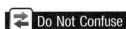

### Do Not Confuse

#### Zantac *with* Zyrtec

An order for Zantac may be confused with Zyrtec. Zantac is a histamine $H_2$ blocker used to decrease secretion of stomach acids, whereas Zyrtec is an antihistamine drug used for allergies.

### Drug Alert!

#### Action/Intervention Alert

Watch for confusion, the most common side effect, when giving histamine $H_2$ blockers.

### Common Side Effects

#### Histamine $H_2$ Blockers

Confusion

Dizziness

Drowsiness

Headache

Nausea/ Vomiting

Give the drug with meals to prolong its therapeutic effects. If the patient is prescribed to take a histamine $H_2$ blocker once a day, give it at bedtime to prolong its effects when there is no food in the stomach and reflux may be worse.

If the patient is to receive an intravenous (IV) drug, be sure to check the IV site at least every 2 to 4 hours for patency and signs of infection.

### What To Do *After* Giving Histamine $H_2$ Blockers

Be sure to review the general nursing responsibilities related to drugs for PUD and GERD (p. 363) in addition to these specific responsibilities after giving histamine $H_2$ blockers.

Because these drugs may cause dizziness or drowsiness, ensure that the call light is within easy reach and remind patients to call for help when getting out of bed.

Watch for other side effects, including nausea or vomiting. Notify the prescriber for any signs of allergic reaction (for example, fever, sore throat, rashes); confusion; black, tarry stools; dizziness; or hallucinations.

### What To *Teach* Patients About Histamine $H_2$ Blockers

Be sure to teach patients about general issues and precautions related to drugs for PUD and GERD (p. 363) in addition to these specific teaching points for histamine $H_2$ blockers.

Advise patients who have been taking over-the-counter histamine $H_2$ blockers for more than 2 weeks to see their prescriber if symptoms have not improved, because these drugs are used for short-term treatment of GERD and ulcers. Signs and symptoms of GERD and PUD are similar to those for stomach cancer, which should be ruled out.

Remind patients that smoking interferes with the action of histamine $H_2$ blockers and encourage them to quit smoking. Because these drugs may cause dizziness or drowsiness, caution patients to avoid driving, operating machines, or engaging in any other activities that require alertness until they know how the drug affects them.

### Life Span Considerations for Histamine $H_2$ Blockers

***Considerations for Pregnancy and Breastfeeding.*** Histamine $H_2$ blockers are pregnancy category B and have not been studied in pregnant women. A woman should always tell her health care provider if she is pregnant or planning to become pregnant. Pregnant women frequently experience heartburn. They should not take any drugs without consulting their health care provider. Instead they should try nonpharmacologic and lifestyle changes first such as limiting spicy foods or foods that cause gas, sitting up for 2 to 3 hours after eating, eating more slowly, and eating more frequent smaller meals. These drugs pass into breast milk and may cause undesired side effects in the breastfeeding infant. They should be avoided while breastfeeding.

***Considerations for Older Adults.*** Older adults are more likely to experience confusion and dizziness because of increased sensitivity to the side effects of histamine $H_2$ blockers when compared to younger adults. Teach family members to watch for changes in cognition or increased confusion. Teach older adults to take special precautions to avoid falls. Instruct them to change positions slowly and to use handrails when going up or down stairs. Suggest that older adults avoid driving or using heavy machinery until they know how the drug affects them.

## PROTON PUMP INHIBITORS

### How Proton Pump Inhibitors Work

Normally the stomach produces acid to help break down food in the process of digestion. When the acid irritates the mucosal lining of the stomach or duodenum, ulceration or bleeding can occur. Proton pump inhibitors (PPIs) work by completely blocking the production of stomach acid. These drugs block the action of "pumps" located in acid-secreting cells, which totally blocks stomach acid secretion.

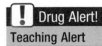

**Drug Alert!**

**Teaching Alert**

Teach patients to notify their prescriber if they have been taking over-the-counter $H_2$ blockers for more than 2 weeks and are still experiencing reflux.

**Clinical Pitfall**

Patients taking histamine $H_2$ blockers should *not* smoke because smoking interferes with the action of these drugs.

**Drug Alert!**

**Action/Intervention Alert**

Monitor older adults closely because they are more likely to experience confusion and dizziness as side effects of histamine $H_2$ blockers.

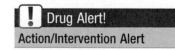

◄ ⊜-Learning Activity 20-5

**Do Not Confuse**

**rabeprazole** *with* **aripiprazole**

An order for rabeprazole may be confused with aripiprazole. Rabeprazole is a PPI used to block gastric secretions, whereas aripiprazole is an antipsychotic drug used for schizophrenia and acute bipolar episodes.

 **Do Not Confuse**

**Prilosec** *with* **Prinivil**

An order for Prilosec may be confused with Prinivil. Prilosec is a PPI used to block stomach acid secretion, whereas Prinivil is an angiotensin-converting enzyme inhibitor used to treat high blood pressure.

**Common Side Effects**

**Proton Pump Inhibitors**

Diarrhea, Constipation,    Headache
Gas, Abdominal pain

 **Drug Alert!**

**Administration Alert**

For best effects PPIs should be given before meals, preferably in the morning.

 **Clinical Pitfall**

Black, tarry stools are *never* normal; they indicate bleeding and should be reported to the prescriber immediately.

PPIs are the most powerful drugs used for treating PUD or GERD and should be used for limited periods of time. They are used when H₂ blockers are not effective. Often PPIs are used in combination with antibiotics to treat *H. pylori* infections in the stomach.

Some are available over the counter; others require a prescription. Common names and doses of drugs for PPIs are listed in the following table. Be sure to consult a drug reference handbook for information on specific PPIs.

**Dosages for Common Proton Pump Inhibitors**

| Drug | Dosage |
|---|---|
| omeprazole (Losec🍁, Prilosec) [TOP 100] | *Adults:* 20-40 mg orally once daily for 4-8 wk |
| lansoprazole (Prevacid) | *Adults:* 15-30 mg orally once daily for 4-8 wk |
| rabeprazole (Aciphex, Pariet🍁) | *Adults:* 20 mg delayed-release tablets orally once daily for 4-8 wk |
| pantoprazole (Protonix) [TOP 100] | *Adults:* 40-80 mg orally once daily |
| esomeprazole magnesium (Nexium) [TOP 100] | *Adults:* 20-40 mg orally once daily for 10 days |

[TOP 100] Top 100 drugs prescribed.

### Intended Responses
- Gastric acid secretion is decreased.
- Acid reflux is decreased.
- Ulcers are healed.

**Side Effects.** Side effects rarely occur with PPIs. The most common side effects are diarrhea, constipation, belching and gas, abdominal pain, and headaches. Some patients report generally feeling ill while taking these drugs.

Lansoprazole (Prevacid), omeprazole (Prilosec), and rabeprazole (Aciphex) also may cause dizziness. In addition, rabeprazole may cause increased sun sensitivity (photosensitivity).

Long-term use of PPIs may lead to stomach infections because these drugs inhibit production of stomach acids that help to kill bacteria. This may also lead to anemia because the loss of stomach acid reduces digestion of protein essential for making new cells.

**Adverse Effects.** Allergic reactions are rare and include itching, dizziness, swollen ankles, muscle and joint pain, blurred vision, depression, and dry mouth.

### What To Do *Before* Giving Proton Pump Inhibitors
Be sure to review the general nursing responsibilities related to drugs for PUD and GERD (p. 363) in addition to these specific responsibilities before giving PPIs.

Give these drugs before meals, preferably in the morning. PPIs can be given with antacids and with or without food.

If the patient is to be given an IV drug, be sure to check the IV site for patency and signs of infection.

### What To Do *After* Giving Proton Pump Inhibitors
Be sure to review the general nursing responsibilities related to drugs for PUD and GERD (p. 363) in addition to these specific responsibilities after giving PPIs.

Report any black, tarry stools to the prescriber immediately. These are indicators of upper GI bleeding, which can lead to severe hemorrhage.

If lansoprazole, rabeprazole, or omeprazole is prescribed, teach the patient to call for help when getting out of bed because these drugs may cause dizziness. Be sure that the call light is within easy reach.

### What To *Teach* Patients About Proton Pump Inhibitors
Be sure to teach patients about general issues and precautions related to drugs for PUD and GERD (p. 363) in addition to these specific teaching points for PPIs.

Instruct patients to take the drug exactly as prescribed and to take it for the full time period, even when they are feeling better. These drugs do not cure the ulcer; they just change the GI environment so that healing is more likely to occur. Stopping the drug too soon can allow a partially healed ulcer to reopen.

Instruct patients to report any black, tarry stools; diarrhea; abdominal pain; or persistent headaches to their prescriber immediately because these are signs of bleeding and possible low blood volume (hypovolemia).

Caution patients prescribed lansoprazole, omeprazole, or rabeprazole to avoid driving or engaging in other activities that require increased alertness. These drugs may cause dizziness.

Teach patients taking rabeprazole about the importance of wearing sunscreen and protective clothing when going outdoors because this drug causes photosensitivity (increased sensitivity of the skin to light and other sources of ultraviolet rays).

### Life Span Considerations for Proton Pump Inhibitors

***Considerations for Pregnancy and Breastfeeding.***  Omeprazole, pantoprazole, and rabeprazole are pregnancy category C drugs and are not safe for use during pregnancy because they may cause harm to the unborn child. The other PPI drugs are pregnancy category B drugs and are considered safe for use during pregnancy, but the benefits must outweigh the risks. PPIs are not recommended for use during breastfeeding. A woman taking a PPI should tell her health care provider if she is pregnant or planning to become pregnant.

***Considerations for Older Adults.***  There is an increased risk for side effects in older adults. PPIs have been associated with an increased risk for hip fractures because of decreased calcium absorption. Some studies have shown that short-term use of PPIs decreases the absorption of vitamin $B_{12}$. Older adults should have more frequent checkups to determine the effectiveness of the drug. In addition, the drug should be stopped in older adults when ulcers or inflammation have healed completely.

## ANTACIDS

### How Antacids Work

Antacids, drugs that neutralize acids in the stomach, are given by mouth to relieve heartburn and indigestion. Many antacids are available over the counter without a prescription.

Common names and doses of a few antacids are listed in the following table. Be sure to consult a drug handbook for information on any specific antacid.

### Dosages for Common Antacids

| Drug | Dosage |
|---|---|
| magnesium hydroxide/aluminum hydroxide/simethicone (Maalox, Milk of Magnesia, Mylanta) | *Adults/Children over 12:* 10-20 mL orally 1 and 3 hr after meals and at bedtime<br>*Children:* Consult the prescriber<br>*Infants:* Consult the prescriber |
| aluminum hydroxide (AlternaGEL, Alugel✚, Amphojel) | *Adults:* 500-1500 mg tablets orally or 5-10 mL liquid orally 3 to 6 times daily |
| calcium carbonate (Calcite✚, Calsan✚, Rolaids, TUMS) | *Adults:* 1-4 chewable tablets orally every hr as needed, but no more than 16 tablets per day |

Antacids are given by mouth to neutralize stomach acids and relieve heartburn and indigestion. Neutralizing stomach acids decreases the irritation and inflammation of the GI mucosa, especially the esophagus. Most antacids use salts of calcium, aluminum, or magnesium to neutralize acid.

### Intended Responses
- Gastric acids are neutralized.
- There is relief from heartburn and indigestion.

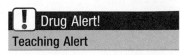

| Table 20-2 | Common Side Effects of Antacids |
|---|---|
| **TYPE OF ANTACID** | **SIDE EFFECTS** |
| Aluminum-containing | Bone pain, constipation, discomfort, loss of appetite, mood changes, muscle weakness, swelling of wrists or ankles, weight loss |
| Calcium-containing | Constipation, decreased respiratory rate, difficult and frequent urination, fatigue, loss of appetite, mood changes, muscle pain, nausea and vomiting, nervousness, restlessness, twitching, unpleasant taste |
| Magnesium-containing | Difficult or painful urination, dizziness, fatigue, irregular heart rhythm, light-headedness, loss of appetite, mood changes, muscle weakness, weight loss |
| Sodium bicarbonate–containing | Decreased respiratory rate, fatigue, frequent urination, headache, loss of appetite, mood changes, muscle pain, nausea or vomiting, nervousness, restlessness, swelling of feet and lower legs, twitching |

- Symptoms of GERD are decreased.
- Ulcers are healing, and pain from ulcers is decreased.

***Side Effects.*** Side effects of antacids are very rare when they are taken as directed. They are more likely to occur if the drug is taken in large doses or over a long period of time or if the patient has kidney disease. The most common side effect of antacids containing calcium or aluminum salts is constipation. The most common side effect of antacids containing magnesium salts is diarrhea. Table 20-2 summarizes the side effects of antacids on the basis of their primary ingredients.

***Adverse Effects.*** Adverse effects have not been reported when these drugs are taken appropriately.

### What To Do *Before* Giving Antacids

Be sure to review the general nursing responsibilities related to drugs for PUD and GERD (p. 363) in addition to these specific responsibilities before giving antacids.

Antacids interfere with absorption of other drugs and should not be taken at the same time. Ensure that antacids are given 1 hour after or 2 hours before any other drug therapy.

### What To Do *After* Giving Antacids

Be sure to review the general nursing responsibilities related to drugs for PUD and GERD (p. 363) after giving antacids. There are no additional specific responsibilities for these drugs.

### What To *Teach* Patients About Antacids

Be sure to teach patients about general issues and precautions related to drugs for PUD and GERD (p. 363) in addition to these specific teaching points for antacids.

Tell patients to contact their prescriber if they have been taking an antacid for more than 2 weeks and have not obtained relief. The excessive use of antacids may cause or worsen kidney problems. Using calcium-based antacids too much may lead to the formation of kidney stones.

Tell patients not to take an aluminum hydroxide or calcium antacid within 1 to 2 hours of other drugs without consulting their prescriber because these drugs affect absorption of other drugs.

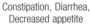
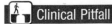 **Drug Alert!**

**Action/Interaction Alert**

Be sure to ask patients about antacid use because these drugs are readily available over the counter.

**Drug Alert!**

**Teaching Alert**

Teach patients to contact their prescriber if they have been taking an antacid for more than 2 weeks and continue to experience signs of reflux or an ulcer.

**Clinical Pitfall**

Patients should *not* take an aluminum hydroxide or a calcium carbonate antacid within 1 to 2 hours of taking other drugs.

Remind patients with heart failure not to take sodium-containing antacids (for example, Alka-Seltzer, Bromo-Seltzer) because they increase sodium and water retention. This problem causes an increase in the workload of the heart and can worsen heart failure.

Be sure to tell patients taking an aluminum hydroxide or a calcium carbonate antacid about the side effect of constipation; patients taking a magnesium-containing antacid should be told about the side effect of diarrhea.

Teach patients that antacids should be avoided if any signs of appendicitis or inflamed bowel are present. Signs include cramping, pain, and soreness in the lower abdomen; bloating; and nausea and vomiting.

### Life Span Considerations for Antacids

***Pediatric Considerations.***    Antacids should not be given to young children unless directed by the prescriber. Excessive amounts of antacids can change the pH of the blood and cause alkalosis.

***Considerations for Pregnancy and Breastfeeding.***    The effects of antacids have not been studied in pregnant women. Magnesium hydroxide antacids (category A, B) are generally considered safe for use during pregnancy. Calcium carbonate and aluminum hydroxide antacids are pregnancy category C drugs. Long-term use of antacids may have negative effects on the fetus, and sodium-containing antacids should not be taken by women who tend to retain body water. Many antacids pass into breast milk, but they have not been reported to cause problems with breastfeeding babies.

***Considerations for Older Adults.***    Older adults should not take aluminum-containing antacids if they have bone problems or Alzheimer's disease because these drugs may cause these conditions to worsen.

### CYTOPROTECTIVE DRUGS

### How Cytoprotective Drugs Work

Cytoprotective (GI coating) drugs decrease acid damage to the stomach by coating the mucosal lining of the stomach and reducing the risk of developing an ulcer. Some cytoprotective drugs such as bismuth subsalicylate (Pepto-Bismol) are available over the counter.

Most of these drugs work by coating some part of the GI mucosa and reducing its exposure to stomach acids. Sucralfate (Carafate) is prescribed to protect open-sore areas in the GI tract and allow ulcers to heal. Sucralfate reacts with stomach acids to form a thick coating that covers the surface of an ulcer. This protects the open area from further damage. It also stops the effects of pepsin (a digestive enzyme that breaks down protein). Interestingly, this drug does not coat the normal stomach mucosa. Bismuth subsalicylate also coats the stomach and intestine protecting the mucosa. In addition, this drug inhibits the activity of *H. pylori* bacteria, helping to decrease GI infections.

The common doses of cytoprotective drugs are listed in the following table. Be sure to consult a drug handbook for more information about any specific cytoprotective drug.

### Dosages for Common Cytoprotective Drugs

| Drug | Dosage |
|---|---|
| bismuth subsalicylate (Pepto-Bismol) | *Adults:* 524 mg orally 4 times daily (30 mL) |
| sucralfate (Carafate, Sulcrate) | *Adults:* Treatment of ulcers—1 g orally 4 times daily 1 hr before meals and at bedtime; Prevention of ulcers—1 g orally twice daily 1 hr before a meal |

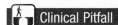
**Clinical Pitfall**

Patients with heart failure should *not* take sodium-containing antacids.

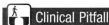
**Clinical Pitfall**

Older adults with bone problems or Alzheimer's disease should *not* take aluminum-containing antacids.

**? Did You Know?**

Sucralfate (Carafate) forms a protective coating over an ulcer but does not coat normal stomach mucosa.

*Intended Responses*
- Ulcers are protected to prevent further tissue damage.
- Ulcers are healed.

*Side Effects.* Side effects are rare with cytoprotective drugs. The most common side effect of sucralfate is constipation. Other side effects include dizziness; drowsiness; diarrhea; dry mouth; rashes; and gastric discomfort such as flatulence (gas), indigestion, and nausea. Side effects of bismuth subsalicylate include constipation, gray-black stools, grayish-colored tongue, stool impaction in infants and debilitated patients, and tinnitus (ringing in the ears).

*Adverse Effects.* No life-threatening adverse effects have been documented with sucralfate. Bismuth subsalicylate contains aspirin, so patients taking bismuth subsalicylate should avoid other drugs containing aspirin because it can increase the effects of anticoagulant drugs such as warfarin (Coumadin).

### What To Do *Before* Giving Cytoprotective Drugs
Be sure to review the general nursing responsibilities related to drugs for PUD and GERD (p. 363) before giving cytoprotective drugs. There are no additional specific responsibilities for these drugs.

### What To Do *After* Giving Cytoprotective Drugs
Be sure to review the general nursing responsibilities related to drugs for PUD and GERD (p. 363) after giving cytoprotective drugs. There are no additional specific responsibilities for these drugs.

### What To *Teach* Patients About Cytoprotective Drugs
Be sure to teach patients about general issues and precautions related to drugs for PUD and GERD (p. 363) in addition to these specific teaching points for cytoprotective drugs.

Instruct patients to take the drug exactly as directed by their prescriber for the full period of time (usually 4 to 8 weeks), even when feeling better.

Teach patients that increased fluid intake, dietary fiber (such as extra fruits, vegetables, and bran), and exercise help to prevent constipation, abdominal pain, and gas.

### Life Span Considerations for Cytoprotective Drugs
*Pediatric Considerations.* Children should not be given bismuth subsalicylate (Pepto-Bismol) because it contains aspirin and can cause Reye's syndrome, a life-threatening condition that affects the liver and central nervous system. It is characterized by vomiting and confusion.

*Considerations for Pregnancy and Breastfeeding.* Sucralfate (pregnancy category B) appears to be safe to use during pregnancy, but extensive studies in pregnant women have not been conducted. Bismuth subsalicylate is pregnancy category C. A woman of childbearing years should be sure to tell her prescriber if she is breastfeeding an infant because it is not known whether sucralfate passes into breast milk.

Teach patients who continue to breastfeed while taking these drugs to follow the tips in Box 1-1 (in Chapter 1) to reduce infant exposure to the drugs.

### PROMOTILITY DRUGS

### How Promotility Drugs Work
When used to treat GERD, promotility drugs increase LES tone and the speed of emptying food out of the stomach. Metoclopramide (Reglan) increases stomach and small intestine contractions (peristalsis), helping to move food through the GI system. When food moves more quickly into the intestinal system, it is less likely

to back up into the esophagus. Promotility drugs are not used to manage gastric or duodenal ulcers.

Metoclopramide is the promotility drug prescribed for treatment of GERD. It is usually given 30 minutes before meals and may be prescribed for 4 to 12 weeks. The common dosages for this drug are listed in the following table.

### Dosages for Common Promotility Drugs

| Drug | Dosage |
| --- | --- |
| metoclopramide (Emex🍁, Maxeran🍁, Octamide, Reglan) | *Adults/Children over 14 years:* Oral—5-10 mg orally 30 min before symptoms are likely to occur (for example, meals and bedtime); IV—10 mg<br>*Children 5-14 years:* Dosage determined by prescriber |

### Intended Responses

- GI peristalsis is increased.
- Digested food moves more rapidly through the GI tract.
- Symptoms of GERD are decreased.

*Side Effects.*   The most common side effects of metoclopramide are fatigue, drowsiness, and restlessness. Other side effects include anxiety, depression, irritability, supraventricular tachycardia, high or low blood pressure, constipation, diarrhea, dry mouth, and nausea. A rare but upsetting side effect for male patients is *gynecomastia* (breast enlargement in men).

*Adverse Effects.*   Adverse effects of this drug include neuroleptic malignant syndrome, a rare and life-threatening condition that causes dangerously high body temperatures. Neuroleptic malignant syndrome is usually caused by the use of drugs that block the neurotransmitter dopamine. Without prompt and expert treatment, this condition can be fatal in as many as 20% of those who develop it. Signs and symptoms include fever, respiratory distress, tachycardia, seizures, diaphoresis, blood pressure changes, pallor, fatigue, severe muscle stiffness, and loss of bladder control. Notify the prescriber immediately for any of these symptoms.

Metoclopramide can also cause tardive dyskinesia, a chronic disorder of the nervous system characterized by involuntary jerky movements of the face, tongue, jaws, trunk, and limbs. Signs and symptoms include uncontrolled rhythmic movement of the mouth, face, or extremities; lip smacking or puckering; puffing of cheeks; uncontrolled chewing; and rapid or wormlike movements of the tongue.

### What To Do *Before* Giving Metoclopramide

Be sure to review the general nursing responsibilities related to drugs for PUD and GERD (p. 363) in addition to these specific responsibilities before giving metoclopramide.

Check the patient's heart rhythm and level of consciousness. Be sure to check baseline electrolyte laboratory values.

### What To Do *After* Giving Metoclopramide

Be sure to review the general nursing responsibilities related to drugs for PUD and GERD (p. 363) in addition to these specific responsibilities after giving metoclopramide.

Watch for signs of side effects or adverse effects, especially malignant neuroleptic syndrome and tardive dyskinesia. Report any signs immediately to the prescriber. Check the patient's level of consciousness and watch for sedation effects, especially with older adults. Monitor intake and output of both food and fluid.

This drug may cause hypotension. Ensure that the call light is within easy reach and instruct the patient to call for help when getting out of bed. Remind the patient to change positions slowly.

**Common Side Effects**
**Metoclopramide**

  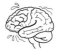

Fatigue      Drowsiness      Restlessness

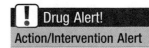 **Drug Alert!**
**Action/Intervention Alert**

Watch the patient taking metoclopramide carefully for signs of neuroleptic malignant syndrome or tardive dyskinesia. Report these signs immediately to the prescriber.

| Box **20-5** | Patient and Family Education for Injury Prevention with Orthostatic Hypotension |

- Change positions slowly.
- If you feel dizzy or light-headed on standing, sit on a chair or the edge of the bed for a few moments before attempting to walk.
- Use the handrails when going up or down stairs.
- If necessary, use a walker or cane for walking.
- Do not drive or operate dangerous equipment the first day you take this drug until you know how it affects you.
- Do not start driving if you feel dizzy or light-headed.
- If you become dizzy or light-headed while driving, pull over immediately.
- Always take the drug with food or just after a meal.
- Make certain to drink enough fluids because low blood pressure is worse when you are dehydrated.
- Ensure that anything spilled on the floor is cleaned up immediately.
- Use adequate lighting at all times, especially at night.

## What To *Teach* Patients About Metoclopramide

Be sure to teach patients about general issues and precautions related to drugs for PUD and GERD (p. 363) in addition to these specific teaching points for metoclopramide.

Because this drug may cause drowsiness, caution the patient to avoid driving or operating machines. Teach older patients and their families about safety precautions for drugs such as metoclopramide, which may cause orthostatic hypotension (Box 20-5).

Remind patients to use frequent mouth hygiene, including mouth rinses, to decrease problems associated with dry mouth.

Teach patients the signs and symptoms of malignant neuroleptic syndrome and tardive dyskinesia. Instruct them to check their body temperature every day and report abnormal signs and symptoms to their prescriber.

Instruct patients to take this drug 30 minutes before meals and at bedtime to help prevent reflux of stomach contents into the esophagus.

## Life Span Considerations for Metoclopramide

*Pediatric Considerations.* Parents must be taught how to read the drug label and correctly give the drug to their child. Unintentional overdoses of metoclopramide have occurred with infants and children. Tardive dyskinesia is more likely to be permanent with excessive doses.

*Considerations for Pregnancy and Breastfeeding.* Metoclopramide is a pregnancy category B drug. Women should check with their prescriber before taking this drug if they are pregnant or planning to become pregnant. Metoclopramide is passed into breast milk and should be avoided while breastfeeding.

*Considerations for Older Adults.* Older adults are more likely to experience side effects such as acute confusion and dizziness. They also are more likely to experience sudden hypotension and are at increased risk for falls. Teach family members to watch for changes in cognition or increased confusion. Teach older adults to take special precautions to avoid falls. Instruct them to change positions slowly and to use handrails when going up or down stairs. Suggest that older adults avoid driving or using dangerous equipment until they know how the drugs affect them.

**ⓔ-Learning Activity 20-7 ▶**

## OTHER DRUGS USED TO TREAT ULCERS

### ANTIBIOTICS FOR *H. PYLORI* INFECTION

Antibiotics are part of the treatment plan for PUD and are used to treat *H. pylori* infections in the GI tract. Common drugs and doses used to treat *H. pylori* infections

---

**! Drug Alert!**

**Teaching Alert**

Teach patients to take metoclopramide 30 minutes before meals and at bedtime.

are listed in the following table. Be sure to consult a drug reference handbook for information about specific antibiotics. See Chapter 9 for additional information on antibiotic drugs.

### Dosages for Common Antibiotics for *H. pylori* Infections

| Drug | Dosage |
| --- | --- |
| clarithromycin (Biaxin) | *Adult:* 500 mg orally every 12 hr for 7-14 days<br>*Children:* 15 mg/kg orally in 2 divided doses |
| metronidazole (Flagyl, Novonidazole🍁, Trikacide🍁) | *Adults:* 250 mg orally 4 times daily when co-administered with bismuth and tetracycline; 500 mg orally twice daily when co-administered with clarithromycin<br>*Children:* Pediatric dosage not established |
| tetracycline (Novotetra🍁, Sumycin, Tetracap) | *Adults:* 250-500 mg orally 4 times daily for 14 days<br>*Children over 8 years:* 25-50 mg/kg/day orally in 4 divided doses (*not* recommended for children under 8 years) |
| amoxicillin (Amoxil, Novamoxin🍁, Trimox) 🔲 | *Adults:* 250-500 mg orally 4 times daily or 1000 mg twice daily for 14 days<br>*Children:* 20-40 mg/kg/day orally in 3 divided doses or 25-45 mg/kg/day in 2 divided doses |

🔲 Top 100 drugs prescribed.

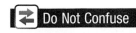

### 🔁 Do Not Confuse

**metronidazole** *with* **metformin**

An order for metronidazole may be confused with metformin. Metronidazole is an antibiotic, whereas metformin is an antidiabetic drug used for management of type 2 diabetes.

# Get Ready for Practice!

## Key Points

- The most common cause of PUD is infection with the *H. pylori* bacteria.
- Complications of ulcers include bleeding, perforation, and gastric obstruction.
- GERD may damage the lining of the esophagus, causing inflammation.
- The cause of GERD is a lower esophageal sphincter that is not working correctly and allows stomach contents to back up (reflux) into the esophagus.
- Complications of GERD include ulcers; bleeding; strictures; and Barrett's esophagus, a pre-cancerous condition that may lead to development of esophageal cancer.
- Histamine H₂ blockers are available in lower doses over the counter for mild heartburn and indigestion. They are also available in higher doses by prescription for moderate-to-severe forms of GERD.
- Watch for confusion, the most common side effect, when giving histamine H₂ blockers.
- Smoking interferes with the action of histamine H₂ blockers.
- Black, tarry stools indicate bleeding and should always be reported to the prescriber.
- Teach patients to take proton pump inhibitors for the full period of time recommended by the prescriber, even if they are feeling better.
- Aluminum hydroxide antacids decrease the absorption of other drugs when taken within 1 to 2 hours.
- Patients with heart failure should not take sodium-containing antacids because they can cause salt and water retention and increase the workload of the heart.

- Teach patients taking any drug that causes constipation to increase fluid intake, eat fiber-containing foods, and exercise to help prevent constipation.
- Children should not be given bismuth subsalicylate (Pepto-Bismol) because it contains aspirin and may cause Reye's syndrome.

## Additional Learning Resources

*e*volve Go to your Evolve website (http://evolve.elsevier.com/Workman/pharmacology/) for the following FREE learning resources:

- eLearning Activities
- Animations
- Video Clips
- Interactive Review Questions
- Audio Key Points
- Audio Glossary
- Audio Glossary—Spanish-English
- Drug Dosage Calculators
- Patient Teaching Handouts

**SG** Go to your Study Guide for additional learning activities to help you master this chapter content.

## Review Questions

1. A patient asks you how histamine H₂ blockers will help prevent GERD. What is your best response?
   A. "It will increase movement of digested food through your bowel."
   B. "It will decrease secretion of acids in your stomach."
   C. "It will coat and protect the stomach lining."
   D. "It will neutralize stomach acids."

2. For which common side effect of histamine H$_2$ blockers must you monitor a patient?

    A. Diarrhea
    B. Confusion
    C. Reflux
    D. Bleeding

3. What must you be sure to do before administering a proton pump inhibitor drug? (Select all that apply.)

    A. Check patient's abdomen for bowel sounds and distention.
    B. Ask the patient about usual bowel habits.
    C. Give a drug to prevent nausea or vomiting.
    D. Give proton pump inhibitors before meals.
    E. Ask about bleeding and reflux.

4. A patient has been taking over-the-counter antacids for over 2 weeks and is still experiencing acid indigestion. What must you instruct the patient to do?

    A. Continue taking the antacids.
    B. Take the antacids more often.
    C. Try a different antacid.
    D. Inform his or her health care provider.

5. Which of the following drugs must not be given to children? (Select all that apply.)

    A. ranitidine (Zantac)
    B. tetracycline (Sumycin)
    C. bismuth subsalicylate (Pepto-Bismol)
    D. amoxicillin (Trimox)
    E. metoclopramide (Reglan)

6. A 14-year-old child with gastroesophageal reflux disease (GERD) has been prescribed ranitidine (Zantac) 1.25 mg/kg/day in 2 divided doses. The child weighs 38 kg. How many milligrams will you give per dose? _____ mg per dose

7. An older adult with a duodenal ulcer is to receive lansoprazole (Prevacid) 30 mg once a day. The pharmacy sends lansoprazole 15 mg/tablet. How many tablets will you give? _____ tablet(s) per dose

8. A patient has been prescribed sucralfate (Carafate) 1 g 4 times a day. Sucralfate comes as an oral suspension of 500 mg in 5 mL. How many milliliters will you give with each dose? _____ mL per dose

## Critical Thinking Activities

Mrs. Freise is a 69-year-old woman admitted to your acute care medical unit with a diagnosis of duodenal ulcer. The health care provider prescribes the following drugs:

Omeprazole (Prilosec) 40 mg orally once a day
Sucralfate (Carafate) 1 g 4 times a day
Clarithromycin (Biaxin) 500 mg twice a day

1. What is the purpose of each of these drugs?

2. When would you give the doses of sucralfate?

3. What would you do if Mrs. Freise had a black, tarry stool?

4. For which adverse effects is Mrs. Freise at risk while taking clarithromycin?

# Drugs for Seizures

## Objectives

*After studying this chapter you should be able to:*

1. Explain how different classes of drugs are used to treat seizures.
2. List the common names, actions, usual adult dosages, possible side effects, and adverse effects of drugs for seizures.
3. Describe what to do before and after giving drugs for seizures.
4. Explain what to teach patients taking drugs for seizures, including what to do, what not to do, and when to call the prescriber.
5. Describe life span considerations for drugs for seizures.

## Key Terms

**absence seizure** (ĂB-sĕns SĒ-zhŭr) (p. 378) A generalized seizure usually lasting less than 20 seconds characterized by a blank stare and sometimes blinking, eye rolling, or chewing movements; also called a petit mal seizure.

**atonic seizure** (ă-TŎN-ĭk SĒ-zhŭr) (p. 378) A seizure characterized by sudden loss of muscle tone for a few seconds followed by confusion.

**aura** (ŎR-ă) (p. 377) Strange sensations such as tingling, smell, or emotional changes that occur before a seizure.

**complex partial seizure** (kŏm-PLĔKS PĂR-shŭl SĒ-zhŭr) (p. 378) A seizure that involves only part of the brain and impairs consciousness; often preceded by a simple partial seizure, aura, or warning.

**epilepsy** (ĔP-ĭl-ĕp-sē) (p. 375) A disorder of the brain that causes recurrent, unprovoked seizures.

**generalized seizure** (JĔN-ŭr-ăl-īzd SĒ-zhŭr) (p. 378) A seizure that involves the entire brain; caused by electrical discharges originating from both sides of the brain.

**myoclonic seizure** (mī-ō-KLŎN-ĭk SĒ-zhŭr) (p. 378) A brief muscle jerk resulting from an abnormal discharge of brain electrical activity; usually involves muscles on both sides of the body, most often the shoulders or upper arms.

**partial seizure** (PĂR-shŭl SĒ-zhŭr) (p. 378) A seizure that starts in one part of the brain. The abnormal electrical activity may remain confined to one area or spread to the entire brain; also called a focal or local seizure.

**postictal phase** (pŏst-ĬK-tŭl FĀZ) (p. 377) "After the seizure" phase often characterized by confusion, headache, sore muscles, and fatigue.

**seizure** (SĒ-zhŭr) (p. 375) Uncontrolled electrical activity in the brain that may produce a physical convulsion, minor physical signs, thought disturbances, or a combination of symptoms.

**seizure disorder** (SĒ-zhŭr dĭs-ŎR-dŭr) (p. 375) A pathologic condition resulting in a sudden episode of uncontrolled electrical activity in the brain.

**status epilepticus** (STĂT-ŭs ĕp-ĭl-LĔP-tĭ-kŭs) (p. 379) A prolonged seizure (usually defined as lasting longer than 30 minutes) or a series of repeated seizures; a continuous state of seizure activity that may occur in almost any seizure type.

**tonic-clonic seizure** (TŎN-ĭk KLŎN-ĭk SĒ-zhŭr) (p. 378) A seizure that lasts 2 to 5 minutes with stiffening or rigidity of the arm and leg muscles and immediate loss of consciousness; also called a grand mal seizure.

◄ -Learning Activity 21-1

## OVERVIEW

A seizure results from excessive or disordered electrical activity in the brain. About 2% of adults experience a seizure at some time during their lives; more than 60% of these adults never have additional seizures. A person with repeated seizures has a seizure disorder, sometimes called epilepsy. Millions of Americans have this brain disorder. Although seizures may begin at any age, most begin during early childhood or late adulthood. Seizures are frightening and can range from minor to life threatening.

> **? Did You Know?**
>
> Although 2% of adults experience a seizure at some time during their lives, about 60% of them never experience another seizure.

## REVIEW OF RELATED PHYSIOLOGY AND PATHOPHYSIOLOGY

When the brain is working normally, electrical impulses are orderly and organized. These impulses help the brain communicate with the spinal cord, nerves, muscles, and other parts of the brain. Abnormal electrical impulses can lead to seizures (Figure 21-1). Often seizures occur when nerve cells fire in a more rapid and less controlled manner (Figure 21-2). Seizures can affect movements, senses, concentration, communication, and level of consciousness. After a seizure, most people experience confusion for a period of time.

### CAUSES OF SEIZURES

Although certain factors are known to cause seizures (Table 21-1), for the most part their cause is unknown. Several risk factors increase the possibility of seizures (Box 21-1). For adults the most common causes include head injury, stroke, and tumor. Certain drugs may lead to seizures (Box 21-2). For children, the most common causes include fever, head injury, central nervous system infection, hypoxia, and electrolyte imbalances.

Stimuli that cause irritation to the brain such as injury, drugs, lack of sleep, infections, and low levels of oxygen may cause a seizure in anyone. However, when a person has a seizure disorder, seizures are more likely to occur during periods of increased emotional or physical stress. Risk factors associated with worsening of a well-controlled seizure disorder include pregnancy and lack of sleep (Box 21-3).

### TYPES OF SEIZURES

Signs and symptoms of a seizure may vary widely, ranging from staring off into space to loss of consciousness and violent jerky movements. The type of seizure

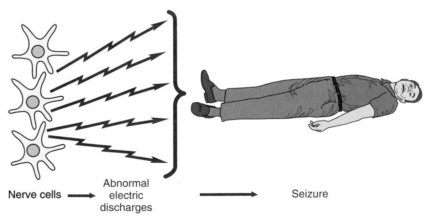

FIGURE 21-1 The cause of seizures.

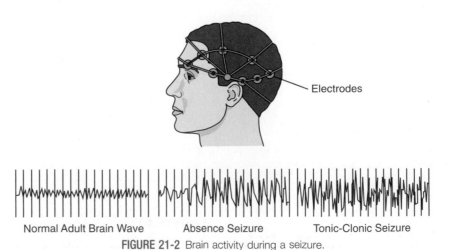

FIGURE 21-2 Brain activity during a seizure.

experienced depends on the part of the brain that is affected, the cause of the seizure, and the person's response. Some people experience an aura, a strange sensation (for example, smell, visual, sound, or taste) that occurs before each seizure. Commonly a seizure consists of an aura followed by the seizure and then a postictal phase usually characterized by confusion, lethargy, and decreased responsiveness

💡 **Memory Jogger**

Before a seizure, a strange sensation called an aura may occur. After a seizure, a period of confusion, lethargy, and decreased responsiveness (postictal phase) usually occurs.

| Table **21-1** | Common Causes of Seizures |

| CAUSE | CHARACTERISTICS |
|---|---|
| Brain injury | Any age—mostly young adults<br>Damage to brain membranes<br>Seizures begin within 2 years of injury |
| Degenerative disorders (for example, dementias) | Mostly affect older adults |
| Developmental/genetic | Condition present at birth<br>Injury near birth; hypoxia at birth<br>Seizures begin during infancy or early childhood |
| Disorders affecting blood vessels (stroke, transient ischemic attacks) | Most common cause of seizures after age 60 |
| Idiopathic (no known cause) | Usually begin between ages 5 and 20<br>Can occur at any age<br>No other neurologic abnormalities present<br>Family history of seizures present |
| Infections (for example, meningitis, encephalitis, brain abscess, immune disorders) | Affect any age<br>Reversible cause of seizures<br>May be caused by acute severe infection in any part of the body<br>Sometimes related to chronic infections |
| Metabolic abnormalities | Affect any age<br>Diabetic complications<br>Electrolyte abnormalities<br>Kidney failure<br>Nutritional deficiencies<br>Phenylketonuria—causes seizures during infancy<br>Metabolic diseases<br>Use of cocaine, amphetamines, alcohol, other illicit drugs<br>Alcohol or drug withdrawal |
| Tumors | Affect any age—most likely after age 30<br>Partial (focal) seizures more common<br>May progress to generalized seizures |

| Box **21-1** | Risk Factors for Seizures |

- Brain infections
- Drugs (see Box 21-2)
- Drug withdrawal
- Emotional stress
- Family history
- Fevers
- Head injury
- Hormone changes
- Hyperventilation
- Lack of food
- Metabolic disorders
- Sensory stimuli (for example, flashing lights)
- Sleep deprivation
- Tumors

| Box **21-2** | Common Seizure-Causing Drugs |

- Antidepressants
- Bupropion alcohol
- Cocaine and other street drugs
- Excessive doses of anti-seizure drugs
- Oral contraceptives
- Phenothiazines
- Theophylline

Box **21-3** Risk Factors for Worsening of Seizures with a Well-Controlled Seizure Disorder

- Illness
- Lack of sleep
- Pregnancy

- Prescribed drugs (see Box 21-2)
- Skipping doses of anti-seizure drugs
- Use of alcohol or street drugs

Table **21-2** Types of Generalized Seizures

| TYPE | SYMPTOMS |
|------|----------|
| Tonic-clonic (grand mal) | Convulsions, muscle rigidity, unconsciousness |
| Tonic | Muscle stiffness, rigidity |
| Atonic | Loss of muscle tone |
| Absence (petit mal) | Brief loss of consciousness |
| Myoclonic | Sporadic (isolated) jerking movements |
| Clonic | Repetitive jerking movements |

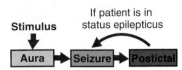

**Stimulus**

If patient is in status epilepticus

Aura → Seizure → Postictal

**FIGURE 21-3** Typical seizure. During status epilepticus the patient experiences a state of continuous seizure.

 **Memory Jogger**

The two major groups of seizures are generalized and partial seizures.

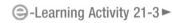 -Learning Activity 21-3 ►

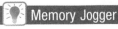 **Memory Jogger**

The six types of generalized seizures are tonic-clonic, tonic, clonic, absence, myoclonic, and atonic.

**Memory Jogger**

The two major types of partial seizures are simple and complex.

(Figure 21-3). Most seizures are brief, lasting a few seconds to a few minutes. *Status epilepticus* is a life-threatening, continuous state of seizure that lasts from 5 to 30 minutes or is a series of repeated seizures without recovery (postictal period). The risk of status epilepticus increases when a seizure is prolonged or when a series of seizures occur.

Seizures are divided into two groups, generalized seizures and partial seizures.

### Generalized Seizures

Generalized seizures affect most or all of the brain. There are six types of generalized seizures (Table 21-2).

Tonic-clonic seizures (also known as grand mal seizures) last 2 to 5 minutes, with stiffening or rigidity of the arm and leg muscles and immediate loss of consciousness. Spasm of the respiratory muscles can cause forced exhalation, sounding like a scream, called the *epileptic cry*. Clonic seizures are characterized by muscle contraction and relaxation. Patients may bite their tongues or become incontinent. Tonic seizures include sudden increase in muscle tone; loss of consciousness; and autonomic signs such as rapid heart rate, sweating, pupil dilation, flushing, and loss of bowel function and bladder control for 30 seconds to several minutes. After the seizure patients are often tired, confused, or lethargic for an hour or more.

Absence seizures (also known as petit mal seizures) are more common in children and tend to occur in families. They are brief (a few seconds) with loss of consciousness and blank staring (a child may appear to be daydreaming). After the seizure the child returns to normal immediately.

A myoclonic seizure involves brief jerking or stiffening of the extremities that lasts a few seconds. It may involve one or more extremities, and the jerking contractions may be asymmetric (stronger on one side of the body) or symmetric (the same on both sides of the body). With an atonic seizure typically there is sudden loss of muscle tone for a few seconds, followed by postictal (after the seizure) confusion.

### Partial Seizures

Partial seizures are also called focal or local seizures. The two major types of partial seizures are simple and complex (Table 21-3). With a simple partial seizure the patient remains conscious. Before the seizure a patient may report an aura. During the seizure the patient remains conscious. One-sided movement of an extremity, unusual sensations, or autonomic changes (heart rate, flushing, epigastric discomfort) may occur. Complex partial seizures cause patients to lose consciousness for 1 to 3 minutes. During a complex partial seizure patients may have *automatisms*

| Table 21-3 | Types of Partial Seizures |
|---|---|
| **TYPE** | **SYMPTOMS** |
| Simple | |
|    Simple partial motor | Head-turning, jerking, muscle rigidity, spasms, |
|    Simple partial sensory | Unusual sensations affecting either vision, hearing, smell, taste, or touch |
|    Simple partial psychologic | Memory or emotional disturbance |
| Complex | Automatisms (for example, chewing, fidgeting, lip smacking, walking and other repetitive involuntary but coordinated movements) |
| Partial with secondary generalization | Symptoms that are initially associated with a preservation of consciousness, which then evolves into a loss of consciousness and convulsions |

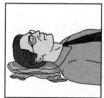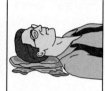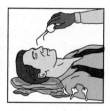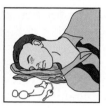

| Help the person to the floor and cushion the head | Loosen any clothing around the neck | Remove any sharp objects | Turn the person on one side |

**FIGURE 21-4** What to do if you witness a generalized or complex partial seizure.

(automatic, unconscious actions) such as lip smacking, patting, or picking at clothes. Often they experience amnesia during the period after a seizure.

**Status epilepticus** is a prolonged seizure (usually defined as lasting longer than 30 minutes) or a series of repeated seizures that may occur in almost any type of seizure. Rapid recognition and treatment of this disorder are essential to prevent brain damage. Actions for treating this life-threatening condition include protecting the airway, providing oxygen, establishing intravenous (IV) access to give 5 to 10 mg of diazepam (Valium) by slow IV injection, and determining and treating the cause.

## TREATMENT OF SEIZURES

Controlling and preventing seizure activity are important for many reasons. During a seizure the patient has no control over motor activities, which can lead to accidents when the person is driving a car or handling heavy or dangerous equipment. Falls are common during a seizure. So the patient having a seizure is at risk for trauma and loss of motor control and could endanger other people. In addition, the confusion and incontinence (common during or after a seizure) reduce a person's productivity and are embarrassing.

Although anti-seizure drugs are a major part of treating and controlling seizures, other important components include precautions such as keeping the airway open, placing a saline lock to give IV drugs, raising side rails, and keeping the bed in its lowest position. Padded tongue blades are no longer used because the jaw may clench as soon as a seizure begins. Forcing a tongue blade into a patient's mouth may cause damage to the teeth and aspiration of tooth fragments. Incorrect tongue blade placement can also cause airway obstruction.

The actions taken during a seizure should be correct for the type of seizure. For example, for a simple partial seizure, watch the patient and document the time the seizure occurred and how long it lasted. For a generalized or complex partial seizure, remove anything that could cause injury to the patient and turn him or her to one side to prevent aspiration and let secretions drain (Figure 21-4).

 **Clinical Pitfall**

Without rapid recognition and treatment, status epilepticus can result in brain damage, coma, and death.

◄ⓔ-Learning Activity 21-4

 **Clinical Pitfall**

Padded tongue blades should *not* be kept at the bedside and should *never* be put into a patient's mouth after a seizure begins.

 **Did You Know?**

The use of padded side rails is controversial because it is not known if they help maintain safety and they may cause the patient and family to feel embarrassed.

## TYPES OF ANTI-SEIZURE DRUGS

Anti-seizure drugs are a major part of the management and control of seizures. These drugs are started one at a time. If a prescribed drug does not work, either the dose may be increased, or another drug may be tried. Sometimes it takes more than one drug to control a patient's seizure disorder. Use of these drugs involves a balance between keeping a therapeutic level of the drug in the blood and avoiding important side effects. Drugs must be taken on time to maintain the blood level and control seizures.

The best outcome for seizure drug therapy is the control and elimination of seizures. The choice of drugs prescribed is based on the type of seizure. Certain drugs are used as first line or first choice for each type of seizure, whereas other drugs are considered as alternatives or second line.

### FIRST-LINE DRUGS FOR PARTIAL AND GENERALIZED SEIZURES

#### How Drugs for Partial and Generalized Seizures Work

The exact action of first-line drugs for partial (simple and complex) or generalized seizures is not known, but they act on the brain and nervous system. Use of these drugs causes a decrease in the voltage, frequency, and spread of electrical impulses within the motor cortex of the brain, which leads to decreased seizure activity.

Commonly prescribed first-line drugs for partial or generalized seizures include carbamazepine (Tegretol), valproic acid (Depakote, Depacon), and phenytoin (Dilantin). The action of valproic acid may be related to increased availability of the neurotransmitter gamma-aminobutyric acid (GABA). Carbamazepine decreases impulse transmission by affecting sodium channels in neurons. Phenytoin (Dilantin) changes ion transport, but the exact action is not known.

Generic names, brand names, and common dosages of these drugs are listed in the following table. Be sure to consult a drug handbook for specific information about each of these drugs.

**Dosages for Common First-Line Drugs for Partial and Generalized Seizures**

| Drug | Dosage |
| --- | --- |
| carbamazepine (Carbamax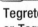, Tegretol) | *Adults:* 600-1600 mg orally daily in 3-4 divided doses<br>*Children less than 6 years:* 10-35 mg/kg/day orally in 3-4 divided doses<br>*Children over 6 years:* 200-1000 mg/day orally in 3-4 divided doses |
| phenytoin (Dilantin) | *Adults:* Oral loading dose—400 mg followed by 300 mg after 2 and 4 hours; maintenance dose—300 mg daily (extended release) or 100 mg 3 times daily (immediate release); IV—15-18 mg/kg loading dose followed by 100 mg 3 times daily<br>*Children:* Oral—5 mg/kg/day in 2-3 divided doses, maximum 300 mg/day; IV—15-20 mg/kg loading dose, then 100 mg every 6-8 hr |
| valproic acid (Depakote; Depacon IV) | *Adults/Children 10 years or older:* Oral and IV—10-15 mg/kg/day in divided doses; can increase by 5-10 mg/kg/day until seizures are controlled; maximum dosage 60 mg/kg/day |

### Intended Responses

- Seizures are controlled and prevented.
- Abnormal electrical impulses are decreased.

***Side Effects.*** Common side effects of drugs for generalized and partial seizures include *ataxia* (loss of coordination, clumsiness), dizziness, light-headedness, and drowsiness. Valproic acid and phenytoin often cause GI symptoms such as indigestion, nausea, and vomiting. Phenytoin also may cause double vision (*diplopia*), rapid involuntary movement of the eyes (*nystagmus*), hypotension, excessive growth of gum tissue *(gingival hyperplasia)*, excessive growth of hair in areas not normally hairy *(hypertrichosis)*, and rashes.

Side effects for which the patient should be instructed to call the prescriber immediately include difficulty coordinating movements; skin rashes; easy bruising; tiny, purple-colored skin spots *(petechiae,* an indication of bleeding beneath the skin); bloody nose; or unusual bleeding. These side effects likely indicate allergic and adverse reactions to these drugs.

*Adverse Effects.* Adverse effects of both carbamazepine and phenytoin include *neutropenia* (a decrease in the number of white blood cells [WBCs] with sore throat, fever, and chills), and *aplastic anemia* (anemia caused by too few red blood cells [RBCs] produced by the bone marrow). A patient who develops neutropenia is at risk for life-threatening infections, whereas a patient with aplastic anemia does not have enough RBCs to carry oxygen to the tissues and cells.

Carbamazepine can also cause *thrombocytopenia* (low platelet count), increasing a patient's risk for severe bleeding. Phenytoin can lead to Stevens-Johnson syndrome, a serious and life-threatening body-wide *(systemic)* allergic reaction with a rash involving burnlike sores on the skin and mucous membranes. This syndrome usually indicates a serious allergic reaction to a drug.

Serious adverse effects of valproic acid include damage to the liver *(hepatotoxicity)* and inflammation of the pancreas *(pancreatitis)*.

### What To Do *Before* Giving First-Line Drugs for Partial and Generalized Seizures

Before giving a first-line drug to prevent partial or generalized seizures, obtain a complete list of drugs the patient is currently taking, including over-the-counter and herbal drugs. These first-line drugs, especially phenytoin, interact with many other drugs. For example, the effects of anticoagulants may be increased, putting the patient at greater risk for bleeding.

If the patient is to receive an IV drug such as phenytoin, make sure to check the IV site for patency and solution compatibility. Use normal saline because this drug *precipitates* (forms solid particles) due to chemical incompatibility with dextrose solutions.

Check a baseline set of vital signs. Be sure to assess the patient's level of consciousness and gait. Ask female patients of childbearing age if they are pregnant, planning to become pregnant, or breastfeeding.

Ask patients to describe the nature of their seizures. Find out whether an aura occurs before each seizure. Instruct patients to notify the nursing staff if they sense that a seizure may occur.

To reduce the risk of injury during a seizure, be sure the patient's bed is in the lowest position and side rails are raised. Ensure that the call light is within easy reach.

### What To Do *After* Giving First-Line Drugs for Partial and Generalized Seizures

After giving a drug to prevent partial or generalized seizures, recheck the patient's level of consciousness. Check his or her gait and vital signs. Remind him or her about the importance of frequent and careful mouth care.

Be sure to ask the patient about nausea and vomiting. If GI symptoms develop, give these drugs with food. Remind the patient to drink plenty of water because these drugs dry the mouth and increase urine excretion.

Because these drugs can cause dizziness or drowsiness, remind the patient to call for help when getting out of bed and make sure that the call light is within easy reach.

Monitor the patient for seizure activity and be prepared to manage a seizure if one occurs (for example, protect the airway and protect the patient from injury). Watch for side effects such as abnormal bleeding and report these to the prescriber.

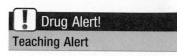

**Teaching Alert**

Teach patients taking drugs for generalized and partial seizures to notify their prescriber immediately for signs of allergic or adverse reactions.

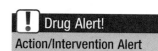

**Action/Intervention Alert**

Drugs for partial and generalized seizures can increase the effects of anticoagulant drugs. Watch for abnormal bleeding.

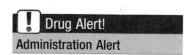

**Administration Alert**

Do *not* use dextrose solutions with IV phenytoin because it causes precipitation as a result of chemical incompatibility.

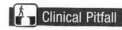

Because drugs for partial and generalized seizures can cause dizziness and drowsiness, a patient should *not* get out of bed without assistance until the effects of the drug are known.

**Drug Alert!**

**Teaching Alert**

Drugs for generalized and partial seizures interfere with the effects of birth control pills. Women may need to use another form of contraception to avoid becoming pregnant.

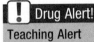

**Clinical Pitfall**

Patients taking drugs to prevent generalized or partial seizures should *not* drink alcohol because it can increase the side effects of dizziness or drowsiness.

**Drug Alert!**

**Teaching Alert**

While taking carbamazepine (Tegretol), patients should avoid grapefruit and grapefruit juice because they may increase the effects of this drug.

**Drug Alert!**

**Teaching Alert**

Patients taking phenytoin (Dilantin) should see their dentist regularly because of extra growth of the gums that occurs while taking this drug.

**Drug Alert!**

**Action/Intervention Alert**

Monitor a patient who is taking valproic acid (Depakote) closely for wound healing and signs of infection.

## What To *Teach* Patients About First-Line Drugs for Partial and Generalized Seizures

For patients taking a first-line drug to prevent partial or generalized seizures, stress the importance of keeping follow-up appointments with the prescriber to monitor control of the seizures. The patient may need to have occasional laboratory tests done to check blood levels of these drugs or to check for liver damage.

Instruct patients to take the drug exactly as prescribed and explain that suddenly stopping the drug may cause seizures to occur. Remind them to take a missed dose as soon as possible but not to take a double dose. Teach about symptoms to report immediately to their prescriber.

Teach female patients of childbearing age that birth control pills may not work effectively while taking these drugs. To prevent pregnancy they may need to use another form of contraception.

Because these drugs can cause dizziness or drowsiness, caution patients to avoid driving, operating machinery, or doing anything that requires mental alertness. Instruct them to get out of bed slowly. Tell them to avoid alcohol while taking these drugs because it can cause increased drowsiness or dizziness.

Suggest that patients wear a medical alert bracelet and carry an identification card with them that states their diagnosis, prescribed drugs, and their prescriber's name.

Carbamazepine (Tegretol) can make skin more sensitive to sunlight. Instruct patients to wear protective clothing and sunscreen and to avoid the use of sun lamps or tanning beds.

Instruct patients to take these drugs with food if GI symptoms occur and to drink plenty of water. Remind patients taking carbamazepine to avoid grapefruit and grapefruit juice because these increase the action of the drug and can lead to more side effects or adverse effects.

Phenytoin (Dilantin) can cause extra growth of gum tissues. Tell patients to visit their dentist regularly and to brush and floss teeth carefully.

Teach patients to take phenytoin at least 2 to 3 hours before or after using antacids. Absorption of phenytoin is decreased by antacids. Valproic acid (Depakote, Depacon) can lead to blood problems that can cause slowed healing and increased risk for infection.

If a patient is to have surgery of any kind, including dental surgery, the surgeon or dentist should be notified about the use of these drugs because of the risk for bleeding.

## Life Span Considerations for First-Line Drugs for Partial and Generalized Seizures

***Pediatric Considerations.*** Phenytoin must be used carefully for children because of extra growth of gums while taking the drug. Children are more likely to have behavioral changes while taking carbamazepine. Adolescents often require increased dosages of anti-seizure drugs because of growth and hormone changes. Adolescents are at risk to stop taking this drug to avoid changes to the skin and gums and to fit in more closely with their peers.

***Considerations for Pregnancy and Breastfeeding.*** Carbamazepine, phenytoin, and valproic acid are pregnancy category D drugs and may be used during pregnancy only if potential benefits outweigh risks to the fetus. A seizure during pregnancy can result in oxygen loss to the fetus or physical injury to the mother or fetus if a fall occurs. Some infants have been born with low birth weight, small head sizes, skull or facial defects, underdeveloped fingernails, and delayed growth when mothers took large doses of this drug during pregnancy. Carbamazepine passes into breast milk.

Safe use of phenytoin (pregnancy category D) during pregnancy or breastfeeding has not been established. Valproic acid (pregnancy category D) during pregnancy has been associated with developmental defects, low IQ, birth defects, congenital anomalies, and damage to the infant's liver. This drug also passes into breast milk and should not be taken while a mother is breastfeeding. Fetal hydantoin syndrome is a rare disorder that is caused by exposure of a fetus to phenytoin. The symptoms of this disorder may include abnormalities of the skull and facial features, growth deficiencies, underdeveloped nails of the fingers and toes, and/or mild developmental delays.

**Considerations for Older Adults.**    Older adults are more sensitive to the effects of these drugs and may experience confusion, restlessness, nervousness, and abnormal heartbeats. Older adults may also experience chest pain. Monitor heart rate and rhythm more frequently. Teach older adults to check their pulse at least once daily and to report abnormal beats to the prescriber. Stress the importance of calling 911 or getting to the nearest emergency department if chest pain occurs, especially if it is accompanied by shortness of breath.

## FIRST-LINE DRUGS FOR ABSENCE SEIZURES

### How Drugs for Absence Seizures Work

First-line drugs for absence seizures include ethosuximide (Zarontin) and valproic acid (Depakote). Ethosuximide depresses the motor cortex and increases the central nervous system (CNS) threshold to stimuli. The action of valproic acid may be related to increased availability of the neurotransmitter GABA.

Generic names, brand names, and common dosages of these drugs are listed in the following table. Be sure to consult a drug handbook for specific information about each of these drugs.

#### Dosages for Common First-Line Drugs for Absence Seizures

| Drug | Dosage |
| --- | --- |
| ethosuximide (Zarontin) | *Adults/Children 6-12 years:* 250 mg orally twice daily; maximum dosage 1.5 g/day <br> *Children 3-6 years:* 250 mg orally daily; maximum dosage 1.5 g/day |
| valproic acid (Depakote; Depacon IV) | *Adults/Children 10 years or older:* Oral and IV—10-15 mg/kg/day in divided doses; can increase by 5-10 mg/kg/day until seizures are controlled; maximum dosage 60 mg/kg/day |

### Intended Responses

- Seizures are controlled and prevented.
- Abnormal electrical impulses are decreased.
- Resistance of CNS to abnormal stimuli is increased.

**Side Effects.**    Common side effects of these drugs include the GI symptoms of nausea, vomiting, and indigestion. They also may cause loss of appetite (anorexia) and weight loss. Valproic acid may cause prolonged bleeding time.

Other side effects of these drugs include mental confusion, drowsiness, dizziness, headaches, constipation, depression, and nervousness.

Patients taking these drugs should notify their prescriber immediately about symptoms of allergic reaction such as rashes, fever, and sore throat. The prescriber should also be notified immediately about signs of bleeding such as easy bruising, petechiae, bloody nose, or any unusual bleeding.

**Adverse Effects.**    Adverse effects of ethosuximide (Zarontin) include a decrease in the number of WBCs *(neutropenia);* reduction in the number of erythrocytes, all types of WBCs, and blood platelets in the circulating blood *(pancytopenia);* and anemia caused by deficient RBC production in the bone marrow *(aplastic anemia).*

Valproic acid can lead to damage or destruction in the liver *(hepatotoxicity),* inflammation of the pancreas *(pancreatitis),* and bone marrow depression. Bone

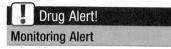

**Monitoring Alert**

Assess older adults who have been prescribed first-line drugs for partial or generalized seizures for abnormal heart rhythms and chest pain. Report these occurrences immediately to the prescriber.

**Common Side Effects**

**First-Line Drugs for Absence Seizures**

Nausea/Vomiting, Indigestion, Decreased appetite, Weight loss

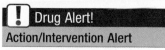

**Action/Intervention Alert**

Report signs of allergic reaction or abnormal bleeding immediately to the prescriber.

marrow depression can result in reduced production of RBCs, which causes anemia; reduced WBCs, which can result in infection; and reduced platelets, which can result in bleeding.

### What To Do *Before* Giving First-Line Drugs for Absence Seizures

Before giving a first-line drug to prevent absence seizures, obtain a complete list of drugs the patient is currently taking, including over-the-counter and herbal drugs. Ask female patients of childbearing age if they are pregnant, planning to become pregnant, or breastfeeding. Check the patient's baseline coagulation laboratory test results.

Check baseline vital signs, level of consciousness, and gait. Obtain a baseline weight for the patient. Be sure the patient's bed is in the lowest position and side rails are raised to prevent injury during an absence seizure. Ensure that the call light is within easy reach.

### What To Do *After* Giving First-Line Drugs for Absence Seizures

After giving a first-line drug to prevent absence seizures, recheck vital signs and level of consciousness. If the patient develops GI distress, give these drugs with food. Check the patient's weight every day.

Instruct the patient to call for help when getting out of bed and make sure that the call light is within easy reach.

Monitor the patient for seizure activity and be prepared to manage a seizure if one occurs (for example, protect the airway and protect the patient from injury). Watch for side effects, including abnormal bleeding, and report these to the prescriber.

### What To *Teach* Patients About First-Line Drugs for Absence Seizures

For patients taking a first-line drug to prevent absence seizures, instruct them to take these drugs exactly as prescribed and to take missed doses as soon as possible but not to take double doses. Tell patients not to stop taking these drugs suddenly because seizures may occur.

Teach patients about side effects, adverse effects, and symptoms to report immediately to their prescriber. Remind them about the importance of follow-up appointments to monitor seizure control and to have ordered laboratory tests done to monitor blood levels of these drugs.

Remind patients to avoid driving or operating machines or doing anything that requires increased alertness. Instruct them to get out of bed slowly because of side effects such as dizziness. Tell them to avoid using alcohol because this can increase the side effects of drowsiness and dizziness.

If a patient is scheduled for surgery, including dental surgery, instruct him or her to notify the surgeon or dentist about the use of these drugs.

Ethosuximide (Zarontin) can make the eyes more sensitive to light. Instruct patients to protect their eyes by wearing dark glasses in bright light.

Suggest that patients wear a medical alert bracelet and carry an identification card stating their diagnosis, prescribed drugs, and their prescriber's name.

### Life Span Considerations for First-Line Drugs for Absence Seizures

*Pediatric Considerations.* Children younger than 2 years of age are at increased risk for liver damage that may lead to death with valproic acid. Safe use of ethosuximide in children younger than 3 years has not been studied or established. Growing children who take drugs for seizures often need dose increases as they grow. Adolescence is a physically and emotionally stressful time with an increased risk for seizure occurrences.

*Considerations for Pregnancy and Breastfeeding.* Safe use of ethosuximide (pregnancy category C) has not been established. Valproic acid (pregnancy category

---

**! Drug Alert!**
**Action/Intervention Alert**

Give drugs for seizures with food if GI symptoms such as nausea, vomiting, and stomach upset develop.

---

**Clinical Pitfall**

Patients should *never* suddenly stop taking seizure drugs because this may cause seizures to occur.

---

**! Drug Alert!**
**Teaching Alert**

Teach patients taking ethosuximide (Zarontin) to wear dark glasses when going out into bright light.

D) during pregnancy has been associated with developmental defects, low IQ, birth defects, congenital anomalies, and damage to the infant's liver. This drug also passes into breast milk and should not be used while a mother is breastfeeding.

***Considerations for Older Adults.***   Valproic acid should be used cautiously in older adults because they may be more sensitive to its side effects such as sleepiness and dizziness. Teach older adults to take special precautions to avoid falls. Instruct them to change positions slowly and to use handrails when going up or down stairs. Suggest that older adults avoid driving or using dangerous machines until they know how the drugs will affect them.

◀ⓔ-Learning Activity 21-5

## SECOND-LINE (ALTERNATIVE) DRUGS FOR SEIZURES

### How Second-Line Drugs for Seizures Work

Phenobarbital (Luminal) and primidone (Mysoline) increase the body's threshold against seizure activity by blocking or slowing the spread of abnormal impulses. The disadvantage of phenobarbital is that it can lead to physical dependence. Primidone is turned into phenobarbital by the body and acts in the same way as phenobarbital. Gabapentin (Neurontin) and lamotrigine (Lamictal) stabilize the membranes of neurons to decrease seizure activity. The action of clonazepam (Klonopin) is not well understood but may be related to inhibition (slowing or stopping) of transmission of abnormal impulses.

Commonly prescribed second-line drugs for seizures are listed in the following table. Be sure to consult a drug handbook for specific information on each of these drugs.

### Dosages for Common Second-Line Drugs for Seizures

| Drug | Dosage |
|---|---|
| clonazepam (Klonopin, Novo-Clonazepam✦, Rivotril) **100** | *Adults:* 1.5 mg orally daily in 3 divided doses; maximum dosage 20 mg/day<br>*Children less than 10 years:* 0.01-0.03 mg/kg orally daily in 3 divided doses; maximum dosage 0.2 mg/kg/day |
| gabapentin (Neurontin) **100** | *Adults/Children over 12 years:* 300-400 mg orally 3 times daily; maximum dosage 1800-2400 mg/day |
| lamotrigine (Lamictal) | With valproic acid:<br>*Adults:* 25 mg orally every day during weeks 1-2; increase to 100-200 mg/day slowly over several weeks; maximum dosage 200 mg/day<br>*Children 2-12 years:* 0.2-1 mg/kg orally daily; increase slowly over several weeks; maximum dosage 5 mg/kg/day<br>With other seizure drugs:<br>*Adults:* 50-500 mg orally daily in 2 divided doses<br>*Children 2-12 years:* 5-15 mg/kg orally daily in 2 divided doses; maximum dosage 400 mg/day |
| phenobarbital (Ancakuxur✦, Barbita, Luminal) | *Adults:* Oral—100-300 mg/day; IV/IM—200-600 mg/day<br>*Children:* Oral, IV—3-8 mg/kg/day<br>*Neonates:* Oral, IV—4 mg/kg/day; maximum dosage 5 mg/kg/day |
| primidone (Mysoline, Primidone✦, Sertan✦) | *Adults/Children 8-12 years:* 250 mg orally daily; maximum dosage 2 g in 2-4 divided doses<br>*Children less than 8 years:* 125 mg orally daily; maximum dosage 1 g in 2-4 divided doses |

**100** Top 100 drugs prescribed.

 **Do Not Confuse**

**Neurontin** *with* **Noroxin**

An order for Neurontin may be confused with Noroxin. Neurontin is an anti-seizure drug, whereas Noroxin is an anti-infective drug.

 **Do Not Confuse**

**Lamictal** *with* **Lamisil**

An order for Lamictal may be confused with Lamisil. Lamictal is an anti-seizure drug, whereas Lamisil is an anti-fungal, anti-infective drug.

 **Do Not Confuse**

**lamotrigine** *with* **lamivudine**

An order for lamotrigine may be confused with lamivudine. Lamotrigine is an anti-seizure drug, whereas lamivudine is an anti-infective, anti-retroviral drug used to treat human immune deficiency virus.

### Intended Responses

- Seizures are controlled and prevented.
- Abnormal electrical impulses are decreased.
- Resistance of CNS to abnormal stimuli is increased.

**Side Effects.** Common side effects of second-line drugs for seizures vary with the prescribed drug. The most common side effects of these drugs are listed in the following table. Be sure to consult a drug handbook for additional information on a specific drug.

**Common Side Effects of Second-Line Drugs for Seizures**

| Drug | Common Side Effects |
|---|---|
| clonazepam (Klonopin) | Appetite changes, ataxia, behavioral changes, diarrhea, dizziness, drowsiness, dry mouth, fatigue, sedation, upset stomach, weakness |
| gabapentin (Neurontin) | Abnormal eye movements, ataxia, blurred vision, clumsiness, cold/flu symptoms, confusion, delusions, dementia, depression, drowsiness, fatigue, hoarseness, lower back or side pain, shaking, swelling in hands and legs, trembling, unsteadiness, weakness, |
| lamotrigine (Lamictal) | Ataxia, blurred vision, clumsiness, diplopia, dizziness, drowsiness, headache, nausea, photosensitivity, poor coordination, rash, rhinitis, somnolence, unsteadiness, vomiting |
| phenobarbital (Luminal) | Depression, dizziness, drowsiness, excitement (especially in children), headache, somnolence, upset stomach, vomiting |
| primidone (Mysoline) | Anorexia, ataxia, clumsiness, dizziness, drowsiness, headache, nausea, sedation, unsteadiness, vertigo, vomiting |

Second-line drugs for seizures are often prescribed with other seizure medications, causing an increased risk for side effects. When seizure drugs are prescribed together, lower doses may be needed. When gabapentin is prescribed for a patient who is taking morphine, increased blood levels of gabapentin can occur, possibly leading to toxicity. A lower dose of gabapentin, morphine, or both may be required to avoid side effects.

Primidone decreases the effects of anticoagulant drugs, so higher doses of an anticoagulant may be needed to achieve therapeutic effects.

**Adverse Effects.** Clonazepam is a benzodiazepine CNS drug with the life-threatening adverse reaction of respiratory depression. Lamotrigine can lead to Stevens-Johnson syndrome, a serious and life-threatening body-wide (systemic) allergic reaction with a rash involving the skin and mucous membranes. It can also lead to toxic epidermal necrolysis, a life-threatening skin disorder characterized by blistering and peeling of the top layer of skin.

Several life-threatening adverse effects are associated with phenobarbital, including closure of the larynx, which blocks the passage of air to the lungs (*laryngospasm*); circulatory collapse (*shock*); and decreased number of WBCs (*neutropenia*). Additional adverse effects include respiratory depression when high doses are prescribed, CNS depression, coma, and death. Swelling similar to that seen in urticaria (hives) can occur beneath the skin instead of on the surface. Other adverse effects include deep swelling around the eyes and lips and sometimes of the hands and feet (*angioedema*) and hypersensitive reaction to the administration of a foreign serum (*serum sickness*), which is characterized by fever, swelling, skin rash, and enlargement of the lymph nodes.

---

**Common Side Effects**

**Second-Line Drugs for Seizures**

Dizziness   Drowsiness   GI upset

Clumsiness, Unsteadiness

---

**⚠ Drug Alert!**

**Interaction Alert**

When a patient takes morphine at the same time as gabapentin (Neurontin), the blood level of gabapentin is increased and could become toxic.

### What To Do *Before* Giving Second-Line Drugs for Seizures

Before giving a second-line drug to prevent seizures, obtain a complete list of drugs the patient is currently taking, including over-the-counter and herbal drugs. Check baseline vital signs, level of consciousness, and gait.

Ask patients about the nature of their seizure activity. Be sure to ask about previous GI problems and symptoms. Make sure that the patient's bed is in the lowest position and side rails are raised.

Remember to schedule at least 2 hours between gabapentin and antacid drugs.

Make sure to ask female patients of childbearing age if they are pregnant, breastfeeding, or planning to become pregnant. Ask about the use of birth control pills.

Ask older adults about the presence of liver or kidney problems.

If the patient is to receive an IV drug form such as phenobarbital, be sure to check that the IV site is patent and the IV solution is compatible with the drug.

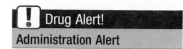

**Drug Alert!**

**Administration Alert**

Antacids interfere with absorption of gabapentin (Neurontin). Schedule at least 2 hours between giving gabapentin and an antacid.

### What To Do *After* Giving Second-Line Drugs for Seizures

After giving a second-line drug to prevent seizures, recheck vital signs, gait, and level of consciousness. Because these drugs can cause dizziness or drowsiness, instruct patients to call for help when getting out of bed and ensure that the call light is within easy reach.

Be sure to assess for and ask about side effects and watch for adverse effects of these drugs. Notify the prescriber if side effects or adverse effects occur. If the patient develops a rash, hold the drug and notify the prescriber immediately. To minimize the risk of severe rashes, the dose of lamotrigine (Lamictal) can be increased very slowly over 6 to 7 weeks. If the patient is taking lamotrigine, skin rash can be the first sign of Stevens-Johnson syndrome or toxic epidermal necrolysis.

Give these drugs with food if the patient develops nausea, vomiting, or stomach upset. Make sure that any ordered laboratory tests are completed.

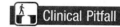

**Clinical Pitfall**

If a patient develops a rash, do *not* give the drug and notify the prescriber immediately.

### What To *Teach* Patients About Second-Line Drugs for Seizures

For patients taking a second-line drug to prevent seizures, teach them about the importance of keeping regular follow-up visits with their prescriber and having laboratory work done to assess control of the seizure disorder. Instruct patients not to suddenly stop taking these drugs because seizures may occur. Tell them to take these drugs exactly as prescribed and not to take double doses. Teach them to ask their prescriber before taking any over-the-counter drugs.

Instruct patients to notify their prescriber immediately about any signs of allergic reactions to these drugs, including skin rashes, fever, flulike symptoms, and swollen glands. They should also notify their prescriber immediately if seizure activity increases.

These drugs may be given with or without food, depending on whether the patient develops GI symptoms such as nausea, vomiting, or upset stomach.

Remind patients that phenobarbital and clonazepam may become habit forming and should only be taken for the period of time prescribed.

When patients taking these drugs are scheduled for surgery (including dental surgery), they should be instructed to notify their surgeon or dentist about their use. Because of side effects such as dizziness and drowsiness, tell patients to avoid driving, operating machinery, or doing anything that requires increased alertness until they know how the drug will affect them.

Phenobarbital and primidone (Mysoline) interfere with the actions of birth control pills. Women taking these drugs should be instructed to use another form of contraception to prevent pregnancy. Remind female patients to notify their prescriber immediately if they are pregnant, breastfeeding, or planning to become pregnant.

Patients taking phenobarbital, primidone, or lamotrigine should be taught to avoid alcohol because it adds to the drowsiness that these drugs may cause.

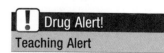

**Drug Alert!**

**Teaching Alert**

Patients should be taught to notify their prescriber immediately if seizure activity increases or changes in any way.

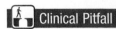
## Clinical Pitfall

Patients should *not* smoke while taking clonazepam (Klonopin).

Tell patients with diabetes that gabapentin may affect a dipstick test for protein in the urine *(proteinuria)*. Gabapentin (Neurontin) should be taken at least 2 hours after an antacid because antacids can decrease absorption of this drug.

Patients taking lamotrigine should be taught to wear sunscreen and protective clothes to prevent photosensitivity reactions. Remind patients about these precautions even if they have dark skin that does not usually get sunburned.

Remind patients who smoke while taking clonazepam (Klonopin) that cigarette smoking may decrease the effectiveness of this drug. If he or she smokes, a higher dose of the drug may be needed to be effective.

Suggest that patients wear a medical alert bracelet and carry an identification card with their diagnosis, drugs in use, and their prescriber's name.

### Life Span Considerations for Second-Line Drugs for Seizures

*Pediatric Considerations.* Children have a higher incidence of rashes with lamotrigine. Gabapentin may cause fever, hyperactivity, and hostile or aggressive behavior in children. They are much more sensitive to the effects of gabapentin and are at increased risk of side effects.

*Considerations for Pregnancy and Breastfeeding.* Women are more likely to experience dizziness when taking lamotrigine (pregnancy category C). These drugs have not been tested in pregnant women. Primidone may cause increased birth defects, and there have been reports of newborns with bleeding problems. If a woman takes lamotrigine during pregnancy, she should also take folic acid. Gabapentin (pregnancy category C) has been associated with bone and kidney problems in pregnant animals but has not been tested in women. Phenobarbital, clonazepam, and primidone are pregnancy category D. In animal studies newborns have been lower weight and have a lower survival rate. These drugs pass into breast milk and should not be taken by a woman who is breastfeeding because they may cause unwanted side effects in infants.

## ! Drug Alert!
**Action/Intervention Alert**

Children and older adults are more sensitive to the effects of second-line anti-seizure drugs and are more likely to develop side effects. Monitor these patients carefully.

*Considerations for Older Adults.* Older adults are also more sensitive to these drugs and more likely to develop side effects. They may develop unusual restlessness or excitement with primidone. Lamotrigine and gabapentin are more slowly eliminated from an older adult's body. Because of this, older adults may need to be started on a lower drug dose.

⊖-Learning Activity 21-6 ▶

# Get Ready for Practice!

## Key Points

- Abnormal electrical impulses in the brain cause seizures to occur.
- The most common ages for onset of seizures are early childhood and late adulthood.
- A typical seizure consists of an aura, the seizure, and a postictal period.
- The two major groups of seizures are generalized and partial.
- Status epilepticus is a prolonged seizure or a series of repeated seizures without enough time for recovery between seizures.
- The exact action of most anti-seizure drugs is not known, but these drugs decrease the voltage, frequency, and spread of abnormal electrical impulses in the brain.

- Many drugs for seizures interfere with the effects of birth control pills, and women should be taught to use an alternative form of contraception to prevent pregnancy.
- Antacids decrease the absorption of anti-seizure drugs and should be given at least 2 to 3 hours before or after taking these drugs.
- Patients who suddenly stop taking anti-seizure drugs are at high risk for having a seizure.
- Patients should be instructed to notify their prescriber immediately if seizure activity increases or changes in any way.

## Additional Learning Resources

evolve Go to your Evolve website (http://evolve.elsevier.com/Workman/pharmacology/) for the following FREE learning resources:

- eLearning Activities
- Animations
- Video Clips
- Interactive Review Questions
- Audio Key Points
- Audio Glossary
- Audio Glossary—Spanish-English
- Drug Dosage Calculators
- Patient Teaching Handouts

**SG** Go to your Study Guide for additional learning activities to help you master this chapter content.

## Review Questions

1. Which drug used to treat seizures increases the availability of the neurotransmitter gamma-aminobutyric acid (GABA)?

   A. phenobarbital (Luminal)
   B. carbamazepine (Tegretol)
   C. valproic acid (Depakote)
   D. phenytoin (Dilantin)

2. For which adverse effects must you watch after giving a patient clonazepam (Klonopin)?

   A. Respiratory depression
   B. Stevens-Johnson syndrome
   C. Aplastic anemia
   D. Thrombocytopenia

3. What safety interventions must you take before giving the first-line drug for seizures phenytoin (Dilantin)? (Select all that apply.)

   A. Obtain a complete list of drugs the patient is currently using.
   B. Ask the patient to describe the nature of previous seizures.
   C. Obtain a baseline patient weight.
   D. Ensure that the call light is within easy reach.
   E. Teach the patient about the importance of frequent mouth care.

4. A patient is taking phenytoin (Dilantin). What must you be sure to teach the patient about this drug?

   A. Visit a dentist regularly.
   B. Avoid grapefruit and grapefruit juice.
   C. Always take the drug on an empty stomach.
   D. Wear protective clothing and a strong sunscreen.

5. Which is an important precaution when administering primidone (Mysoline) to an older adult?

   A. They may develop high fevers.
   B. They will have a higher incidence of rashes.
   C. They may develop hostile, aggressive behavior.
   D. They may develop unusual restlessness or excitement.

6. A patient has been prescribed carbamazepine (Tegretol) 600 mg per day in 3 divided doses. How many milligrams do you give with each dose? _____ mg

7. An infant is to be given phenobarbital 4 mg/kg in an oral suspension. The infant weighs 5 kg. How many milligrams do you give? _____ mg

## Critical Thinking Activities

Jimmy P. is 9 years old. His teacher notices that he often stares off into space and appears to be daydreaming. She states that his grades have gone down and he sometimes does not seem to be paying attention in class.

1. What type of seizure is this child experiencing?

2. What would you expect to happen after a child has this type of seizure?

3. What drugs would you expect to be prescribed for this child?

## Objectives

*After studying this chapter you should be able to:*

1. Explain how different classes of drugs are used to treat depression, anxiety, and psychosis.
2. List the common names, actions, usual adult dosages, possible side effects, and adverse effects of drugs for depression and anxiety.
3. Describe what to do before and after giving drugs for depression and anxiety.
4. Explain what to teach patients taking drugs for depression and anxiety, including what to do, what not to do, and when to call the prescriber.
5. Describe life span considerations for drugs for depression and anxiety.
6. List the common names, actions, usual adult dosages, possible side effects, and adverse effects of drugs for psychosis.
7. Describe what to do before and after giving drugs for psychosis.
8. Explain what to teach patients taking drugs for psychosis, including what to do, what not to do, and when to call the prescriber.
9. Describe life span considerations for drugs for psychosis.

## Key Terms

**antianxiety drug** (ăn-tē-ăng-ZĪ-ĕ-tē DRŬG) (p. 400) A drug that eases anxiety; also known as an anxiolytic.

**antidepressant drug** (ăn-tē-dē-PRĔS-sĕnt DRŬG) (p. 394) A drug used to treat the symptoms of depression.

**antipsychotic drug** (ăn-tē-sī-KŎT-ĭk DRŬG) (p. 405) A drug used to treat psychosis; also called major tranquilizers and neuroleptics.

**anxiety** (ăng-ZĪ-ĕ-tē) (p. 398) A multiple-system response sometimes described as a feeling of dread about a perceived threat or danger thought to be unique to humans.

**benzodiazepine** (bĕn-zō-dī-ĂZ-ĕ-pēn) (p. 401) A type of drug commonly used to treat anxiety, produce sedation, or relax muscles.

**bipolar disorder** (bī-PŌ-lŭr dĭs-ŌR-dŭr) (p. 392) A psychiatric disorder characterized by alternating episodes of mania and depression; also called bipolar illness, or manic-depressive illness.

**depression** (dĕ-PRĔSH-ŭn) (p. 391) An illness characterized by feelings of sadness, despair, loss of energy, and difficulty dealing with normal daily life.

**delusions** (dĕ-LŪ-zhŭnz) (p. 404) Fixed false beliefs or opinions that are held despite a lack of supporting evidence and are resistant to reason or fact.

**dysthymia** (dĭs-THĪ-mē-ă) (p. 391) A chronic but less severe form of depression that is characterized by moods that are persistently low.

**generalized anxiety disorder (GAD)** (JĔN-ŭr-ăl-īzd ăng-ZĪ-ĕ-tē dĭs-ŌR-dŭr) (p. 398) Excessive, almost daily anxiety and worry for longer than 6 months.

**hallucinations** (hăl-lū-sĭ-NĀ-shŭnz) (p. 404) The perception of something such as sounds or visual images that are not actually present except in the mind; they may involve sight, hearing, smell, taste, or touch.

**illusions** (ĭl-LŪ-zhŭnz) (p. 404) Incorrect mental representations of misinterpreted events such as hearing the food cart coming down the hall and believing it is a stampede of animals.

**major depression** (MĀ-jŭr dē-PRĔSH-ŭn) (p. 391) A disabling mental disorder marked by a persistent low mood, lack of pleasure in life, and increased risk of suicide, which is diagnosed based on the presence of symptoms of depression for 2 or more weeks.

**mania** (MĀ-nē-ă) (p. 392) An extremely elevated mood state that occurs as part of bipolar disorder and is characterized by mental and physical hyperactivity and possibly psychosis.

**obsessive-compulsive disorder (OCD)** (ŏb-SĔS-ĭv kŏm-PŬL-sĭv dĭs-ŌR-dŭr) (p. 400) A psychiatric disorder characterized by obsessive thoughts and compulsive actions such as cleaning, checking, counting, or hoarding.

**panic disorder** (PĂN-ĭk dĭs-ŌR-dŭr) (p. 398) An anxiety disorder characterized by attacks of anxiety or terror, often but not always occurring unexpectedly and without reason and lasting 15 to 30 minutes.

**post-traumatic stress disorder (PTSD)** (PŌST tră-MĂT-ĭk STRĔS dĭs-ŌR-dŭr) (p. 400) An anxiety disorder caused by serious traumatic events; characterized by symptoms of survivor guilt, reliving the trauma in dreams, numbness and lack of involvement with reality, or recurrent intrusive thoughts and images.

**psychosis** (sī-KŌ-sĭs) (p. 404) An illness that prevents a person from being able to distinguish between the real world and the imaginary world; it commonly includes delusions or hallucinations.

**selective serotonin reuptake inhibitors (SSRIs)** (sĕ-LĔK-tĭv sĕr-ō-TŌ-nĭn rē-ŪP-tāk ĭn-HĬB-ĭ-tŭrz) (p. 394)

Antidepressant drugs that act by blocking the reuptake of serotonin, making more serotonin available to act on receptors in the brain.

**tricyclic antidepressants (TCAs)** (trī-SĬK-lĭk ăn-tē-dē-PRĔS-sĕnts) (p. 394) Antidepressant drugs that act by blocking the reuptake of norepinephrine and serotonin and making more of these substances available to act on receptors in the brain.

◄ ⊖-Learning Activity 22-1

## OVERVIEW

Psychiatric disorders are a broad group of illnesses that may include affective or emotional instability, behavioral problems, and cognitive dysfunction or impairment. Specific illnesses include major depression, generalized anxiety disorder, bipolar disorder, and schizophrenia. Mental illness may be of biologic (for example, anatomic, chemical, or genetic) or psychologic (for example, trauma or conflict) origin and may affect a person's ability to function in society or relationships.

Major mental illnesses are the most common cause of disability in the United States. About 23% of North American adults experience a clinically diagnosable mental illness each year. Between 9% and 13% of children younger than age 18 experience serious emotional disturbance with functional impairment, whereas 5% to 9% have serious emotional disturbance with extreme functional impairment caused by a mental illness.

Depression, anxiety, and psychosis are major psychiatric illnesses. As many as 30% of patients in the United States report symptoms of depression, but only about 10% experience major depression. Anxiety affects as much as 3% of the population in the United States each year. The incidence of schizophrenia, a major psychotic disorder, is about 1% worldwide. The chronic nature of these illnesses presents many challenges for treatment.

**? Did You Know?**

As many as 30% of patients in the United States report symptoms of depression, and about 10% experience major depression.

## DEPRESSION

**Depression** is an illness characterized by persistent feelings of sadness, despair, loss of energy, and difficulty dealing with normal daily life. It involves the body, mood, and thoughts and affects how a person eats and sleeps, how he or she feels about himself or herself and relates to others, and how he or she thinks about things. Each year around 10% of American adults (1.8 million) suffer from depression. It interferes with the ability to function normally and causes pain and suffering for patients with this disorder and their loved ones. Figure 22-1 gives some examples of depression.

Depression can occur at any age but typically develops in the middle teens, 20s, or 30s. Women are twice as likely as men to experience depression, but men are less likely than women to seek treatment. Because depression is often mistaken for a normal part of aging, many older adults with depression may be undiagnosed or untreated. Children and adolescents with depression often pretend to be sick, refuse to go to school, get into trouble in school, have negative outlooks, and feel misunderstood. Many people with depression do not seek treatment because they do not recognize the condition as a treatable illness.

There are three forms of depressive disorders: major depression, dysthymia, and bipolar disorder. **Major depression** is a disabling mental disorder marked by a persistent low mood, lack of pleasure in life, and increased risk of suicide. Diagnosis is based on the presence of five or more depression symptoms that last 2 weeks or more (Box 22-1). Major depression may occur just once or several times during a lifetime.

**Dysthymia** is a chronic but less severe form of depression characterized by moods that are persistently low. The symptoms may be daunting but are not disabling. A person with dysthymia may experience episodes of major depression.

**? Did You Know?**

Women are twice as likely as men to experience depression; men are less likely to seek treatment.

◄ ⊖-Learning Activity 22-2

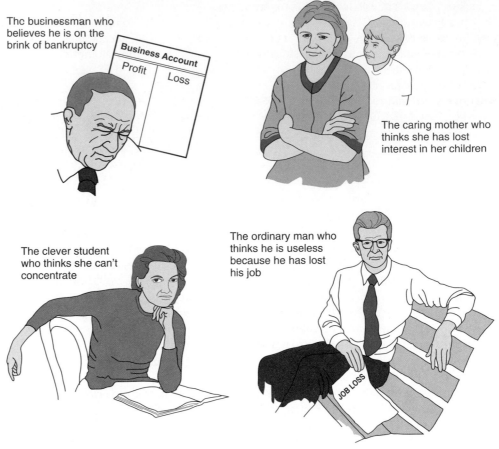

**FIGURE 22-1** Examples of depression.

---

**Box 22-1**    Symptoms of Depression

- Abrupt changes in eating habits
- Chronic fatigue; being slowed down
- Decreased ability to perform normal daily tasks
- Decreased appetite and/or weight loss or overeating and weight gain
- Difficulty concentrating, remembering, or making decisions
- Feelings of hopelessness or pessimism
- Inability to experience pleasure in hobbies and activities that were once enjoyed
- Insomnia, early morning awakening, or oversleeping
- Irritability
- Numb or empty feeling or absence of any feelings at all
- Persistent feeling of worthlessness, guilt, helplessness, or sadness
- Persistent physical symptoms that do not respond to treatment (for example, headaches, digestive disorders, chronic pain)
- Recurrent thoughts of death or suicide
- Restlessness

---

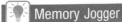 **Memory Jogger**

Bipolar disorder is characterized by cycling moods—from severe highs to severe lows.

**Bipolar disorder,** formerly called manic-depression, is characterized by cycling moods from severe highs **(mania)** to severe lows (depression). Mood changes may be sudden and dramatic, or they may be gradual. During a low cycle the person has symptoms of depression (see Box 22-1). During a high cycle he or she may be overactive, overly talkative, and full of energy. Mania can affect thought processes, judgment, and social behavior. Box 22-2 summarizes symptoms of mania. Untreated mania may progress to psychosis.

Diagnosis of depression is based on identifying symptoms (see Box 22-1). A complete physical examination is important to rule out physical disorders such as thyroid disease, anemia, and viral infections. Neurologic examinations can rule out

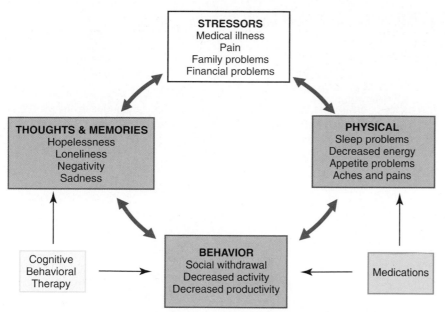

**FIGURE 22-2** The cycle of depression.

---

**Box 22-2** Symptoms of Mania

- Abnormal or excessive elation
- Decreased need for sleep
- Grandiose notions
- Inappropriate social behavior
- Increased sexual desire

- Increased talking
- Markedly increased energy
- Poor judgment
- Racing thoughts
- Unusual irritability

---

neurologic disorders. Several short questionnaires have been developed to assist with screening for depression and mania (for example, Goldberg Depression Questionnaire [18 questions] or The Wakefield Questionnaire for Depression [12 questions]). These questionnaires can indicate the need for further evaluation. A detailed history by a qualified health care professional is important to discover specific factors in a patient's life that may contribute to depression.

The most common treatments for depression include counseling or psychotherapy and antidepressant drugs. Depression treatment is individualized, taking into account the severity and cause of the depression episode. Most patients with depression are treated as outpatients; however, when a person has suicidal thoughts (also called *suicidal ideation*) and particularly if the person has a suicide plan, hospitalization may be required. With treatment symptoms can be well controlled. Figure 22-2 shows the cycle of depression, including how and when to intervene for effective treatment with medications and psychotherapy.

### REVIEW OF RELATED PHYSIOLOGY AND PATHOPHYSIOLOGY

The exact cause of depression is not known, but theories include heredity, changes in neurotransmitter levels, altered neuroendocrine function, and psychosocial factors. Table 22-1 summarizes factors often associated with depression.

Research suggests that depression may be caused by an imbalance of brain chemicals called *neurotransmitters* (for example, serotonin, dopamine, and norepinephrine). Communication between neurons in the brain occurs by the movement of these chemicals across a small gap called the *synapse*. Neurotransmitters are released from one neuron at the presynaptic nerve terminal and then cross the synapse, where they may be accepted by the next neuron at a specialized site called a *receptor* (Figure 22-3). When neurotransmitter levels decrease or become imbalanced, the neurons may be less able to communicate with each other, which may lead to depression and other mood changes.

**Clinical Pitfall**

When a patient with depression has suicidal thoughts and a suicide plan, hospitalization may be required for the patient's safety.

◄ ⊖-Learning Activity 22-3

Table 22-1 Factors Associated with Depression

| FACTOR | EXAMPLES | FACTOR | EXAMPLES |
|---|---|---|---|
| Chemicals | Dopamine<br>Norepinephrine<br>Serotonin | Heredity | First-degree relatives (for example, mother, father) |
| Physical factors | Environmental conditions<br>Extreme stress<br>Trauma | Physical illness | Acquired immune deficiency syndrome<br>Adrenal disorders<br>Brain tumors |
| Drugs | Abuse of alcohol or amphetamines<br>Antipsychotics<br>Beta blockers<br>Corticosteroids<br>Reserpine | | Multiple sclerosis<br>Parkinson's disease<br>Stroke<br>Thyroid disorders |
| | | Psychosocial factors | Abuse<br>Introversion<br>Separations or losses |
| Gender | Postmenopause<br>Postpartum<br>Thyroid dysfunction<br>Women twice as susceptible as men | Seasonal | Climates with long, severe winter |

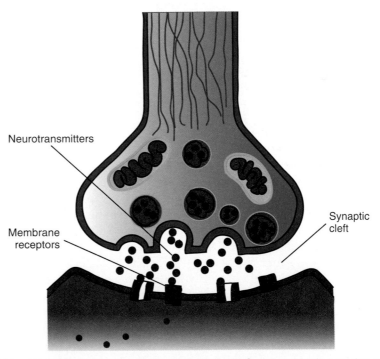

**FIGURE 22-3** Neurotransmitters carry signals across the synapse from a neuron to receptors on the next neuron.

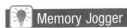 Memory Jogger

The two most common groups of drugs to treat depression are SSRIs and TCAs.

# TYPES OF DRUGS FOR DEPRESSION

## ANTIDEPRESSANTS

### How Antidepressants Work

Antidepressant drugs are used to treat people with depression. Prescription and use of these drugs can lead to the improvement of symptoms, particularly when patients also receive some form of psychotherapy or counseling.

The two most common groups of drugs used to treat depression are selective serotonin reuptake inhibitors (SSRIs), and tricyclic antidepressants (TCAs). SSRIs have fewer side effects than TCAs. With most of these drugs, it can take as long as

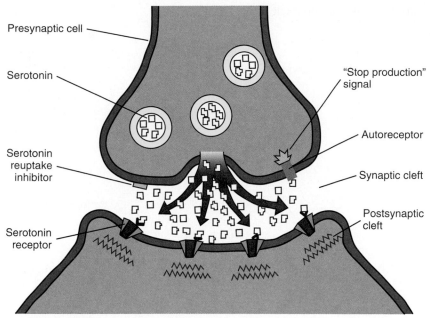

**FIGURE 22-4** Selective serotonin reuptake inhibitor drugs increase the amount of serotonin in the brain by blocking reuptake of neurotransmitters by neurons.

8 weeks for symptoms of depression to improve. Often depression is chronic, and patients must continue to take antidepressants even when they have no symptoms to keep the depression from returning.

SSRIs work by increasing the amount of serotonin in the brain by inhibiting reuptake (Figure 22-4). TCAs inhibit the reuptake of the neurotransmitters norepinephrine, dopamine, or serotonin by nerve cells. The effects of these drugs occur immediately, but the patient's symptoms often do not respond for 2 to 8 weeks. Other drugs such as norepinephrine and dopamine reuptake inhibitors (NDRIs) (for example, bupropion [Wellbutrin]) correct the imbalance of the neurotransmitters dopamine and norepinephrine.

Generic names, trade names, and dosages of common antidepressants are listed in the following table. Be sure to consult a drug handbook for specific information about any drug used to treat depression.

### Dosages for Common Antidepressant Drugs

| Drug | Dosage |
|------|--------|
| *SSRIs* | |
| citalopram (Celexa) | *Adults:* 20 mg orally once daily; may increase by 20 mg per week up to 60 mg/day; usual dosage is 20-40 mg/day |
| escitalopram (Lexapro) 🔳 | *Adults:* 10 mg orally once daily; may increase to 20 mg after 1 week |
| fluoxetine (Prozac, Prozac Weekly) 🔳 | *Adults:* 20 mg orally daily in the morning; may increase by 20 mg every 4 weeks up to 80 mg; doses over 20 mg/day should be given in 2 divided doses; 90 mg once a week<br>*Children (8-18 years):* 10-20 mg orally daily; may increase to 20 mg/day after 1 week |
| paroxetine (Paxil, Paxil CR) 🔳 | *Adults:* 20 mg orally daily, may increase by 10 mg per week up to 50 mg/day; controlled-release (CR)—12.5 mg/day, may increase by 12.5 mg per week to a maximum dosage of 62.5 mg/day |

*Continued*

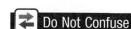 **Do Not Confuse**

**Lexapro** *with* **Loxitane**

An order for Lexapro may be confused with Loxitane. Lexapro is an SSRI drug used to treat depression, whereas Loxitane is a central nervous system (CNS) drug used to treat psychotic disorders.

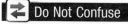 **Do Not Confuse**

**Celexa** *with* **Zyprexa or Celebrex**

An order for Celexa may be confused with Zyprexa or Celebrex. Celexa is an SSR! drug used to treat depression, whereas Zyprexa is an antipsychotic drug used to treat psychotic disorders. Celebrex is a nonsteroidal anti-inflammatory drug (NSAID) used to treat osteoarthritis and rheumatoid arthritis.

## Do Not Confuse

**sertraline** *with* **Soriatane**

An order for sertraline may be confused with Soriatane. Sertraline is an SSRI drug used to treat depression, whereas Soriatane is a skin agent used to treat severe psoriasis.

## Do Not Confuse

**buPROPion** *with* **busPIRone**

An order for bupropion can be confused with buspirone. Bupropion is an antidepressant drug, whereas buspirone is an anti-anxiety drug.

## Do Not Confuse

**Wellbutrin SR** *with* **Wellbutrin XL**

An order for Wellbutrin SR can be confused with Wellbutrin XL. Both drugs are norepinephrine and dopamine reuptake inhibitors used to treat depression. But Wellbutrin SR is a slow-release form of the drug given twice a day, whereas Wellbutrin XL is an extended-release form of the drug given once a day.

## Do Not Confuse

**trazodone** *with* **tramadol**

An order for trazodone may be confused with tramadol. Trazodone is a combined reuptake inhibitor and receptor blocker used to treat depression, whereas tramadol is an analgesic used to treat moderate-to-moderately severe pain.

## Common Side Effects

### Antidepressants

 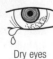 

Hypotension    Headache    Dry eyes

Dizziness    Drowsiness

### Dosages for Common Antidepressant Drugs—cont'd

| Drug | Dosage |
|------|--------|
| sertraline (Zoloft) **TOP 100** | *Adults:* 50 mg orally daily; may increase by 25 mg/day each week; maximum dosage 200 mg/day<br>*Children (13-17 years):* 50 mg orally once daily<br>*Children (6-12 years):* 25 mg orally once daily |
| **TCAs** | |
| amitriptyline (Apo-Amitriptyline🍁, Elavil) **TOP 100** | *Adults:* 75 mg orally daily in divided doses; may increase to 150 mg/day |
| desipramine (Norpramin, Pertofrane🍁) | *Adults:* 100-200 mg orally daily; may increase to 300 mg/day<br>*Children (>12 years):* 25-50 mg orally daily; may increase to 100 mg/day over 1-2 weeks<br>*Children (6-12 years):* 1-5 mg/kg orally daily in 2-3 divided doses |
| imipramine (Impril🍁, Nofranil, Novo Pramine🍁, Tofranil) | *Adults:* 25-50 mg orally 3-4 times daily; maximum dosage 300 mg/day; may give total dosage at bedtime<br>*Children (>12 years):* 25-50 mg orally daily in divided doses; maximum dosage 75 mg/day<br>*Children (6-12 years):* 25 mg orally daily in divided doses; maximum dosage 50 mg |
| nortriptyline (Aventyl, Pamelor) | *Adults:* 25 mg orally 3-4 times daily up to 150 mg/day |
| *Serotonin and Norepinephrine Reuptake Inhibitors* | |
| duloxetine (Cymbalta) | *Adults:* 20-30 mg orally twice daily |
| venlafaxine (Effexor) **TOP 100** | *Adults:* 75 mg orally daily in 2-3 divided doses, maximum dosage 375 mg/day in 3 divided doses; extended release (XR)—75 mg once daily |
| *Norepinephrine and Dopamine Reuptake Inhibitors* | |
| buPROPion (Wellbutrin) **TOP 100** | *Adults:* 100 mg orally twice daily; maximum dosage 450 mg in 3 divided doses |
| *Combined Reuptake Inhibitors and Receptor Blockers* | |
| mirtazapine (Remeron) | *Adults:* 15 mg orally daily in single bedtime dose; maximum dosage 45 mg/day |
| nefazodone | *Adults:* 100 mg orally twice daily; maximum dosage 600 mg/day in 2 divided doses |
| trazodone (Desyrel) **TOP 100** | *Adults:* 150 mg orally daily in 3 divided doses; maximum dosage 600 mg/day in divided doses |

**TOP 100** Top 100 drugs prescribed.

### Intended Responses
- Depression is corrected.
- Symptoms of depressed mood are decreased.

**Side Effects.** Common side effects of SSRIs include insomnia, nausea, diarrhea, apathy, anxiety, nervousness, dizziness, drowsiness, fatigue, confusion, headache, weakness, abdominal pain, anorexia, dry mouth, dyspepsia, flatulence, increased saliva, increased sweating, decreased interest in sexual activity, and tremors.

Common side effects of TCAs include lethargy, sedation, drowsiness, fatigue, blurred vision, dry eyes, dry mouth, hypotension, and constipation.

**Adverse Effects.** TCAs such as amitriptyline (Elavil), desipramine (Norpramin), imipramine (Tofranil), and nortriptyline (Aventyl) may cause serious adverse cardiac effects, including unstable ventricular dysrhythmias (abnormal heart rhythms) or asystole (absence of a heart rhythm).

Venlafaxine (Effexor), duloxetine (Cymbalta), and buPROPion (Wellbutrin) may cause seizures. Mirtazapine (Remeron) can lead to neutropenia (decreased white blood cells [WBCs]), which increases the risk of infection. Nefazodone has been known to cause liver failure or liver toxicity.

Thoughts of suicide may increase in children, adolescents, and young adults when taking antidepressants; a warning appears on all labels for these drugs.

Signs of allergic reactions to antidepressants include chest pain, increased or irregular heart rhythm, shortness of breath, fever, hives, rash, itching, difficulty breathing or swallowing, swelling, decreased coordination, shaking hands (tremors), dizziness, light-headedness, and thoughts of hurting oneself.

## What To Do *Before* Giving Antidepressants

Always obtain a complete list of drugs the patient is currently taking, including over-the-counter and herbal drugs. Check baseline blood pressure and heart rate and rhythm.

Assess the patient's mental status and ask about suicidal thoughts. Ask about usual bowel pattern, fluid intake, and diet. Ask whether the patient has a family history of depression.

If a patient is taking a TCA, ask about smoking because smoking cigarettes may decrease the effectiveness of these drugs.

Wellbutrin may be prescribed as Wellbutrin SR, the sustained-release form, which is administered in two doses at least 8 hours apart. Wellbutrin XL extended-release tablets should be taken once a day in the morning. Wellbutrin SR and XL tablets should be swallowed whole and never chewed, divided, or crushed.

## What To Do *After* Giving Antidepressants

Recheck the patient's blood pressure and heart rate and rhythm and monitor for decreased blood pressure and abnormal heart rhythms. Reassess the patient's mental status to determine his or her response to drugs. Monitor the patient for drug side effects, adverse effects, or allergic reactions and report them to the prescriber. Ask patients about suicidal thoughts and determine if they have a suicide plan. Immediately report suicidal thoughts or plans to the prescriber.

Because of the risk of dizziness, instruct patients to call for assistance when getting out of bed and ensure that the call light is within easy reach.

## What To *Teach* Patients About Antidepressants

Instruct patients to take these drugs exactly as directed by their prescriber. Explain that their prescriber may start with a low drug dose and gradually increase it until therapeutic antidepressant effects are achieved. Tell patients about the importance of keeping follow-up appointments to monitor the progress of treatment.

Remind patients that antidepressants can control the symptoms of depression but will not cure depression. Teach them that it may take 1 to 8 weeks before symptoms of depression improve. Remind patients to take their antidepressant even when feeling well.

If an antidepressant dose is missed, tell the patient to take the dose as soon as possible unless it is almost time for the next dose. Remind him or her not to double the doses of these drugs.

Tell patients to report any side effects to their prescriber immediately. Remind them to continue taking these drugs while waiting to talk to their prescriber. Antidepressants may need to be discontinued gradually to avoid adverse effects.

Teach patients that Wellbutrin works by correcting the imbalance of the neurotransmitters dopamine and norepinephrine and that it may be prescribed as Wellbutrin SR (sustained-release form, which is administered in two doses at least 8 hours apart) or Wellbutrin XL (extended-release tablets that should be taken once a day in the morning). Instruct patients that Wellbutrin SR and XL tablets should be swallowed whole and never chewed, divided, or crushed.

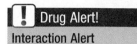

**Interaction Alert**

Be sure to ask a patient about the use of St. John's wort, an herbal product used to treat depression. It should not be taken with antidepressant drugs.

**Drug Alert!**

**Interaction Alert**

Ask patients taking a TCA drug about smoking because smoking cigarettes may decrease the effectiveness of these drugs.

**Clinical Pitfall**

Immediately report any suicidal thoughts or suicide plans to the prescriber.

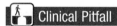

**Teaching Alert**

Be sure to teach patients who are taking an antidepressant that it may take 1 to 8 weeks before symptoms of depression improve.

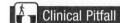

**Clinical Pitfall**

Instruct patients *not* to stop taking an antidepressant without first talking to their prescriber.

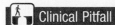
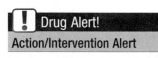
Caution patients to avoid driving, operating machines, or doing anything requiring alertness because of drowsiness, dizziness, and impaired (blurred) vision until the effects of the drug are known. Remind them to change positions slowly because of hypotension and dizziness.

Teach patients that frequent mouth rinses and good oral hygiene can minimize the effects of dry mouth.

Remind women of childbearing age to notify their prescriber if they are pregnant, plan to become pregnant, or are breastfeeding.

Tell patients to avoid alcohol while taking antidepressants because alcohol may increase drowsiness.

Instruct patients taking an SSRI to take the dose once a day in the morning or evening.

Caution patients taking a monoamine oxidase inhibitor (MAOI) and transitioning to an SSRI, TCA, or other antidepressant that these drugs should not be used for at least 14 days after discontinuing MAOI drugs because of a life-threatening drug interaction called *serotonin syndrome*. Symptoms include confusion, agitation, restlessness, stomach disturbances, sudden elevated temperature, extremely high blood pressure, and severe seizures.

Remind patients to tell their health care providers about taking antidepressant drugs before having any surgical procedures, including dental surgery.

Advise patients to wear a medical alert bracelet or carry an identification card stating the name of the drug and the reason for taking it.

### Life Span Considerations for Antidepressants

***Pediatric Considerations.*** SSRIs, TCAs, and other antidepressant drugs should be used with caution in depressed children and adolescents because the risk of suicidal thoughts or actions may increase while taking these drugs. Fluoxetine (Prozac) may cause unusual excitement, restlessness, irritability, or trouble sleeping in children because they are more sensitive to the effects of this drug. Venlafaxine (Effexor) may slow growth and weight gain in children. A child's growth should be monitored carefully while taking this drug.

***Considerations for Pregnancy and Breastfeeding.*** SSRIs (pregnancy category C) have not been tested during pregnancy. Paroxetine (Paxil) should be avoided in pregnancy. Some of these drugs pass through breast milk and may have unwanted effects such as drowsiness, decreased feeding, and weight loss on the breastfeeding infant. TCAs are pregnancy category C (amitriptyline, desipramine) or D (nortriptyline, imipramine).

***Considerations for Older Adults.*** Older adults may require lower doses of SSRIs because of possible increased reaction to the effects and side effects of these drugs and slower metabolism of drugs such as escitalopram (Lexapro). Older patients with kidney disease or liver failure should be given lower doses of these drugs because they are metabolized by the liver and kidneys.

⊜-Learning Activity 22-4 ▶

## ANXIETY

**Anxiety** is a feeling of apprehension, fear, or worry. It can occur without a cause and may not be based on a real-life situation. Symptoms of anxiety vary with the form of anxiety disorder (Box 22-3).

Common anxiety disorders include panic disorder, generalized anxiety disorder, phobic disorder, obsessive-compulsive disorder, and post-traumatic stress disorder (PTSD). **Panic disorders** are separate and intense periods of fear or feelings of doom that develop over a short period of time such as 10 minutes. A panic attack, the main symptom of panic disorder, is characterized by anxiety or terror and usually lasts between 15 and 30 minutes. **Generalized anxiety disorder (GAD)** is when a person experiences excessive, almost daily anxiety and worry for more than 6 months. It

Box **22-3**   Symptoms of Anxiety

**PANIC DISORDER**
- Chest pain
- Chills or hot flashes
- Dizziness
- Feeling of being detached from the world (derealization)
- Fear of dying
- Nausea
- Numbness and tingling
- Palpitations
- Sense of choking
- Shortness of breath
- Sweating
- Trembling

**GENERALIZED ANXIETY DISORDER**
- Difficulty concentrating
- Easy fatigue
- Excessive, unrealistic worry
- Irritability
- Muscle tension
- Restlessness
- Sleep disturbance

**PHOBIC DISORDER**
- Intense, persistent, recurrent fear of certain objects (for example, snakes, spiders, blood)
- Intense, persistent, recurrent fear of certain situations (for example, heights, speaking in front of a group, public places)
- Panic attack possibly triggered by objects and situations

**OBSESSIVE-COMPULSIVE DISORDER**
- Obsessive thoughts such as:
  - Excessive focus on religious or moral ideas
  - Fear of being contaminated by germs or dirt or contaminating others
  - Fear of causing harm to yourself or others
  - Fear of losing or not having things you might need
  - Intrusive sexually explicit or violent thoughts and images
  - Order and symmetry—the idea that everything must line up "just right."
  - Superstitions—excessive attention to something considered lucky or unlucky
- Compulsive behaviors such as:
  - Accumulating "junk" such as old newspapers, magazines, empty food containers, or other things for which you don't have a use
  - Counting, tapping, repeating certain words, or doing other senseless things to reduce anxiety
  - Excessively double checking things such as locks, appliances, and switches
  - Ordering or making groups of things even or arranging things "just so"
  - Praying excessively or engaging in rituals triggered by religious fear
  - Repeatedly checking in on loved ones to make sure they're safe
  - Spending a lot of time washing or cleaning

**STRESS DISORDERS (POST-TRAUMATIC STRESS DISORDER)**
- Avoiding activities, places, or people associated with the triggering event
- Being hypervigilant
- Difficulty concentrating
- Difficulty sleeping
- Feeling a general sense of doom and gloom along with decreased positive emotions and hopes for the future

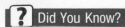

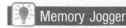

affects about 3% of the population in the United States. Women are twice as likely as men to be affected. GAD most often begins during childhood or adolescence, but it may begin at any age.

*Phobic disorders* are intense, persistent, recurrent fears of certain objects (for example, snakes) or situations (for example, speaking in front of a group) that can cause a panic attack. Obsessive-compulsive disorder (OCD) is characterized by obsessive thoughts and compulsive actions. The person with OCD becomes trapped in a pattern of repetitive thoughts and behaviors that do not make sense and are distressing but are very difficult to overcome. Post-traumatic stress disorder (PTSD) leads to anxiety and is caused by exposure to death or near-death experiences such as floods, fires, earthquakes, shootings, automobile accidents, or war. The traumatic experience recurs in thoughts and dreams.

Diagnosing a patient with anxiety involves a comprehensive health history and physical examination with close attention to blood pressure, heart rate, and respiratory rate. The health care provider asks questions about the feeling of anxiety and may order diagnostic tests such as a complete blood count (CBC), thyroid function test, and electrocardiogram (ECG). Often he or she will refer the patient to a psychiatrist or clinical psychologist to determine the cause of the anxiety.

Treatment of anxiety depends on the cause. Short-term anxiety attacks can be treated at home with interventions such as talking with a supportive person, meditating, taking a warm bath, resting in a dark room, or performing deep-breathing exercises. Strategies for coping with anxiety and stress include eating a well-balanced diet, getting enough sleep, exercising regularly, limiting caffeine and alcohol, avoiding nicotine and recreational drugs, using relaxation techniques, and balancing fun activities with responsibilities. Group therapy may be useful for anxieties such as fear of flying. Physical conditions may be treated with drugs or surgery. An example of a physical cause for anxiety is a tumor called a *pheochromocytoma*, which causes the adrenal glands to produce excessive amounts of adrenaline. Surgical removal of this tumor can resolve the symptom of anxiety. Symptoms of hyperthyroidism include anxiety. Careful diagnosis is essential because many of the symptoms of hyperthyroidism are also found in anxiety disorder. Hyperthyroidism and anxiety are often confused. Medical or surgical treatment of hyperthyroidism can also resolve the anxiety. Counseling or psychotherapy may also be helpful. Antianxiety drugs are often prescribed to control the symptoms of anxiety.

⊖-Learning Activity 22-5 ►

## REVIEW OF RELATED PHYSIOLOGY AND PATHOPHYSIOLOGY

Anxiety that is perceived as out of proportion with what is normal or expected may escalate through a feedback circle (Figure 22-5). Physical symptoms may affect the heart (increased rate, pounding), lungs (increased rate and depth, shortness of breath), and nervous system (tremors, headaches). Emotional symptoms of anxiety include apprehension, dread, irritability, restlessness, and difficulty concentrating. Causes and factors associated with anxiety include mental conditions, physical conditions, the effects of drugs, or a combination of these causes. Box 22-4 summarizes the causes of the mental condition and the external factors associated with anxiety.

## TYPES OF DRUGS FOR ANXIETY

### ANTIANXIETY DRUGS

#### How Antianxiety Drugs Work

Mild anxiety is a common experience and usually requires no treatment. Moderate-to-severe anxiety is a symptom of psychiatric disorders such as phobia, panic disorder, OCD, and PTSD.

Chronic and severe anxiety are treated with antianxiety drugs, also called *anxiolytics* or *minor tranquilizers*. Most drugs used to treat anxiety also cause sedation or sleep and are likely to cause *dependence* (the psychologic craving for, or physiologic reliance on, a chemical substance) when taken for an extended period.

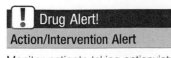

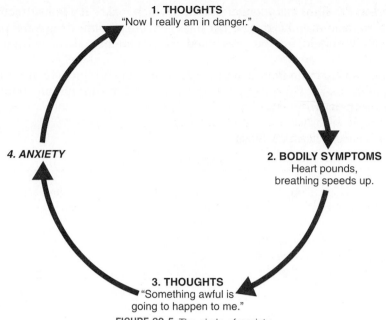

**1. THOUGHTS**
"Now I really am in danger."

**2. BODILY SYMPTOMS**
Heart pounds,
breathing speeds up.

*4. ANXIETY*

**3. THOUGHTS**
"Something awful is
going to happen to me."

**FIGURE 22-5** The circle of anxiety.

---

**Box 22-4** | **Causes and External Factors Associated with Anxiety**

- Financial stress
- Lack of oxygen such as high-altitude sickness, emphysema, and pulmonary embolus
- Side effect of medication
- Stress at work
- Stress from a serious medical illness
- Stress from emotional trauma such as death of a loved one
- Stress from school
- Stress in personal relationships such as marriage
- Symptoms of a medical illness
- Use of illicit drugs such as cocaine

---

In the past **benzodiazepines** were the most commonly prescribed drugs for treatment of anxiety. When taken as directed, these drugs allow many patients with anxiety to lead nearly normal lives. Buspirone (BuSpar) and SSRIs such as sertraline (Zoloft), paroxetine (Paxil), fluoxetine (Prozac), and venlafaxine (Effexor) are now prescribed to treat anxiety more commonly than benzodiazepines because they have milder side effects and patients are less likely to become dependent on them. The major benefit of benzodiazepines is that they act within 30 minutes and may be given as needed, whereas it may take SSRIs 3 to 5 weeks to control anxiety. Benzodiazepines also decrease symptoms of alcohol withdrawal and prevent delirium tremens.

Benzodiazepines are CNS depressants that increase the inhibitory actions of gamma-aminobutyric acid (GABA) in the brain. GABA is a neurotransmitter that transmits messages from brain cell to brain cell. It sends a message to the brain neurons to slow down or stop firing. This quiets the brain and decreases anxiety.

SSRIs relieve anxiety by affecting the action of the neurotransmitter serotonin in the brain. Serotonin stays in the synaptic gap longer, and transmission of impulses is slowed. It is also theorized that these drugs may affect the limbic system, which is the part of the brain associated with emotions. They calm and relax people with anxiety; however, they may take several weeks to become effective.

Buspirone (BuSpar) binds the neuroreceptors for serotonin and dopamine in the brain and increases norepinephrine metabolism to relieve anxiety. Binding the neurotransmitters slows the transmission of impulses and quiets the brain to relieve anxiety.

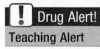

**! Drug Alert!**

**Teaching Alert**

Teach patients that it may take SSRI drugs 3 to 5 weeks to control anxiety.

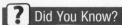

Diazepam (Valium) has a longer half-life, which makes it a less attractive choice than other benzodiazepine drugs. Because benzodiazepine drugs are potentially addictive, they should not be prescribed for a patient with a substance abuse disorder.

Generic names, trade names, and dosages of drugs for anxiety are listed in the following table. Be sure to consult a drug handbook for information about any specific antianxiety drug.

**Dosages for Common Antianxiety Drugs**

| Drug | Dosage |
| --- | --- |
| *Benzodiazepines* | |
| alprazolam (Apo-Alpraz🍁, Nu-Alpraz🍁, Xanax) | *Adults:* 0.25-0.5 mg orally 2-3 times daily, do not exceed 4 mg/day; extended release (XR)—1-10 mg once daily |
| clonazepam (Gen-Clonazepam🍁, Klonopin, Novo-Clonazepam🍁) | *Adults:* 0.125-0.25 mg orally twice daily |
| clorazepate (Novo-Clopate🍁, Tranxene) | *Adults:* 5 mg orally daily at bedtime; maximum dosage 60 mg/day |
| chlordiazepoxide (Librium, Novopoxide🍁) | *Adults:* Oral—7.5-10 mg as a single dose at bedtime or as 2-3 divided doses daily, maximum dose 60 mg daily; IM/IV—50-100 mg first dose, then 25-50 mg 3-4 times daily<br>*Children (>6 years):* Oral—5 mg 2-4 times daily<br>*Children (>12 years):* IM/IV—25-50 mg per dose |
| diazepam (Valium, Vivol🍁) 🔲TOP100 | *Adults:* Oral—2-10 mg/day in 2-4 divided doses; IM/IV—2-10 mg, repeat every 3-4 hr as needed |
| lorazepam (Ativan, Nu-Loraz🍁) 🔲TOP100 | *Adults:* 2-6 mg orally per day in divided doses; maximum dosage 10 mg/day |
| oxazepam (Novoxapam🍁, Serax) | *Adults:* 10-30 mg orally 3-4 times daily |
| *Anxiolytics* | |
| busPIRone (BuSpar) | *Adults:* 7.5-15 mg orally daily in divided doses; maximum dosage 60 mg/day |

🔲TOP100 Top 100 drugs prescribed.

### Intended Responses
- Anxiety is relieved without too much sedation.
- Symptoms of anxiety are decreased.
- Sense of well being is improved.

***Side Effects.*** The most common side effects of benzodiazepines are related to their CNS effects. They include sedation, sleepiness, depression, lethargy, apathy, fatigue, hypoactivity, light-headedness, memory impairment, disorientation, amnesia, dizziness, delirium, headache, slurred speech, behavioral changes, ataxia, unsteadiness, euphoria, dysarthria, inability to perform complex mental functions, nervousness, irritability, difficulty concentrating, "glassy-eyed" appearance, changes in heart rate and blood pressure, changes in bowel function, and skin rashes. With chlordiazepoxide (Librium), there is pain at intramuscular sites after injection.

Common side effects of busPIRone include dizziness and drowsiness. Others may include excitement, fatigue, headache, insomnia, nervousness, weakness, blurred vision, nasal congestion, sore throat, tinnitus, chest pain, palpitations, tachycardia, nausea, rash, myalgia, lack of coordination, numbness, paresthesia, clammy skin, and sweating.

***Adverse Effects.*** Life-threatening adverse effects of benzodiazepines include seizures and coma. BusPIRone can result in hallucinations and heart failure.

**Common Side Effects**

**Antianxiety Drugs**

Dizziness  Drowsiness  Headache

Fatigue  Rash

Suddenly stopping a benzodiazepine can cause a potentially life-threatening reaction of withdrawal symptoms, including nervousness, restlessness, tremulousness, weakness, and seizures. The patient may become dehydrated or delirious or may develop insomnia, confusion, and visual or auditory hallucinations.

Suicidal ideation (creating a plan to carry out suicide) may occur with patients taking clonazepam (Klonopin).

### What To Do *Before* Giving Antianxiety Drugs

Obtain a complete list of drugs the patient is currently taking, including over-the-counter and herbal drugs. Check baseline blood pressure, heart rate, and respiratory rate. If an anxiety drug is to be given intravenously, assess the site and ensure that it is patent.

Assess the patient's baseline level of anxiety and mental status. Assess for the presence of suicidal thoughts. Assess an older adult patient's risk for falls and apply precautions against falls if needed.

### What To Do *After* Giving Antianxiety Drugs

Recheck the patient's blood pressure, heart rate, and respiratory rate. Monitor him or her for dizziness, drowsiness, or light-headedness. Report changes to the prescriber. Watch for side effects and adverse effects. Assess gait for steadiness. Continue to monitor level of anxiety to assess the effectiveness of the drug. Assess and monitor the patient for suicidal ideation.

Because of the tendency to become dependent on benzodiazepines, give these drugs only as prescribed. Observe for signs of dependency while patients are taking them and report them to the prescriber.

Instruct the patient to call for help when getting out of bed and ensure that the call light is within easy reach.

### What To *Teach* Patients About Antianxiety Drugs

Instruct patients to take these drugs, especially benzodiazepines, exactly as prescribed to decrease the chance of dependence. Remind patients about the importance of making and keeping follow-up appointments to monitor the effectiveness of anxiety treatment. Tell patients not to skip or double the doses of these drugs.

Remind patients that their prescriber may want to wean them off of these drugs gradually because stopping suddenly can cause withdrawal symptoms such as sweating, vomiting, muscle cramps, tremors, or seizures.

Teach patients about the signs of dependence and instruct them to report these signs immediately to their prescriber.

Urge patients to tell their health care provider or surgeon about the use of these drugs before having surgical procedures or medical tests.

Caution patients to avoid driving, operating machines, or doing anything that requires increased alertness while taking these drugs. Teach patients to avoid alcohol and other CNS depressants while taking benzodiazepines because of the added sedative effects.

Tell women of childbearing age to inform their prescriber if they are pregnant, plan to become pregnant, or are breastfeeding.

Teach patients not to take benzodiazepines with antacids because antacids decrease their absorption. Instruct patients to take these drugs 1 hour before or 2 hours after an antacid.

Remind patients taking alprazolam (Xanax), diazepam (Valium), midazolam (Versed), triazolam (Halcion), or busPIRone (BuSpar) to avoid drinking grapefruit juice while taking these drugs because grapefruit juice slows their metabolism and causes increased blood concentration.

Advise patients to wear a medical alert bracelet or carry an identification card stating the name of the drug and the reason for taking it.

---

**Clinical Pitfall**

Patients should *not* stop taking benzodiazepine drugs suddenly because of the risk for life-threatening withdrawal symptoms, including nervousness, restlessness, tremulousness, weakness, and seizures.

---

**Drug Alert!**

**Teaching Alert**

Be sure to teach patients to take benzodiazepines exactly as prescribed to decrease the risk of developing dependence on these drugs.

---

**Drug Alert!**

**Teaching Alert**

Teach patients that the signs of dependence on benzodiazepines include:

- Strong desire or need to continue taking the drug.
- Need to increase the dose to feel the effects of the drug.
- Withdrawal effects after the drug is stopped (for example, irritability, nervousness, trouble sleeping, abdominal cramps, trembling, or shaking)

---

**Drug Alert!**

**Teaching Alert**

Teach patients taking a benzodiazepine to take the drug 1 hour before or 2 hours after an antacid.

---

**Drug Alert!**

**Teaching Alert**

Teach patients who take alprazolam, diazepam, midazolam, triazolam, or busPIRone to *avoid* drinking grapefruit juice.

---

◀ ⊖-Learning Activity 22-6

### Life Span Considerations for Antianxiety Drugs

*Pediatric Considerations.*   Children are more sensitive to the effects of benzodiazepines and more likely to experience side effects. Using clonazepam (Klonopin) during childhood may cause decreased mental and physical growth. Clonazepam should not be used in children younger than 18 years with panic disorders because safety and effectiveness have not been established.

*Considerations for Pregnancy and Breastfeeding.*   Benzodiazepines (pregnancy category D/X) should not be used during pregnancy. Chlordiazepoxide (Librium) and diazepam have caused birth defects when used during the first trimester of pregnancy. Use of benzodiazepines during pregnancy causes the fetus to become dependent on these drugs and can cause withdrawal symptoms after birth. These drugs should not be taken when a woman is breastfeeding because they can cause drowsiness, difficulty with feeding, and weight loss in the infant. Physical dependence and withdrawal symptoms may also occur in breastfed infants.

*Considerations for Older Adults.*   Older adults are more sensitive to the effects of benzodiazepines and are more at risk for side effects. Older adults should be monitored for respiratory depression. Benzodiazepines may cause daytime drowsiness, falls, and injuries. Teach older adults to change positions slowly and to use handrails when going up or down stairs. Instruct family members to assess older adults who are taking benzodiazepines for changes in cognition or reduced mental alertness. Low doses of benzodiazepines should be used with these patients because they are more sensitive to the effects and side effects of these drugs. Drowsiness may be much more intense in older adults. Instruct older adults not to drive or use dangerous equipment until they know how the drug will affect them. Chlordiazepoxide and clorazepate (Tranxene) are not recommended for older adults because they have a long half-life. BusPIRone should be started at 5 mg twice a day for these patients.

## PSYCHOSIS

**Psychosis** is a loss of contact with reality that may be brief or long term. Common symptoms of psychosis include **delusions** (false ideas about what is occurring or personal identity), **illusions** (mistaken perceptions), and **hallucinations** (seeing or hearing things that are not there). Other symptoms of psychosis are listed in Box 22-5. An example of a delusion is when a person exaggerates his or her sense of self-importance and is convinced that he or she has special powers, talents, or abilities. The person may believe that he or she is a famous movie star or a saint. An example of an illusion is when a person thinks that he or she hears voices in the wind. The most common type of hallucination is hearing imaginary voices (*auditory hallucination*) that give commands, make comments, or warn of impending danger. A visual hallucination occurs when a person sees something that is not there, such as a bright light, a shape, or a human figure. A person who is experiencing a psychotic episode may be unaware that anything is wrong and unable to ask for help.

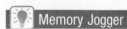

**Clinical Pitfall**

Benzodiazepines should *not* be used during pregnancy because the fetus can become dependent on these drugs and experience withdrawal symptoms after birth.

**Drug Alert!**

**Teaching Alert**

Teach family members to watch for changes in cognition or decreased mental alertness in older adults taking antianxiety drugs.

**Memory Jogger**

Psychotic disorders include delusions, illusions, and hallucinations.

| Box **22-5**   Symptoms of Psychosis |
| --- |
| • Confusion<br>• Depression and sometimes suicidal thoughts<br>• Disorganized thoughts or speech<br>• Emotion exhibited in an abnormal manner<br>• Extreme excitement (mania)<br>• False beliefs (delusions)<br>• Loss of touch with reality<br>• Mistaken perceptions (illusions)<br>• Seeing, hearing, feeling, or perceiving things that are not there (hallucinations)<br>• Unfounded fears or suspicions |

Diagnosing a patient with psychosis involves psychologic evaluation and testing, usually done by a psychiatrist or psychologist. Questions about symptoms, lifestyle, and family history are important. Magnetic resonance imaging (MRI) of the brain and blood tests for drugs or physical conditions that may cause psychosis may also be performed.

Treatment of psychosis includes psychologic therapies such as counseling, guided discussion, and cognitive behavior therapy to help change or eliminate unwanted thoughts or beliefs. Antipsychotic drugs help to decrease auditory hallucinations and delusions and stabilize thinking and behavior. Hospital care may be needed to ensure a patient's safety because a person with psychosis may harm himself or herself or others. Many symptoms of psychosis can be controlled with long-term treatment.

## REVIEW OF RELATED PHYSIOLOGY AND PATHOPHYSIOLOGY

The exact cause of psychotic disorders is not known. One theory is that these disorders develop because the brain overreacts to neurotransmitters (substances that carry messages between nerves) in the brain. Heredity may also play a part in the development of psychotic disorders such as schizophrenia, which tends to run in families. Psychosis may be caused by a variety of medical or psychiatric problems. Box 22-6 summarizes potential causes of psychosis.

## TYPES OF DRUGS FOR PSYCHOSIS

### ANTIPSYCHOTICS

#### How Antipsychotics Work

Sometimes called neuroleptics or major tranquilizers, antipsychotic drugs are prescribed to treat and control the symptoms of psychosis such as hallucinations and delusions. These drugs produce a tranquillizing effect that helps to relax the CNS, allowing patients to function appropriately and effectively. They also control the symptoms of other psychiatric disorders that may lead to psychosis such as bipolar disorder.

All antipsychotic drugs tend to block dopamine receptors in the dopamine pathways in the brain. The normal effect of releasing the neurotransmitter dopamine is decreased. Transmission of impulses is decreased, which in turn decreases the symptoms of hallucinations, illusions, and delusions. However, patients should be taught that several days to weeks may pass before the therapeutic effects of these drugs begin.

Major tranquilizers are the most commonly prescribed drugs for psychosis. Other drugs used to treat psychosis include lithium carbonate (Lithonate) and thiothixene (Navane).

Antipsychotic drugs are occasionally used to treat acute delirium. The danger of using these drugs is prolonged or worsening agitation, especially when using older drugs such as haloperidol (Haldol). These drugs should no longer be prescribed for patients with dementia unless the patient is agitated, aggressive, or showing psychotic behavior that is distressing to patients or dangerous to others. Antipsychotic drugs should never be used at the whim of a caregiver for the sole purpose of restraining patients who wander, have insomnia, or do not cooperate.

> **Memory Jogger**
>
> Major tranquilizers are the drugs most commonly prescribed to treat psychosis.

> **Clinical Pitfall**
>
> Antipsychotic drugs should never be used to restrain patients who wander, have insomnia, or are uncooperative.

◄ⓔ-Learning Activity 22-7

---

**Box 22-6** | Potential Causes of Psychosis

- Alcohol and other drugs
- Bipolar disorders (manic depression)
- Brain tumors
- Dementia (Alzheimer's and other degenerative brain disorders)
- Epilepsy
- Psychotic depression
- Schizophrenia
- Stroke

Generic names, trade names, and doses of drugs for psychosis are listed in the following table. Be sure to consult a drug handbook for information about a specific antipsychotic drug.

**Dosages for Common Drugs for Psychosis**

| Drug | Dosage |
|---|---|
| *Antipsychotics* | |
| chlorproMAZINE (Chlorpromanyl✦, Largactil✦, Thorazine) | *Adults:* Oral—10-25 mg 2-4 times daily, usual dosage 300 mg/day in divided doses; IM—25-50 mg, maximum dosage 400 mg every 3-12 hr as needed<br>*Children:* Oral—0.55 mg/kg every 4-6 hr as needed; IM—0.55 mg/kg every 6-8 hr as needed |
| clozapine (Clozaril) | *Adults:* 25 mg orally 1-2 times daily; gradually increase to target dosage of 300-450 mg/day |
| olanzapine (Zyprexa) | *Adults:* 5-10 mg orally once daily; increase to 10-15 mg/day; maximum dosage 20 mg/day |
| prochlorperazine (Compazine, Provazin✦, Stemetil✦) | *Adults/Children >12 years:* 5-10 mg orally 3-4 times daily up to 150 mg/day<br>*Adults:* IM—10-20 mg every 2-6 hr up to 200 mg/day<br>*Children 2-12 years:* IM—132 mcg/kg; not to exceed 10 mg per dose |
| quetiapine (Seroquel) | *Adults:* 25 mg orally twice daily; maximum dosage 800 mg/day |
| risperidone (Risperdal) | *Adults:* 1-3 mg orally twice daily; maximum dosage 6 mg/day |
| *Other Drugs* | |
| lithium carbonate (Carbolith✦, Eskalith, Lithizine✦, Lithonate) | *Adults/Children >12 years:* 300-600 mg orally 3 times daily<br>*Children <12 years:* 15-20 mg orally daily in 3-4 divided doses; maximum dose 2400 mg daily |
| thiothixene (Navane) | *Adults:* Oral—2 mg 3 times daily or 5 mg twice daily, maximum dosage 60 mg/day; IM—4 mg 2-4 times daily, maximum dosage 30 mg/day |

### Do Not Confuse

**chlorproMAZINE** *with* **chlorproPAMIDE**

An order for chlorpromazine may be confused with chlorpropamide. Chlorpromazine is an antipsychotic drug used to treat psychosis, whereas chlorpropamide is a sulfonylurea used to treat type 2 diabetes.

### Do Not Confuse

**Clozaril** *with* **Colazal**

An order for Clozaril may be confused with Colazal. Clozaril is an antipsychotic drug used to treat psychotic disorders, whereas Colazal is a GI anti-inflammatory drug used to treat mild-to-moderate ulcerative colitis.

### Do Not Confuse

**Zyprexa** *with* **Celexa** or **Zyrtec**

An order for Zyprexa may be confused with Celexa or Zyrtec. Zyprexa is used to treat psychotic disorders, whereas Celexa is an SSRI drug used to treat depression. Zyrtec is an antihistamine used to treat allergies.

### Common Side Effects

**Antipsychotics**

Drowsiness    Dizziness    Hypotension

Blurred vision    Dry mouth

### Intended Responses

- Signs and symptoms of psychosis, including hallucinations and delusions, are decreased.
- Behavior is improved (or there is less antisocial behavior).
- Schizophrenic behavior is decreased.
- Suicidal behavior is decreased.

**Side Effects.** Early in treatment common side effects of antipsychotic drugs include sedation and drowsiness, dizziness, agitation, headache, hypotension, tachycardia, restlessness, muscle spasms, tremor, weakness, dry mouth, dry eyes, blurred vision, constipation, weight gain, photosensitivity, diarrhea, constipation, and nausea.

**Adverse Effects.** Several life-threatening adverse effects can occur with antipsychotic drugs. Tardive dyskinesia, a disorder characterized by involuntary movements most often affecting the mouth, lips, and tongue and sometimes the trunk or other parts of the body such as arms and legs, can be caused by all antipsychotics. However, this adverse effect is much more common with first-generation drugs.

Several drugs sometimes cause seizures, including clozapine, haloperidol, olanzapine, quetiapine, and lithium.

Neuroleptic malignant syndrome is a rare, potentially life-threatening disorder involving dysfunction of the autonomic nervous system. The autonomic nervous system is the branch of the nervous system responsible for regulating such involuntary actions as heart rate, blood pressure, digestion, and sweating. Muscle tone becomes rigid with tremors, body temperature and respiratory rate are markedly elevated, heart rate is tachycardic, blood pressure may be elevated or decreased, and consciousness is also severely affected. All antipsychotic drugs can cause this syndrome.

Neutropenia (decreased WBCs) can result from taking clozapine or prochlorperazine. Clozapine can also cause myocarditis (inflammation of the heart muscle).

Quetiapine (Seroquel) and risperidone (Risperdal) cause increased risk of death in older adults with dementia.

### What To Do *Before* Giving Antipsychotics

Obtain a complete list of drugs the patient is currently taking, including over-the-counter and herbal drugs. Check the patient's baseline blood pressure, heart rate and rhythm, and respiratory rate. Monitor fluid intake and urine output. Obtain a baseline weight.

Assess baseline mental status and level of psychosis. Check orientation, mood, and behavior. Ask patients about suicidal thoughts and start suicide precautions if necessary. Be sure to observe that patients swallow these drugs.

Check older patients for risk of falls and, if appropriate, initiate fall precautions. If the drug is to be given intravenously, assess the site and ensure that it is patent.

Ask women of childbearing age if they are pregnant, plan to become pregnant, or are breastfeeding.

Ask patients about smoking because smoking may decrease the effectiveness of olanzapine and clozapine.

### What To Do *After* Giving Antipsychotics

Recheck the patient's heart rate and rhythm, blood pressure, and respiratory rate. Monitor intake and output and daily weight. Monitor bowel function. Report constipation to the prescriber and encourage the patient to drink extra fluids.

Watch for signs of side effects or life-threatening adverse effects and report these to the charge nurse and prescriber.

Instruct patients to call for help getting out of bed and ensure that the call light is within easy reach.

Reassess the patient's mental status, monitoring orientation, mood, and behavior for changes. Watch for sedation. Ask the patient about suicidal thoughts.

Give antipsychotic drugs with food if the patient develops GI upset symptoms.

### What To *Teach* Patients About Antipsychotics

Tell patients to take these drugs exactly as prescribed and to continue to take them even if they are feeling well. Remind them about the importance of making and keeping follow-up appointments to monitor the progress of treatment. Instruct them to avoid stopping these drugs suddenly, skipping drug doses, or doubling doses. Tell them to ask their prescriber before taking any over-the-counter drugs.

Teach patients that their prescriber may start with a low dose and gradually increase it to achieve therapeutic effects.

Be sure to teach patients about the side effects and adverse effects of these drugs and to notify their prescriber if any of these symptoms occur. Tell them to immediately report sore throat, unusual bleeding or bruising, rash, or tremors.

Remind patients about the importance of psychotherapy to help keep psychosis under control.

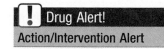

**Drug Alert!**
**Action/Intervention Alert**

Before giving an antipsychotic, be sure to ask the patient about suicidal thoughts and initiate suicide precautions if needed.

◄ ⊖-Learning Activity 22-8

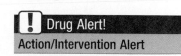

**Drug Alert!**
**Action/Intervention Alert**

Discuss with patients the importance of psychotherapy in addition to antipsychotic drug therapy to help keep their psychosis under control.

Remind patients to change positions slowly. Caution them to avoid driving, operating machines, or doing anything that requires increased alertness while taking these drugs until the drug effects are clear. Remind them to avoid alcohol and other CNS depressants while taking these drugs.

Tell patients to increase activity, fluid intake, and bulk foods to prevent constipation. Remind them to take these drugs and antacids at least 2 hours apart to prevent decreased absorption. Instruct them to take these drugs with food if GI upset occurs.

Let patients know that some of these drugs may cause urine to be abnormally colored (for example, prochlorperazine may turn urine pink or reddish-brown).

Protective clothing, hats, and sunscreens should be used to protect against *photosensitivity* (sensitivity to light). Frequent mouth rinses and oral care can help minimize dry mouth.

Patients should notify their surgeons about the use of these drugs before any surgical procedures, including dental surgery.

Remind women of childbearing age to notify their prescriber immediately if they become pregnant, plan to become pregnant, or are breastfeeding.

Instruct patients taking quetiapine (Seroquel) to avoid temperature extremes because this drug impairs body temperature regulation.

Teach patients taking quetiapine (Seroquel) or olanzapine (Zyprexa) to avoid grapefruit and grapefruit juice during therapy. Grapefruit can interfere with metabolism of the drug, causing increased blood levels and increased risk for side effects or adverse effects.

Encourage patients to wear a medical alert bracelet or carry an identification card stating the name of the drug and the reason for taking it.

### Life Span Considerations for Antipsychotics

*Pediatric Considerations.* Side effects and adverse effects are more likely in children because they are more sensitive to the effects of these drugs.

*Considerations for Pregnancy and Breastfeeding.* Drugs for psychosis (pregnancy category C) should be avoided during pregnancy. These drugs may cross the placenta and cause unwanted side effects such as involuntary movements on the newborn infant. Lithium is pregnancy category D and should be avoided during pregnancy and breastfeeding. They should usually not be taken during breastfeeding.

*Considerations for Older Adults.* Side effects and adverse effects are more likely in older adults because they are more sensitive to the effects of these drugs. They should start with lower doses of all antipsychotic drugs. Older adults with renal insufficiency should also be started with lower doses.

Most of the antipsychotic drugs, especially chlorpromazine (Thorazine) can cause a rapid fall in blood pressure when changing from a sitting to a standing position (orthostatic hypotension). Teach older adults to change positions slowly and to sit on the edge of the bed for a few moments before standing. Remind them to always use handrails when going up or down stairs.

Lithium can cause excessive urination and quickly lead to dehydration, especially in older adults. Remind older adults to drink daily about the same amount of fluid they lose in urination. Also remind them to notify the prescriber if they are too nauseated and cannot take in as much fluid as they should.

**Drug Alert!**
**Teaching Alert**

Tell patients taking prochlorperazine (Compazine) that it may turn their urine pink or reddish-brown.

**Drug Alert!**
**Teaching Alert**

Instruct patients taking quetiapine (Seroquel) to avoid temperature extremes because this drug impairs body temperature regulation.

**Drug Alert!**
**Teaching Alert**

To prevent falls, teach older adults to change positions slowly while taking chlorpromazine (Thorazine) because it can cause a rapid drop in blood pressure.

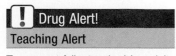-Learning Activity 22-9 ▶

## Get Ready for Practice!

### Key Points

- Mental illness can be caused by biologic or psychologic factors.
- Women are twice as likely as men to develop depression, but men are less likely to seek treatment for depression.
- Depression can be mistaken as part of the aging process, and many older adults go undiagnosed and untreated.
- Many people with depression do not seek treatment because they do not recognize that it is a treatable illness.
- Anxiety may occur without a cause or may be based on a real-life situation.
- Physical reactions such as increased heart rate, sweating, trembling, fatigue, and weakness often occur with anxiety.
- A person experiencing a psychotic disorder may be unaware that anything is wrong and unable to ask for help.
- Treatment for depression, anxiety, and psychosis includes psychotherapy, counseling, and medications.
- It may take up to 8 weeks for improvement of depression symptoms after an antidepressant drug is prescribed.
- Be sure to ask a patient with a mental disorder about suicidal thoughts.
- Instruct patients not to stop taking these drugs without talking with their prescriber.
- Assess a patient with an anxiety disorder for physical signs such as changes in blood pressure, heart rate, and respiratory rate.
- Teach patients taking benzodiazepines to take the drugs exactly as prescribed to decrease the risk of developing drug dependence.

### Additional Learning Resources

evolve Go to your Evolve website (http://evolve.elsevier.com/Workman/pharmacology/) for the following FREE learning resources:

- eLearning Activities
- Animations
- Video Clips
- Interactive Review Questions
- Audio Key Points
- Audio Glossary
- Audio Glossary—Spanish-English
- Drug Dosage Calculators
- Patient Teaching Handouts

SG Go to your Study Guide for additional learning activities to help you master this chapter content.

### Review Questions

1. How do tricyclic antidepressants (TCAs) work to treat depression?

   A. By inhibiting the reuptake of the neurotransmitters norepinephrine, dopamine, or serotonin by nerve cells
   B. By inhibiting the actions of gamma-aminobutyric acid (GABA) in the brain
   C. By affecting the action of the neurotransmitter serotonin in the brain
   D. By inhibiting the activity of monoamine oxidase preventing the breakdown of monoamine neurotransmitters

2. For which signs of dependence must you teach patients to watch when they have been prescribed a benzodiazepine drug for anxiety? (Select all that apply.)

   A. A strong desire or need to continue taking the drug
   B. Dry mouth, constipation, and blurred vision
   C. A need to increase the dose to receive the effects of the drug
   D. Withdrawal symptoms when the drug is stopped
   E. Increased heart rate, blood pressure, and respiratory rate

3. A patient who has been taking amitriptyline (Elavil) to treat depression has developed an irregular heart rate of 112 beats per minute. What is your best first action?

   A. Hold the dose and notify the patient's health care provider.
   B. Have the patient take slow deep breaths.
   C. Give the patient's beta blocker drug early.
   D. Assist the patient out of bed and up into a chair.

4. A patient prescribed the SSRI sertraline (Zoloft) asks why diazepam (Valium) wasn't prescribed instead. What is your best response?

   A. "Sertraline works directly on the neurotransmitters, and diazepam works on the receptors."
   B. "Sertraline has milder side effects and is less likely to cause dependence than diazepam."
   C. "Diazepam is more likely to cause dangerously high blood pressure, and sertraline has no effect on blood pressure."
   D. "Diazepam interacts with other drugs and food, whereas sertraline can be taken without regard to other drugs or food."

5. Which antidepressant drug may slow growth and weight gain in children?

   A. fluoxetine (Prozac)
   B. sertraline (Zoloft)
   C. venlafaxine (Effexor)
   D. duloxetine (Cymbalta)

6. The patient prescribed chlorpromazine (Thorazine) has developed rigid muscle tone, an elevated temperature of 101° F, and confusion. What is your best action?

   A. Send urine and blood samples to the laboratory for culture and sensitivity tests.
   B. Administer acetaminophen (Tylenol) as ordered.
   C. Document these findings as expected and common side effects.
   D. Hold the drug and notify the prescriber immediately

7. For what do you assess in a patient before and after giving a drug to treat psychosis?

   A. Increased blood pressure
   B. Suicidal thoughts
   C. Level of consciousness
   D. Pain control

8. The patient prescribed chlorpromazine (Thorazine) tells you that his urine has turned reddish brown. What do you teach this patient?

   A. "Chlorpromazine often turns a patient's urine pink or reddish-brown."
   B. "This drug may cause blood loss in your urine, which is why it is reddish-brown."
   C. "Always notify your prescriber when a drug causes the color of your urine to change."
   D. "Be sure to drink more fluids whenever your urine appears dark in color."

9. How can the intake and output of an older adult be affected by prescribed lithium (Lithonate)?

   A. Lithium can cause an increase in thirst so the older adult drinks more fluids.
   B. Lithium can cause excessive urination, which can lead to dehydration.
   C. Lithium can cause a decrease in urination, which can lead to fluid overload.
   D. Lithium can cause decreased thirst, which can lead to fluid volume deficit.

10. The prescriber orders fluoxetine (Prozac) 60 mg in 2 divided doses. Fluoxetine comes in scored 20-mg tablets.

    a. How many mg do you give for each dose? _____ mg
    b. How many tablets would you give for each dose? _____ tablet(s)

11. The prescriber's order for a patient with generalized anxiety disorder is for diazepam (Valium) 5 mg IM every 6 hours as needed. Diazepam is available as 10 mg/mL. How many milliliters do you give for each dose? _____ mL

## Critical Thinking Activities

Mr. Thorne is a 74-year-old man admitted to the psychiatric floor after stating that a voice told him to drive his car over the neighbor's cat because the cat was evil.

1. What is Mr. Thorne's diagnosis?

2. What is Mr. Thorne experiencing?

3. The range of beginning doses of chlorpromazine (Thorazine) is 10 to 25 mg. Why would you expect his starting dose to be low?

4. Mr. Thorne tells you that he has not had a bowel movement for the past 2 days. What would you instruct him to do?

5. Mr. Thorne is ready for discharge. He tells you that he's feeling much better and asks if he really needs to continue to see the psychiatrist every week. What would you be sure to tell him?

# Drugs for Alzheimer's and Parkinson's Disease

## Objectives

*After studying this chapter you should be able to:*

1. Explain how different classes of drugs are used to treat Alzheimer's disease and Parkinson's disease.
2. List the names, actions, usual adult dosages, possible side effects, and adverse effects of drugs for Alzheimer's disease.
3. Describe what to do before and after giving drugs for Alzheimer's disease.
4. Explain what to teach patients and their families or caregivers about drugs for Alzheimer's disease, including what to do, what not to do, and when to call the prescriber.
5. Describe life span considerations for drugs for Alzheimer's disease.

6. List the names, actions, usual adult dosages, possible side effects, and adverse effects of drugs for Parkinson's disease.
7. Describe what to do before and after giving drugs for Parkinson's disease.
8. Explain what to teach patients and their families or caregivers about drugs for Parkinson's disease, including what to do, what not to do, and when to call the prescriber.
9. Describe life span considerations for drugs for Parkinson's disease.

## Key Terms

**Alzheimer's disease** (ĂLZ-hī-mŭrz dĭz-ĒZ) (p. 411) A progressive, incurable condition that destroys brain cells, gradually causing loss of intellectual abilities such as memory and extreme changes in personality and behavior.

**dementia** (dĕ-MĔN-chă) (p. 412) The loss of intellectual functions (such as thinking, remembering, and reasoning) of sufficient severity to interfere with a person's daily functioning.

**neuron** (NYŪR-ŏn) (p. 411) A unique type of cell found in the brain and body that is specialized to process and transmit information.

**neurotransmitter** (nyŭr-ō-TRĂNZ-mĭt-tŭr) (p. 411) A chemical substance such as acetylcholine or dopamine that transmits nerve impulses across a synapse.

**Parkinson's disease** (PĂR-kĭn-sŭnz dĭz-ĒZ) (p. 415) A progressive disorder of the nervous system marked by muscle tremors, muscle rigidity, decreased mobility, stooped posture, slowed voluntary movements, and a masklike facial expression.

◄ⓔ-Learning Activity 23-1

## OVERVIEW

Alzheimer's disease and Parkinson's disease are progressive neurologic disorders that become common as people age. Alzheimer's disease is the most common form of dementia. Parkinson's disease is a neurodegenerative disease with slow and progressive degeneration of the nervous system. Both illnesses involve interrupted transmission of nerve impulses. Transmission of these impulses is normally helped by the presence of neurotransmitters (for example, dopamine, acetylcholine), which are chemicals that transmit messages from one nerve cell (neuron) to another (see Figure 22-3 in Chapter 22).

## ALZHEIMER'S DISEASE

Alzheimer's disease is a progressive and incurable condition that destroys brain cells, with gradual loss of intellectual abilities such as memory and extreme changes in personality and behavior. It is the most feared and common form of dementia.

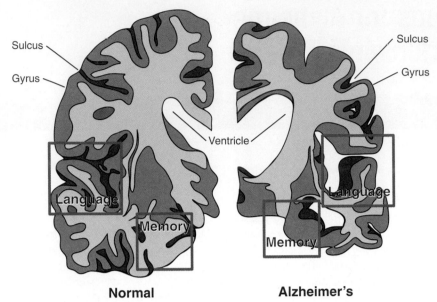

**FIGURE 23-1** Cross sections of a normal brain and a brain affected by Alzheimer's disease. Neurons die in areas of the brain important to memory and language.

**Dementia** is a brain disorder that seriously affects a person's ability to perform activities of daily living (ADLs), including loss of intellectual functions (for example, thinking, remembering, and reasoning). About 4.5 million people in the United States have Alzheimer's disease, and it affects about 20 million people worldwide. About 10% of people over age 65 are affected, and as many as 50% of people over age 85 have Alzheimer's disease.

## REVIEW OF RELATED PHYSIOLOGY AND PATHOPHYSIOLOGY

There are two main pathologic changes in Alzheimer's disease. First is the presence of large amounts of the protein beta-amyloid (Abeta), which clumps together and forms plaques between cells in the brain. Second, other proteins twist and form tangles within the neurons. As a result, neurons die in the areas of the brain that are important to memory and other essential mental abilities (Figure 23-1). Connections between nerve cells are also disrupted. Levels of chemicals (for example, acetylcholine and acetylcholinesterase) in the brain that carry messages between nerve cells are lower.

No single cause has been established for Alzheimer's disease. Instead, a combination of factors has been proposed. Age is the greatest risk factor. Genetics may play a role in development of this condition. People with Down syndrome, a common disorder involving an extra chromosome number 21 (trisomy 21), have an increased risk of Alzheimer's disease by ages 50 to 60 years. A person who has a severe head injury or whiplash injury may also be at increased risk of developing dementia. People who smoke or have high blood pressure or high cholesterol levels also seem to have a higher risk for Alzheimer's disease.

Alzheimer's disease symptoms begin very slowly (Table 23-1). In the early stage the first symptom may be mild forgetfulness, which can be confused with age-related memory changes. People may have difficulty remembering recent events, activities, or the names of familiar people and things. They may also have difficulty solving simple mathematics problems. As the disease progresses symptoms are more noticeable, and family members seek medical help. In the middle stage people forget how to perform simple tasks (for example, brushing teeth, combing hair). The patient no longer thinks clearly and fails to recognize familiar people or places. Problems with speaking, understanding, reading, or writing can begin. In the late stage a patient can become anxious or aggressive and can wander away from home. As the disease progresses the patient eventually needs total care to prevent complications of immo-

| Table 23-1 | Symptoms of Alzheimer's Disease |
| --- | --- |

| STAGE | SYMPTOMS |
| --- | --- |
| Early | Forgetfulness<br>• Difficulty recalling events and activities<br>• Difficulty remembering names of familiar people and things<br>• Inability to solve simple mathematics problems |
| Middle | Beginning to have difficulty speaking, understanding, reading, and writing<br>Failure to recognize familiar people and places<br>Forgetting how to perform simple tasks such as brushing teeth and combing hair<br>Inability to think clearly |
| Late | Aggressiveness<br>Anxiety<br>Need for total care<br>Wandering away from home |

bility, aspiration, urinary tract infections, pneumonia, and pressure ulcers, which commonly lead to death in these patients.

There is no test that diagnoses Alzheimer's disease. The only absolute way to confirm that a patient has this illness is to see the plaques and tangles in the brain tissue, which can be done only by autopsy after the patient dies. Diagnosis is made by excluding other possible causes (for example, thyroid problems, drug reactions, depression, brain tumors, and blood vessel diseases). On the basis of symptom assessment, health history, tests of memory and problem solving, and brain scan, a diagnosis of probable Alzheimer's disease can be made.

There is no cure for Alzheimer's disease. Early diagnosis is important because it helps patients and families plan for the future, makes it possible for the patient with dementia to benefit from drugs that can slow the progress of the disease, and helps the patient and family to identify sources of advice and support. No treatment can stop the progression of Alzheimer's disease. Drug therapy may help prevent symptoms from becoming worse for a limited time and allow the patient to continue performing some daily activities for a longer period. Drugs may also be prescribed to help control behavioral symptoms such as sleeplessness, agitation, wandering, anxiety, and depression.

## TYPES OF DRUGS FOR ALZHEIMER'S DISEASE

### CHOLINESTERASE/ACETYLCHOLINESTERASE INHIBITORS AND MEMANTINE

#### How Drugs for Alzheimer's Disease Work

No drug has been developed that protects neurons from the changes that occur with Alzheimer's disease. Drug treatments have been developed that can temporarily slow the progression of symptoms in some patients.

Cholinesterase/acetylcholinesterase inhibitors reduce the activity of the enzyme acetylcholinesterase that breaks down acetylcholine in the synapses of neurons. This action keeps levels of acetylcholine higher. The three drugs in this category, donepezil (Aricept), rivastigmine (Exelon), and galantamine (Reminyl), are the main ones used for Alzheimer treatment. The effects of these drugs are only temporary.

Memantine (Namenda) blocks the amino acid glutamate at N-methyl-D-aspartate receptors in the brain, preventing overstimulation (overstimulation of these receptors damages neurons and appears to be one cause of Alzheimer's disease). It can be effective in helping modify dementia (temporarily) in some patients with moderate-to-severe Alzheimer's disease.

Generic names, trade names, and common dosages of these drugs are listed in the following table. Be sure to consult a drug reference for specific information about any drugs used for Alzheimer's disease.

**? Did You Know?**

The only way to absolutely diagnose Alzheimer's disease is to look for plaques and tangles in brain tissue by autopsy after the patient's death.

**Memory Jogger**

Drugs prescribed for Alzheimer's disease and Parkinson's disease can help control the symptoms but *cannot* cure the disease.

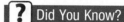 ◄ @-Learning Activity 23-2

**⇄ Do Not Confuse**

**Aricept** *with* **Aciphex**

An order for Aricept may be confused with Aciphex. Aricept is an acetylcholinesterase inhibitor used for Alzheimer's disease, whereas Aciphex is a proton pump inhibitor used to treat gastroesophageal reflux disease (GERD) and gastric ulcers.

**Common Side Effects**

**Drugs for Alzheimer's Disease**

Nausea/ Vomiting, Diarrhea    Dizziness    Headache

Fatigue    Insomnia

**Drug Alert!**

**Administration Alert**

Assess a patient's ability to swallow before giving drugs for Alzheimer's disease because he or she may be at risk for aspiration.

**Memory Jogger**

If a patient has a seizure, documentation should include:
- The time of seizure onset.
- The time of seizure termination.
- The total duration of the seizure.
- Characteristics of the seizure, including tonic movement location, clonic movement location, pupil changes, cyanosis, incontinence, and the patient's orientation after the seizure.

**Dosages for Common Drugs for Alzheimer's Disease**

| Drug | Dosage |
|---|---|
| donepezil (Aricept) | *Adults:* 5 mg orally at bedtime; increase to 10 mg after 4-6 weeks |
| galantamine (Reminyl🍁, Razadyne) | *Adults:* 4 mg orally twice daily with food, increase at 4-week intervals to 12 mg twice daily; extended-release—8 mg once daily in the morning, increase at 4-week intervals to 24 mg daily |
| memantine (Namenda, Ebixa🍁) | *Adults:* 5 mg orally daily; increase to 5 mg twice daily, then 5 mg in AM and 10 mg in PM; maximum dosage 10 mg twice daily |
| rivastigmine (Exelon) | *Adults:* Oral—1.5 mg twice daily with food, increase at 2-week intervals to 6 mg twice daily; Patch—apply 1 patch (4.6 mg) at a different body site once daily, may increase to a 9.5-mg patch |

*Intended Responses*
- Dementia with Alzheimer's disease decreases temporarily.
- Degradation of acetylcholine is inhibited.
- Progression of Alzheimer's disease symptoms is slowed.
- Cognitive function in patients with Alzheimer's disease is improved.

*Side Effects.* The most common side effects of cholinesterase/acetylcholinesterase inhibitors are nausea, vomiting, diarrhea, stomach cramps, headaches, dizziness, fatigue, weakness, insomnia, and loss of appetite *(anorexia).*

Less common side effects include syncope, hypotension, frequent urination, incontinence, and weight loss.

*Adverse Effects.* Adverse effects of cholinesterase/acetylcholinesterase inhibitors include abnormal heart rhythms such as bradycardia and atrial fibrillation. Although uncommon, all of these drugs may cause GI bleeding. Two additional uncommon but serious adverse effects include difficulty urinating and seizures.

Symptoms of overdose with these drugs include upset stomach, vomiting, drooling, sweating, slow heartbeat (bradycardia), difficulty breathing, muscle weakness, and seizures. Report these effects to the prescriber immediately.

**What To Do *Before* Giving Drugs for Alzheimer's Disease**
Obtain a complete list of drugs currently being used by the patient, including over-the-counter and herbal products. Assess the patient for baseline cognitive function (for example, memory, attention, reasoning, language, and ability to perform simple tasks).

Obtain a baseline weight. Check baseline blood pressure and heart rate and rhythm. Ask about recent nausea, vomiting, loss of appetite, and weight loss. Have the patient or caregiver tell you about usual urinary output pattern.

Assess swallowing because patients may develop difficulty as the disease progresses and be at risk for aspiration. Drugs may need to be crushed or given in liquid form. Do not crush time-released pills or open time-released capsules.

Ask about a history of liver or kidney problems that may affect metabolism of these drugs. Also ask about previous problems with GI bleeding or ulcers.

**What To Do *After* Giving Drugs for Alzheimer's Disease**
Reassess the patient's cognitive function often. Watch for changes in memory, attention, reasoning, language, and ability to perform simple tasks. Cognitive assessment is a long-term task because changes may take time to appear.

Recheck and monitor the patient's heart rate and rhythm and blood pressure. Monitor intake and output and daily weights. Continue to monitor the patient's swallowing ability. Watch him or her for potential seizure activity.

Because these drugs may cause dizziness and fatigue, instruct the patient to call for help when getting out of bed and ensure that the call light is within easy reach.

Ask the patient about nausea, vomiting, and GI discomfort. Check stools or emesis for signs of GI bleeding. Notify the prescriber if side effects occur.

### What to *Teach* Patients About Drugs for Alzheimer's Disease

Always include the person providing home care for the patient when teaching about these drugs. Include information about safe dosage and proper storage. Patients with difficulty swallowing may need medications crushed or in liquid form. Remind caregivers not to crush extended-release drugs.

Remind patients and caregivers that these drugs should be taken exactly as instructed by their prescriber. Tell them about the importance of keeping follow-up appointments to monitor the progress of controlling the symptoms of the disease. Instruct them to report side effects and signs of allergic or toxic reactions to their prescriber immediately.

Caution patients and caregivers that these drugs may cause dizziness, weakness, and fatigue. Teach them about the side effects of these drugs and the importance of notifying their prescriber for any signs of bleeding.

Teach patients and their caregivers to administer donepezil (Aricept) at bedtime and galantamine (Reminyl, Razadyne) and rivastigmine (Exelon) twice a day with food.

Instruct patients and caregivers about the desired outcomes of temporary improved memory, attention, reasoning, language, and ability to perform simple tasks. Remind patients and caregivers to notify their prescriber about any changes in cognitive function.

### Life Span Considerations for Drugs for Alzheimer's Disease

*Considerations for Older Adults.*   All of these drugs should be used cautiously in patients with histories of GI bleeding, liver disease, kidney disease, or heart disease. Rivastigmine should also be used cautiously for patients with asthma or chronic obstructive pulmonary disease (COPD). Older, frail women should not take more than 5 mg/day of donepezil because the drug has been associated with significant weight loss. This drug should be used with caution in any older adult with a low body weight.

Because these drugs increase urination, the older adult, especially one who is confused, may have more episodes of incontinence. Remind family members to ensure that the older adult has the opportunity to use the bathroom every 2 hours while awake and at least once during the night.

## PARKINSON'S DISEASE

Parkinson's disease is a slow, progressive, degenerative disease of the nervous system. In the United States about one million people are affected by this disease. It affects 1 in 100 people older than 65 and commonly begins between the ages of 50 and 79.

The exact cause of Parkinson's disease is not known; many factors may play a part. Age, especially age 50 and older, is a major risk factor. Genetic and environmental factors may cause development of this condition. Two abnormal genes have been identified in people affected by Parkinson's disease before age 40. Environmental factors such as exposure to weak toxins over a long period of time are thought to lead to Parkinson's disease in genetically predisposed people. Several drugs have caused secondary Parkinson's disease (Table 23-2).

## REVIEW OF RELATED PHYSIOLOGY AND PATHOPHYSIOLOGY

Normally, when the brain initiates an impulse to move a muscle, the impulse passes through the basal ganglia. The function of the basal ganglia is to make muscle

**[!] Drug Alert!**
**Action/Intervention Alert**

Because acetylcholinesterase inhibitors may cause GI bleeding, monitor the patient carefully for any signs of bleeding.

**[!] Drug Alert!**
**Administration Alert**

Give galantamine (Reminyl, Razadyne) and rivastigmine (Exelon) twice a day with food to minimize the GI upset that is common with these drugs.

**[!] Drug Alert!**
**Teaching Alert**

Teach care providers to remind patients to use the bathroom every 2 hours to avoid incontinence episodes while taking drugs for Alzheimer's disease.

◄ⓔ-Learning Activity 23-3

Table 23-2 | Drugs That Cause Secondary Parkinson's Disease

| CATEGORY | DRUG NAME |
| --- | --- |
| Antiemetics | prochlorperazine (Compazine) |
| Antihypertensives | reserpine (Serpasil) |
| Antipsychotics | chlorpromazine (Thorazine) |
| | fluphenazine (Prolixin) |
| | haloperidol (Haldol) |
| | mesoridazine (Serentil) |
| | perphenazine (Trilafon) |
| | risperidone (Risperdal) |
| | thioridazine (Mellaril) |
| | trifluoperazine (Stelazine) |
| GI motility drugs | metoclopramide (Reglan) |
| Illicit drugs | methcathinone—a psychoactive stimulant |
| | N-MPTP (1-methyl-4-phenyl-1,2,3,6-tetrahydropyridine)— a contaminant found in illicit drugs |

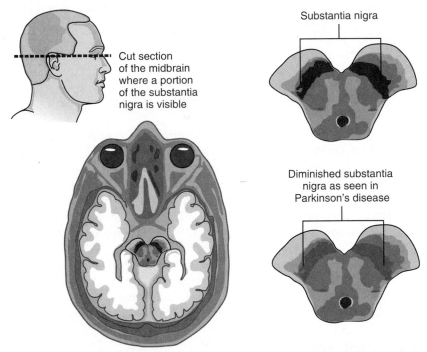

FIGURE 23-2 In Parkinson's disease, nerve cells in the substantia nigra degenerate and less dopamine is produced. This results in fewer connections between the nerve cells in the basal ganglia and in decreased smooth movements.

**Memory Jogger**

The four major symptoms of Parkinson's disease are:
• Tremor at rest.
• Rigidity.
• Bradykinesia (slow movements and difficulty starting to move).
• Abnormal gait.

movements smooth and coordinate changes in posture. Basal ganglia release chemical messengers called *neurotransmitters* (for example, dopamine) that trigger the next nerve cell in the pathway to send an impulse. In Parkinson's disease nerve cells degenerate in a part of the basal ganglia called the *substantia nigra* (Figure 23-2). This causes a decrease in the production of dopamine and the number of connections between nerve cells in the basal ganglia. As a result the basal ganglia are less able to produce smooth movements. These changes cause symptoms of increased tremor, lack of coordination, and slowed or reduced movements *(bradykinesia)*. Parkinson's disease begins subtly and progresses gradually. Symptoms appear when the amount of dopamine decreases in the brain.

The symptoms appear gradually and increase in severity as the disease progresses. Symptoms may be motor or nonmotor (Box 23-1). For many patients the initial symptom is a coarse, rhythmic *tremor* of the hand while the hand is at rest, also called *pill-rolling tremor*. Other early symptoms include decreased sense of smell,

**Box 23-1** Symptoms of Parkinson's Disease

| MOTOR SYMPTOMS | NONMOTOR SYMPTOMS |
|---|---|
| • Bradykinesia | • Constipation |
| • Decreased arm swing when walking | • Decreased sense of smell |
| • Difficulty rising from a chair | • Depression |
| • Difficulty turning in bed | • Drooling |
| • Lack of facial expression | • Increased sweating |
| • Micrographia (small handwriting) | • Low voice volume |
| • Postural instability | • Male erectile dysfunction |
| • Rigidity and freezing in place | • Painful foot cramps |
| • Stooped, shuffling gait | • Sleep disturbance |
| • Tremor | • Urinary frequency and urgency |

decreased body movements, difficulty walking, and lack of facial expression. As the disease progresses muscles become rigid, movements become slow and difficult to initiate, and stiffness occurs. Stiffness and decreased mobility lead to difficulty with daily tasks such as buttoning shirts or tying shoes. When the disease is advanced, the patient may suddenly stop walking, quicken his or her steps, or stumble-run to avoid falling. Posture becomes stooped, and balance becomes difficult to maintain.

There is no specific test or marker for diagnosing Parkinson's disease. Diagnosis is based on symptoms. Early mild disease can be difficult to diagnose because the symptoms are subtle. Diagnosis can also be difficult in older adults because aging can cause some of the same changes that occur with Parkinson's disease such as loss of balance, muscle stiffness, slow movements, and stooped posture. A diagnosis of Parkinson's disease is probable if drug therapy improves symptoms and other diseases have been ruled out.

There is no cure for Parkinson's disease. Goals of drug therapy include minimizing disability, reducing possible side effects of drug therapy, and helping the patient maintain a high quality of life. Drug therapy may make movement easier and prolong normal function for several years. Changes in the home should include safety measures to prevent falls (for example, removing throw rugs, installing railings in bathrooms). Tasks such as buttoning or tying laces can be made easier by replacing buttons or ties with Velcro fasteners.

## TYPES OF DRUGS FOR PARKINSON'S DISEASE

### DOPAMINERGIC/DOPAMINE AGONISTS, COMT INHIBITORS, MAO-B INHIBITORS, ANTICHOLINERGICS

#### How Drugs for Parkinson's Disease Work

No drugs have been developed that will reverse the progression of Parkinson's disease. However, certain drugs can be used effectively to control the symptoms of the disease.

Drugs are prescribed to improve movement and enable patients to function effectively. The period of time that drugs for Parkinson's disease remain effective varies. For some patients they may work for several years, whereas for others they may work for only a short period.

Dopaminergic and dopamine agonist drugs increase the amount of dopamine activity in the brain, thereby reducing tremor and muscle rigidity and improving movement. Carbidopa prevents levodopa from being converted to dopamine before it reaches the brain. When carbidopa is added to levodopa, lower doses of levodopa can be used, leading to reduced side effects such as nausea and vomiting. Dopamine agonist drugs stimulate dopamine receptors to relieve symptoms and delay onset of motor complications.

Catechol-*o*-methyltransferase (COMT) inhibitors allow a larger amount of levodopa to reach the brain, which raises dopamine levels in the brain. They help provide a more stable, constant supply of levodopa, which makes its beneficial effects last longer.

 **Memory Jogger**

The goals of treatment for Parkinson's disease are to minimize disability, reduce possible side effects of drug therapy, and help the patient maintain a high quality of life.

◄ ⊖-Learning Activity 23-4

**Memory Jogger**

Drug classes for Parkinson's disease are:
- Dopaminergic/dopamine agonists.
- COMT inhibitors.
- MAO-B inhibitors.
- Anticholinergic drugs.

Monoamine oxidase B (MAO-B) inhibitors inhibit the enzyme that breaks down dopamine in the brain. As a result, more dopamine is available, and the progression of Parkinson's disease is slowed.

Anticholinergic drugs are effective against tremors and rigidity. These drugs block cholinergic nerve impulses that help control the muscles of the arms, legs, and body. They also restrict the action of acetylcholine, an important chemical messenger in the brain that helps regulate muscle movement, sweat gland function, and intestinal function.

Generic names, trade names, and dosages of the most commonly prescribed drugs are listed in the following table. Be sure to consult a drug reference for specific information about any drug used to treat Parkinson's disease.

### Dosages for Common Drugs for Parkinson's Disease

| Drug | Dosage (Adults only) |
| --- | --- |
| *Dopaminergic/Dopamine Antagonists* | |
| apomorphine (Apokyn) | Subcutaneous—0.2 mL; can be increased by 0.1 mL; each dose should not exceed 0.6 mL |
| bromocriptine (Apo-Bromocriptine❦, Parlodel) | 1.25-2.5 mg orally twice daily with meals; increase at 14- to 28-day intervals by 2.5 mg/day to a maximum dosage 100 mg/day in divided doses; always give with meals |
| carbidopa/levodopa (Sinemet, Sinemet CR) | 25 mg carbidopa/100 mg levodopa orally 3-4 times daily; extended-release—50 mg carbidopa/200 mg levodopa twice daily |
| pramipexole (Mirapex) | 0.125 mg orally 3 times daily initially; dosage range 1.5-4.5 mg/day in 3 divided doses |
| ropinirole (Requip) | 0.25 mg orally 3 times daily for 1 week, then gradually increase at weekly intervals up to 24 mg/day; extended-release—2 mg once daily, increase at 1-2 week intervals by 2 mg/day, maximum dosage 24 mg/day |
| *COMT Inhibitors* | |
| entacapone (Comtan) | 200 mg orally given with each dose of carbidopa/levodopa; maximum dosage 1600 mg/day (8 doses) |
| tolcapone (Tasmar) | 100 mg orally 3 times daily given with each dose of carbidopa/levodopa; may increase to 200 mg 3 times daily |
| *MAO-B Inhibitors* | |
| rasagiline (Azilect) | 1 mg orally once daily; 0.5-1 mg once daily when combined with levodopa |
| selegiline (Eldepryl, Novo-Selegiline❦, Zelapar) | 5 mg orally twice daily with breakfast and lunch; oral dissolving tablet—1.25 mg dissolved in mouth once daily (in the morning before breakfast) for 6 weeks, then may increase to 2.5 mg once daily |
| *Anticholinergic Drugs* | |
| benztropine (Apo-Benztropine❦, Cogentin) | 1-2 mg orally per day in 1-2 divided doses |
| trihexyphenidyl (Apo-Trihex❦, Artane, Novohexidyl❦, Trihexane) | 1 mg orally day 1, 2 mg day 2, then increase by 2 mg every 3-5 days up to 6-10 mg/day in 3 divided doses; maximum dosage 15 mg/day |

**Do Not Confuse**

**Mirapex** *with* **MiraLax**

An order for Mirapex can be confused with MiraLax. Mirapex is a DOPamine agonist used to treat the symptoms of Parkinson's disease, whereas MiraLax is an osmotic laxative used to treat constipation.

### Intended Responses
- Signs and symptoms of Parkinson's disease are decreased.
- Tremor and rigidity of Parkinson's disease are relieved.

*Side Effects.*   The most common side effects of drugs to treat Parkinson's disease are dizziness, nausea, and hypotension. Common side effects of these drugs are summarized by drug or drug group in the following table.

### Common Side Effects of Drugs for Parkinson's Disease

| Drugs or Drug Groups | Side Effects |
|---|---|
| Anticholinergic drugs | Blurred vision, constipation, dizziness, dry eyes, dry mouth, nervousness, sedation |
| carbidopa-levodopa (Sinemet) | Involuntary movements (dyskinesia), nausea and vomiting |
| COMT inhibitors | Constipation, diarrhea, dyskinesia, dystonia (slow movement or extended spasm in a group of muscles), headache, sleep disorder |
| Dopamine agonists | Amnesia, chest pain, constipation, dizziness, dry mouth, dyskinesia, dyspepsia, flushing, hallucinations, hypotension, nausea and vomiting, pallor, rhinorrhea (runny nose), somnolence, sweating, weakness, yawning |
| MAO-B inhibitors | Confusion, dizziness, dry mouth, nausea, vivid dreams and hallucinations |

**Common Side Effects**

**Drugs for Parkinson's Disease**

Dizziness     Nausea     Hypotension

*Adverse Effects.*   Serious adverse effects of carbidopa-levodopa (Sinemet) include depression with suicidal tendencies; neutropenia (decreased number of white blood cells), and neuroleptic malignant syndrome (dysfunction of the autonomic nervous system, the branch of the nervous system responsible for regulating involuntary actions such as heart rate, blood pressure, digestion, and sweating; muscle tone; body temperature; and consciousness).

Apomorphine (Apokyn) can cause life-threatening central nervous system (CNS) depression, including respiratory depression, coma, and cardiac arrest.

Bromocriptine (Parlodel) may lead to shock, or acute myocardial infarction. Pramipexole (Mirapex) can cause sleep attacks (*narcolepsy*).

COMT inhibitors can cause neuroleptic malignant syndrome or rhabdomyolysis, a serious and potentially fatal effect involving destruction or degeneration of skeletal muscle. Signs and symptoms of this disorder include muscle aches; muscle weakness; and dark, cola-colored urine.

**! Drug Alert!**

**Administration Alert**

Always ask patients taking COMT inhibitor drugs about muscle aches or weakness—symptoms of rhabdomyolysis and an adverse effect of these drugs.

### What To Do *Before* Giving Drugs for Parkinson's Disease

Obtain a complete list of drugs currently being used by the patient, including over-the-counter and herbal products. Check blood pressure, heart rate, and respiratory rate for a baseline. Assess baseline neurologic and mental status. Check for baseline dyskinesia, rigidity, tremors, and gait. Assess swallowing ability.

Ask women of childbearing age if they are pregnant or planning to become pregnant. Ask the patient about kidney or liver disease, which may affect metabolism of these drugs.

Teach patients and their caregivers that extended-release forms of these drugs must be swallowed whole and not chewed or split in half. Be sure to give apomorphine (Apokyn) subcutaneously and not intravenously.

 **Clinical Pitfall**

Be sure to give apomorphine subcutaneously and *not* intravenously because intravenous drugs are immediately absorbed and act very rapidly.

### What To Do *After* Giving Drugs for Parkinson's Disease

Regularly reassess the patient's vital signs, including blood pressure, heart rate, and respiratory rate every 4 to 8 hours. Because of side effects such as dizziness and hypotension, instruct the patient to call for help when getting out of bed and ensure that the call light is within easy reach. Tell the patient to change positions slowly.

Reassess the patient's mental status and watch for confusion or hallucinations. Watch the patient taking ropinirole (Requip) for episodes of falling asleep suddenly

| Table 23-3 | Signs and Symptoms of Adverse Effects of Drugs Used to Treat Parkinson's Disease | | |
|---|---|---|---|
| **ADVERSE EFFECT** | **SIGNS AND SYMPTOMS** | **ADVERSE EFFECT** | **SIGNS AND SYMPTOMS** |
| Neuroleptic malignant syndrome | Changes in cognition, including agitation, delirium, and coma<br>High fever<br>Muscle rigidity<br>Muscle tremors<br>Pharyngitis<br>Unstable blood pressure | Rhabdomyolysis | Dark red or cola-colored urine<br>Fatigue<br>Generalized weakness<br>Joint pain<br>Muscle stiffness or aching<br>Muscle tenderness<br>Seizures<br>Unintentional weight gain<br>Weakness of the affected muscle(s) |
| Neutropenia | Anal ulcers<br>Decreased immune response<br>Fever<br>Increased risk of bacterial infections<br>Painful mouth ulcers<br>Sore throat | | |

**! Drug Alert!**

**Action/Intervention Alert**

Immediately report episodes of narcolepsy to the prescriber for a patient taking ropinirole (Requip).

**! Drug Alert!**

**Action/Intervention Alert**

To determine the effectiveness of drug therapy for Parkinson's disease, regularly reassess the patient for dyskinesia, rigidity, tremors, and gait.

**! Drug Alert!**

**Teaching Alert**

Patients should be taught to notify their prescriber *immediately* if symptoms of Parkinson's disease (for example, shaking, stiffness and slow movement) become worse.

(narcolepsy). Report this immediately to the prescriber because the drug may need to be discontinued.

Ask the patient about side effects such as nausea and vomiting. Watch for side effects or adverse effects and report them immediately to the prescriber. Signs and symptoms of such adverse effects as neutropenia, neuroleptic malignant syndrome, and rhabdomyolysis are summarized in Table 23-3. Observe the patient for signs of drug allergic reactions such as rashes, hives, or changes in respiratory status.

After giving these drugs, be sure to monitor the patient's intake and output and assess for bladder distention because some drugs can cause urine retention. Monitor the patient for difficulty swallowing, which could increase the risk for aspiration.

Keep track of bowel movements and check bowel sounds because some drugs for Parkinson's disease can cause constipation or diarrhea.

Reassess dyskinesia, rigidity, tremors, and gait while the patient is taking drugs for Parkinson's disease.

### What To *Teach* Patients About Drugs for Parkinson's Disease

Always include the person providing home care when teaching about these drugs. Instruct the caregiver to report any changes in swallowing ability to the prescriber because of the increased risk of aspiration.

Instruct patients to take drugs for Parkinson's disease exactly as prescribed and stress the importance of keeping follow-up appointments to monitor the progress of treatment. Remind them to notify the prescriber if symptoms of Parkinson's disease (for example, shaking, stiffness, and slow movement) become worse. Teach them to report any side effects immediately to their prescriber. Tell them to consult their prescriber before taking any over-the-counter or herbal products.

Missed doses of drugs for Parkinson's disease should be taken as soon as possible. However, if it is almost time for the next dose, teach patients to skip the missed dose to avoid taking a double dose of these drugs.

Tell patients that some drugs for Parkinson's disease are started at lower doses and gradually increased by the prescriber to best control the symptoms. Remind them that these drugs can be used to control symptoms but do not cure the disease. Instruct them to avoid stopping these drugs suddenly because symptoms may become much worse.

| Box 23-2 | Foods to Avoid When Taking MAO Inhibitors |
|---|---|

- Aged cheeses
- Avocadoes
- Bananas, figs
- Beer
- Broad beans
- Dried sausage
- Fish
- Liver
- Meats prepared with tenderizer
- Pickled herring
- Poultry
- Raisins
- Red wine
- Salami
- Sauerkraut
- Sour cream
- Soy sauce
- Yeast extract
- Yogurt

Teach patients to be careful not to overdo physical activities but to gradually increase activities to avoid falls and injuries.

Remind patients to always notify their surgeons or dentists that they are taking these drugs before having any surgical procedure.

Drugs such as selegiline (Carbex) may cause photosensitivity. Tell patients to wear protective clothing and sunscreen and to avoid excessive sun exposure. Because of side effects such as dizziness and drowsiness, caution patients to avoid driving, operating machines, or doing anything that requires increased alertness. Teach them to avoid alcohol or other CNS depressants because they can add to the drowsiness sometimes caused by these drugs. Instruct them to change positions slowly because of the possible side effect of hypotension.

Tell patients to take drugs that cause GI upset with food or milk. Teach patients prescribed anticholinergic drugs to have regular eye examinations because these drugs can cause blurred vision. Dry mouth can be kept to a minimum by frequent mouth care, ice chips, or sugarless candy.

Tell patients who are prescribed entacapone (Comtan) that this drug may change urine to a brownish-orange color and explain that this side effect is not harmful.

Instruct patients who are prescribed an MAO-B inhibitor such as selegiline (Carbex) or rasagiline (Azilect) to avoid the foods listed in Box 23-2 while taking these drugs and for 2 weeks after stopping them. Teach them also to avoid large amounts of chocolate, coffee, tea, or colas with caffeine. These foods contain tyramine, an amino acid that can cause a hypertensive crisis in patients receiving MAO inhibitor therapy.

Anticholinergic drugs can cause decreased perspiration. Caution patients taking these drugs to be careful about overheating in hot weather.

Inform patients taking the combination of carbidopa-levodopa (Sinemet) that this drug can cause darkening of urine or perspiration. Caution them to report any changes in skin lesions immediately to the prescriber because carbidopa-levodopa can activate malignant melanoma. This drug may be contraindicated in patients with a history of melanoma.

Patients prescribed apomorphine (Apokyn) at home need special teaching about how to give the subcutaneous injections and how to care for the special dosing pen used to give this drug. Include the caregiver in your teaching because the patient's muscle rigidity and tremors may make it impossible to self-inject.

### Life Span Considerations for Drugs for Parkinson's Disease

*Considerations for Pregnancy and Breastfeeding.*   Bromocriptine (Parlodel) is usually not recommended during pregnancy or breastfeeding. It stops the production of breast milk. Most drugs for Parkinson's disease are pregnancy category C. They have not been tested in pregnancy or breastfeeding and should not be used unless the benefits outweigh the risks.

*Considerations for Older Adults.*   Older adults should be aware that they may experience confusion, hallucinations, and uncontrolled body movements because they are more sensitive to the effects of these drugs.

The older adult with Parkinson's disease is already unstable when walking and is at increased risk for falls. The drugs can cause a rapid decrease in blood pressure.

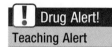

**Drug Alert!**

**Teaching Alert**

While taking selegiline (Carbex) or rasagiline (Azilect), patients should *avoid* foods that contain tyramine.

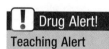

**Drug Alert!**

**Teaching Alert**

Teach patients taking anticholinergic drugs to remain indoors in an air-conditioned setting during hot weather.

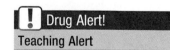

**Drug Alert!**

**Teaching Alert**

Because carbidopa-levodopa may activate malignant melanoma, instruct patients to watch for and report any changes in skin lesions to their prescriber immediately.

◄ⓔ-Learning Activity 23-5

Remind older adults to sit on the side of the bed for a few moments before attempting to stand and to change positions slowly. Instruct them to wear shoes, rather than slippers, for better stability and to use handrails when going up or down stairs. Assess the older adult's need for assistive devices, such as a cane or a walker for ambulating.

Ⓔ-Learning Activity 23-6 ▶

## Get Ready for Practice!

### Key Points

- Alzheimer's disease and Parkinson's disease are both progressive neurologic disorders that occur more often with aging.
- There is no cure for either Alzheimer's disease or Parkinson's disease. Treatment focuses on controlling symptoms.
- Alzheimer's disease is the most common form of dementia and affects a person's ability to perform activities of daily living.
- With Alzheimer's disease neurons essential to memory and cognitive function die.
- Mild forgetfulness, the first symptom of Alzheimer's disease, can be confused with age-related memory changes.
- With Parkinson's disease there is a deficit of chemical messengers called *neurotransmitters* that facilitate transmission of brain impulses.
- The major symptoms of Parkinson's disease are tremor at rest, rigidity, bradykinesia, and abnormal gait. (Tremor is often the initial symptom.)
- The goals of treatment for Parkinson's disease are minimizing disability, reducing possible side effects of drug therapy, and helping the patient to maintain a high quality of life.
- Patient safety is a major concern for patients with Parkinson's disease and Alzheimer's disease.
- Teach a patient to report worsening of Parkinson's disease symptoms immediately to his or her prescriber.

### Additional Learning Resources

**evolve** Go to your Evolve website (http://evolve.elsevier.com/Workman/pharmacology/) for the following FREE learning resources:
- eLearning Activities
- Animations
- Video Clips
- Interactive Review Questions
- Audio Key Points
- Audio Glossary
- Audio Glossary—Spanish-English
- Drug Dosage Calculators
- Patient Teaching Handouts

**SG** Go to your Study Guide for additional learning activities to help you master this chapter content.

### Review Questions

1. How do drugs used for Alzheimer's disease work?
   - A. They prolong the availability of dopamine.
   - B. They inhibit the breakdown of acetylcholine.
   - C. They inhibit transmission of abnormal nerve impulses.
   - D. They act in the brain to degrade dopamine more rapidly.

2. The spouse of a patient with Alzheimer's disease asks the nurse how donepezil (Aricept) will help his wife. What is your best response?
   - A. "Donepezil will protect the neurons in your wife's brain from the changes caused by this disease."
   - B. "This drug treatment will cure your wife's Alzheimer's disease."
   - C. "The action of donepezil will slow the progression of the disease by keeping levels of acetylcholine higher."
   - D. "This drug will not cure your's wife's disease, but it will prevent it from getting worse."

3. What must you include in a cognitive assessment before and after giving a drug for Alzheimer's disease? (Select all that apply.)
   - A. Language skills
   - B. Memory
   - C. Attention span
   - D. Advanced mathematics skills
   - E. Ability to perform simple tasks

4. What do you teach the spouse and the patient who has been prescribed rivastigmine (Exelon) to prevent common side effects?
   - A. "Give this drug twice a day with food."
   - B. "Check the patient's blood pressure before giving the drug."
   - C. "Be sure to monitor urine output and bowel movements."
   - D. "The drug is best when given on an empty stomach."

5. What is the maximum dose of donepezil (Aricept) that can be given to an older, frail female patient with Alzheimer's disease?
   - A. 1 mg/day
   - B. 3 mg/day
   - C. 5 mg/day
   - D. 7 mg/day

6. Which patient response indicates to you that carbidopa-levodopa (Sinemet) therapy for Parkinson's disease is effective?

   A. Reduced tremor and muscle rigidity
   B. Improved memory and attention span
   C. Increased ability to perform simple tasks
   D. Prevention of seizures

7. For which dangerous side effect must you monitor in a patient who is taking carbidopa-levodopa (Sinemet)?

   A. GI hemorrhage
   B. Suicidal thoughts
   C. Rhabdomyolysis
   D. Respiratory depression

8. Why do you teach patients taking MAO inhibitors for Parkinson's disease to avoid foods that contain tyramine?

   A. They will cause an upset stomach.
   B. They may lead to rhabdomyolysis.
   C. They may cause a hypertensive crisis.
   D. They will lead to decreased sweating.

9. About which safety measure do you instruct the older adult who has been prescribed carbidopa-levodopa for Parkinson's disease?

   A. Apply sunscreens and wear protective clothing whenever outdoors.
   B. Always take this medication at bedtime to prevent serious adverse effects.
   C. Monitor fluid intake and urine output to prevent dehydration.
   D. Sit on the side of the bed for a few minutes before getting up.

10. A patient with Alzheimer's disease is prescribed rivastigmine (Exelon) 6 mg twice a day. The drug comes in 1.5 mg per tablet. How many tablets do you give for each dose? _____ tablet(s)

11. A patient with Parkinson's disease is ordered apomorphine (Apokyn) 2 mg subcutaneously. The drug comes in 10 mg/1 mL. How many milliliters do you inject for each dose? _____ mL

## Critical Thinking Activities

Mr. Wright is a 69-year-old man who has recently been diagnosed with Parkinson's disease. The health care provider prescribes carbidopa-levodopa (Sinemet) orally 4 times a day and selegiline (Carbex) 5 mg orally twice a day.

1. List four serious side effects of carbidopa-levodopa for which you should monitor.

2. What should you tell Mr. Wright when he asks why he must take two drugs?

3. About what precaution would you instruct Mr. Wright when he tells you how much better he is feeling since he started taking these drugs?

## Objectives

*After studying this chapter you should be able to:*

1. List the names, actions, usual adult dosages, possible side effects, and adverse effects of drugs for thyroid problems.
2. Describe what to do before and after giving drugs for thyroid problems.
3. Explain what to teach patients taking drugs for thyroid problems, including what to do, what not to do, and when to call the prescriber.
4. Describe life span considerations for drugs for thyroid problems.
5. List the names, actions, usual adult dosages, possible side effects, and adverse effects of drugs for perimenopausal hormone replacement.
6. Explain what to teach patients taking perimenopausal hormone replacement drugs, including what to do, what not to do, and when to call the prescriber.

## Key Terms

**endocrine gland** (ĔN-dō-krĭn GLĂND) (p. 425) A gland that secretes one or more hormones that are carried to target tissue or tissues by the blood rather than by a duct.

**estrogen** (ĔS-trō-jĕn) (p. 434) The main female sex hormone secreted by the ovaries and adrenal glands.

**follicle-stimulating hormone** (FŎL-ĭ-kŭl STĬM-yū-lā-tĭng HŌR-mōn) (p. 435) Hormone secreted by the pituitary gland that causes the ovary to secrete estrogen and allows one ovum each month to complete maturation.

**goiter** (GŌY-tŭr) (p. 426) An enlarged thyroid gland that can be seen as a distinct swelling in the neck. It can occur with either hypothyroidism or hyperthyroidism.

**hyperthyroidism** (hī-pŭr-THĪ-rōyd-ĭz-ŭm) (p. 431) An abnormal increase in thyroid gland activity, causing high blood levels of thyroid hormones and symptoms of increased metabolism.

**hypothyroidism** (hī-pō-THĪ-rōyd-ĭz-ŭm) (p. 426) An abnormally low level of thyroid gland activity, causing low blood levels of thyroid hormones and symptoms of decreased metabolism.

**menarche** (mĕn-ĂRSH) (p. 434) The beginning of the years of menstruation in an adolescent female.

**menopause** (MĔN-ō-pŏz) (p. 435) The cessation of menstrual periods and ovulation. Natural menopause occurs as a result of age-related changes in the ovary, causing it to no longer respond to hormone stimulation by secreting estrogen and ovulation.

**menstruation** (mĕn-strū-Ā-shŭn) (p. 434) The periodic shedding of the uterine lining that occurs as a result of the cyclic changes of hormone levels in females.

**metabolism** (mĕ-TĂB-ō-lĭz-ŭm) (p. 425) The energy use of each cell and the work performed within the body.

**perimenopause** (pĕr-ē-MĔN-ō-pŏz) (p. 435) The transition time in a woman from having regular hormone cycles with menstrual periods to the time when menstrual periods have stopped for a full year.

**progesterone** (prō-JĔS-tŭr-ōn) (p. 435) The female hormone that supports pregnancy by maintaining the thickened uterine lining.

**target tissue** (TĂR-gĕt TĬSH-ū) (p. 425) A tissue or organ that is affected or controlled by a specific hormone.

**thyroid crisis** (THĪ-rōyd CRĪ-sĭs) (p. 431) Severe hyperthyroidism, also known as thyroid storm, that occurs when the disease is not treated or when the patient is very stressed. The symptoms (fever; high blood pressure; and rapid, irregular heart rate) can develop quickly and lead to seizures or heart failure.

**thyrotoxicosis** (thī-rō-tŏks-ĭ-KŌ-sĭs) (p. 431) Another name for hyperthyroidism, causing the symptoms of an increased metabolic rate in all cells.

e-Learning Activity 24-1 ►

## OVERVIEW

An **endocrine gland** secretes one or more hormones that are carried to tissues by the blood rather than by a duct. This process is different from that of nonendocrine glands such as the salivary glands, which use a duct to connect the gland to certain tissues. Endocrine glands release their secretions (hormones) into the blood, which then circulate everywhere. Once in the blood, the hormone is carried to its target tissue. The **target tissue** is a tissue or organ that is affected or controlled by the hormone. For example, the target tissues of estrogen are the uterine lining and certain breast cells. The target tissue of glucagon, a hormone made by the pancreas, is the liver. Thyroid hormones affect all body cells, so the entire body is their target tissue.

## HYPOTHYROIDISM

### REVIEW OF RELATED PHYSIOLOGY AND PATHOPHYSIOLOGY

The thyroid gland is located in the front of the neck just below the Adam's apple (Figure 24-1). It is one of the most important endocrine glands in the body. It has a rich blood supply, and its small follicle cells produce two thyroid hormones: thyroxine ($T_4$) and triiodothyronine ($T_3$). Table 24-1 lists the normal blood levels for all thyroid hormones. $T_3$ and $T_4$ are made from the amino acid tyrosine and the mineral iodine. For the thyroid gland to make correct amounts of both hormones, the diet must contain enough protein and iodine.

When $T_3$ and $T_4$ leave the thyroid gland and enter other body cells, they bind to receptors inside the cell and activate the genes for metabolism. **Metabolism** is the energy use of each cell and the amount of work performed in the body. These hormones increase the rate of metabolism in any cell that they enter. In other words,

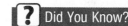

**? Did You Know?**

The most common dietary sources of iodine are saltwater fish and table salt to which iodide is added.

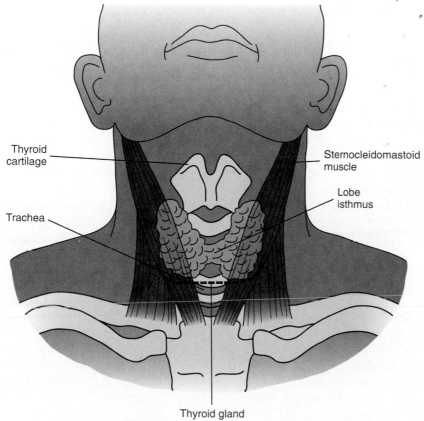

Thyroid cartilage

Sternocleidomastoid muscle

Lobe isthmus

Trachea

Thyroid gland

**FIGURE 24-1** Location of the thyroid gland.

| Table 24-1 | Blood Values for Thyroid Function | |
|---|---|---|
| **TEST** | **NORMAL RANGE** | **MEANING OF ABNORMAL VALUES** |
| T$_3$ | 70-205 ng/dL | *Increased:* Hyperthyroidism *Decreased:* Hypothyroidism |
| T$_4$ | 4-12 mcg/dL | *Increased:* Hyperthyroidism *Decreased:* Hypothyroidism |
| Thyroid antibodies | Titer <1:100* | *Increased:* Hypothyroidism |
| TSH receptor antibodies (TSH-RABs) | Titer <130%* | *Increased:* Graves' disease |
| Thyroid-stimulating hormone (TSH) | 2-10 microunits/mL | *Increased:* Main hypothyroidism; hyperthyroidism caused by brain or pituitary problems *Decreased:* Main hyperthyroidism; hypothyroidism caused by brain or pituitary problems, and Graves' disease |

*Low levels have no meaning.

they speed up the energy use and work output of each cell. Important functions controlled by thyroid hormones include:

- Assisting in brain development before birth and during early childhood.
- Maintaining brain function throughout the life span.
- Helping maintain the ability to think, remember, and learn.
- Maintaining heart and skeletal muscle function.
- Maintaining bone formation and reducing bone density loss.
- Ensuring continued production of other hormones.
- Maintaining effective respiratory function and cell uptake of oxygen.

**Hypothyroidism** is a condition of low thyroid function, causing low blood levels of thyroid hormones (THs) and symptoms of slow metabolism. This health problem is also called an *underactive thyroid*. Thyroid cells may fail to produce enough thyroid hormones because they have been damaged by infection, trauma, or immune problems and no longer function. Other causes include a diet in which a person does not eat enough iodine or tyrosine to make thyroid hormones. Damage to the anterior pituitary gland and other brain areas also can reduce thyroid function.

When the production of T$_3$ and T$_4$ is too low or absent, the blood levels decline, and the patient's entire body metabolism is slowed, sometimes to dangerously low levels. In an effort to increase thyroid hormone production, the thyroid gland cells can divide, making the whole thyroid gland larger, forming a goiter. Figure 24-2 shows a patient with a goiter, which can be seen as a distinct swelling in the neck. Box 24-1 lists other common symptoms of hypothyroidism.

A confusing issue is that a goiter can form with both hypothyroidism and hyperthyroidism. The presence of a goiter indicates that the patient has a thyroid problem but does not help determine whether the problem is caused by an underactive or overactive thyroid.

The most common causes of hypothyroidism are infections of the thyroid gland, too little iodine or tyrosine in the diet, failure of the thyroid gland to form completely during fetal life, brain tumors, and treatment (surgery or radiation) for hyperthyroidism. Some drugs can also reduce thyroid gland function. The most common one is lithium (Eskalith, Lithonate, Lithotabs). If left untreated, hypothyroidism can slow metabolism to such a low level that the heart stops and death occurs. This severe type of hypothyroidism is called *myxedema* and requires immediate medical attention. Hypothyroidism is much more common in women than in men. Figure 24-3 shows a woman with severe hypothyroidism. Figure 24-4 shows an infant with hypothyroidism.

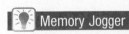

**Memory Jogger**

A goiter can be present when the thyroid gland is overactive or underactive.

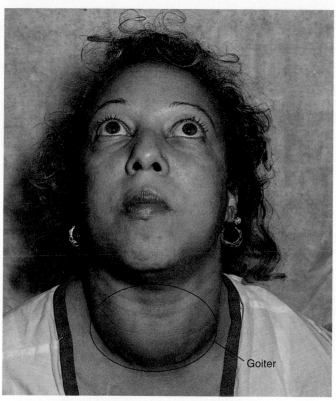

Goiter

**FIGURE 24-2** Woman with a goiter.

---

**Box 24-1**   Signs and Symptoms of Hypothyroidism

**INFANTS AND CHILDREN**
- Constipation
- Excess facial and body hair
- Mental retardation
- Poor eater
- Protruding tongue
- Short stature
- Sleeps excessively

**ADULTS**
- Constipation
- Decreased scalp hair, increased body hair
- Edema of the face, around the eyes, and on shins

- Feels cold all the time
- Lacks energy, sleeps excessively
- Lower than normal body temperature
- Menstrual irregularities
- No interest in sex
- Slow heart rate
- Slow respiratory rate
- Speaks slowly
- Thickened, waxy-feeling skin
- Thick tongue
- Thinks slowly
- Weight gain

---

◀ 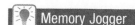-Learning Activity 24-2

# TYPES OF THYROID HORMONE REPLACEMENT DRUGS

## LEVOTHYROXINE AND LIOTHYRONINE

### How Thyroid Hormone Replacement Drugs Work

The hormones that the thyroid gland makes are essential for life. Keeping thyroid hormone function at the right level is important for overall health. The goal of drug therapy is to ensure that the patient's whole body metabolism is as close to normal as possible. If the thyroid is not making these hormones at all or not making enough, the person's entire metabolism becomes slower and slower until it finally stops. At that point death occurs. Replacement of thyroid hormones is needed to keep all cells, tissues, and organs functioning at the proper level. Usually, when a person has an underactive thyroid gland causing hypothyroidism, he or she must take thyroid hormone replacement drugs for the rest of his or her life.

**Memory Jogger**

The goal of drug therapy for thyroid problems is to ensure that the patient's entire body metabolism is as close to normal as possible.

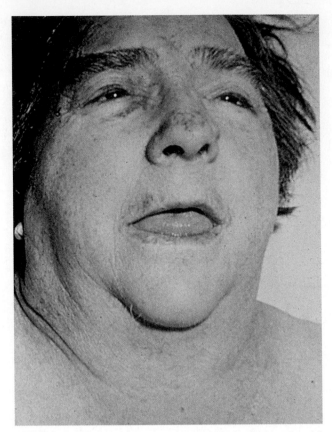

**FIGURE 24-3** Facial appearance of a woman with severe hypothyroidism.

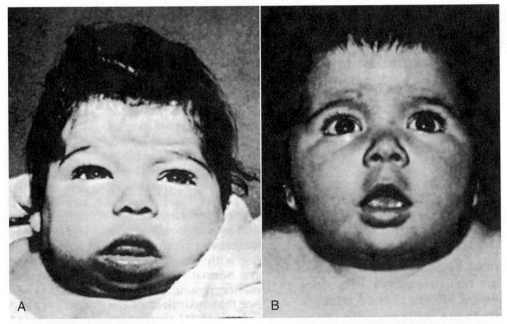

**FIGURE 24-4** Facial appearance of an infant with hypothyroidism before treatment **(A)** and after thyroid hormone replacement therapy **(B).**

Thyroid hormone replacement drugs work just like the patient's own thyroid hormones. They enter the blood and go into all cells. Once inside the cell, the drug binds to receptors and activates the genes for metabolism. Just like $T_3$ and $T_4$, these drugs increase the rate of metabolism in any cell they enter, speeding up the energy use and work output of each cell.

At one time thyroid hormone replacements were only available from other animals. Today most patients taking these drugs take a synthetic hormone drug, which is more consistent for dosage than the natural hormones. The drugs listed in the following table are those most commonly prescribed for thyroid hormone replacement. Be sure to consult a drug reference for information about other thyroid hormone replacement drugs.

### Dosages for Common Thyroid Hormone Replacement Drugs

| Drug | Dosage |
|---|---|
| levothyroxine sodium [synthetic] **TOP 100** (Eltroxin🍁, Levothroid, Levoxyl, Synthroid **TOP 100**, Unithroid) | *Adults:* Oral—25-250 mcg daily; IV—12.5-150 mcg daily <br> *Children:* Oral—2-15 mcg/kg daily; IV—1-7.5 mcg/kg daily |
| liothyronine sodium [synthetic] (Cytomel, Triostat) | *Adults:* 25-75 mcg orally daily <br> *Children 1-3 years:* Oral/IV—5-50 mcg daily |

**TOP 100** Top 100 drugs prescribed.

## *Intended Responses*

- Body temperature is normal.
- Level of activity is normal.
- Heart rate, blood pressure, and respiratory rate are normal for the patient's age and size.
- Body weight is maintained when the patient takes in the amount of calories needed for his or her age, size, and activity level.
- The patient is mentally alert; he or she is able to remember people, places, and events from the recent and distant past.
- Bowel movement pattern is normal.

**Side Effects.**   Thyroid hormone replacement drugs have few side effects. In general, the side effects are really those of an overdose of the drug, and the symptoms are those of hyperthyroidism. They include rapid heart rate and high blood pressure, warm skin, a sensation of feeling too warm, sweating, difficulty sleeping, weight loss, and an increase in the number of bowel movements each day.

**Adverse Effects.**   The most serious adverse effect of thyroid hormone replacement drugs is an increase in the activity of the cardiac and nervous systems. The increase in cardiac activity can overwork the heart and lead to angina pain, a heart attack, and heart failure.

In the nervous system the increased activity can lead to seizures. Seizures are rare and can occur in any patient taking high doses of thyroid hormone replacement drugs but are more likely to occur in the patient who already has a seizure disorder.

Thyroid hormone replacement drugs enhance the action of drugs that reduce blood clotting (anticoagulants), especially warfarin (Coumadin). This action can lead to excessive bruising and bleeding.

### What To Do *Before* Giving Thyroid Hormone Replacement Drugs

Check the patient's blood pressure and heart rate and rhythm. The side effects and adverse effects of thyroid hormone replacement drugs increase metabolic rate and cardiac activity. Checking these vital signs before giving the drug establishes a baseline to determine whether the drug is working correctly or causing an overdose effect.

Check the dose and the specific drug name carefully. Thyroid hormone replacement drugs are not interchangeable because the strength of each drug varies. In fact, if the patient has been on a specific brand of the drug at home, he or she should be prescribed to take the same brand when in another health care setting.

The drug is given just once daily, usually in the morning. However, a patient may have routinely been taking it at another time of day. If this is the case, discuss the timing with the prescriber and try to keep the patient on the same drug schedule in your setting that is usually followed at home. This action reduces the chances for unexpected changes in the patient's response to the drug.

### What To Do *After* Giving Thyroid Hormone Replacement Drugs

Check the patient's blood pressure and heart rate and rhythm to determine whether the drug is working and if there are side effects. Ask the patient whether he or she has any chest pain or discomfort. This symptom may be the first indication of an adverse cardiac effect.

If the patient also takes a drug that affects blood clotting, especially warfarin (Coumadin), check at least once each shift for any sign of increased bleeding. Look for bleeding from the gums; unusual or excessive bruising anywhere on the skin; bleeding around IV sites or for more than 5 minutes after discontinuing an IV; and for the presence of blood in urine, stool, or vomitus.

### What To *Teach* Patients About Thyroid Hormone Replacement Drugs

When a patient is diagnosed with hypothyroidism and is first prescribed a thyroid hormone replacement drug, the dose for the first several weeks is low. Usually it is increased slowly every 2 to 3 weeks until the patient has normal blood levels of TH and signs of normal metabolism. Teach patients not to increase the dose beyond what is prescribed for them. Increasing the drug too quickly can lead to adverse effects such as a heart attack or seizures. Teach them to check their own pulse each morning before taking the drug and again each evening before going to bed. If the pulse rate becomes 20 beats higher than the normal rate for 1 week or if it becomes consistently irregular, they should notify their prescriber. Tell them to go to the emergency department immediately if they start to have chest pain.

Teach patients that they need to take the drug daily to maintain normal body function. If the patient is ill and cannot take the drug orally, instruct him or her to contact the prescriber to get a parenteral dose of the drug. Remind patients not to stop the drug suddenly or to change the dose (up or down) without contacting their prescriber.

Taking the drug with a fiber supplement reduces the absorption of the drug. Teach patients to take it 2 to 3 hours before taking a fiber supplement or at least 4 hours after taking the supplement.

Remind patients who also take warfarin (Coumadin) to keep all follow-up appointments and appointments for blood-clotting tests because these drugs increase the effectiveness of warfarin. Teach them to avoid situations that can lead to bleeding and other drugs (such as aspirin) that can make bleeding worse.

### Life Span Considerations for Thyroid Hormone Replacement Drugs

*Pediatric Considerations.*    Children may develop hypothyroidism or may have been born without a thyroid gland. In either case, they must take thyroid hormone replacement drugs for their entire life. During infancy and early childhood when the patient is going through periods of rapid growth, he or she actually needs a *higher* drug amount per kilogram of body weight than does an adult! For an infant who does not have thyroid function, not taking the drug leads to mental impairment and stunted physical growth.

*Considerations for Pregnancy and Breastfeeding.*    Thyroid hormone replacement drugs are pregnancy category A and safe to take during pregnancy. In fact, for a pregnant woman who has hypothyroidism, not taking the drug can lead to problems with the pregnancy and the fetus. Pregnant women often need a *higher* dose of the drug. Because thyroid hormone replacement drugs can enter breast milk

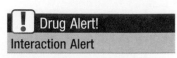

and increase the infant's metabolism, the mother taking these drugs should not breastfeed.

***Considerations for Older Adults.*** Older adults may develop hypothyroidism as part of the aging process or may have had hypothyroidism for many years. Either way, the metabolism of older adults is more sensitive to thyroid hormone replacement drugs, and they are more likely to have adverse cardiac and nervous system effects. For this reason older adults who need these drugs are usually prescribed a lower dose than younger adults. Older adults should be seen by their prescriber every 3 to 6 months and have their cardiac function monitored closely. In addition, older adults are more likely to have diabetes. Thyroid hormone replacement drugs change the effectiveness of insulin and other drugs for diabetes, and often drugs for diabetes need to be increased to prevent high blood sugar levels (*hyperglycemia*). Teach older adults with diabetes and hypothyroidism to check their blood glucose levels more frequently.

◀ⓔ-Learning Activity 24-3

## HYPERTHYROIDISM

### REVIEW OF RELATED PHYSIOLOGY AND PATHOPHYSIOLOGY

**Hyperthyroidism** is an increase in thyroid gland activity causing high blood levels of thyroid hormones ($T_3$ and $T_4$) and symptoms of increased metabolism. This health problem is also called an *overactive thyroid*. Thyroid cells may produce excessive thyroid hormones for several reasons, but the most common type of hyperthyroidism is Graves' disease. With this problem the body makes antibodies to thyroid-stimulating hormone (TSH) receptors on thyroid cells. When these antibodies bind to the TSH receptors, they act as agonists and turn on the thyroid cells, causing the cells to divide, forming a goiter and producing excessive amounts of $T_3$ and $T_4$. As a result the patient's body metabolism is much faster than normal.

Another name for hyperthyroidism is **thyrotoxicosis** because the side effects of excessive thyroid hormones can cause toxic side effects to some organs. Symptoms of hyperthyroidism from any cause are listed in Box 24-2. Additional symptoms that occur only with hyperthyroidism caused by Graves' disease include bulging or protruding eyes (*exophthalmos*) (Figure 24-5) and blurred vision. Other causes of hyperthyroidism include tumors in the thyroid gland, excessive growth of thyroid tissue, and excessive intake of iodine. In addition, tumors in the brain or pituitary gland can send chemical signals that make the thyroid gland bigger and more active than normal. Hyperthyroidism is more common in women than in men.

When hyperthyroidism is severe, it is called **thyroid crisis** or *thyroid storm*. This condition is an extreme state of hyperthyroidism in which all symptoms are more severe and life threatening. The patient has a fever; dangerously high blood pressure; and a rapid, irregular heartbeat. Symptoms can develop quickly; if not treated, this problem can lead to seizures and heart failure. Thyroid crisis also can occur when

> **Memory Jogger**
>
> *Agonists* activate receptors leading to increased cell activity.

---

**Box 24-2** Signs and Symptoms of Hyperthyroidism

| **GENERAL SYMPTOMS** | • Rapid heart rate |
|---|---|
| • Diarrhea | • Sweating |
| • Difficulty sleeping | • Thinning of scalp hair |
| • Feeling too warm most of the time | • Weight loss |
| • Fine tremors of the hands | |
| • Heartbeat irregularities | **ADDITIONAL SYMPTOMS SPECIFIC TO GRAVES'** |
| • High blood pressure | **DISEASE ONLY** |
| • Higher than normal body temperature | • Blurred vision |
| • Menstrual irregularities | • Bulging or protruding eyes (exophthalmia) |

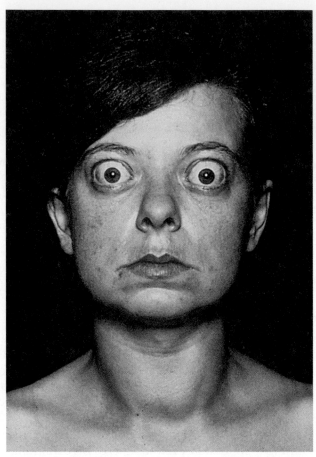

**FIGURE 24-5** Facial appearance of a woman with hyperthyroidism from Graves' disease. Note the bulging eyes, goiter, and lack of body fat.

the patient is severely stressed (such as during pregnancy, after trauma or serious infection, or during diabetic acidosis).

For a person whose thyroid gland is overactive, causing hyperthyroidism, the excess thyroid hormones increase the metabolism of all cells above normal levels. This problem makes every organ work harder than it should, especially the heart. If metabolism remains high, death can occur from heart failure.

## TYPES OF THYROID-SUPPRESSING DRUGS

### METHIMAZOLE AND PROPYLTHIOURACIL

#### How Thyroid-Suppressing Drugs Work

Most of the time hyperthyroidism is a permanent health problem that is treated by destroying all or part of the thyroid gland by surgically removing either some or all of it *(thyroidectomy)* or using radiation to destroy thyroid cells. Drug therapy to reduce thyroid production of hormones is often used before surgery. If the patient is too ill for surgery or radiation, thyroid-suppressing drugs may be used long term in place of these treatments.

Thyroid-suppressing drugs enter the thyroid gland and combine with the enzyme responsible for connecting iodine (iodide) with tyrosine to make active $T_3$ and $T_4$. This action keeps the enzyme so busy working on the drug that it does not have the opportunity to make thyroid hormones. These drugs do not affect the hormones already formed and stored in the thyroid gland, so it may take as long as 3 or 4 weeks for a person to use all of the thyroid hormones made before the drug was started. Until that time the person continues to have symptoms of hyperthyroidism.

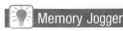
**Memory Jogger**

The effects of thyroid-suppressing drugs are usually not seen until 3 to 4 weeks after they have been taken daily.

## Dosages for Common Thyroid-Suppressing Drugs

| Drug | Dosage |
|------|--------|
| methimazole (Tapazole) | *Adults:* Initial dose—15-60 mg orally in 1-3 divided doses at 8-hr intervals; maintenance dosage—5-15 mg orally at 8-hr intervals<br>*Children:* Initial dose—0.5-0.7 mg/kg orally in 1-3 divided doses at 8-hr intervals; maintenance dosage—usually one-half the initial dose |
| propylthiouracil (Propacil, Propyl-Thyracil🍁, PTU) | *Adults:* Initial dose—100-150 mg orally every 8 hr; maintenance dosage—50 mg orally every 8 hr<br>*Children:* Initial dose—50 mg orally every 8 hr; maintenance dosage—determined by response |

### Intended Responses

- Body temperature is normal.
- Level of activity is normal.
- Heart rate, blood pressure, and respiratory rate are normal for the patient's age and size.
- Body weight is maintained when the patient takes in the amount of calories needed for his or her age, size, and activity level.
- Bowel movement pattern is normal.

*Side Effects.* Thyroid-suppressing drugs have many minor side effects. These include rash, loss of taste sensation, headache, muscle and joint aches, itchiness, drowsiness, nausea, vomiting, lymph node enlargement, and swelling of the feet and ankles.

*Adverse Effects.* A major adverse effect of thyroid-suppressing drugs is bone marrow suppression, which reduces the amount of blood cells. As a result the patient is less resistant to infection and more likely to be anemic.

These drugs, especially propylthiouracil, can be hepatotoxic. (Propylthiouracil has a black box warning for liver damage.) These drugs can also damage the kidneys, but this occurs more rarely.

Thyroid-suppressing drugs enhance the action of drugs that reduce blood clotting (anticoagulants), especially warfarin (Coumadin). This action increases the risk for excessive bruising and bleeding.

### What To Do *Before* Giving Thyroid-Suppressing Drugs

Check the patient's liver function tests before giving these drugs. Both thyroid-suppressing drugs are hepatotoxic. If a patient already has a liver problem, the effects of the drugs on the liver are worse and occur at lower doses.

Check the dose and the specific drug name carefully. Although methimazole and propylthiouracil work in the same way, they are not interchangeable because the strength of each drug varies.

### What To Do *After* Giving Thyroid-Suppressing Drugs

Check patients who also take a drug that affects blood clotting, especially warfarin (Coumadin), at least once each shift for any sign of increased bleeding. Look for bleeding from the gums; unusual or excessive bruising anywhere on the skin; bleeding around IV sites or for more than 5 minutes after discontinuing an IV; and the presence of blood in urine, stool, or vomitus.

Check the patient daily for yellowing of the skin or sclera (jaundice), which is a symptom of liver problems. The best places to check are the whites of the eyes closest to the iris, the roof of the mouth, and the skin on the chest. Avoid checking the soles of the feet or palms of the hands, especially in patients with darker skin, because these areas often appear yellow even when the patient is not jaundiced.

Check the patient's white blood cell count (WBC). Adverse effects of thyroid-suppressing drugs are bone marrow suppression, which reduces the WBC count and increases the risk for infection.

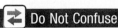

**Do Not Confuse**

**methimazole** *with* **metolazone**

An order for methimazole can be confused with metolazone. Methimazole is a thyroid-suppressing drug, whereas metolazone is a diuretic.

**Do Not Confuse**

**propylthiouracil** *with* **Purinethol**

An order for propylthiouracil can be confused with Purinethol. Propylthiouracil is a thyroid-suppressing drug, whereas Purinethol is a cancer chemotherapy drug.

**Common Side Effects**

**Thyroid-Suppressing Drugs**

Rash    Nausea    Headache

Muscle aches

**Clinical Pitfall**

Do not substitute methimazole for propylthiouracil. Methimazole is 10 times stronger than propylthiouracil.

### What To *Teach* Patients About Thyroid-Suppressing Drugs

Teach patients taking warfarin (Coumadin) to keep all follow-up appointments and appointments for blood-clotting tests because these drugs increase the effectiveness of warfarin. Instruct them to avoid situations that can lead to bleeding and other drugs that can make bleeding worse.

Remind patients taking thyroid-suppressing drugs to avoid crowds and people who are ill because these drugs suppress the production of white blood cells in the bone marrow. This effect reduces the patient's immunity and resistance to infection.

Teach patients to check the color of the roof of the mouth and the whites of the eyes every day for the presence of a yellow tinge. These drugs can cause liver damage and lead to jaundice. Teach patients to report jaundice to their prescriber as soon as possible.

### Life Span Considerations for Thyroid-Suppressing Drugs

***Pediatric Considerations.*** Thyroid-suppressing drugs are used with caution on a short-term basis in children. Adverse effects are rare in children, and side effects occur in children at about the same rate as they occur in adults.

***Considerations for Pregnancy and Breastfeeding.*** Thyroid-suppressing drugs are pregnancy category D drugs and can cause miscarriages and birth defects. These drugs should not be given during pregnancy unless the benefits of treatment are thought to outweigh the risk in a life-threatening situation or when other treatments are not available. Women taking thyroid-suppressing drugs should not breastfeed.

***Considerations for Older Adults.*** Older adults taking thyroid-suppressing drugs are more likely to have an adverse effect, and adverse effects are more likely to be severe. The older patient's resistance to infection is already lower than that of a younger adult because of age-related changes that occur in the immune system. Decreased bone marrow activity makes this problem worse. Urge adults to get an annual flu shot and a vaccination against pneumonia. Many older adults also take warfarin (Coumadin). The effects of warfarin are increased when the patient also takes a thyroid-suppressing drug. Remind patients taking both types of drugs to see their prescriber more frequently and have clotting studies, especially the international normalized ratio (INR), checked as often as every week.

## MENOPAUSE

## REVIEW OF RELATED PHYSIOLOGY AND PATHOPHYSIOLOGY

The cyclic hormone changes that occur during adolescence and continue throughout a woman's menstruating years promote conception and pregnancy. Conception occurs when a mature egg *(ovum)* is released from a woman's ovary and is fertilized by a sperm *(spermatozoon)* during sexual intercourse. When the fertilized egg successfully implants in the uterus, pregnancy results. The maturation of an egg and proper preparation of the uterine lining to support pregnancy depend on the presence and timing of specific hormones.

**Menstruation** is the periodic shedding of the uterine lining that occurs as a result of the cyclic changes of hormone levels in females. **Menarche** is the beginning of the years of menstruation in an adolescent female. It occurs as a result of the secretion of *gonadotropin-releasing hormone (GnRH)* in the brain. These hormones start to be secreted in both females and males at the beginning of puberty. Their job is to trigger sex hormone secretion in females and males so physical changes occur that lead to interest in sexual activity *(libido)* and the ability to perform sexual intercourse. **Estrogen** is the main female sex hormone secreted by the ovaries and adrenal glands.

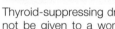 **Clinical Pitfall**

Thyroid-suppressing drugs should not be given to a woman who is pregnant or breastfeeding.

-Learning Activity 24-4 ▶

 **Memory Jogger**

GnRH is secreted by the hypothalamus of both males and females to start the hormone changes needed for puberty.

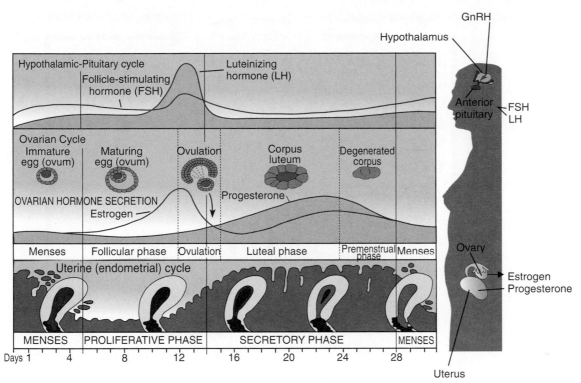

**FIGURE 24-6** Hormone interactions for ovulation and menstruation. *GnRH*, Gonadotropin-releasing hormone.

In females the secretion of GnRH stimulates the release of two hormones from the pituitary gland: follicle-stimulating hormone (FSH) and luteinizing hormone (Figure 24-6).

**Follicle-stimulating hormone** causes the ovary to secrete estrogen and allows one ovum in the ovary to complete maturation each month. As estrogen levels rise in the blood, the lining of the uterus grows and thickens (see Figure 24-6). After about 14 days of lining growth, it is thick enough to support the implantation of a fertilized egg. At this optimum midcycle time, GnRH triggers the pituitary gland to release *luteinizing hormone,* which causes secretion of progesterone by the ovary and allows the release of a mature ovum. This process is known as *ovulation.* The outer covering *(corpus luteum)* from the released ovum also secretes progesterone. **Progesterone** supports any pregnancy that occurs by maintaining the thickened uterine lining and allowing it to secrete nutrients needed by the early embryo. If fertilization and pregnancy do not occur, the outer covering from the released ovum degenerates in about 12 days, and circulating levels of estrogen and progesterone drop. The loss of these hormones allows the lining of the uterus to stop growing and to shed as menstruation. Figure 24-7 shows the feedback loops controlling the secretion of estrogen and progesterone.

**Menopause** is the cessation of menstrual periods and ovulation. Natural menopause occurs as a result of age-related changes in the ovary in which glandular cells shrink and become nonfunctional, a process called *involution.* The ovaries become smaller and no longer respond to hormones by secreting estrogen and releasing mature eggs. Natural menopause occurs gradually, over months to years. (Menopause caused by surgery or drug therapy can be sudden.) **Perimenopause** is the transition in a woman from having regular hormone cycles with menstrual periods to the time when menstrual periods have stopped for a full year. During this time hormone levels change, causing the woman to have a variety of uncomfortable but usually minor symptoms. Perimenopause often spans 1 to 2 years but may be as long as 5 or more years.

 **Memory Jogger**

Estrogen causes the uterine lining to thicken during the first half of the menstrual cycle. Progesterone maintains the lining and causes it to secrete nutrients during the second half of the cycle. The drop in the level of these hormones allows menstruation to occur.

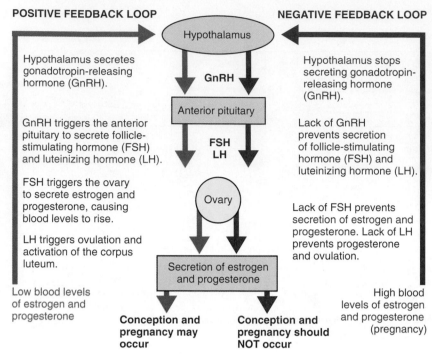

FIGURE 24-7 Positive and negative feedback control over estrogen and progesterone secretion.

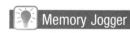

**Memory Jogger**

Menopause symptoms are caused by low levels of estrogen and high levels of FSH.

When the glandular cells of the ovary shrink, they no longer produce normal levels of estrogen. The decreased blood levels of estrogen trigger the brain to secrete GnRH, which then triggers the pituitary gland to secrete FSH (see Figure 24-7). Before menopause the FSH acts on the ovary and causes ovarian cells to secret estrogen, which then inhibits the pathway through negative feedback. With nonfunctional ovarian cells unable to respond to FSH by increasing estrogen secretion, this pathway is disrupted for a time. The continued low blood levels of estrogen constantly stimulate the brain to secret GnRH in large amounts, resulting in the secretion of very large amounts of FSH (Figure 24-8). This extra FSH is useless because the ovary cannot respond to it and it has effects on other body tissues. Box 24-3 lists the symptoms associated with decreased estrogen levels and increased FSH levels.

High levels of FSH act on blood vessels, making them dilate suddenly, resulting in the woman experiencing sudden whole-body flushes and radiant heat. These are commonly called *hot flashes* or *hot flushes*. They may occur as often as every hour or as infrequently as once a week. During the flushes the woman feels intensely and uncomfortably warm. At night these flushes are often followed by excessive sweating that leaves night clothes and bedding wet. Low estrogen levels cause unpleasant changes in the skin and vaginal tissues. They also allow an increased rate of bone loss (osteoporosis) in women who have other risk factors for this chronic health problem.

## TYPES OF PERIMENOPAUSAL HORMONE REPLACEMENT DRUGS

### CONJUGATED ESTROGENS

#### How Perimenopausal Hormone Replacement Therapy Works

*Hormone replacement therapy (HRT)* is the replacement of naturally secreted estrogen and progesterone with exogenous hormones during the perimenopausal period. Providing low doses of estrogen increases blood estrogen levels, which helps with perimenopausal symptoms in two ways. First it relieves the direct problems from low estrogen levels (see Box 24-3). It also inhibits the feedback system and lowers the levels of FSH. This reduces the side effects of high FSH levels (see Box 24-3).

**Positive but ineffective feedback loop**

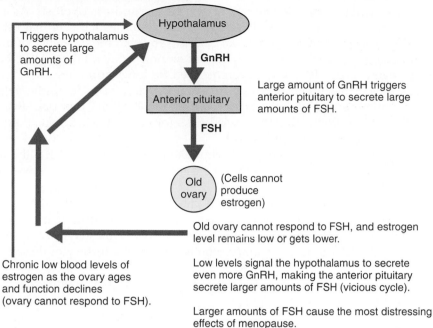

FIGURE 24-8 Mechanism for hot flushes and night sweats associated with menopause. *FSH,* Follicle-stimulating hormone; *GnRH,* gonadotropin-releasing hormone.

---

| Box **24-3** | Common Perimenopausal Symptoms |
| --- | --- |

| **SYMPTOMS RELATED TO REDUCED ESTROGEN LEVELS** | **SYMPTOMS RELATED TO HIGH FOLLICLE-STIMULATING HORMONE LEVELS** |
| --- | --- |
| • Atrophy of vaginal tissue | • Decreased mental concentration |
| • Dry skin | • Hot flushes |
| • Increased rate of osteoporosis | • Night sweats |
| • Painful intercourse | • Sleep difficulties |
| • Reduced cervical mucus | |

## Dosages for Common Perimenopausal Hormone Replacement Therapy Drugs

| Drug | Dosage (Adults Only) |
| --- | --- |
| conjugated estrogens (Cenestin, C.E.S.✦, Enjuvia, Premarin) | 0.3 mg, 0.45 mg, or 0.625 mg orally once daily, given cyclically or continuously, alone in women without a uterus, in combination with a progestin in women with a uterus |
| conjugated estrogens; medroxyPROGESTERone | |
| (Premphase) | 0.625 mg of conjugated estrogens orally once daily on days 1-14, then 1 light-blue tablet (0.625 mg conjugated estrogens/5 mg medroxyPROGESTERone acetate) orally once daily on days 15-28 |
| (Prempro) | 0.3 mg or 0.45 mg along with medroxyPROGESTERone acetate 1.5 mg/day, or 0.625 mg/2.5 mg and the 0.625 mg/5 mg for those not responding to lower doses |

### Intended Responses
• The number and severity of hot flushes and night sweats are reduced.
• Vaginal dryness is reduced.

***Side Effects.*** Common side effects of perimenopausal HRT include breast tenderness, breakthrough bleeding, fluid retention, weight gain, and acne. These occur with conjugated estrogen alone and when combined with progesterone. Fluid retention can cause or worsen hypertension.

 **Do Not Confuse**

**Premphase** *with* **Prempro**

An order for Premphase can be confused with Prempro. Although both drugs are used for perimenopausal hormone replacement therapy, the dosages of the combined hormones are different.

**Common Side Effects**

**Perimenopausal Hormone Replacement Therapy**

Acne

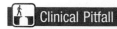

**Clinical Pitfall**

Patients taking perimenopausal HRT should not smoke.

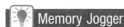

**Memory Jogger**

Taking perimenopausal HRT drugs more often than prescribed or not following instructions for timing increases the risk for excessive uterine bleeding.

*Adverse Effects.* For years estrogen-based HRT during and after menopause was thought to reduce the risk for coronary artery disease and osteoporosis. As a result many women were on long-term HRT. More recent studies indicate that estrogen-based HRT does not protect against heart disease and that the incidence of myocardial infarction (heart attack) is slightly higher among women taking HRT. For this reason estrogen-based HRT is not recommended for long-term therapy.

Drugs for perimenopausal HRT increase blood clotting, placing the patient at risk for thrombosis and emboli. Cigarette smoking worsens this risk. Results of increased clot formation include increased risks for heart attack, stroke, pulmonary embolism, and deep vein thrombosis.

In women who have a uterus and who take perimenopausal HRT, the uterine lining can become excessively thick, increasing the risk for excessive uterine bleeding.

The hormones in perimenopausal HRT can increase the growth of cancers that are hormone sensitive such as cervical, breast, ovarian, and uterine cancers. These drugs should not be used in women who have a history of these types of cancer and should be used with caution in women who have a family history of these types of cancer.

These hormones also increase the risk for liver impairment, gallbladder disease, and pancreatitis.

### What To *Teach* Patients About Perimenopausal Hormone Replacement Therapy

Teach women to take drugs for perimenopausal HRT exactly as prescribed with regard to dosage and timing.

Encourage women to have annual screenings for breast, cervical, uterine, and ovarian cancer while taking these drugs.

Urge patients who smoke to either quit or reduce smoking during the time that they take these drugs.

Teach patients to check the color of the roof of the mouth and the whites of the eyes every day for the presence of a yellow tinge. These drugs can cause liver damage and lead to jaundice. Tell them to report jaundice to their prescriber as soon as possible.

Teach patients to seek medical attention immediately if they have chest pain or difficulty breathing, swelling in one leg, or symptoms of stroke. Stroke symptoms include facial drooping, blurred vision, difficulty speaking, and muscle weakness on one side of the body.

e-Learning Activity 24-5 ►

## Get Ready for Practice!

### Key Points

- Proper thyroid function is essential for life. Both an underactive thyroid gland (causing hypothyroidism) and an overactive thyroid gland (causing hyperthyroidism) must be treated.
- Thyroid problems are 5 to 10 times more common in women than men.
- Side effects and adverse effects of thyroid hormone replacement drugs resemble hyperthyroidism.
- Infants and young children may need a *higher* dose (in terms of micrograms per kilogram of body weight) of thyroid hormone replacement drugs than adults and older adults need.
- Thyroid crisis (or thyroid storm) is an emergency situation. The death rate for thyroid crisis is about 30%, even when the patient is treated correctly.

- Teach patients taking thyroid hormone replacement drugs not to stop the drug suddenly or change the dose of the drug without consulting their prescriber.
- When thyroid hormone replacement drugs are first started, the dose is low and is increased slowly until the patient gets to the dose that keeps metabolism at a normal level.
- Thyroid hormone replacement drugs increase a patient's blood sugar level; patients with diabetes may need higher doses of insulin or other antidiabetic drugs.
- Both thyroid hormone replacement drugs and thyroid-suppressing drugs increase the effectiveness of warfarin (Coumadin), increasing a patient's risk for bleeding.
- The effects of thyroid-suppressing drugs may not be seen until 2 to 4 weeks after therapy has started because of the existing thyroid hormones stored in the gland.

- Drugs for perimenopausal hormone replacement should be taken only short term to reduce the symptoms of menopause.
- Drugs for perimenopausal HRT increase blood clot formation, increasing the risks for heart attack, stroke, pulmonary embolism, and deep vein thrombosis.

## Additional Learning Resources

**evolve** Go to your Evolve website (http://evolve.elsevier.com/Workman/pharmacology/) for the following FREE learning resources:

- eLearning Activities
- Animations
- Video Clips
- Interactive Review Questions
- Audio Key Points
- Audio Glossary
- Audio Glossary—Spanish-English
- Drug Dosage Calculators
- Patient Teaching Handouts

**SG** Go to your Study Guide for additional learning activities to help you master this chapter content.

## Review Questions

1. Which condition indicates that drug therapy for a patient with hypothyroidism is effective?
   A. The patient is thirsty.
   B. The patient's weight has been the same for 3 weeks.
   C. The patient's total white blood cell count is 6000 cells/mm$^3$.
   D. The patient has had a bowel movement every day for 1 week.

2. A patient prescribed methimazole (Tapazole) is also taking warfarin (Coumadin). What is the most important action to take after giving this drug?
   A. Checking IV sites for oozing and the skin for bruising
   B. Checking the skin and whites of the eyes for jaundice
   C. Checking bowel sounds for signs of obstruction
   D. Teaching the patient to drink plenty of water

3. For which condition or side effect should you teach the patient prescribed a thyroid hormone replacement drug to seek medical assistance immediately?
   A. Dry, waxy skin
   B. Facial flushing
   C. Chest pain
   D. Insomnia

4. A patient is newly pregnant and tells you that she has been taking levothyroxine (Synthroid) for the last 12 years for hypothyroidism. She asks you whether she should take this drug during pregnancy and while breastfeeding. What is your best response?
   A. "This drug should not be taken during pregnancy or while breastfeeding."
   B. "This drug can be taken during pregnancy but not while breastfeeding."
   C. "This drug can be taken during pregnancy and while breastfeeding."
   D. "This drug should not be taken during pregnancy but can be taken while breastfeeding."

5. A patient has all of the following health problems or conditions. Which one alerts you as a reason for not taking perimenopausal hormone replacement therapy?
   A. Mastectomy 3 years ago for breast cancer
   B. Broken hip 1 year ago from osteoporosis
   C. Gestational diabetes during her last pregnancy
   D. Gastroesophageal reflux disease for the last year

6. Which activity must you advise the patient to avoid while taking perimenopausal hormone replacement therapy?
   A. Smoking cigarettes
   B. Having sexual intercourse
   C. Drinking alcoholic beverages
   D. Engaging in moderate-to-heavy exercise

7. A 6-year-old child is being started on levothyroxine (Synthroid) intravenously and is prescribed 5 mcg/kg of body weight. The child weighs 28 kg. The drug vial contains 100 mcg/mL.
   a. How many micrograms will this patient receive based on body weight? _____ mcg
   b. How many milliliters of drug will be drawn up to equal this dose? _____ mL

8. A patient is to receive 5 mg of methimazole (Tapazole) orally every 8 hours. You have on hand 10-mg tablets of methimazole (Tapazole). How many 10-mg tablets do you give for the correct dose? _____ tablet(s)

## Critical Thinking Activities

The patient is a 34-year-old woman who has been taking liothyronine (Cytomel) 50 mcg PO daily for the past year. She tells you that she has been constipated, has no "pep," and has gained 15 lb in the past 2 months.

1. What type of drug is liothyronine?

2. What are the side effects of this drug?

3. Are the problems she describes side effects of this drug?

4. What is the most likely cause of her health problems?

# Drugs for Diabetes

evolve

http://evolve.elsevier.com/Workman/pharmacology/

## Objectives

*After studying this chapter you should be able to:*

1. Explain the causes, symptoms, and complications of diabetes.
2. List the names, actions, usual dosages, possible side effects, and adverse effects of insulin.
3. Describe what to do before and after giving insulin.
4. Describe what to teach patients taking insulin, including what to do, what not to do, and when to call the prescriber.
5. Describe the steps for subcutaneous insulin administration.
6. Explain the correct way to mix different types of insulin in the same syringe.
7. Describe life span considerations for insulin therapy.
8. List the names, actions, usual adult dosages, possible side effects, and adverse effects of commonly prescribed oral antidiabetic drugs.
9. Describe what to do before and after giving oral antidiabetic drugs.
10. Explain what to teach patients taking oral antidiabetic drugs, including what to do, what not to do, and when to call the prescriber.
11. Describe life span considerations for oral antidiabetic drugs.
12. List the names, actions, usual adult dosages, possible side effects, and adverse effects of incretins and amylin, and what to teach patients about drugs that increase them.

## Key Terms

**adenosine triphosphate (ATP)** (ă-DĔN-ō-sēn trī-FŎS-fāt) (p. 442) The main chemical energy substance that drives all the cellular reactions of the body.

**diabetes mellitus** (dī-ĕ-BĒ-tĕs MĔL-lĭ-tŭs) (p. 444) A metabolic disease that results from either the loss of the ability to make insulin or the loss of receptor sensitivity to the presence of insulin.

**euglycemia** (yū-glī-SĒ-mē-ă) (p. 442) A fasting blood glucose level that is in the normal range (70 to 110 mg/dL).

**glucagon** (GLŪ-kă-gŏn) (p. 443) The hormone released by alpha cells of the pancreas that prevents hypoglycemia by breaking down glycogen from the liver into glucose.

**glucose** (GLŪ-kōs) (p. 442) The most common simple carbohydrate and the main fuel for the human body. Once inside cells, glucose is used to make the chemical energy substance adenosine triphosphate (ATP).

**glycogen** (GLĪ-kō-jĕn) (p. 442) A human starch that serves as the storage form of extra glucose.

**hyperglycemia** (hī-pŭr-glī-SĒ-mē-ă) (p. 442) A blood glucose level above normal (higher than 110 mg/dL when fasting).

**hypoglycemia** (hī-pō-glī-SĒ-mē-ă) (p. 443) A blood glucose level below normal (lower than 70 mg/dL).

**insulin** (ĬN-sŭl-ĭn) (p. 442) The hormone produced by the beta cells of the pancreas that prevents blood glucose levels from becoming too high.

**ketoacidosis** (kē-tō-ăs-ĭ-DŌ-sĭs) (p. 445) An excessive buildup of ketone bodies that occurs when cells use fat rather than glucose for fuel. Ketone bodies are formed as a byproduct of fat metabolism.

ⓔ-Learning Activity 25-1 ▶

## OVERVIEW

The pancreas is one of the most important endocrine glands of the body. As discussed in Chapter 24, an endocrine gland is a tissue that secretes at least one hormone directly into the blood, which then circulates to its target tissue. The *target tissue* is a tissue or organ that is affected or controlled by the hormone. This chapter focuses on the hormones of the pancreas. Figure 25-1 shows the body location of the pancreas.

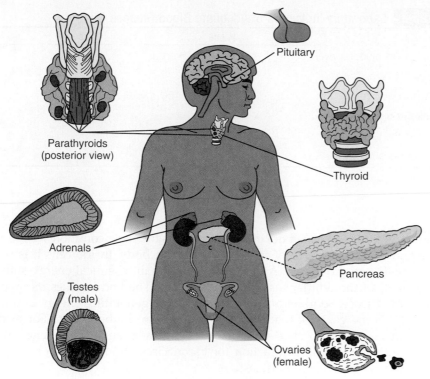

**FIGURE 25-1** Location of the pancreas.

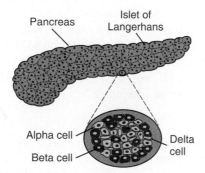

**FIGURE 25-2** Close-up view of the pancreas showing the islets of Langerhans that contain the glucagon-secreting alpha cells and the insulin-secreting beta cells.

The pancreas makes two hormones, insulin and glucagon, that are important for using the right "fuel" in the body. The beta cells of the pancreas make insulin, and the alpha cells of the pancreas make glucagon (Figure 25-2). The target tissues of insulin are skeletal muscle and fat cells. The target tissue of glucagon is the liver. Together insulin and glucagon ensure that the right amount of glucose is always present to provide enough energy for proper body *metabolism* (the energy use by each cell and amount of work performed within the body).

## REVIEW OF RELATED PHYSIOLOGY AND PATHOPHYSIOLOGY

### NORMAL PHYSIOLOGY

People need to eat to provide the materials that cells use to function. Food contains three main types of nutrients: carbohydrates, proteins, and fats. Proteins and fats make cell structures and all the hormones and enzymes that the body needs daily. Although both proteins and fats can make fuel to run the actions of the body, the main source of fuel is carbohydrate. People eat carbohydrates as sugars and starches. Once inside the digestive tract, the body converts most of the carbohydrates that are

| Table 25-1 | Laboratory Indicators of Adequate Blood Glucose Control |
|---|---|
| **TEST** | **VALUE** |
| Fasting blood glucose level | 70 to 110 mg/dL |
| Hemoglobin A1c | 4% to 6% |
| Spot blood glucose level* | Less than 150 mg/dL |
| Blood ketone body level | Negative |
| Urine glucose level | Negative |
| Urine ketone body level | Negative |

*Random, not fasting.

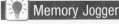

**Memory Jogger**

Body cells need glucose and oxygen to make enough adenosine triphosphate (ATP) to perform all bodily functions.

eaten into glucose (also called dextrose). **Glucose** is the most common simple carbohydrate and the main source of fuel for the human body. Inside cells it is used to form **adenosine triphosphate (ATP)**, which is the main chemical energy substance that drives all of the cellular reactions of the body. The body makes its own ATP, mostly from glucose. So glucose is the main fuel for generating energy in the form of ATP. ATP is the gasoline that makes the engine in the body run. For example, ATP provides skeletal muscle contraction for movement and maintenance of body temperature, heart muscle contraction for blood circulation, neuron excitation for thinking, and GI work for food digestion.

As you can see, people need a constant supply of glucose in the blood ready to enter cells so that enough ATP can be made to ensure good body function. In fact, some cells, such as brain cells, die within a few minutes if blood glucose levels become too low. To be fully functional the brain needs a constant supply of glucose. Other problems develop if blood glucose levels become and remain too high. The right balance of insulin and glucagon, along with food intake, ensure that we always have the right amount of glucose in the blood. **Euglycemia** is a normal fasting blood glucose level (between 70 and 110 mg/dL). Table 25-1 lists the laboratory values that indicate that control of glucose is adequate.

### Insulin

**Insulin** is the hormone produced by the beta cells of the pancreas to prevent blood glucose levels from becoming too high. A blood glucose level above normal is called **hyperglycemia.** Insulin is made and released from the beta cells into the blood whenever blood glucose levels start to rise above normal levels. So the trigger for insulin secretion is hyperglycemia, and its action is to restore normal blood glucose levels by moving blood glucose into cells. The insulin binds to insulin receptors on the membranes of many cells. The result of having insulin bound to its receptor is that the cell membrane becomes more open to glucose, allowing the blood glucose to enter the cell (Figure 25-3). As glucose from the blood enters the cells, the blood glucose level returns to normal (euglycemia). The glucose in the cell then can be used immediately to make ATP if the cell needs more chemical energy. If the cell already has enough ATP, the glucose is made into glycogen and stored for later use in the liver and muscle. The important thing to remember is that insulin lowers blood glucose levels.

Insulin is called the *hormone of plenty* because in the healthy person eating well makes blood levels of carbohydrates, proteins, and fats rise. When you have more than enough glucose to meet your energy needs, insulin allows the extra glucose to be converted to glycogen. **Glycogen** is human starch that serves as the storage form of extra glucose. Molecules of glucose are linked together to form the trunk and branches of glycogen "trees" (Figure 25-4). In addition to keeping blood glucose levels from rising too high, insulin also helps control protein and fat metabolism. Box 25-1 lists the controlling effects of insulin.

**Memory Jogger**

The trigger for insulin secretion is hyperglycemia, and its action is to restore normal blood glucose levels by allowing blood glucose to move into cells.

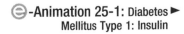

-Animation 25-1: Diabetes ►
Mellitus Type 1: Insulin

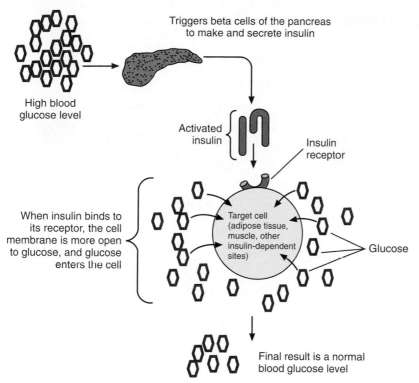

FIGURE 25-3 Action of insulin.

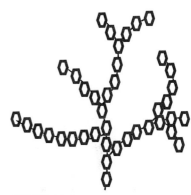

**FIGURE 25-4** One glycogen "tree" with 40 molecules of glucose stored in it.

| Box 25-1 | Effects of Insulin |

- Prevents blood glucose levels from rising too high
- Prevents muscle breakdown
- Stores fats inside fat cells
- Builds glycogen (stored form of glucose) in the liver and muscle
- Improves protein digestion and use in the body
- Increases the amount of energy produced in the cells
- Induces cell division for growth and wound healing
- Maintains blood levels of cholesterol and other fats within normal limits

## Glucagon

If insulin were the only hormone controlling blood glucose levels, the body would be at risk for having blood glucose levels below normal, a condition called **hypoglycemia.** Low blood glucose levels reduce body metabolism because not enough glucose enters cells to make adequate amounts of ATP. If hypoglycemia is severe enough, it can quickly lead to death. So how does a person have a blood glucose level that is constantly in the normal range without eating every hour? The answer is the action of the hormone glucagon.

Glucagon is the hormone released by the alpha cells of the pancreas that prevents hypoglycemia by breaking down glycogen into glucose. It is released whenever blood glucose starts to fall below normal levels. The trigger for glucagon secretion is hypoglycemia, and its action is to raise the blood glucose level back up to normal. Glucagon travels to the liver and other storage sites of glycogen, binds to liver cells, and removes glucose from glycogen trees. This action releases free glucose into the blood (Figure 25-5), bringing the level back to normal (euglycemia).

Glucagon is the "hormone of starvation" because it is triggered when blood glucose levels are low such as when you are sleeping (and not eating). Thanks to the action of glucagon, a person can go 10 to 12 hours without eating and not become so hypoglycemic that cells die. So glucagon and insulin have opposite actions.

 **Memory Jogger**

Hypoglycemia (low blood glucose levels) can rapidly lead to death.

 **Memory Jogger**

The trigger for glucagon secretion is hypoglycemia, and its action is to restore the blood glucose level back to normal.

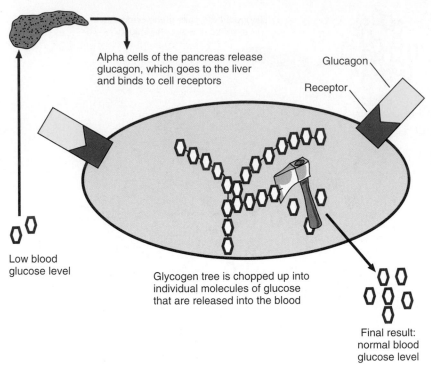

**FIGURE 25-5** Action of glucagon.

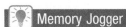

Blood glucose is controlled by insulin and glucagon. Insulin causes blood glucose levels to decrease, preventing hyperglycemia. Glucagon causes blood glucose levels to rise, preventing hypoglycemia.

Control of blood glucose levels is critical for good health. The balance between insulin and glucagon action keeps blood glucose levels in the normal range. Although the cell types for insulin and glucagon secretion are both in the pancreas, problems occur much more often with the cells that secrete insulin.

## PATHOPHYSIOLOGY

One of the most common endocrine problems in the United States is diabetes mellitus, also called "sugar" diabetes. **Diabetes mellitus** is a metabolic disease that results from either the loss of the ability to make insulin or the loss of receptor sensitivity to the presence of insulin. The first result of either of these problems is increased blood glucose levels (hyperglycemia). The two most common forms of diabetes mellitus are type 1 and type 2. They differ in cause, usual age of onset, degree of insulin secretion remaining, and how they are treated. The two types have many of the same symptoms, and the long-term complications are the same.

### Type 1 Diabetes

Type 1 diabetes also has been called *juvenile diabetes* and *insulin-dependent diabetes mellitus*. With this form of diabetes, the beta cells of the pancreas no longer make and secrete any insulin. The most common cause of type 1 diabetes is inflammation and destruction of the beta cells after a viral infection. Other causes of type 1 diabetes remain unknown. Without insulin the patient's blood glucose level becomes very high, but glucose cannot enter many cells. As a result, the body switches from using glucose to using fat to make ATP. Overall the body has less ATP available; and metabolism of carbohydrates, proteins, and fats becomes abnormal. Because insulin is no longer produced, patients who have type 1 diabetes must use insulin daily for the rest of their lives or receive a pancreas transplant.

Usually the onset of type 1 diabetes is sudden. Although the disease can occur at any age, it most commonly begins in children and young adults. The first symptoms are caused by hyperglycemia. These include excessive hunger and eating (*polyphagia*), thirst, drinking more fluids than usual throughout the day (*polydipsia*), urinating more (*polyuria*), weight loss, and fatigue. The fasting blood glucose level is above 110 mg/dL, and often glucose is present in the urine.

Patients with type 1 diabetes do not make their own insulin and must use insulin from other sources.

Symptoms of untreated diabetes include excessive hunger, thirst, polydipsia, polyuria, weight loss, and fatigue.

| Box 25-2 | Signs and Symptoms of Ketoacidosis |

- Abdominal pain
- Blood glucose level greater than 300 mg/dL
- Blood pH less than 7.35
- Dehydration
- "Fruity" odor of the breath
- Intense thirst (if alert)
- Ketone bodies in the blood even after dilution
- Kussmaul's respirations (deep and rapid)
- Lethargy to coma
- Nausea
- Urine glucose positive
- Urine ketone bodies positive
- Warm, dry skin

If type 1 diabetes is not treated with insulin, hyperglycemia worsens, and the body uses more fat for fuel. When fat is used to make ATP, a byproduct is the formation of ketoacids. If these ketoacids form faster than they are eliminated, the patient develops *diabetic ketoacidosis (DKA)*, a serious complication that can result in coma and death. Ketoacidosis is the excessive buildup of ketone bodies when cells use fat instead of glucose for fuel. The signs and symptoms of this emergency condition are listed in Box 25-2. Triggers of DKA in a person who has type 1 diabetes include illness, infection, stress, excessive carbohydrate intake, and not taking the proper amount of insulin.

### Type 2 Diabetes

Type 2 diabetes also has been called *adult-onset diabetes* and *noninsulin-dependent diabetes mellitus*. It is much more common than type 1 diabetes. The cause of type 2 diabetes appears to be genetic, although not everyone with the gene mutation develops the disease. If a person has one parent with type 2 diabetes, his or her risk for developing the disease is about 30%. The biggest risk factors for developing the disease are obesity and a sedentary lifestyle. Although people of all races and ethnicities can develop type 2 diabetes, it is very common in American Indian and Hispanic populations. In the past, type 2 diabetes did not develop until people were at least 40 years old. Now, however, with severe obesity present in childhood, type 2 diabetes is occurring at any age, even in children.

With type 2 diabetes the person still has beta cells that make some insulin. In fact, some people who have type 2 diabetes have normal levels of insulin; however, the insulin receptors are not very sensitive to insulin. As a result, insulin does not bind as tightly to its receptors as it should, and less glucose moves from the blood into the cells. So hyperglycemia is present with type 2 diabetes.

Because some insulin continues to be made and used with type 2 diabetes, the symptoms are much more gradual in onset than those of type 1 diabetes. In addition, because some glucose does get into the cells, fat is not used for fuel in type 2 diabetes, and the person usually does not make excessive ketone bodies. Many people have type 2 diabetes for 10 years or more without being aware of it.

### Long-Term Complications of Diabetes

Insulin is important for all types of metabolism, not just for glucose control. Without adequate amounts of insulin the person with either type of diabetes has major changes in blood vessels that lead to organ damage, serious health problems, and early death. Box 25-3 lists many of the serious complications of untreated or poorly controlled diabetes. The long-term complications of the disease are the same for both types 1 and 2 diabetes. More than 50,000 people in the United States die directly from diabetes each year. Another 1 million patients with diabetes die annually from heart attacks, strokes, and kidney failure caused by diabetes. Diabetes is the main cause of foot and leg amputations and new cases of blindness.

 Memory Jogger

Patients with type 2 diabetes make some of their own insulin, but the insulin receptors are resistant to binding with the insulin. This problem is most common among people who are overweight.

◄ ⊖-Learning Activity 25-2

> **Box 25-3**   Complications of Poorly Controlled Diabetes
>
> - Blindness
> - Early death
> - Erectile dysfunction
> - High blood cholesterol levels
> - High blood triglyceride levels
> - Hypertension
> - Increased risk for heart attack
>
> - Increased risk for infection
> - Increased risk for stroke
> - Loss of touch sensation (peripheral neuropathy)
> - Kidney failure
> - Poor wound healing (especially on the feet and legs, leading to amputation)

**Memory Jogger**

Complications from untreated or poorly controlled diabetes include blindness; kidney failure; foot and leg amputations; hypertension; and increased risk for infection, heart attacks, and strokes.

**Memory Jogger**

Insulin only controls diabetes; it does not cure the disease.

**Memory Jogger**

Because insulin is destroyed by stomach acids and intestinal enzymes, it cannot be used as an oral drug. Most commonly it is injected subcutaneously.

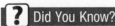

**Did You Know?**

All mammals and rodents make insulin that is very similar to human insulin.

## TYPES OF DRUGS FOR DIABETES

Drug therapy for diabetes reduces the risks for many long-term complications and extends life. Patients who are able to control blood glucose levels with a combination of drug therapy, diet, and regular exercise also live longer, healthier lives. Helping patients with diabetes understand the disease and its drug therapy is an important nursing responsibility.

The three major groups of drugs used to manage diabetes are insulin from other sources, oral antidiabetic drugs, and drugs that increase the amounts of other hormones (incretins and amylin) that work with insulin. All patients with type 1 diabetes must receive insulin therapy as hormone replacement for the rest of their lives because they no longer make their own insulin.

For the patient who has type 2 diabetes and still makes some insulin, other drugs can help maintain normal blood glucose levels in a variety of ways. Usually these drugs are used in combination with diet and exercise for best control of blood glucose levels and prevention of long-term complications of diabetes.

### INSULIN THERAPY

The goals of insulin therapy for type 1 diabetes are to maintain blood glucose levels within the normal range, avoid ketoacidosis, and prevent or delay the blood vessel changes that lead to organ damage. Because people with type 1 diabetes do not make and secrete insulin, they must use insulin therapy to control blood glucose levels for the rest of their lives. Insulin is a small protein and is destroyed by stomach acids and intestinal enzymes.

#### Types of Insulin

Insulin that could be injected and used as a drug was first discovered in 1922. The first insulin commonly used as therapy for patients with diabetes was extracted from the pancreases of pigs and cows and then purified for human use. This insulin was not quite the same as insulin made by the human pancreas but was similar enough to control blood glucose levels when injected into humans. Today, although some insulin is still used from beef and pork sources, most of it is synthetic and is identical to the insulin secreted by humans. Regardless of insulin type, it is a *high-alert drug*, meaning that it can cause serious harm if the wrong dose is given, if a dose is given to a patient for whom it was *not* prescribed, or if a dose is *not* given to a patient for whom it was prescribed.

For most patients with diabetes, insulin is injected subcutaneously using a special syringe with a short, thin needle (Figure 25-6). Special internal and external insulin pumps also can be used to deliver insulin either continuously as needed or hourly. Although both of these methods have advantages over regular injections, they are expensive and have some complications. Thus most patients with type 1 diabetes use standard insulin syringes to inject insulin from once to as many as 8 or 10 times each day.

Many different types of insulin are available as therapy for type 1 diabetes, although all insulin works in the same way at the cellular level. Insulin types vary by how fast they work, how long the effects last (duration), and whether they are

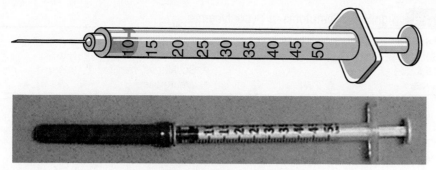

**FIGURE 25-6** An insulin syringe.

## Table 25-2 Types and Durations of Insulin

| PREPARATION | TRADE NAME | ONSET (hr) | PEAK (hr) | DURATION (hr) |
|---|---|---|---|---|
| **RAPID-ACTING** | | | | |
| Insulin aspart | NovoLog | 0.25 | 1-3 | 3-5 |
| Insulin glulisine | Apidra | 0.3 | 0.5-1.5 | 3-4 |
| Insulin lispro injection | Humalog | 0.25 | 0.5-1.5 | 5 |
| **SHORT-ACTING** | | | | |
| Regular human insulin injection | Humulin R | 0.5 | 2-4 | 5-7 |
| | Novolin R | 0.5 | 2.5-5 | 8 |
| **INTERMEDIATE-ACTING INSULIN** | | | | |
| Isophane Insulin NPH injection | Humulin N | 1.5 | 4-12 | 10-16 or |
| | Novolin N | | | longer |
| Insulin detemir injection | Levemir | 1 | None | 5.7-24 |
| 70% human insulin isophane suspension/30% human regular insulin injection | Humulin 70/30 | 0.5 | 6-10 | 10-16 |
| | Novolin 70/30 | 0.5 | 6-10 | 10-16 |
| 50% human insulin isophane suspension/50% human insulin injection | Humulin 50/50 | 0.5 | 3-5 | 10-16 or longer |
| 70% insulin aspart protamine suspension/30% insulin aspart injection | Novolog Mix 70/30 | 0.25 | 1-4 | 18-24 |
| 75% insulin lispro protamine suspension/25% insulin lispro injection | Humalog Mix 75/25 | 0.25 | 1-2 | 18-24 |
| **LONG-ACTING INSULIN** | | | | |
| Insulin glargine injection | Lantus | 2 | None | 24 |

synthetic or come from animal sources. Table 25-2 lists the most common types of insulin for general injection and their features. Be sure to consult a drug reference for more information about a specific insulin.

## How Insulin Therapy Works

Just like the insulin the body makes, insulin injected into the body binds to insulin receptors on the membranes of many cells. The result of having the injected insulin bound to its receptor is that the cell membrane becomes more open to glucose, allowing glucose to leave the blood and enter cells (see Figure 25-3). As glucose from the blood enters the cells, the blood glucose level is reduced to normal (euglycemia).

 Memory Jogger

Insulin injected into the body works in exactly the same way as insulin secreted by the pancreas.

| Box 25-4 | Signs and Symptoms of Hypoglycemia |
|---|---|

- Anxiety, confusion, loss of consciousness
- Cool, clammy skin
- Headache
- Hunger
- Increased sweating
- Rapid, pounding heart rate
- Shakiness, tremors
- Weakness

### Intended Responses

- Blood glucose levels are in the normal range.
- There is no glucose or acetone in the urine.
- Blood lipid levels are at or close to the normal range.

**Side Effects.** Insulin as a drug has few side effects. Side effects are usually related to having repeated subcutaneous injections at one site or body area. These problems include injection site infections, swelling of fat tissue (*lipohypertrophy*) from repeated injections, and uneven loss of fat tissue (*lipoatrophy*) resulting from tissue responses to impurities in beef or pork insulin.

**Adverse Effects.** The main adverse effect of insulin is the lowering of blood glucose levels *below* normal (*hypoglycemia*). This action, sometimes called *insulin shock*, is dangerous because brain cells are very sensitive to low blood glucose levels and the patient can become nonresponsive very quickly. If the problem is not corrected quickly, the patient can die. The signs and symptoms of hypoglycemia are listed in Box 25-4.

Allergic reactions have occurred with the use of insulin. These reactions are more common for insulin made from beef or pork and insulin that contains substances such as zinc.

### Insulin Regimens

The goal of insulin therapy for patients with type 1 diabetes is to keep blood glucose levels within the normal range at all times. Better overall blood glucose control occurs with multiple injections of insulin each day.

An *insulin regimen* or program is the insulin injection schedule used to prevent hyperglycemia. The most effective regimens are those that provide insulin in a pattern that closely resembles the way insulin normally is released from the healthy pancreas. The normal pancreas releases a constant (*basal*) amount of insulin that keeps blood glucose levels normal between meals by balancing liver glucose production with whole-body glucose use. The normal pancreas also is stimulated by eating food to produce additional insulin to prevent blood glucose levels from rising too high after meals.

The total amount of insulin needed and how often it is needed for blood glucose control varies among patients. A usual starting dose is between 0.5 and 1 unit/kg of body weight per day. Usually the patient injects long-acting insulin at the beginning of the day for a basal dose. Shorter-acting insulin is taken before meals and snacks. The amount of insulin needed and injected is based on blood glucose levels. The patient checks his or her blood glucose level 2 to 12 times each day based on insulin regimen, activity level, age, the total amount of calories needed in a day, and how his or her blood glucose level responds to the insulin. Some standard insulin regimens (injection programs) are shown in Figure 25-7.

**Single Daily Injection Regimen.** Some patients inject insulin only once daily. Usually a once-a-day regimen includes only intermediate-acting insulin or combined short- and intermediate-acting insulin. Often a single dose of insulin may not match the blood insulin level with food intake, and the person has periods of hyperglycemia.

**Memory Jogger**

Insulin side effects are:
- Injection site infections.
- Lipohypertrophy.
- Lipatrophy.

**Memory Jogger**

Hypoglycemia is *always* a potential adverse effect of insulin therapy.

**Memory Jogger**

True allergic reactions to insulin are rare but can occur with beef, pork, or zinc insulins.

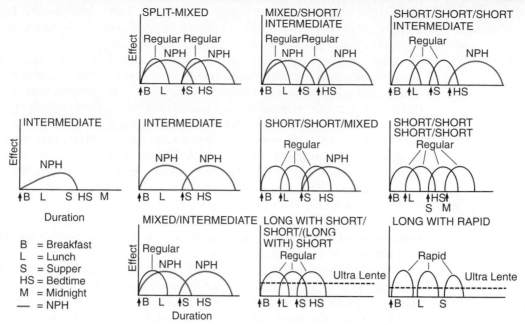

FIGURE 25-7 Examples of different insulin dosing schedules.

***Two-Dose Injection Regimen.***   Combinations of short- and intermediate-acting insulin are injected twice daily. Usually two thirds of the daily dose is given before breakfast, and one third before the evening meal.

***Three-Dose Injection Regimen.***   A combination of short- and intermediate-acting insulin is given before breakfast, short-acting insulin is given before the evening meal, and intermediate-acting insulin is given at bedtime. Giving intermediate-acting insulin at bedtime lowers fasting and after-breakfast blood glucose levels.

***Four-Dose Injection Regimen.***   Giving short-acting insulin 30 minutes before meals allows the greatest amount of insulin to be present during the time of greatest insulin need. Basal insulin is provided by twice-daily injections of intermediate-acting insulin or a once-daily injection of long-acting insulin. Injection of before-meal short-acting insulin allows some patients to have more flexibility in meal timing and size. The short-acting insulin should be given within 15 minutes of eating a meal.

***Intensified Insulin Regimens.***   Intensified regimens include a basal dose of intermediate- or long-acting insulin and multiple-bolus doses of short- or rapid-acting insulin designed to bring the next blood glucose value into the target range. Insulin dosage is based on the patient's blood glucose patterns. Usually the patient must check the blood glucose levels at least eight times per day. Blood glucose testing 1 to 2 hours after meals and within 10 minutes before the next meal helps to determine how effective the bolus dose is.

Patients on intensified insulin regimens have much responsibility for their own diabetic health. They need clear patient education to achieve target blood glucose levels. Patients must know how to self-monitor blood glucose levels and adjust insulin doses and must understand nutrition therapy to maintain target blood glucose values.

### What To Do *Before* Injecting Insulin

*Insulin drug errors are common and have serious consequences, including death.* The many different types of insulin increase the risk for errors. It is important not to interchange insulin types and to ensure that the dose prescribed is the one given.

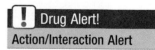

**Drug Alert!**

**Action/Interaction Alert**

Whenever insulin is given *before* a meal, it is critical that the patient eat a meal of sufficient calories within 30 minutes of the insulin injection.

**Memory Jogger**

Intensified insulin regimens provide the best control over blood glucose levels but require many more "sticks" each day than other insulin injection regimens.

◄ ⊖-Learning Activity 25-3

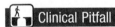
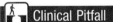
Test the patient's blood glucose level before giving insulin and make sure that the patient can and will eat within 15 to 30 minutes of the insulin injection. If the meal is delayed, he or she could become hypoglycemic. It is best to ensure that the meal is actually on the unit before giving the insulin.

Check the order carefully for the exact type and amount of insulin to be injected. Do not interchange insulin types. Insulin preparations are available in U-50, U-100, and U-500 concentrations. The most commonly used preparation is U-100 insulin (100 units per mL). When doses are less than 50 units, they are usually administered with a U-50 syringe (50 units per 0.5 mL). This drug is available in a concentration of 50 units on a 0.5-mL volume. U-100 insulin provides 100 units of insulin in 1 mL of drug. Some insulin is available in U-500 strength, which provides 500 units of insulin in 1 mL of drug. To give the correct amount of insulin, the syringe must be calibrated in the same units as the drug. So if a patient is to receive 15 units of U-50 insulin, use a U-50 insulin syringe. As you can see, giving U-50 insulin in a U-500 syringe would result in too little insulin and hyperglycemia. Giving U-500 insulin in a U-50 syringe could result in a huge overdose, severe hypoglycemia, and death.

Check the insulin vial for color and clarity. Some insulin is supposed to be clear and colorless. This includes rapid-acting insulin, short-acting insulin, insulin glargine (Lantus), and insulin detemir (Levemir). If particles are present or if the liquid is cloudy, discard the insulin and open a new vial. All other insulin types have a cloudy appearance after they have been gently rotated.

Gently roll the insulin vial (or pen, cartridge, syringe, or other prefilled injection device) between your hands to mix and warm the insulin. Do not shake the vial because bubbles will form and the dose may not be accurate.

Needles on insulin syringes are small gauge (28 gauge, 29 gauge, and 30 gauge) and vary in length from ½ inch to ⁵⁄₁₆ inch. Use shorter needles for thinner patients and longer needles for patients who have greater amounts of subcutaneous tissue.

Check and recheck that the amount and type of insulin you have drawn up into the syringe is the amount ordered. If possible, have another nurse also check the syringe volume and insulin type.

Select an appropriate site for the injection. Recommended sites are shown in Figure 25-8. If the patient is just starting on insulin therapy, the abdomen is the preferred site (except for a 2-inch circle around the umbilicus). If the patient has been self-injecting insulin, use the same site that he or she normally uses but use a different area within that site. Absorption of insulin after injection varies from site to site and can make the peak action of insulin less predictable.

Cleanse the site with an alcohol swab and grasp a fold of skin in your nondominant hand. Insert the needle at a 90-degree angle (a 45-degree angle if the patient is very thin) and inject the insulin without pulling back on the plunger. (It is not necessary to check for a blood return, and pulling tissue back into the needle can cause bruising and other tissue damage.)

After the injection is complete, withdraw the needle rapidly while supporting the skin. Do not massage the site because doing so can change the rate that insulin is absorbed from the tissues.

If the patient is to receive two different types of insulin at the same time, it may be possible to mix the two types together in the same syringe so the patient is only injected once. Check whether the two prescribed types can be mixed together. Some insulin cannot be mixed with any other solution. For example, neither insulin glargine (Lantus) nor insulin detemir (Levemir) can be mixed with other insulin. If the prescribed types can be mixed, follow the directions in Box 25-5, which describes the correct technique to mix 10 units of regular insulin with 20 units of NPH insulin.

### What To Do *After* Injecting Insulin

Check the patient hourly for signs and symptoms of hypoglycemia. These include confusion, cool and clammy skin, tremors, headache, hunger, and sweating (see Box 25-4). Keep a simple sugar (such as orange juice and sugar packets) on the unit.

| Box 25-5 | Guide for Mixing Two Types of Insulin |
| --- | --- |

**10 UNITS OF REGULAR INSULIN WITH 20 UNITS OF NPH INSULIN:**

- After checking to make sure that you have the correct concentration and types of insulin, clean the rubber stoppers of each bottle with separate alcohol swabs.
- Draw up 20 units of air and inject it into the NPH bottle with the bottle in its normal, upright position. Always inject the air into the intermediate-acting insulin bottle first. The amount of air injected is the same amount as the insulin to be removed.
- Draw up 10 units of air and inject it into the regular insulin (short-acting insulin) bottle with the bottle in its normal, upright position. The amount of air injected is the same as the amount of insulin to be removed.
- Without removing the needle, turn the bottle upside down and withdraw 10 units of regular insulin; then withdraw the needle from the bottle. Always withdraw the shorter-acting insulin first. Make sure that the syringe is free from air bubbles.
- Now place the same needle with the syringe attached into the NPH bottle, invert the bottle, and withdraw 20 units of NPH insulin into the same syringe with the regular insulin. Take care not to inject any regular insulin into the NPH bottle.
- Check the syringe for the volume of insulin. For this example there should be 30 units in the syringe.

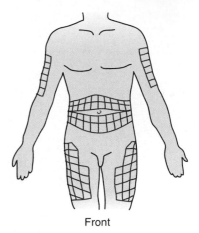

Front

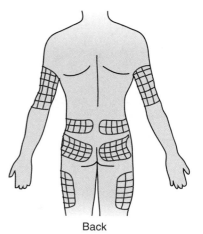

Back

**FIGURE 25-8** Common insulin injection sites.

Ensure that the patient's meals or between-meal snacks are on time and that he or she eats them.

Check the patient's response to insulin. Check blood glucose levels as often as ordered and document the results. Compare results with pretherapy blood glucose levels to determine whether the dose and regimen are effective.

### What To *Teach* Patients About Insulin

Stress that insulin does not cure diabetes but only helps to manage blood glucose levels. Help the patient understand that insulin is only part of the therapy to slow or prevent diabetes complications.

Most patients worry about being able to self-inject insulin. Many are concerned that they will be unable to "stick" themselves with a needle. The whole process of drawing up and injecting the correct amount of insulin without contaminating the drug or the needle may be a very frightening thought. A team approach to patient education, including a diabetes educator, can be very helpful. If a diabetes educator is involved, you should hear what this person actually tells the patient and family so you will be able to reinforce the teaching. Usually teaching a patient how to self-inject insulin takes more than one teaching session and requires that he or she is alert enough to learn; can see well enough to ensure safe drug administration; and has good use of the arms, hands, and fingers to be able to perform the physical actions involved. Follow the principles for patient teaching discussed in Chapter 3.

Teach patients to use the steps in Box 25-6 to self-administer insulin. To begin teaching, use normal saline solution and the same type of insulin syringe that the patient will use at home. Demonstrate how to correctly draw up insulin into the syringe and inject it. You can use a raw chicken leg or a teaching injection pad to demonstrate the actual injection. Have the patient, and whomever the patient designates as a helper, demonstrate the techniques back to you. Praise him or her when techniques are correct. Repeat the demonstration of any techniques that need improvement.

Teach patients to always have a spare bottle of each type of insulin that they use. Teach them about how to store insulin between uses. Most insulin should be refrigerated but never frozen. When a bottle of insulin has been opened, it can be stored in the refrigerator or kept at room temperature out of the refrigerator for up to 28 days. Temperatures higher than 86 degrees and exposure to sunlight can cause the insulin to degrade more rapidly. Prefilled insulin syringes, cartridges, or pens should be stored upright with the needle pointing upward rather than lying flat. For prefilled pens and cartridges of insulin detemir (Levemir), the in-use cartridges should not

**⚠ Drug Alert!**

**Teaching Alert**

Insulin therapy without diet control and regular exercise is not as effective at preventing complications.

**⚠ Drug Alert!**

**Teaching Alert**

Teach patients that it is important that at least one other family member, friend, companion, or neighbor also know how to inject insulin safely.

---

**Box 25-6** Patient Education Guide for Self-Injection of Insulin

- Wash your hands.
- Inspect the insulin container for the type of insulin and the expiration date.
- For rapid-acting insulin, short-acting insulin, insulin glargine, or insulin detemir, inspect the bottle for color and clarity. If particles are present or if the insulin is cloudy, discard the bottle and open a new one.
- For other insulin, gently rotate the bottle or container between the palms of your hands to mix the insulin.
- Clean the bottle stopper with an alcohol sponge (leave out this step if you are using a prefilled pen or cartridge).
- Remove the cover from the needle and pull back the plunger to draw in the same amount of air into the syringe as the amount of insulin you will be withdrawing from the bottle.
- Push the needle through the rubber stopper and inject the air into the insulin bottle with the bottle in the upright position (do not let the air bubble into the insulin).
- With the needle still in the bottle stopper, turn the bottle upside down and withdraw the same amount of insulin from the bottle as the air you put into the bottle.
- Make sure that the tip of the plunger is on the line of the syringe for your insulin dose.
- If air bubbles are present, tap the syringe while holding it upside down, letting the bubbles come to the top of the syringe where the needle is attached. Push out any air bubbles and recheck to ensure that the tip of the plunger is on the same line as your insulin dose.
- Remove the needle from the bottle stopper and recap the needle until you are ready to inject the insulin.
- Select an area within your usual injection site that has not been injected within the past 2 weeks.
- Cleanse the skin area with an alcohol swab.
- Remove the cap from the needle on the insulin syringe.
- Pinch up a fold of skin in the area you cleaned and push the needle in at a 90-degree angle.
- Push the plunger all the way down to ensure that the entire insulin dose is injected.
- Release the fold of skin and remove the needle straight out quickly.
- Do not rub or massage the spot where you injected the insulin.
- Place the syringe with the needle (without recapping it) into a puncture-proof container.

---

be stored in a refrigerator but should be kept at room temperature. In addition, the in-use cartridges should not be stored with the needle in place.

Advise patients not to share used needles or prefilled syringes, cartridges, or pens with another person, even a family member who also has diabetes. Sharing needles increases the risk for bloodborne diseases.

Teach patients to check the injection site daily for any signs or symptoms of infection (warmth, redness, firmness to the touch, presence of drainage, pain in and around the area). The presence of any symptom indicating infection should be reported immediately to their prescriber.

Teach patients the signs and symptoms of hypoglycemia (see Box 25-4). Urge them not to skip or delay meals. Tell them to always carry a simple sugar (such as candy, a sugar packet, or glucose tablets or paste) in a pocket or purse and to eat it at the first sign of hypoglycemia.

Stress to patients who are using insulin on a one-dose, two-dose, three-dose, or four-dose injection regimen the importance of keeping to the schedule for insulin injection and meals. For patients using insulin on an intensified injection regimen, there is more flexibility of meal timing because the injections are timed to the meals and blood glucose levels.

Remind patients that blood glucose control to prevent complications works best when insulin therapy is combined with diet control and regular exercise.

### Life Span Considerations for Insulin

*Pediatric Considerations.* Many children have type 1 diabetes and require insulin injections and blood testing of glucose levels. Most children dislike being stuck with needles and being different from their friends. In addition, a child may have daily differences in the amount or type of food eaten and the amount of exercise experienced. These differences can make having good control over blood glucose levels a

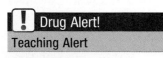

**Drug Alert!**

**Teaching Alert**

Teach patients the signs and symptoms of hypoglycemia (confusion, cool and clammy skin, tremors, headache, hunger, sweating). Urge patients not to skip or delay meals after taking insulin.

real challenge. Because the complications of hyperglycemia begin even in childhood, good glucose control is needed at any age. Best control is achieved using the intensified injection regimen with short-acting insulin; however, because of the large number of needlesticks per day, this regimen may be the one least acceptable to the child.

Depending on age, a child can learn to manage blood glucose testing and insulin injections. However, a parent or other adult living with the child also needs to know how to test blood glucose levels, inject insulin, and manage hypoglycemia.

***Considerations for Pregnancy and Breastfeeding.*** The disease is often more difficult to control during this physically stressful time. In addition, some patients who do not have diabetes may have problems with hyperglycemia only during pregnancy. This condition is called *gestational diabetes*. Untreated diabetes during pregnancy increases health problems in the mother and can cause birth defects in the infant, especially if the mother develops diabetic ketoacidosis (DKA). Hypoglycemia during pregnancy can also have severe consequences for both mother and infant.

Although insulin is a pregnancy category B or C drug, it is the treatment of choice for diabetes during pregnancy. Insulin needs change during pregnancy and often increase during the last 6 months. Usually the best control is achieved with the use of an intensified insulin injection schedule. This schedule helps prevent extreme hyperglycemia and DKA and also reduces the risk for hypoglycemia. Reassure patients who use additional insulin injections during pregnancy that the extra injections usually are not needed once the pregnancy is over.

Injected insulin is also thought to enter breast milk but should not cause hypoglycemia in the infant. Diabetes may be more difficult to control when breastfeeding. Mothers with diabetes who wish to breastfeed their infants should do so under the direction of their endocrinologists and pediatricians.

***Considerations for Older Adults.*** Type 1 diabetes is managed with insulin, and insulin use in an older adult can pose some special problems. Many older adults with type 1 diabetes have some degree of reduced vision and a decreased sense of touch as a result of the disease. These problems increase the risk for errors in insulin dosing, injection, and self-monitoring of blood glucose levels. Older patients may benefit from the use of prefilled insulin syringes, cartridges, or pens. However, these specialty items cost more than standard insulin supplies, and many older adults are on fixed incomes. Urge older adults with vision problems to use magnifying glasses and good light when testing blood glucose levels or withdrawing insulin.

The risk for hypoglycemia is increased in older adults, especially if they also take beta-adrenergic blocking drugs, warfarin (Coumadin), or other drugs that increase the hypoglycemic response. In addition, hypoglycemia may be harder to recognize in older adults. The older adult may eat less than a younger adult and must understand how to match insulin dosage and scheduling with food intake.

## ORAL ANTIDIABETIC DRUGS

Drugs for type 2 diabetes used to be called *oral hypoglycemic agents*. However, because the goal of therapy is to help the person become euglycemic rather than hypoglycemic, this term is not accurate. The better term is *antidiabetic drug*. These drugs are oral agents with different mechanisms of action. Because they work in different ways to control blood glucose levels, two or more drugs may be used together for best control. In addition, some patients with type 2 diabetes require insulin therapy occasionally when the disease is made worse by temporary health problems or other drugs. Over time diabetes may progress to the point at which not enough beta cells remain and insulin therapy becomes permanent.

The drugs for treating type 2 diabetes are classified by their chemical structures or their actions. The five major classes of antidiabetic drugs are the sulfonylureas, the meglitinides, the biguanides, the alpha-glucosidase inhibitors, and the thiazolidinediones. The mechanism of action for each class of drugs is somewhat different. The decision to use one type of drug with or instead of another type is based on how much beta cell function is left, how the patient responds to the drug, and the patient's

 **Memory Jogger**

Controlling type 1 diabetes in children is more difficult because of day-to-day variations in the amount and types of food eaten and in the amount of exercise experienced.

 **Memory Jogger**

Insulin is the preferred drug to manage diabetes during pregnancy.

 **Drug Alert!**
**Interaction Alert**

The risk for hypoglycemia with insulin is increased when patients also take beta-adrenergic blocking drugs, warfarin (Coumadin), or other drugs that increase the hypoglycemic response.

◀ -Learning Activity 25-4

 **Memory Jogger**

The goal of drug therapy for type 2 diabetes is to have normal blood glucose levels, reduced blood fat levels, and normal body weight.

**Do Not Confuse**

**glipiZIDE** *with* **glyBURIDE**

An order for glipizide can be confused with glyburide. Although both drugs are oral antidiabetic drugs from the second-generation sulfonylurea class, the dosages are very different.

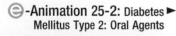
-Animation 25-2: Diabetes ▶
Mellitus Type 2: Oral Agents

**Do Not Confuse**

**Amaryl** *with* **Reminyl**

An order for Amaryl can be confused with Reminyl. Amaryl is an oral antidiabetic drug, whereas Reminyl is a drug for Alzheimer's disease.

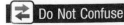

**Do Not Confuse**

**Diabeta** *with* **Zebeta**

An order for Diabeta can be confused with Zebeta. Diabeta is an oral antidiabetic drug, whereas Zebeta is an antihypertensive drug.

overall health. In addition, the dosages for these drugs are not based on body size. Instead they are based on how the patient responds to the drug.

Regardless of what drug or drugs are used for type 2 diabetes, the best control occurs in combination with diet and exercise. These lifestyle changes can be hard for the patient to make, but they help to reduce the risk for complications. Keeping body weight at or near the ideal level and participating in moderate exercise at least three times each week can delay the vascular changes that can cause severe organ damage.

### How Oral Antidiabetic Drugs Work

*Sulfonylureas* were the first oral antidiabetic agents. These early drugs are called first-generation sulfonylureas, and today are seldom used. The newer second-generation sulfonylureas are similar chemically to the sulfonamide antibacterial drugs. They work to lower blood glucose levels by triggering pancreatic beta cells to release the small amount of preformed insulin present in the beta cells. Information about sulfonylureas in this section is based on these second-generation drugs.

*Meglitinide* drugs act directly on the beta cells of the pancreas. These drugs stimulate a brief, burstlike release of insulin from the beta cells, usually within 30 to 60 minutes of taking the drug. Because the drug is taken right before every meal, the brief burst of insulin more closely resembles how the normal pancreas responds to a meal.

*Biguanides (metformin)* lower blood glucose levels to the normal range by several mechanisms. Unlike sulfonylureas and meglitinides, they do *not* act directly on the beta cells of the pancreas. Instead they act on the liver to reduce release of glucose from stored glycogen. They also increase the sensitivity of the insulin receptor to the binding of naturally secreted insulin, which improves the movement of glucose from the blood into the cells. In addition, this class of drugs reduces the absorption of glucose from the intestinal tract into the blood. As a result, the biguanides lower blood glucose levels to normal without causing hypoglycemia.

*Alpha-glucosidase inhibitors* work by slowing the digestion of dietary starches and other complex carbohydrates by inhibiting an enzyme that breaks them down into glucose. The result of this action is that blood glucose does not rise as far or as fast after a meal. Drugs from this class do not cause hypoglycemia when taken as the only therapy for diabetes. Often these drugs are used in combination with other antidiabetic drugs for best blood glucose control.

*Thiazolidinedione* drugs, often called *glitazones*, work with the patient's own insulin to reduce blood glucose levels by making the insulin receptor more sensitive to insulin. When receptors are sensitive to insulin, insulin binds to them better and longer. The longer insulin is bound to receptors, the longer the cell membranes allow glucose from the blood to enter cells, reducing blood glucose levels. This action also reduces the amount of glucose the liver releases from glycogen breakdown.

### Intended Responses
- Blood glucose levels are in the normal range.
- There is no glucose in the urine.

### Dosages for Common Oral Antidiabetic Drugs

| Drug | Dosages (Adults Only) |
|---|---|
| *Second-Generation Sulfonylureas* | |
| glimepiride ❶ (Amaryl, Apo-Glimepiride♣, Novo-Glimepiride♣) | 1-8 mg orally daily at breakfast or first meal of the day |
| glipiZIDE 🔲 ❶ (Glucotrol) | Immediate-release: 5-40 mg orally once or 5-20 mg orally twice daily |
| (Glucotrol XL) | Extended-release: 5-20 mg orally once daily |
| glyBURIDE 🔲 ❶ (Apo-Glyburide♣, Diabeta, Gen-Glybe♣, Euglucon♣, Micronase) | 1.25-20 mg orally daily in 1-2 divided doses |
| glyBURIDE, micronized ❶ (Glynase Pres-Tab) | 0.75-12 mg orally daily in 1-2 divided doses |

## Dosages for Common Oral Antidiabetic Drugs—cont'd

| Drug | Dosages (Adults Only) |
| --- | --- |
| **Meglitinides** | |
| nateglinide ❶ (Starlix) | 60-120 mg orally within 15-30 min of every meal |
| repaglinide ❶ (GlucoNorm🍁, Prandin) | 0.5-4 mg orally within 15-30 min of every meal |
| **Biguanides** | |
| metformin 🔲❶ (Apo-Metformin🍁, Fortamet, Glucophage, Glumetza🍁, Glycon🍁, Riomet) | Immediate-release: 500-850 mg orally 3 times daily with meals |
| (Glucophage XR) | Extended-release: 500-2000 mg orally once daily with evening meal |
| **Alpha-Glucosidase Inhibitors** | |
| acarbose (Prandase🍁, Precose) | 25-100 mg orally 3 times daily with first bite of a meal |
| miglitol (Glyset) | 25-100 mg orally 3 times daily with first bite of a meal |
| **Thiazolidinediones** | |
| pioglitazone ❶ (Actos 🔲, Apo-Pioglitazone🍁, Novo-Pioglitazone🍁) | 15-45 mg orally daily |
| rosiglitazone ❶ (Avandia)🔲 | 2-4 mg orally once or twice daily |

🔲 Top 100 drugs prescribed; ❶ High-alert drug.

**Side Effects.** Side effects common to most of the oral antidiabetic drugs include nausea, vomiting, diarrhea, and rashes.

*Sulfonylureas* also may cause increased sun sensitivity (photosensitivity), blurred vision, fluid retention, and anemia.

*Meglitinides* also may cause dizziness, back pain, upper respiratory infections, and flulike achiness.

*Metformin* (Glucophage) and the *alpha-glucosidase inhibitors* also may cause bloating, flatulence, indigestion, abdominal pain, and headache.

*Thiazolidinedione drugs* also may cause upper respiratory infections, headaches, muscle aches, fluid retention, weight gain, and anemia.

**Adverse Effects.** The most common adverse effect for oral antidiabetic drugs is severe hypoglycemia. Some drugs, such as the sulfonylureas and the meglitinides, cause this effect individually. For others the risk for hypoglycemia occurs only when the drugs are used in combination. Sulfonylureas and meglitinides force the beta cells to release more insulin. Unlike natural insulin release, the drug-induced insulin release does not occur in response to a high blood sugar level. The release can occur at any time, even when the patient's blood glucose level is normal. This action would lead to hypoglycemia.

*Metformin* can cause lactic acidosis, which is the buildup of lactic acid in tissues when not enough oxygen is present to allow metabolism to occur normally. Lactic acid also is produced when not enough glucose is made in the liver. Signs and symptoms of lactic acidosis are muscle aches; fatigue; drowsiness; abdominal pain; hypotension; and a slow, irregular heartbeat. Lactic acidosis is more likely to occur when other conditions are present that reduce blood flow or movement of oxygen into the tissues, including dehydration, sepsis, heart failure, and respiratory problems leading to hypoxia. Drinking alcohol, having liver disease, or having kidney problems increases the risk for lactic acidosis.

Tests that involve the use of radio-opaque dye (such as urograms, angiograms, and other scans) can lead to kidney failure with metformin, usually within 48 hours. A patient who takes metformin may take the dose before receiving the dye but should not resume the drug again until 48 hours after testing with dye or surgery with anesthesia, or until good urine output has been reestablished.

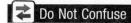

### Do Not Confuse

**Micronase** with **Microzide**

An order for Micronase can be confused with Microzide. Micronase is an oral antidiabetic drug, whereas Microzide is a diuretic.

### Do Not Confuse

**Prandin** with **Avandia**

An order for Prandin can be confused with Avandia. Prandin is an oral antidiabetic drug from the meglitinide class, whereas Avandia is an oral antidiabetic drug from the thiazolidinedione class.

### Do Not Confuse

**metformin** with **metronidazole**

An order for metformin can be confused with metronidazole. Metformin is an oral antidiabetic drug from the biguanide class, whereas metronidazole is an oral antibiotic drug.

### Do Not Confuse

**Precose** with **Precare**

An order for Precose can be confused with Precare. Precose is an oral antidiabetic drug from the alpha-glucosidase inhibitor class, whereas Precare is a chewable prenatal vitamin.

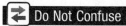

### Do Not Confuse

**Actos** with **Actonel**

An order for Actos can be confused with Actonel. Actos is an oral antidiabetic drug from the thiazolidinedione class, whereas Actonel is a drug that prevents calcium loss from bones.

### Common Side Effects

**Oral Antidiabetic Drugs**

Nausea/Vomiting, Diarrhea    Rash

**Memory Jogger**

Oral antidiabetic drugs that, when used alone, can cause hypoglycemia are the sulfonylureas and meglitinides.

**Clinical Pitfall**

Metformin (Glucophage) can cause lactic acidosis. Do not give this drug within 48 hours to anyone who has had testing with dye or surgery with anesthesia.

**Clinical Pitfall**

Do not give the thiazolidinediones to a patient with severe heart failure.

**Drug Alert!**

**Action/Intervention Alert**

Give oral antidiabetic drugs with food (preferably with a meal) to reduce the risk for hypoglycemia.

**Clinical Pitfall**

Do not give metformin to a patient with a serum creatinine higher than 1.4 mg/dL (females) or 1.5 mg/dL (males).

**Clinical Pitfall**

Do not crush metformin (Glucophage XR) tablets.

*Alpha-glucosidase inhibitors* and *thiazolidinedione drugs* can cause liver problems, leading to jaundice, higher-than-normal liver enzymes, and difficulty digesting fatty meals. This problem is more likely to happen in a patient who also has kidney problems because the drug remains in the body longer.

*Thiazolidinedione drugs,* especially rosiglitazone, may lead to heart failure as a result of water retention. In fact, rosiglitazone (Avandia) has a black box warning indicating that it should not be prescribed for anyone who has or who is at risk for heart failure. This problem is more common in a patient who has had a myocardial infarction in the past or who already has another cardiac problem.

### What To Do *Before* Giving Antidiabetic Drugs

If the patient is just being started on a sulfonylurea, ask about any allergies to the sulfonamide type of antibacterial drugs. The sulfonylurea drugs are similar to the sulfonamides, and an allergy to one usually is associated with an allergy to the other.

Make sure that the patient's meal is actually on the unit before giving the drug and that he or she is able to eat the meal within a few minutes of taking the drug. This action prevents hypoglycemia. In the case of alpha-glucosidase drugs, the drug should be given with the first bite of a meal because it acts by inhibiting carbohydrate digestion in the intestinal tract.

Check to see whether the patient is also taking any other drug that can make hypoglycemia worse. Observe the patient closely for hypoglycemia if he or she also is taking aspirin, nonsteroidal anti-inflammatory drugs (NSAIDs), warfarin (Coumadin), beta-adrenergic blockers, fluoroquinolone antibiotics, probenecid, or azole antifungal drugs.

*Metformin* (a biguanide) requires many nursing actions before giving the drug. Check to see if the patient is scheduled for surgery or a scan test involving dye during the next 48 hours because the prescriber may hold the drug for 48 hours after the procedure to reduce the risk for kidney failure.

Check the patient's vital signs (including temperature, mental status, heart rate, and blood pressure) before starting metformin. Use this information as a baseline to determine whether any side effect or adverse effect is present.

Check the patient's daily urine output and current laboratory work, especially blood urea nitrogen (BUN) and serum creatinine levels because kidney problems increase the effects of the drug and the risk for lactic acidosis.

If metformin (Glucophage XR) is prescribed, do not crush the tablet. Crushing the tablet destroys its time-release properties and may allow too much drug to enter the patient's bloodstream at one time. In addition, instead of having an extended effect, the drug leaves the body too quickly.

Give the patient a full glass of water to drink with metformin to prevent dehydration, which would increase the risk for lactic acidosis.

With *alpha-glucosidase inhibitors* and *thiazolidinedione drugs,* check the patient's most recent laboratory tests, especially liver enzyme levels. These drugs are contraindicated for patients with liver disease. In addition, these levels can be used as a baseline to determine whether liver problems are developing.

With *thiazolidinedione drugs,* check the patient's vital signs (especially heart rate, blood pressure, and respiratory rate) and pulse oximetry. These vital signs serve as a baseline and can be used to help determine if a problem with heart failure is developing.

Check the patient's weight and indications of edema formation to use as a baseline to determine whether water retention occurs as a result of taking a thiazolidinedione.

### What To Do *After* Giving Oral Antidiabetic Drugs

Check the patient hourly for signs and symptoms of hypoglycemia. These include confusion, cool and clammy skin, tremors, headache, hunger, and sweating (see Box 25-4). Keep a simple sugar (such as orange juice and sugar packets) on the unit. Ensure that the patient's meals are on time and that he or she is able to eat them.

Monitor the patient's fasting blood glucose levels daily to determine the effectiveness of the drug in managing the disease.

With *alpha-glucosidase inhibitors* and *thiazolidinediones,* monitor liver function tests for elevations. Check the patient daily for jaundice by looking at the skin, roof of the mouth, or whites of the eyes. If these signs appear, notify the prescriber.

With *metformin,* check the patient's vital signs (including temperature, heart rate, and blood pressure) and mental status at least every 4 hours for symptoms of lactic acidosis. Urge the him or her to drink plenty of water throughout the day and night to prevent dehydration.

With *thiazolidinediones,* weigh the patient daily and compare the results with his or her initial weight. Weight gain of more than ½ lb in 1 day or 3 lb in 1 week is usually a result of water retention, which is an indication of heart failure. Check the patient's ankles for edema formation, which may indicate water retention or heart failure.

Check the patient's heart rate and blood pressure at least once each shift. Also listen to his or her lungs. Monitoring these vital signs can help identify a heart failure problem early.

### What To *Teach* Patients About Oral Antidiabetic Drugs

Teach patients the signs and symptoms of hypoglycemia (see Box 25-4). Urge them not to skip or delay meals. Tell them to always carry a simple sugar (such as candy, a sugar packet, or glucose tablets or paste) in a pocket or purse and to eat it at the first sign of hypoglycemia.

Instruct patients to avoid drinking alcohol because it is likely to induce hypoglycemia. In addition, if the patient is drinking alcohol, he or she may be less likely to recognize the symptoms of hypoglycemia. If alcohol is used, it should be limited to one serving and taken either with food or right after a meal is completed.

*Sulfonylureas* increase sun sensitivity (photosensitivity) and greatly increase the risk for sunburn, even for people who have dark skin.

*Meglitinides* are given right before any meal or substantial snack. For most patients the drug is taken three times a day. If the patient has more than three meals in a day, the drug should also be taken with each of the extra meals. Teach patients to prevent hypoglycemia by taking the drug no sooner than 15 to 30 minutes before a meal.

*Metformin* should be taken with food. Teach patients not to chew or crush Glucophage XR tablets. Teach them that metformin can cause lactic acidosis, which can be avoided by drinking plenty of water (day and night), avoiding alcoholic beverages, and avoiding dehydration.

With *alpha-glucosidase inhibitors,* tell patients not to remove the drug from the foil wrapper until it is time to take it. The foil helps prevent the drug from deteriorating.

With *alpha-glucosidase inhibitors* or *thiazolidinediones,* teach patients the symptoms of liver impairment (jaundice of the skin and sclera, nausea and lack of appetite, dark urine, pale stools) and to report these to their prescriber.

With *thiazolidinediones,* teach patients to check for signs of water retention and heart failure. Patients should weigh themselves daily at the same time each day wearing the same amount of clothing. They should also check their pulse rates twice a day, noting the rate and the quality of the pulse. If a patient does not know how to take a pulse, show him or her exactly how and have him or her demonstrate this skill back to you. Instruct patients to keep a written record of daily weights and heart rates. Teach the patient that a weight gain of more than three pounds in 1 week, especially if the ankles are also swollen, should be reported to their prescriber. A heart rate that increases in rate over time and is harder to feel may indicate heart failure. Remind him or her to report this change to the prescriber. If the patient becomes increasingly short of breath over time, tell the patient to report this symptom to his or her prescriber.

---

**! Drug Alert!**
**Action/Intervention Alert**

Because thiazolidinediones (especially rosiglitazone [Avandia]) can cause or worsen cardiac complications, weigh the patient daily and monitor heart rate and rhythm, blood pressure, and lung sounds every 8 hours.

**! Drug Alert!**
**Teaching Alert**

Teach patients the signs and symptoms of hypoglycemia: confusion, cool and clammy skin, tremors, headache, hunger, and sweating. Urge patients not to skip or delay meals.

**! Drug Alert!**
**Teaching Alert**

Teach patients taking a sulfonylurea to avoid direct sunlight, use sunscreen, and wear protective clothing (including a hat) whenever sun exposure is likely to occur to prevent a severe sunburn.

**! Drug Alert!**
**Teaching Alert**

Meglitinide drug doses are matched to meals. If a meal is missed, that drug dose must also be missed to prevent hypoglycemia.

Remind women that thiazolidinediones may reduce the effectiveness of oral contraceptives and can stimulate ovulation. This action increases the risk for preg-nancy, even among women undergoing menopause.

### Life Span Considerations for Oral Antidiabetic Drugs

**Pediatric Considerations.**   Oral antidiabetic drugs from the sulfonylurea, alpha-glucosidase inhibitor, and thiazolidinedione classes are not recommended for use in children who have type 2 diabetes.

Metformin and meglitinides are prescribed for children with type 2 diabetes who are over 10 years of age. The dose for a child is not based on his or her size or body weight but on how he or she responds to the drug and may be the same as for an adult with type 2 diabetes.

**Considerations for Pregnancy and Breastfeeding.**   Diabetes is often more difficult to control during this physically stressful time. In addition, some patients who do not have diabetes may have problems with hyperglycemia only during pregnancy. This condition is called gestational diabetes.

Insulin is the drug of choice for treating hyperglycemia during pregnancy. The oral antidiabetic drugs should be avoided. Because these drugs appear to enter breast milk and may cause side effects in the infant, they should not be taken by nursing mothers.

**Considerations for Older Adults.**   Oral antidiabetic drugs should be used with caution in older adults. The risk for hypoglycemia is increased in these patients, especially if they are also taking beta-adrenergic blocking drugs or warfarin (Coumadin). In addition, hypoglycemia may be harder to recognize in older adults. Often the dose prescribed for older adults, especially if they are malnourished, is *lower* than for younger adults.

*Metformin* must be used with caution in adults older than age 65. The older adult is more likely to have heart failure, poor circulation, kidney disease, or liver disease. All of these problems greatly increase the risk for the complication of lactic acidosis. If the drug is prescribed for an older adult, more careful monitoring of kidney and heart function is needed. Metformin is not recommended for patients older than age 80.

*Alpha-glucosidase inhibitors* should be used with caution in older adults and should not be used at all in those who are malnourished, have difficulty digesting or absorbing food, or have liver or intestinal tract problems. The intestinal side effects of the drugs may be worse in older adults.

*Thiazolidinedione drugs* are prescribed for older adults who have type 2 diabetes and do not have either liver impairment or cardiac problems. Because the cardiac status of older adults is likely to change more rapidly than younger adults, it is important to emphasize the signs and symptoms of heart failure.

### ORAL COMBINATION DRUGS

Often type 2 diabetes is best controlled using more than one antidiabetic drug. To simplify drug therapy, some oral drugs have been combined. The patient may not understand that a single tablet contains more than one drug. Be sure to teach the patient about the side effects, adverse effects, and issues that should be reported to their prescriber for both drugs contained in a combination tablet.

**Common Oral Combination Drugs for Type 2 Diabetes**

| Drug Name | Contains |
| --- | --- |
| Metaglip | glipiZIDE and metformin |
| Glucovance | glyBURIDE and metformin |
| Avandamet | metformin and rosiglitazone |
| Avandaryl | rosiglitazone and glimepiride |

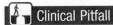

## DRUGS THAT INCREASE INCRETINS AND AMYLIN

New drugs for type 2 diabetes increase the amount of natural hormones that work with insulin to keep blood glucose levels within the normal range. The three classes of drugs that have this effect are the incretin analogs, amylin analogs, and DDP-IV inhibitors.

Incretins are a type of natural "gut" hormones that, in addition to insulin, also lower plasma glucose levels. In the person who does not have diabetes, they are released by the intestine throughout the day in response to food intake and have multiple effects on the stomach, liver, pancreas, and brain to work together to regulate blood glucose. Amylin is a naturally occurring hormone produced by beta cells in the pancreas that works with and is co-secreted with insulin in response to blood glucose elevation. Amylin levels are deficient in patients with type 1 diabetes and in patients with type 2 diabetes who are also deficient in insulin.

### How Drugs That Increase Incretin and Amylin Work

*Exenatide* (Byetta) and *liraglutide* (Victoza) are similar to the incretin hormone glucagon-like peptide-1 (GLP-1), which is made in the intestinal tract whenever a meal is eaten. Just like GLP-1, these drugs trigger the pancreas to release insulin to handle any glucose or other carbohydrates eaten at a meal. They also make the person feel full *(satiety)*, reduce the sensation of hunger (so the person eats less), and slow the rate of stomach emptying. These actions all lower blood glucose levels and help the person lose weight. The actions of these drugs rely on pancreatic insulin production. These drugs are not to be used for patients who have type 1 diabetes. They are usually used along with either a sulfonylurea antidiabetic drug or metformin (Glucophage) for best glucose control in patients with type 2 diabetes.

*Pramlintide* (Symlin) is chemically similar to natural amylin. The drug delays gastric emptying and lowers after-meal blood glucose levels; triggers satiety in the brain; and suppresses glucagon action, which prevents liver release of glucose. When used along with metformin, the drug reduces insulin needs by as much as 50%. It is used for treatment of types 1 and 2 diabetes.

*Sitagliptin* (Januvia) inhibits the enzyme DDP-IV, which normally breaks down and inactivates the incretin hormones, especially GLP-1 and glucose-dependent insulinotropic peptide. By inhibiting this enzyme, sitagliptin slows the inactivation of the incretin hormones. Thus it increases the active incretin hormone levels in the body, reducing both before- and after-meal blood glucose levels. It works only when blood glucose is elevated. In addition, sitagliptin appears to improve beta cell function, increasing the amount of insulin produced by these cells. Sitagliptin also is available as a single tablet in combination with metformin (Janumet).

### Dosages for Common Drugs That Increase Incretins and Amylin

| Drug | Dosage (Adults Only) |
| --- | --- |
| *Incretin Analog* | |
| exenatide ❶ (Byetta) | 5-10 mcg subcutaneously twice daily before the two largest meals |
| liraglutide ❶ (Victoza) | Initially 0.6 mg subcutaneously daily; gradually increase to 1.8 mg subcutaneously daily |
| *Amylin Analog* | |
| pramlintide ❶ (Symlin) | Type 1 diabetes: 15-60 mcg subcutaneously with meal 3-4 times daily |
| | Type 2 diabetes: 60-120 mcg subcutaneously with meal 3-4 times daily |
| *DDP-IV Inhibitor* | |
| sitagliptin (Januvia) | 100 mg orally once daily with or without food |

❶ High-alert drug.

### Intended Responses

- Blood glucose levels are in the normal range.
- There is no glucose in the urine.
- The patient loses weight.

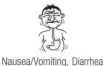

**Common Side Effects**

**Drugs That Increase Incretins and Amylin**

Nausea/Vomiting, Diarrhea

*Side Effects.* The most common side effects of the drugs that increase incretins and amylin are nausea, vomiting, and diarrhea. *Exenatide, liraglutide,* and *pramlintide* may also cause irritation at the injection site. Additional side effects for sitagliptin include runny nose, sore throat, and increased incidence of upper respiratory infections.

*Adverse Effects.* The drugs that increase incretins and amylin can cause hypoglycemia, especially in patients who are also taking a sulfonylurea antidiabetic drug. In fact, pramlintide carries a black-box warning for insulin-induced severe hypoglycemia. (A *black-box warning* means that studies have shown that a drug may produce serious or even life-threatening effects in some people in addition to its beneficial effects.) The hypoglycemic risk is higher in patients with type 1 diabetes and usually occurs within 3 hours of injection. The black box also warns against the risk of hypoglycemia while driving or operating heavy equipment.

*Sitagliptin* may cause serious allergic reactions, including anaphylaxis, angioedema, and Stevens-Johnson syndrome, although these problems are rare. In addition, the drug is excreted by the kidneys, making side effects worse in patients who have any degree of kidney impairment.

### What To *Teach* Patients About Exenatide and Liraglutide

Teach patients the signs and symptoms of hypoglycemia (see Box 25-4), especially if a sulfonylurea drug is also part of their therapy.

Exenatide and liraglutide come in a prefilled pen that contains a full 1-month supply of doses (Figure 25-9). Instruct patients how to activate the pen, attach the needle, and self-inject subcutaneously. Demonstrate these actions to patients and families and have patients (and at least one family member) demonstrate the actions

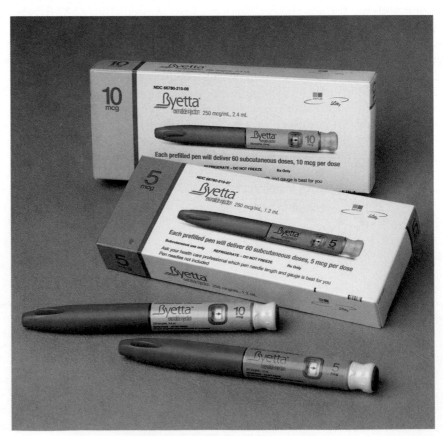

**FIGURE 25-9** The Byetta injection system.

back to you. Stress the importance of having at least one other person at home who can give the drug safely to patients.

Tell patients that the drug works with the intestinal tract to prevent blood glucose levels from becoming too high as a result of eating a meal. Teach them that this drug should be taken before the two main meals of the day, not after a meal, so it has the best chance of working properly.

Instruct patients to store the drug in the refrigerator and never to freeze it. Warm temperatures, freezing temperatures, and exposure to light can all make the drug lose its effectiveness.

Remind patients that weight loss is a positive action of the drug. The drug dose does not need to be changed as a result of weight loss.

Advise patients not to share the pen or needles with other people, even a family member who has diabetes. Sharing needles increases the risk for bloodborne diseases.

Teach patients to check the injection site daily for any signs or symptoms of infection. Any symptom indicating infection should be reported immediately to their prescriber.

### What To *Teach* Patients About Pramlintide

The issues about drawing up the pramlintide, selecting a site, and self-injection of the drug are the same as those for insulin. Use the teaching directions on pp. 451-452 for insulin self-injection to teach patients about self-injecting pramlintide. A U-100 syringe is used to administer the drug; however, it is necessary to convert the microgram dosage to insulin syringe unit increments (for example, 15 mcg is equal to 2.5 units on a U-100 insulin syringe). Teach patients to inject pramlintide into a site different from an insulin injection site.

Teach patients to always have a spare bottle of pramlintide. Between uses it should be refrigerated but never frozen. Just as for insulin and exenatide, advise patients not to share used needles or prefilled syringes or pen injectors with another person.

Teach patients to check the injection site daily for any signs or symptoms of infection (warmth, redness, skin firm to the touch, presence of drainage, pain in and around the area). The presence of any symptom indicating infection should be reported immediately to their prescriber.

Teach patients the signs and symptoms of hypoglycemia (see Box 25-4). Urge them not to skip or delay meals. Instruct patients who are just beginning to use pramlintide to check their blood sugar more often, especially before and after meals, to reduce the risk for hypoglycemia.

Pramlintide slows stomach emptying and absorption of other drugs. Teach patients who are taking other oral drugs requiring a rapid onset of action (for example, analgesics) that it is important to take these drugs either 1 hour before or 2 hours after eating.

### What To *Teach* Patients About Sitagliptin

Teach patients the signs and symptoms of hypoglycemia (see Box 25-4). Instruct them to avoid drinking alcohol because alcohol is likely to induce hypoglycemia. In addition, if the patient is drinking alcohol, he or she may be less likely to recognize the symptoms of hypoglycemia. If alcohol is used, it should be limited to one serving and taken either with food or right after a meal is completed.

Teach patients to take a missed dose as soon as soon as possible. If it is almost time for the next dose, they should take only that dose and not take the drug more than once a day or double the dose.

Teach patients to stop the drug and notify their prescriber as soon as possible if an allergic reaction occurs (rash, itching or hives, swelling of the face, lips, or tongue). Instruct them to go to the emergency department or call 911 immediately if breathing problems develop or if they should feel faint or light-headed.

---

**[!] Drug Alert!**

**Teaching Alert**

Exenatide (Byetta) doses are matched to the two main meals of the day. If a meal is missed, that drug dose must also be missed to prevent hypoglycemia.

---

**[!] Drug Alert!**

**Teaching Alert**

Teach patients taking exenatide (Byetta) to check the injection site daily for symptoms of infection (warmth, redness, skin firm to the touch, presence of drainage, pain in and around the area) and to report any of these to their prescriber.

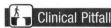

### Life Span Considerations for Drugs That Increase Incretins and Amylin

*Pediatric Considerations.*   All four drugs that increase incretins and amylin are newly approved and have not been tested in children. They currently are not recommended for use in children under 18 years of age.

*Considerations for Pregnancy and Breastfeeding.*   These drugs are not recommended for treatment of diabetes during pregnancy or while breastfeeding. (Insulin is the drug of choice for treating hyperglycemia during pregnancy.)

*Considerations for Older Adults.*   Drugs to increase incretins and amylin may be taken by older adults; but they are at even greater risk for hypoglycemia, especially when a drug to increase an incretin or amylin is used along with a sulfonylurea. The risk is greater if the patient also takes another drug that enhances the effect of sulfonylureas such as beta-adrenergic blocking drugs or warfarin (Coumadin). In addition, hypoglycemia may be harder to recognize in the older adult. Teach older adults to test their blood glucose level more frequently and to always carry a simple sugar source with them.

Older patients are also at greater risk for infection. Teach older adults using exenatide, liraglutide, or pramlintide to check the injection site daily for any signs or symptoms of infection (warmth, redness, skin firm to the touch, presence of drainage, pain in and around the area). The presence of any symptom indicating infection should be reported immediately to their prescriber.

The dose of sitagliptin should be reduced for older adults who have any degree of kidney impairment. Kidney function tests, especially BUN, and creatinine should be monitored closely (see Chapter 1, Table 1-5).

e-Learning Activity 25-6 ►

## Get Ready for Practice!

### Key Points

- Body cells use glucose and oxygen to make the chemical energy substance ATP to use as fuel for cellular work in the body.
- Hypoglycemia can lead to brain cell dysfunction and death.
- A patient with type 1 diabetes can't make insulin because of destruction of the beta cells of the pancreas.
- A patient with type 2 diabetes still makes some insulin. The insulin does not interact well with its receptor.
- Complications from untreated or poorly controlled diabetes include blindness; kidney failure; foot and leg amputations; hypertension; and increased risk for infection, heart attacks, and strokes.
- The goals of insulin therapy for type 1 diabetes are to maintain blood glucose levels within the normal range, avoid ketoacidosis, and prevent or delay the blood vessel changes that lead to organ damage.
- Check the order carefully for the exact type and amount of insulin to be injected. Do not interchange insulin types.
- Use an insulin syringe that is marked off in the same concentration units as the insulin you are injecting.
- Rotate the area for injection within one injection site.
- Administer insulin as a subcutaneous injection, not an intramuscular injection.

- Do not pull back on the plunger before injecting the insulin and do not rub or massage the injection site.
- When mixing two different type of insulin in the same syringe, inject both bottles with the amount of air equal to the dose of that insulin. Draw up the short-acting insulin first.
- Keep simple sugars (sugar packets, orange juice, glucose tables, glucose paste) and glucagon on the unit whenever a person with diabetes is a patient on the unit.
- Determine how well an older adult who is to self-inject insulin can see the markings on the syringe and reach the injection site.
- Because the different types of antidiabetic drugs work in different ways, a patient may be prescribed to take more than one type.
- After giving an oral antidiabetic drug that can cause hypoglycemia, check the patient hourly for the signs and symptoms of hypoglycemia.
- Drugs that are likely to increase the effectiveness of antidiabetic drugs and increase the risk for hypoglycemia include aspirin, other nonsteroidal anti-inflammatory drugs (NSAIDs), warfarin (Coumadin), beta-adrenergic blockers, ciprofloxacin (Cipro), probenecid, and miconazole (Micatin).
- Remind patients to limit alcohol intake and drink only with or after a full meal to prevent hypoglycemia.

- Meglitinide drugs should be taken right before a meal or a substantial snack. If a meal is skipped, that drug dose should also be skipped.
- Ensure that metformin (Glucophage) is not given to a patient within 48 hours after having a test involving dye or surgery requiring anesthesia (the drug increases the risk for lactic acidosis).
- Signs and symptoms of lactic acidosis include muscle aches; fatigue; abdominal pain; hypotension; and a slow, irregular heartbeat.
- Do not crush Glucophage XR tablets.
- Alpha-glucosidase inhibitor drugs must be given with the first bite of food.
- Pramlintide is an injectable drug given to work with insulin in lowering blood glucose levels. It should not be mixed with insulin, nor should it be injected within 2 inches of the site of an insulin injection.

## Additional Learning Resources

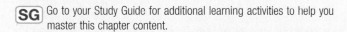 Go to your Evolve website (http://evolve.elsevier.com/Workman/pharmacology/) for the following FREE learning resources:

- eLearning Activities
- Animations
- Video Clips
- Interactive Review Questions
- Audio Key Points
- Audio Glossary
- Audio Glossary—Spanish-English
- Drug Dosage Calculators
- Patient Teaching Handouts

**SG** Go to your Study Guide for additional learning activities to help you master this chapter content.

## Review Questions

1. What is the basic underlying pathology of diabetes mellitus?

   A. A disruption of the cellular glycolytic pathway
   B. An inability of the liver to catabolize glycogen
   C. A failure to synthesize and/or use insulin
   D. An inhibition of the conversion of protein to amino acids

2. Which side effect is unique to insulin as an antidiabetic drug?

   A. Lipoatrophy
   B. Ketoacidosis
   C. Hypoglycemia
   D. Hyperglycemia

3. In bringing an insulin dose to administer to a patient with diabetes, you find the patient to be sweaty and confused. What is your best first action?

   A. Inject the insulin as prescribed.
   B. Inject 20% glucose immediately.
   C. Check the patient's identification.
   D. Check the patient's blood glucose level.

4. What must you tell a patient using prefilled insulin syringes with regular insulin at home about storing these devices?

   A. "Keep them flat and do not attach the needles until you are ready to use a syringe."
   B. "Keep them in the upright position with the needle pointing toward the ceiling."
   C. "Keep them in the upright position with the needle pointing toward the floor."
   D. "Storage position is unimportant as long as they are kept in the refrigerator."

5. When starting to draw up and administer a dose of NPH insulin, you find that the insulin in the vial is uniformly cloudy. What is your best action?

   A. Shake the vial vigorously
   B. Draw up the medication
   C. Add normal saline
   D. Open a new vial

6. A patient is prescribed to take 10 units of regular insulin and 15 units of NPH insulin each morning. How do you instruct this patient to self-administer the prescribed doses of insulin?

   A. "First draw up the regular insulin and then draw up the NPH insulin in the same syringe."
   B. "First draw up the NPH insulin and then draw up the regular insulin in the same syringe."
   C. "First draw up and administer the regular insulin and then draw up and administer the NPH insulin."
   D. "First draw up and administer the NPH insulin. Wait at least 15 minutes and then draw up and administer the regular insulin."

7. Which patient issue for diabetes is more common among older adults who are on insulin therapy?

   A. Problems of accuracy in drawing up the correct insulin dose
   B. Tissue damage from injections as a result of insufficient subcutaneous tissue
   C. Dependent edema as a result of the high sodium content of synthetic insulin
   D. Increased risk for systemic allergic reactions to insulin because of altered immune function

8. A patient with type 2 diabetes is now prescribed to change her oral antidiabetic agent from glyburide (Diabeta) to acarbose (Precose). She asks you why she need not be worried about the new drug making her hypoglycemic. What is your best answer?

   A. "Because your pancreatic function is improving, it does not need as much stimulation. Acarbose is not as powerful as glyburide."
   B. "Acarbose increases glucose uptake by the cells without the need for insulin, so you cannot become hypoglycemic even if you miss a meal on this medication."
   C. "Glyburide is actually an oral form of insulin, and too much could make your blood sugar drop quickly. Acarbose reduces blood sugar by suppressing pancreatic release of glucagon."
   D. "Glyburide stimulates your pancreas to secrete insulin, increasing your risk for hypoglycemia. Acarbose does not stimulate insulin secretion; it reduces your intestinal uptake of sugar."

9. You remain alert for hypoglycemia after giving which of the following drugs alone as therapy for diabetes? (Select all that apply.)

   A. Alpha-glucosidase inhibitors
   B. Metformin (Glucophage)
   C. Exenatide (Byetta)
   D. Meglitinides
   E. Sulfonylureas
   F. Thiazolidinediones

10. The patient prescribed rosiglitazone (Avandia) tells you that he has gained 5 pounds this week and that his ankles are swollen. What is your best action?

    A. Tell the patient to call the prescriber immediately.
    B. Tell the patient to go to the nearest emergency department.
    C. Tell the patient to stop the drug for 2 days and check whether these new symptoms have improved.
    D. Reassure the patient that this is an expected and normal side effect of rosiglitazone.

11. An older adult patient with type 2 diabetes who has been taking rosiglitazone (Avandia) for 1 month tells you that her urine is the color of coffee. What is your best action?

    A. Document this patient report as the only action
    B. Encourage the patient to drink more water
    C. Test the patient's urine for ketone bodies
    D. Notify the prescriber immediately

12. Which precaution is most important to teach a patient prescribed exenatide (Byetta) for the treatment of type 2 diabetes?

    A. Avoiding drinking alcoholic beverages to prevent liver problems
    B. Being sure to eat a full meal within 30 minutes of taking the drug
    C. Reporting any weight loss of more than 5 lb to the prescriber immediately
    D. Avoiding crowds and people who are ill because resistance to infection is now lower

13. A patient is prescribed to receive 750 mg of metformin (Glucophage) oral solution through an NG tube. You have on hand the oral solution with a concentration of 100 mg/mL. How many milliliters will you administer through the tube? _____ mL

14. You are to mix 20 units of NPH insulin (U-100) with 15 units of regular insulin (U-100) in the same syringe. What will the total number of units be for the correct amounts of both types of insulin? _____ units

## Critical Thinking Activities

A patient who came back to the floor from the recovery room after an emergency appendectomy under general anesthesia also has type 2 diabetes and hypertension. She took a Glucophage XR 500-mg tablet and a Toprol 50-mg tablet orally about 4 hours before her emergency surgery. She now tells you that the muscles of her legs and arms ache, her abdomen hurts (not over the incision site), and she feels so sleepy that she cannot keep her eyes open. When you take her vital signs, her blood pressure is 90/60, and her heart rate is 56 with about 20 skipped beats per minute.

1. Are these vital signs consistent with shock?

2. What type of drug is Glucophage?

3. What type of drug is Toprol?

4. Are the side effects or adverse effects of either of these drugs likely to be causing her problems, or are they just the expected responses to surgery?

# Drugs for Glaucoma

evolve

http://evolve.elsevier.com/Workman/pharmacology/

## Objectives

*After studying this chapter you should be able to:*

1. Describe the proper technique to administer eye drops and eye ointments.
2. Explain the causes, symptoms, and complications of glaucoma.
3. List the names, actions, usual adult dosages, possible side effects, and adverse effects of drugs for glaucoma.
4. Describe what to do before and after giving drugs for glaucoma.
5. Explain what to teach patients taking drugs for glaucoma, including what to do, what not to do, and when to call the prescriber.
6. Describe life span considerations for drugs for glaucoma.

## Key Terms

**anterior chamber** (ăn-TĒR-ē-ŭr CHĂM-bŭr) (p. 467) The part of the anterior eye segment that extends from the iris to the cornea.

**anterior segment** (ăn-TĒR-ē-ŭr SĔG-mĕnt) (p. 467) The front of the eye that extends from the lens to the cornea and contains the anterior and posterior chambers.

**aqueous humor** (ŎK-wē-ŭs HYŪ-mŭr) (p. 468) The clear fluid made continuously by the ciliary body of the eye that circulates from the posterior chamber through the pupil and into the anterior chamber, where it drains. This fluid helps maintain the pressure and shape of the eyeball.

**conjunctiva** (kŏn-JŬNK-tĭ-vă) (p. 466) A thin, clear membrane containing blood vessels that lines the eyelids and covers the front of the eye.

**glaucoma** (glŏ-KŌ-mă) (p. 468) A condition in which the aqueous humor does not drain normally out of the eye, causing a rise in intraocular pressure to levels that may damage the optic nerve.

**intraocular pressure (IOP)** (ĭn-trŭ-ŎK-yū-lŭr PRĔSH-ŭr) (p. 468) The fluid pressure inside the eyeball that helps to maintain the correct shape of the eye. The normal range for IOP is 10 to 20 mm Hg.

**miosis** (mī-Ō-sĭs) (p. 466) Constriction of the pupil, making the opening smaller and letting less light into the eye.

**mydriasis** (mĭ-DRĒ-ă-sĭs) (p. 466) Dilation of the pupil, making the opening larger and letting more light into the eye.

**photoreceptors** (fō-tō-rē-SĔP-tŭrz) (p. 466) Special nerve endings that react to light and change it into electrical impulses that are perceived as images by the brain.

**posterior chamber** (pŏs-TĒR-ē-ŭr CHĂM-bŭr) (p. 467) The part of the anterior segment of the eye between the lens and the iris.

**posterior segment** (pŏs-TĒR-ē-ŭr SĔG-mĕnt) (p. 467) The entire back part of the eye from the lens to the area of the sclera where the optic nerve leaves the eye.

**punctum** (PŬNK-tŭm) (p. 470) The opening at the inner corner of the eye to the tube that drains tears into the nasolacrimal sac. It can be blocked by lightly pressing on it.

**retina** (RĔT-ĭn-ă) (p. 466) The lining of the back part of the eye, opposite the pupil, that contains photoreceptors.

**sclera** (SKLĔR-ă) (p. 466) The tough white outer layer of the entire eye; also called the white of the eye.

◄ -Learning Activity 26-1

## OVERVIEW

The eye, along with the brain, is the organ that allows sight (vision). Sight is one of the five senses and is important for communicating with the world. We use sight to assess surroundings; be independent; be warned of danger; and work, play, and interact with others.

Sight can be reduced by many disorders. Some such as glaucoma can be controlled if found and treated early, allowing the patient to continue to have effective vision.

### Memory Jogger

The five main senses are sight, hearing, smell, touch, and taste.

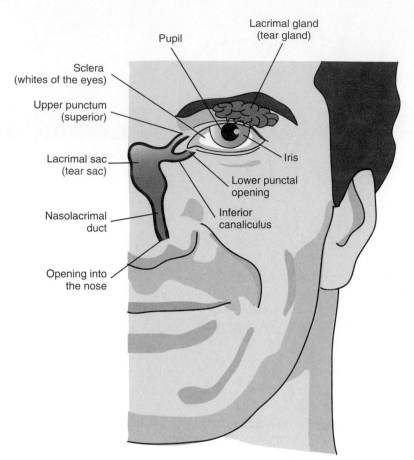

**FIGURE 26-1** Features of the external eye (front view) along with the tear gland and duct system.

## REVIEW OF RELATED PHYSIOLOGY AND PATHOPHYSIOLOGY

### PHYSIOLOGY

The eyes are able to change light into nerve impulses that are sent to the brain, where images are "seen." Figure 26-1 shows the features of the eye from the front (looking at a person directly in the face). The eye is a hollow ball made up of several layers. The whole outer layer of the eye is the **sclera**, the tough white layer that is also called the *white* of the eye. The sclera has few blood vessels. (The blood vessels seen on the sclera are in the conjunctiva.) The **conjunctiva** is a thin, clear membrane containing blood vessels that lines the eyelids and covers the front of the eye.

At the front of the eye is the *cornea*, the clear portion of the sclera that covers the front section of the eye and allows light to enter. Although the cornea is where contact lenses are placed, the cornea is *not* the lens of the eye. The *iris* is the ring of color that surrounds the pupil. The *pupil* is a round opening in the center of the iris that lets light into the eye. It dilates to increase in size, letting more light into the eye, and constricts to decrease in size, letting less light into the eye. **Miosis** is constriction of the pupil, making the opening smaller and letting less light into the eye. **Mydriasis** is dilation of the pupil, making the opening larger and letting more light into the eye (Figure 26-2).

The hollow eyeball is filled with clear substances that allow light to bend and penetrate all the way from the front of the eye to the back wall of the eye to the retina. The **retina** is the lining of the back part of the eye, opposite the pupil, that contains light-sensitive photoreceptors. **Photoreceptors** are special nerve endings that react to light and changes it into electrical impulses that are perceived as images by the brain. These are the true sense organs for vision. They allow images to been "seen" in the brain. Figure 26-3 shows a cut-away side view of the eye. The optic

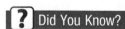

**Did You Know?**

When an eye is "bloodshot," the blood vessels you can see are in the conjunctiva and not the sclera.

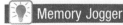

**Memory Jogger**

Constriction of the pupil is miosis (small word, small pupil size). Dilation of the pupil is mydriasis (larger word, larger pupil size).

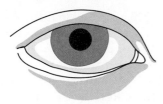

A  Normal pupil slightly dilated for moderate light.

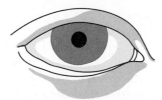

B  Miosis—pupil constricted when exposed to increased light or close work, such as reading. (Smaller word, smaller opening.)

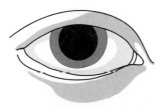

C  Mydriasis—pupil dilated when exposed to reduced light or when looking at a distance. (Larger word, larger opening.)

**FIGURE 26-2** Miosis and mydriasis.

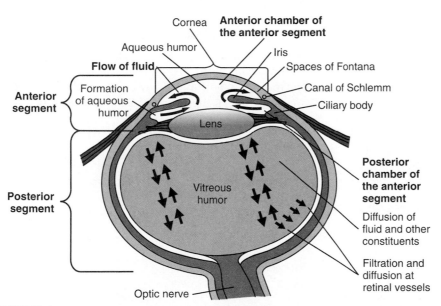

**FIGURE 26-3** Side view (cut-away) of the internal features of the eye and flow of aqueous humor.

nerve connects the photoreceptors in the retina to the brain and sends impulses that are changed to images in the brain.

The eye is divided into two segments, the posterior segment and the anterior segment (see Figure 26-3). The **posterior segment** is the entire back part of the eye from the lens to the area of the sclera where the optic nerve leaves the eye. It contains the *vitreous body (vitreous humor),* which is the gel-like filling of the eye. The **anterior segment** is the front of the eye that extends from the lens to the cornea and contains the anterior and posterior chambers. It is filled with a small amount of clear fluid known as *aqueous humor.* The **anterior chamber** is the part of the anterior eye segment that extends from the iris to the cornea. The **posterior chamber** is the part of the anterior eye segment between the lens and the iris.

Because the eye is hollow and needs to retain a ball-shape for vision, the gel in the posterior segment (vitreous body) and the fluid in the anterior segment (aqueous humor) must be present in set amounts that apply pressure inside the eye to keep it round. This pressure is known as intraocular pressure (IOP), and it has to be just right. If the pressure is too low, the eyeball is soft and collapses, preventing light from striking the photoreceptors in the back of the eye. If the pressure is too high, it compresses blood vessels in the eye, reducing blood flow and oxygen delivery to the photoreceptors. Without enough oxygen, the photoreceptors die, and sight is lost permanently.

How does the pressure become too high? The gel-like vitreous body is made as the eyes form and grow. It does not change in volume once eye growth is complete. However, the aqueous humor is made continuously from blood plasma. Aqueous humor is the clear fluid made continuously by the ciliary body that circulates from the posterior chamber through the pupil and into the anterior chamber, where it drains (see Figure 26-3). At the outer edges of the iris, beneath the cornea, there are blood vessels (the *trabecular network*) that collect this fluid and drain it through the Canal of Schlemm, returning it to the blood. About 1 mL of aqueous humor is always present in each eye, but it is continuously made and reabsorbed at a rate of about 5 mL daily. When fluid is made at the same rate that it is reabsorbed, the pressure inside the eye remains within the normal range (10 to 20 mm Hg). When fluid is reabsorbed too slowly, the amount in the eye increases, and so does the IOP.

## PATHOPHYSIOLOGY

Glaucoma is a condition of increased IOP caused by an increase in the amount of aqueous humor. Both eyes can have the problem, or it may affect only one eye. There are many types and causes of glaucoma (Table 26-1). The most common type is a chronic condition related to aging called *primary open-angle glaucoma (POAG)*, which affects both eyes. Although we usually think of glaucoma as a disorder of older adults, children can also have it. In children the problem most often is caused by eye trauma that blocks the canal of Schlemm and usually only affects one eye.

> **Memory Jogger**
>
> Keeping the IOP within the normal range (10 to 20 mm Hg) is important to maintain vision.

### Table 26-1   Types and Causes of Glaucoma

| TYPE | CAUSES |
|---|---|
| **PRIMARY OPEN-ANGLE GLAUCOMA** Chronic problem in which aqueous humor is not reabsorbed well because of thickening of blood vessels in the trabecular meshwork; the most common type of glaucoma; has no pain or other warning signs | Increasing age Blockage of central eye vein Diabetes Heredity Hypertension Severe nearsightedness |
| **ACUTE CLOSED-ANGLE GLAUCOMA** Sudden movement of the iris forward against the cornea, preventing fluid in the posterior chamber from reaching the anterior chamber where reabsorption occurs; usually occurs only in one eye with pain around the eye, headache, nausea, and vomiting; sight in the affected eye is rapidly reduced; this condition is an emergency | Head or eye trauma Moving from a low-light area to an area with extremely bright light |
| **SECONDARY GLAUCOMA** Caused by another problem in the eye; usually when the other problem is treated successfully, glaucoma is reduced or may go away completely | Blood vessel diseases Eye surgery Infections of the deep structures of the eye Tumor in the eye or brain |

POAG occurs when aqueous humor is made at the normal rate but reabsorption is reduced, leading to an increase in the amount of fluid and pressure inside the eye. This type of glaucoma is painless and has no early symptoms. The damage occurs so slowly that the patient may not even be aware that sight is being lost. Usually side vision (also known as *peripheral vision*) is lost first. Once photoreceptors die, they cannot be replaced. Without treatment, glaucoma leads to blindness.

## GENERAL ISSUES FOR LOCAL EYE DRUG THERAPY

Drugs placed directly into the eye are *local* eye drug therapy. Eye drops are thin, sterile, liquid drugs that are squeezed as a small drop or drops from a small container. Eye ointments are thick, greasy drugs that stay in contact with the eye surface longer than drops. They can deliver a high concentration of drug and blur vision for minutes to hours after instillation.

Although drugs for eye problems can be taken orally or by another systemic method, they most often are administered as eye drops or eye ointments. Other routes include eye injections and placing drug disks on or in the eye. The following section discusses information about the correct use of eye drops and eye ointments, regardless of their specific actions or why they are prescribed.

Many different drug types can be delivered as eye drops or eye ointments. Each type has different actions and effects, along with some common actions and effects. General nursing responsibilities for the common effects of eye drops and eye ointments are listed in the following paragraphs. Specific nursing responsibilities are listed with each individual drug class.

### What To Do *Before* Giving Eye Drugs

Check the order to see which eye is to receive the drug. A problem may affect only one eye, and the drug should be applied only to that eye. To avoid confusion, issues related to the right eye are indicated by writing "right eye" rather than using the Latin abbreviation "OD" *(oculus dexter)*. Issues related to the left eye are indicated as "left eye" rather than "OS" *(oculus sinister)*. Issues related to both eyes are indicated as either "both eyes" or "left and right eyes" rather than "OU" *(oculus uterque)*. When eye drugs are prescribed, the prescriber should indicate which eye or eyes are to be treated, and the pharmacist indicates this information on the drug bottles. If the eye drop bottle or eye ointment tube is not labeled with this information, the nurse labels it to correspond to the eye or eyes being treated.

Always wash your hands. Although the eye is not sterile, aseptic technique is used when touching the eye or placing drugs into the eye because it is not well protected by the immune system and can be infected easily.

Many eye drugs come in different strengths. Always check the strength prescribed with that of the drug you have on hand to be sure that you are giving the correct dose.

Check to be sure that a tube of ointment is for ophthalmic (eye) use. Some drugs for the eye are also available as regular topical ointments, but these contain larger particles that should not be placed in the eye.

Check to see whether any other eye drops are to be administered. If so, wait at least 10 minutes after instilling the first set and before instilling the second set of eye drops. If more than two drugs are to be instilled, wait at least 10 minutes between each set.

If a patient wears contact lenses, ask him or her to remove them before instilling the drop into the eye. Contact lenses can absorb some drugs or the preservative in them and become cloudy or discolored. In addition, contact lenses can keep the drug from spreading evenly across the eye. For some drugs the contact lens can be replaced 15 minutes after the drug is instilled. For other drugs, especially ointments, contact lenses should not be worn until drug therapy is complete.

Inspect the eye for redness, drainage, or open areas. If open areas are present, check to determine whether the drug can be instilled. Some drugs should not be

**Memory Jogger**

Drug therapy for glaucoma does not cure the problem; it only controls it.

◄ⓔ-Learning Activity 26-2

**Clinical Pitfall**

*Avoid* the use of the Latin terms for right eye (OD), left eye (OS), and both eyes (OU).

**Drug Alert!**

**Interaction Alert**

Always wait at least 10 minutes between instilling different eye drops to prevent a drug interaction or dilution of drug concentration.

◄ⓔ-Video 26-1: Administering Eye Medications

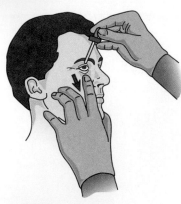

**FIGURE 26-4** Correct technique for instilling eye drops.

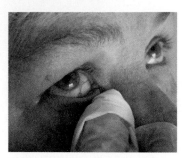

**FIGURE 26-5** Applying punctal occlusion to prevent systemic absorption.

> ⚠ **Drug Alert!**
>
> **Teaching Alert**
>
> Using more eye drops than prescribed leads to systemic side effects. Teach patients to use eye drops exactly as prescribed and not to administer extra drops.

> ⚠ **Drug Alert!**
>
> **Teaching Alert**
>
> If infants or young children need eye drugs, demonstrate drug instillation to the parent or guardian and teach them to obtain the assistance of another adult.

> ⚠ **Drug Alert!**
>
> **Teaching Alert**
>
> Teach patients using eye drugs for any eye problem to immediately call their prescriber or go to the emergency department if a sudden reduction or loss of vision occurs.

instilled into an eye with open areas because the drug is rapidly absorbed into systemic circulation when applied to an open area and the side effects are widespread. For other drugs this is not a problem.

For ointments, after removing the cap from the ointment tube, squeeze a small amount out onto a tissue (without touching the tip of the tube or letting it come into contact with the tissue) and discard this ointment. This action reduces the chance of instilling contaminated ointment into the patient's eye.

Follow the steps in Box 26-1 for placing eye drops or ointments into another person's eye. Figure 26-4 shows a common technique for instilling eye drops or ointments.

### What To Do *After* Giving Eye Drugs

For any eye drop that can have systemic side effects, apply gentle pressure to the punctum in the corner of the eye nearest the nose for about 1 minute (Figure 26-5). The **punctum** is the opening of the tube at the inner corner of the eye that drains tears into the nose and mouth (see Figure 26-1). This area is also called the *inner canthus* and can be blocked by lightly pressing on it. Applying pressure to this area immediately after drops are instilled lets the drug coat the entire eye before any of it leaves the area. This action is called *punctal occlusion* and reduces systemic absorption of the drug.

Instruct patients to keep the eye closed for about 1 minute after instilling the drug to ensure that it spreads evenly across the eye.

### What To *Teach* Patients About Eye Drugs

Teach patients to use eye drugs exactly as prescribed. Some people, especially older adults, may not consider eye drops to be a true drug. They also may believe that "if one drop is good, 10 drops will be better." Explain that using more drops than prescribed increases the chance that the drug will be absorbed into the blood and result in systemic effects. In addition, the effect of the drug on the eye may be too strong when extra drug is applied. Take as much time as needed to help the patient understand that using the right dose is critical for eye (and general) health.

Teach patients the steps in Box 26-1 for correctly instilling drops into one or both eyes. Using saline eye drops for practice, demonstrate the steps to patients and have patients demonstrate them back to you. If a patient has physical problems or is confused and cannot instill the eye drops, teach a family member, friend, or neighbor how to do this correctly.

Teach patients how to use punctal occlusion by applying pressure over the punctum immediately after instilling the drops. This action keeps the drug on the eye longer and helps to prevent systemic effects.

Administering eye drugs to an infant or child can be difficult. Sudden head movement can cause the tip of the bottle or tube to scratch the eye.

Many patients have more difficulty placing ointments in the eye than using eye drops. It may be helpful to demonstrate the steps to a family member or other responsible person.

Older adults may have more difficulty self-administering eye drops because of physical limitations. Adaptive devices are available that hold the bottle of eye drops and help keep the eyelids open. When the device is placed around the eye, the tip of the bottle lines up directly over the center of the eye (Figure 26-6). The patient then only has to trigger the right number of drops. Although this method does not place the drops in a lid pocket, it is acceptable.

Instruct patients not to share the eye ointment with anyone else to prevent spreading eye infections from one person to another.

Remind patients not to drive or use heavy equipment while the drug is in their eye and vision is blurred.

Regardless of the reason that eye drugs are prescribed, a sudden decrease in vision is always a problem and needs immediate attention.

## Box **26-1**  How to Instill Eye Drops or Ointments

**SELF-ADMINISTRATION**
1. Check the name, strength, expiration date, color, and clarity of the eye drops to be instilled. If the drug is an ointment, be sure that it is an ophthalmic (eye) preparation and not a general topical ointment.
2. Check to see whether only one eye is to have the drug or if both eyes are to receive the drug.
3. If both eyes are to receive the same drug and one eye is infected, use two separate bottles or tubes and carefully label each with "right" or "left" for the correct eye.
4. Wash your hands.
5. Remove the cap from the bottle or tube, keeping the cap upright to prevent contaminating it.
6. Tilt your head backward, open your eyes, and look up at the ceiling.
7. Using your nondominant hand, gently pull the lower lid down against your cheek, forming a small pocket.
8. Hold the eye drop bottle or ointment tube (with the cap off) like a pencil with the tip pointing down with your dominant hand.
9. For ointment, squeeze a small amount out onto a tissue (without touching the tip to the tissue) and discard this ointment.
10. Rest the wrist that is holding the bottle or tube against your mouth or upper lip.
11. For eye drops, gently squeeze the bottle and release the prescribed number of drops into the pocket that you have made with your lower lid. Do not touch any part of the eye or lid with the tip of the bottle. For ointment, gently squeeze the tube and release a small amount of ointment into the pocket that you have made with your lower lid. Do not touch any part of the eye or lid with the tip of the tube.
12. Gently release the lower lid.
13. Close the eye gently (without squeezing the lids tightly) and roll your eye under the lid to spread the drug across the eye.
14. For eye drops, gently press and hold the corner of the eye nearest the nose to close off the punctum and prevent the drug from being absorbed systemically.
15. Without pressing on the lid, gently blot or wipe away any excess drug or tears with a tissue.
16. Gently release the lower lid.
17. Keep the eye closed for about 1 minute.
18. Place the cap back on the bottle or tube.
19. Wash your hands again.
20. Do not drive or operate heavy machinery while your vision is blurry.

**ADMINISTERING DRUGS TO ANOTHER PERSON**
1. Follow self-administration steps 1 through 5.
2. Put on gloves if secretions are present in or around the eye.
3. Explain the procedure to the patient.
4. Have the patient sit in a chair and the person applying the drug stand behind the patient (or alternatively stand in front of the patient who is sitting in a chair or over the patient who is lying in bed).
5. Ask the patient to tilt the head backward, with the back of the head resting against the body of the person applying the drug (or against the back of the chair) and looking up at the ceiling.
6. Gently pull the lower lid down against the patient's cheek, forming a small pocket.
7. Hold the eye-drop bottle or ointment tube (with the cap off) like a pencil, with the tip pointing down.
8. For ointment, squeeze out and discard a small amount of ointment as described in step 9.
9. Follow steps 11 through 16.
10. Tell the patient to keep his or her eyes closed for a minute.
11. Remove your gloves.
12. Place the cap back on the bottle or tube.
13. Wash your hands again.
14. Remind the patient not to drive or operate heavy machinery while his or her vision is blurry.

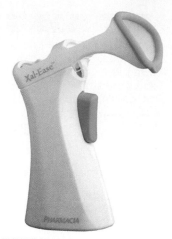

**FIGURE 26-6** The Xal-Ease adaptive device for self-administering eye drops.

◄ ⊖-Learning Activity 26-3

# TYPES OF DRUGS FOR GLAUCOMA

Drugs for glaucoma improve the reabsorption of aqueous humor and/or reduce the amount that is made. These actions restore good blood flow inside the eye and keep the remaining photoreceptors healthy. Most glaucoma drugs are administered as eye drops. For sudden-onset glaucoma (acute closed-angle glaucoma), systemic drugs may be used.

## PROSTAGLANDIN AGONISTS

### How Prostaglandin Agonists Work

The prostaglandin agonists are very effective but are newer and more expensive. Advantages include that most are used only once a day and seem to have fewer systemic side effects than other drugs. Prostaglandin agonists bind to prostaglandin receptor sites in the eye and relax blood vessel smooth muscles. These drugs cause the blood vessels in the trabecular network of the eye, where the aqueous humor is reabsorbed, to dilate and collect more fluid. This allows the fluid to leave the eye more quickly and lowers the IOP. Generic names, trade names, and usual dosages of these drugs are listed in the following table. Be sure to consult a drug reference book for specific information about glaucoma drugs.

### Dosages for Common Prostaglandin Agonists

| Drugs | Dosage (Adults and Children) |
| --- | --- |
| bimatoprost (Lumigan) | 1 gtt in affected eye or eyes daily in the evening |
| latanoprost (Xalatan) TOP100 | 1 gtt in affected eye or eyes daily in the evening |
| travoprost (Travatan) | 1 gtt in affected eye or eyes daily in the evening |

TOP100 Top 100 drugs prescribed.

### Intended Responses
- IOP is reduced.
- There is no further loss of sight.

*Side Effects.* The most common side effects of prostaglandin agonists are eye itching, eye redness, a permanent change in the iris color from lighter colors to brown (Figure 26-7), thickening and lengthening of the eyelashes, and darkening of the skin on the eyelids. Less common side effects include eye inflammation, dry eyes, swelling of the eyelids, headache, colds, and other upper respiratory infections.

**Common Side Effects**

**Prostaglandin Agonists**

Itchiness, Redness

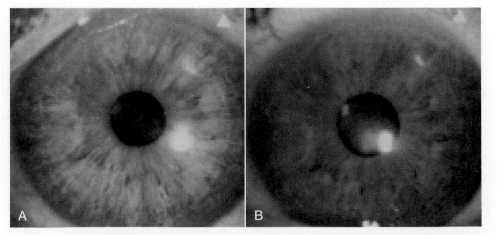

**FIGURE 26-7** Changes in iris color associated with prostaglandin agonist drug therapy for glaucoma. **A,** Before treatment. **B,** After treatment.

*Adverse Effects.*   Adverse effects related to systemic absorption of prostaglandins inhibitors are rare. These include muscle weakness, hypotension, elevated liver enzymes, and an increase in body hair.

## What To Do *Before* Giving Prostaglandin Agonists

Be sure to review the general nursing responsibilities related to eye drug therapy (pp. 469-470) in addition to these specific responsibilities before giving prostaglandin antagonists.

Inspect the eye for any corneal abrasions or other signs of trauma. These drugs should not be used if the surface of the eye is not intact.

## What To Do *After* Giving Prostaglandin Agonists

Be sure to review the general nursing responsibilities related to eye drug therapy (p. 470) after giving prostaglandin agonists.

## What To *Teach* Patients About Prostaglandin Agonists

Be sure to teach patients the general care needs and precautions related to eye drugs (pp. 470-471) in addition to these specific points for prostaglandin antagonists.

Remind patients that using higher doses than prescribed can reduce the effectiveness of the drug in controlling glaucoma.

Tell patients that eye and eyelid color can change over time and that the lashes can become thicker and longer. If only one eye has glaucoma, the color and lash changes will occur only in that eye. Stress that the drug should *not* be used in the eye that does not have glaucoma.

Remind patients to report any new symptoms (general or specific to the eye) to their prescriber as soon as possible. Stress that they should call their prescriber or go to the emergency department immediately if they have a sudden loss or reduction of vision.

### Life Span Considerations for Prostaglandin Antagonists

*Pediatric Considerations.*   The safety and effectiveness of these drugs have not been established in children. However, glaucoma in children that does not respond well to other drugs may be treated with a prostaglandin agonist. Teaching the child, the parent, or any other caregiver how to instill eye drops safely is critical (see Box 26-1). It is also important to stress that, if only one eye is affected, which is common when glaucoma is the result of trauma, the drugs must only be placed in the affected eye.

*Considerations for Pregnancy and Breastfeeding.*   Prostaglandin agonists for glaucoma therapy are pregnancy category C drugs. Unless the risk for sight loss is severe, these drugs should be avoided during the first trimester of pregnancy and used with caution during the later 6 months of pregnancy. Breastfeeding is not recommended while taking prostaglandin agonists.

*Considerations for Older Adults.*   Focus on correct technique for administering eye drops. Teach older adults with physical limitations how to use adaptive devices for eye drop administration.

## BETA-ADRENERGIC BLOCKING AGENTS

Beta-adrenergic blocking agents, more commonly known as *beta blockers*, bind to adrenergic receptor sites and act as antagonists. They block the receptor and prevent the naturally occurring adrenalin from binding to it. This response slows or inhibits the normal actions of the cells. Generic names, trade names, and common dosages of these drugs are listed in the following table. Be sure to consult a drug reference for specific information about glaucoma drugs.

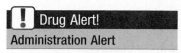

**Drug Alert!**

**Administration Alert**

Do not instill prostaglandin agonists into an eye that does not have an intact surface.

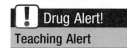

**Drug Alert!**

**Teaching Alert**

Remind patients using a prostaglandin agonist for glaucoma in only one eye not to place the drops in the unaffected eye even though their eye colors may now be different.

Dosages for Common Beta-Adrenergic Blocking Drugs

| Drugs | Dosage (Adults) |
|---|---|
| betaxolol hydrochloride (Betoptic) | 1-2 gtts in affected eye every 12 hr |
| carteolol (Cartrol, Ocupress) | 1 gtt in affected eye every 12 hr |
| levobunolol (Betagan) | 0.25%—1-2 gtts in affected eye every 12 hr; 0.5%—1-2 gtts in affected eye daily |
| timolol ❶ (Betimol, Istalol, Timoptic) | 1 gtt in affected eye every 12 hr |
| timolol GFS ❶ (gel-forming solution) (Timoptic-XE, timolol-GFS) | 1 gtt in affected eye daily |

❶ High-alert drug.

### How Beta-Adrenergic Blocking Agents Work

Selectively blocking beta-adrenergic receptors in the eye causes less aqueous humor to be produced by the ciliary bodies. These drugs also cause fluid to be absorbed slightly.

### Intended Responses
- IOP is reduced.
- There is no further loss of sight.

***Side Effects.*** Common side effects for beta blockers used in the eye include tearing, blurred vision, and a mild burning sensation within the first few minutes after the drug is instilled. Later tear production is reduced; and the eyes are dry, itchy, and red. The pupil is constricted (*miosis*). The eyelids can become inflamed and crusty.

***Adverse Effects.*** Long-term use of beta blockers can increase the risk for *cataracts*, a disorder in which the normally clear eye lens becomes cloudy and reduces vision. The most serious adverse effects occur when these drugs are absorbed systemically. They can block beta receptors in the heart, slowing the heart rate, and may even lead to heart failure. In the lungs beta blockers can make the airways narrower, making asthma and bronchitis worse.

### What To Do *Before* Giving Beta-Adrenergic Blocking Agents

Be sure to review the general nursing responsibilities related to eye drug therapy (pp. 469-470) in addition to these specific responsibilities before giving beta blockers.

Check the patient's vital signs (especially blood pressure, heart rate, respiratory rate, and pulse oximetry). Use these data as a baseline to determine whether an adverse reaction occurs.

Check to see whether the patient is also taking an oral beta blocker for control of blood pressure or heart rhythm problems. An oral drug taken along with beta-blocking eye drops could make the adverse effects more severe.

Check the patient's record to determine whether the patient has asthma, chronic obstructive pulmonary disease (COPD), or heart failure. Beta blockers should be used cautiously in patients with any of these problems.

### What To Do *After* Giving Beta-Adrenergic Blocking Agents

Be sure to review the general nursing responsibilities related to eye drug therapy (p. 470) in addition to these specific responsibilities after giving beta blockers.

Be sure to apply pressure over the punctum for at least 1 full minute immediately after instilling the eye drop to reduce the risk for systemic side effects.

Tell the patient to call you immediately if wheezing develops or dizziness is present. Check his or her blood pressure, heart rate, respiratory rate, and pulse oximetry at least every 4 hours for the presence of an adverse effect. Notify the

**Common Side Effects**

**Beta-Adrenergic Blocking Agents**

Miosis, Itchiness, Redness

**Memory Jogger**

When beta-blocking eye drops are absorbed systemically, they can worsen asthma and heart failure.

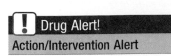

**Drug Alert!**

**Action/Intervention Alert**

Notify the prescriber immediately if heart rate drops or difficulty breathing develops after a beta blocker has been instilled in the eye.

prescriber if the heart rate drops below 60 beats per minute, wheezes develop, or the pulse oximetry reading drops below 92%.

### What To *Teach* Patients About Beta-Adrenergic Blocking Agents

Be sure to teach patients the general care needs and precautions related to eye drugs (pp. 470-471) in addition to these specific points for beta blockers.

Remind patients to use the drug exactly as prescribed and not to use more drops or take the drug more often. The risk for heart and breathing problems increases if more drug is used.

Tell patients to use good light when reading and to be careful in darker rooms. The pupil of the eye will not open further to let in more light, and it may be harder to see objects in dim light. This problem can increase the risk for falls.

Remind patients with diabetes that drugs from this class can mask the symptoms of hypoglycemia if the drug is absorbed systemically.

Remind patients to report any new eye or general symptoms to the prescriber as soon as possible. Stress to patients to call their prescriber or go to the emergency department immediately if they have a sudden loss or reduction of vision.

### Life Span Considerations for Beta-Adrenergic Blocking Agents

*Pediatric Considerations.*   Even though glaucoma is rare in children, teaching the child, parent, or other caregiver how to safely instill eye drops is critical. It is also important to stress that only the prescribed dose should be used.

*Considerations for Pregnancy and Breastfeeding.*   Beta blockers are pregnancy category C drugs when given for glaucoma. Unless the risk for sight loss is severe, these drugs should be avoided during the first trimester of pregnancy and used with caution during the later 6 months of pregnancy. Breastfeeding is permitted with the use of a beta blocker for glaucoma.

*Considerations for Older Adults.*   Focus on preventing severe systemic side effects. With high doses systemic absorption is possible, and the effects on the cardiac and respiratory systems can be severe. Heart failure and bronchospasms can become worse. The risk for hypoglycemia increases among patients with diabetes. Thus these drugs should either not be used or used cautiously in older adults who have heart failure, asthma, COPD, other respiratory problems, or diabetes. If they are used, stress the importance of using the right dose and the need to occlude the punctum after administration.

Take as much time as needed to help older adults understand that using the right dose is critical for their eye and general health. Teach them how to apply gentle pressure on the punctum to prevent systemic absorption. Stress the importance of using only the prescribed number of drops. Urge them to keep a record of any new symptoms or worsening of existing health problems and to notify their prescriber as soon as possible.

## ADRENERGIC AGONISTS

### How Adrenergic Agonists Work

Adrenergic agonists bind to receptor sites that usually bind to naturally occurring adrenalin. This action "turns on" the receptor and reduces the amount of aqueous humor produced by the ciliary bodies. They also dilate the pupil and improve fluid flow through it. These actions reduce the amount of fluid in the eye, lowering the IOP.

When used as eye drops, the effects of these drugs should be present only in the eye. They are normally used for short-term therapy to prevent or reduce pressure after eye surgery. Although adrenergic agonists can be used systemically, the eye-drop form of the drug is used for glaucoma therapy. Generic names, trade names, and common dosages of these drugs are listed in the following table. Be sure to consult a drug reference for specific information about glaucoma drugs.

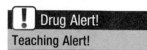

**Drug Alert!**

**Teaching Alert!**

Ensure that the patient understands the importance of taking only the correct dose of the drug and occluding the punctum immediately after placing the drops in his or her eye.

Dosages for Common Adrenergic Agonists

| Drug | Dosage |
|------|--------|
| apraclonidine (Iopidine) | 1-2 gtts in affected eye every 8 hr |
| brimonidine tartrate (Alphagan P) | 1 gtt in affected eye every 8 hr |
| dipivefrin hydrochloride (Propine) | 1 gtt in affected eye every 12 hr |

### Intended Responses
- IOP is reduced.
- There is no further loss of sight.

**Side Effects**    Common side effects are tearing and blurred vision for a few minutes after instilling the drug. The pupil dilates *(mydriasis)* and remains dilated, even when there is plenty of light. The sclera may also be red and itchy. Less common side effects include eyelid crusting, eye discharge, and nasal dryness.

**Adverse Effects.**    If the drug is absorbed systemically, the patient may become drowsy. Blood pressure can decrease, and the heart rate can become slow and irregular. Usually these symptoms occur only when the drug is overused.

### What To Do *Before* Giving Adrenergic Agonists
Be sure to review the general nursing responsibilities related to eye drug therapy (pp. 469-470) in addition to these specific responsibilities before giving adrenergic agonists.

Check the patient's vital signs, especially blood pressure and heart rate. Use this information as a baseline to determine whether an adverse reaction is occurring.

Check to see whether the patient also takes a monoamine oxidase (MAO) inhibitor drug. Adrenergic agonists are contraindicated for use in these patients.

### What To Do *After* Giving Adrenergic Agonists
Be sure to review the general nursing responsibilities related to eye drug therapy (p. 470) in addition to these specific responsibilities after giving adrenergic agonists.

Check the patient's vital signs at least once per shift to determine whether the drug is having an effect on blood pressure or heart rate.

Check the patient's level of consciousness hourly for the first several hours after the first dose to determine whether the patient becomes drowsy. If drowsiness occurs, remind the patient to call for assistance when getting out of the bed.

Most adrenergic agonists should be protected from light and heat. The container is a solid color that doesn't allow light to enter. Refrigerate these drugs, but do not allow them to freeze.

### What To *Teach* Patients About Adrenergic Agonists
Be sure to teach patients the general care needs and precautions related to eye drugs (pp. 470-471) in addition to these specific points for beta blockers.

Teach patients to store the drug properly and protect it from light.

If patients become drowsy on this drug, remind them to avoid operating dangerous equipment or driving when the drug has its peak effect.

Because the pupil is dilated, patients have increased sensitivity to light. Teach them to wear sunglasses when in the sunlight or other bright light conditions.

Remind patients to report any new eye or general symptoms to their prescriber as soon as possible. Stress that patients should call their prescriber or go to the emergency department immediately if they have a sudden loss or reduction of vision.

If the patient has been prescribed to use the drug for a limited time such as 1 week, remind him or her not to continue the drug beyond that time period. These drugs not only lower elevated IOP, but they can also lower normal IOP, which can cause problems.

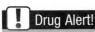

**Common Side Effects**

**Adrenergic Agonists**

Tearing, Blurred vision, Itchiness, Redness

**① Drug Alert!**

**Interaction Alert**

Adrenergic-agonist eye drops for glaucoma should not be administered to anyone who is taking an MAO inhibitor or who has taken a drug from this class within the last 14 days.

**① Drug Alert!**

**Teaching Alert**

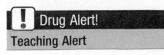
Remind patients using adrenergic agonists to wear sunglasses when in bright light conditions.

## Life Span Considerations for Adrenergic Agonists

*Pediatric Considerations.*   When glaucoma is present in a child, the drugs are used because the disorder can lead to blindness. Teaching the child, parent, or other caregiver how to instill eye drops safely is critical. It is also important to stress that only the prescribed dose should be used.

*Considerations for Pregnancy and Breastfeeding.*   Adrenergic agonists for glaucoma therapy are pregnancy category C drugs. Unless the risk for sight loss is severe, these drugs should be avoided during the first trimester of pregnancy and used with caution during the later 6 months of pregnancy. Breastfeeding is *not* recommended while taking adrenergic agonists for glaucoma.

*Considerations for Older Adults.*   Focus on correct technique for eye drop administration and preventing severe systemic side effects. Teach older adults who have physical limitations how to use adaptive devices for eye drop administration.

If an older adult has other health problems, especially heart or respiratory problems, these conditions can be made worse by systemic absorption of adrenergic agonists. Teach older adults how to apply gentle pressure on the punctum to prevent systemic absorption. Stress the importance of using only the prescribed number of drops. Urge older adults to keep a record of any new symptoms or worsening of existing health problems and to notify their prescriber as soon as possible.

## CHOLINERGIC DRUGS

### How Cholinergic Drugs Work

There are two main types of cholinergic drugs. Both types cause a response similar to the response that occurs when the naturally produced substance, acetylcholine, binds to its receptor sites and turns them on. One type of cholinergic drug is an acetylcholine agonist and acts just like acetylcholine. The other type of cholinergic drug works on the enzyme that destroys acetylcholine. The result of this action is that there is more natural acetylcholine around to bind to the acetylcholine receptor.

By either acting like acetylcholine or allowing it to remain in higher concentrations, the cholinergic drugs lower IOP by decreasing the amount of aqueous humor produced and improving its flow. These drugs make the pupil smaller (miosis) but at the same time make more room between the iris and the lens, allowing the fluid to flow better through the pupil even though it is smaller. Generic names, trade names, and common dosages of these drugs are listed in the following table. Be sure to consult a drug reference for specific information about glaucoma drugs.

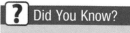

**? Did You Know?**

Cholinergic drugs are named after acetylcholine.

### Dosages for Common Cholinergic Drugs

| Drugs | Dosage |
|---|---|
| carbachol (Carboptic, Isopto Carbachol) | 2 gtts in affected eye every 8 hr |
| echothiophate (Phospholine Iodide) | 1 gtt in affected eye once or twice daily |
| pilocarpine (Adsorbocarpine, Akarpine, Isopto Carpine, Ocu-Carpine, Ocusert, Piloptic, Pilopine, Pilostat) | 2 gtts in affected eye every 6 to 8 hr, depending on strength of solution and patient response to the drug |

### Intended Responses

- IOP is reduced.
- There is no further loss of sight.

*Side Effects.*   The local side effects of cholinergic drugs for the eye include miosis, tearing, a mild burning sensation, blurred vision, and eye redness. These drugs are absorbed easily through the mucous membranes of the eyelids and can cause systemic effects such as headache, flushing, increased saliva, and sweating.

**Common Side Effects**

**Cholinergic Drugs**

Miosis, Tearing, Itchiness, Redness

***Adverse Effects.*** When larger amounts of the drug are absorbed into the blood, systemic adverse effects are possible. These include asthma, hypotension, heart block and other rhythm problems, abdominal cramps, diarrhea, incontinence of urine, vomiting, and dizziness.

### What To Do *Before* Giving Cholinergic Drugs

Be sure to review the general nursing responsibilities related to eye drug therapy (pp. 469-470) in addition to these specific responsibilities before giving cholinergic drugs.

Check the patient's vital signs, especially blood pressure, heart rate, respiratory rate, and pulse oximetry. Use these data as a baseline to determine whether an adverse reaction is occurring.

Check to see whether the patient is also taking an oral cholinergic drug for other health problems (such as urinary retention or myasthenia gravis). An oral drug taken along with the eye-drop form of a cholinergic drug could make adverse effects more severe.

Check the patient's record to determine whether he or she has asthma, COPD, or heart failure. Cholinergic drugs should be used cautiously in patients with any of these problems because the drugs can make them worse.

### What To Do *After* Giving Cholinergic Drugs

Be sure to review the general nursing responsibilities related to eye drug therapy (p. 470) in addition to these specific responsibilities after giving cholinergic drugs.

Be sure to apply pressure over the punctal area for at least 1 full minute immediately after instilling the eye drop to reduce the risk for systemic side effects.

If excess drug is present on the patient's skin, wipe it off immediately to prevent systemic side effects (these drugs can be absorbed through the skin).

Check the patient's blood pressure, heart rate, respiratory rate, and pulse oximetry at least every 4 hours for the presence of an adverse effect. Notify the prescriber if the heart rate drops below 60 beats per minute, wheezes develop, or the pulse oximetry reading drops below 92%.

Tell the patient to call you immediately if he or she develops wheezing or notes an increase in drooling or sweating or if dizziness is present.

Remind the patient that the pupils will not open as wide when light is low. He or she may need more light to read and see easily.

If any drug has come into contact with your skin, wash it off immediately because it can be absorbed by the skin and cause side effects.

### What To *Teach* Patients About Cholinergic Drugs

Be sure to teach patients the general care needs and precautions related to eye drugs (pp. 470-471) in addition to these specific points for cholinergic drugs.

Remind patients to use the drug exactly as prescribed and not to use more drops or take the drug more frequently. The risk for heart, breathing, and nervous system problems greatly increase if more drug is used.

Tell patients to use good light when reading and be careful in darker rooms. The pupil of the eye will not open wider to let in more light, and it may be harder to see objects in dim light. This problem can increase the risk for falls.

Remind patients to report any new eye or general symptoms to the prescriber as soon as possible. Stress to them that if they have a sudden loss or reduction of vision to call their prescriber or go to the emergency department immediately.

Tell patients to report an increase in drooling or sweating to their prescriber immediately because these are often the symptoms of drug overdose.

### CARBONIC ANHYDRASE INHIBITORS

#### How Carbonic Anhydrase Inhibitors Work

Carbonic anhydrase inhibitors (CAIs) are a type of diuretic that also can lower IOP. These drugs work by reducing production of aqueous humor by as much as 60%.

---

**⚠ Drug Alert!**
**Action/Intervention Alert**

Wipe any excess drug from the patient's skin to prevent systemic side effects.

---

**⚠ Drug Alert!**
**Action/Intervention Alert**

Notify the prescriber immediately if the heart rate drops below 60 or if breathing problems develop after a cholinergic drug has been administered.

They do not affect the flow or absorption of the fluid. They can be taken orally and as eye drops to control glaucoma. Generic names, trade names, and common dosages of these drugs are listed in the following table. Be sure to consult a drug reference for specific information about glaucoma drugs.

### Dosages for Common Carbonic Anhydrase Inhibitors

| Drug | Dosage (Adults) |
|------|-----------------|
| acetaZOLAMIDE (Diamox) | 250 mg orally 1 to 4 times daily (sustained-release capsules) |
| brinzolamide (Azopt) | 1 gtt in affected eye every 8 hr |
| dorzolamide (Trusopt) | 1 gtt in affected eye every 8 hr |
| methazolamide (Neptazane) | 50-100 mg orally every 8 to 12 hr |

### Intended Responses
- IOP is reduced.
- There is no further loss of sight.

**Side Effects.**  When carbonic anhydrase inhibitors are used as eye drops, the most common side effect is blurred vision briefly after instilling the drug. The sclera may also become red and itchy.

When these drugs are given systemically, there are many more side effects such as changes in blood glucose levels (up or down), headache, fever, nausea, vomiting, and diarrhea.

**Adverse Effects.**  Carbonic anhydrase inhibitors are related to the sulfonamide antibacterial drugs ("sulfa" drugs). If a patient has an allergy to sulfonamides, he or she may also have an allergy to carbonic anhydrase inhibitors, even when they are used as eye drops.

When taken systemically, these drugs can cause acidosis; severe skin reactions; electrolyte imbalances; dizziness; confusion; and numbness of the hands, feet, and face. Carbonic anhydrase inhibitors also interact with many drugs. Be sure to check a drug handbook or the package insert before administering any of these drugs by mouth or as an injection.

### What To Do *Before* Giving Carbonic Anhydrase Inhibitors

Be sure to review the general nursing responsibilities related to eye drug therapy (pp. 469-470) in addition to these specific responsibilities before giving carbonic anhydrase inhibitors.

Ask the patient whether he or she is allergic to sulfonamide antibacterial drugs. Because carbonic anhydrase inhibitors are a type of sulfonamide, the patient may also have an allergy to these drugs. If he or she has a known allergy to sulfonamides, report this to the prescriber before administering the eye drops.

Follow the general directions for eye drop administration. Shake the bottle well before administering the eye drops. Then follow the steps listed in Box 26-1.

### What To Do *After* Giving Carbonic Anhydrase Inhibitors

Be sure to review the general nursing responsibilities related to eye drug therapy (p. 470) in addition to these specific responsibilities after giving carbonic anhydrase inhibitors.

When giving the first dose of a drug from this class, check the patient's vital signs every hour for the first 2 hours. Also ask the patient whether any shortness of breath, dizziness, or general skin itchiness is occurring. These are all symptoms of an allergic reaction.

If another drug is also to be administered in the eye, wait at least 10 minutes before instilling it.

If the patient wears contact lenses, they may be reinserted 15 minutes after the drops have been instilled.

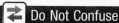

**Do Not Confuse**

**acetaZOLAMIDE** *with* **acetoHEXAMIDE**

An order for acetaZOLAMIDE can be confused with acetoHEXAMIDE. AcetaZOLAMIDE is a drug to treat glaucoma, whereas acetoHEXAMIDE is a drug for type 2 diabetes.

**Do Not Confuse**

**Diamox** *with* **Diabinese**

An order for Diamox can be confused with Diabinese. Diamox is a diuretic drug to treat glaucoma, whereas Diabinese is a drug for type 2 diabetes.

**Common Side Effects**

**Carbonic Anhydrase Inhibitors**

Blurred vision, Itchiness, Redness

**Drug Alert!**

**Administration Alert**

Do not administer a carbonic anhydrase inhibitor to a patient who has a "sulfa drug" allergy.

### What To *Teach* Patients About Carbonic Anhydrase Inhibitors

Be sure to teach patients the general care needs and precautions related to eye drugs (pp. 470-471) in addition to these specific points for carbonic anhydrase inhibitors.

Teach patients to shake the bottle well before instilling the drug.

Remind patients to report any new eye or general symptoms to their prescriber as soon as possible. Stress that they should call their prescriber or go to the emergency department immediately if they have a sudden loss or reduction of vision.

### Life Span Considerations for Carbonic Anhydrase Inhibitors

*Pediatric Considerations.* Carbonic anhydrase inhibitors are not used in children with glaucoma because these drugs slow growth when used long term.

*Considerations for Pregnancy and Breastfeeding.* Carbonic anhydrase inhibitors are known to cause birth defects in animals. Unless the risk for sight loss is severe, these drugs should be avoided during pregnancy. Carbonic anhydrase inhibitors are not recommended during breastfeeding.

*Considerations for Older Adults.* The use of carbonic anhydrase inhibitors can increase the risk for acidosis. Other health problems that are more common among older adults and also increase the risk for acidosis include renal impairment (kidney disease) and any type of chronic pulmonary problem, especially emphysema and COPD. The risk for acidosis is low when the patient is taking the drug in eye-drop form. However, misuse or overuse of the drug can lead to acidosis and other systemic problems.

> **Clinical Pitfall**
>
> Do not give carbonic anhydrase inhibitors to children or women who are pregnant or breastfeeding.

ⓔ-Learning Activity 26-4 ▶

## Get Ready for Practice!

### Key Points

- Use aseptic technique when instilling eye drugs because the eye can easily become infected.
- Apply only ointments that are labeled "for ophthalmic use" in the eye.
- Place eye drops or eye ointments only in the affected eye.
- If both eyes are to be treated and one eye is infected, use a separate bottle or tube for each eye.
- Place the drops or ointment into a pocket created by gently pulling the lower lid downward.
- Never touch any part of the patient's eye with the tip of the bottle or tube.
- Drugs administered as eye drops can enter the blood and cause systemic effects.
- When instilling eye drops that can have systemic effects, apply gentle pressure to the corner of the eye nearest the nose (the inner canthus where the drainage ducts are located) for 1 to 2 minutes after instilling the drops.
- Teach the patient to use eye drops or ointments exactly as directed and never to use more drug than prescribed.
- Glaucoma can occur at any age and can affect one or both eyes.
- Untreated glaucoma leads to blindness.
- The goal of glaucoma therapy is to keep the IOP within normal range and prevent loss of photoreceptors.
- Most drugs for glaucoma come in different strengths; be sure to check the strength of the drug that you have on hand with that of the prescription to prevent overdosing or underdosing.

- Adrenergic agonists cause the pupils to dilate and the eye to be more sensitive to light. Urge patients to wear dark glasses or a hat with a brim in bright conditions.
- Beta blockers and cholinergic drugs make the pupil smaller even in low-light conditions. Teach patients to be more cautious in dim lighting to avoid falls and to use more light to read or do close work.
- Beta blockers and cholinergic drugs, if absorbed systemically, can slow the heart rate, lower blood pressure, and cause asthma. Be sure to warn patients about these side effects and tell them to notify their prescriber if symptoms appear or worsen.
- Warn patients with diabetes that beta blockers can mask the symptoms of hypoglycemia. Blood glucose levels may need to be checked more often.
- Over time the prostaglandin agonist eye drops change the color of the iris to brown, darken the eyelids, and increase the number and length of eyelashes.

### Additional Learning Resources

ⓔvolve Go to your Evolve website (http://evolve.elsevier.com/Workman/pharmacology/) for the following FREE learning resources:

- eLearning Activities
- Animations
- Video Clips
- Interactive Review Questions
- Audio Key Points
- Audio Glossary

- Audio Glossary—Spanish-English
- Drug Dosage Calculators
- Patient Teaching Handouts

**SG** Go to your Study Guide for additional learning activities to help you master this chapter content.

## Review Questions

1. You are teaching a family member to apply eye drops before a patient's surgery. Into which exact area do you instruct the drops to be instilled?
   A. The corner of the eye nearest the nose
   B. The corner of the eye nearest the side of the head
   C. The center of the eye where the pupil is located
   D. The pocket created by pulling down the lower lid

2. A patient asks you why untreated glaucoma leads to blindness. What is your best response?
   A. "The lens dries out, becomes compacted, and loses its clarity."
   B. "The cornea bulges outward, and the light rays are focused on the 'blind spot.'"
   C. "The blood vessels of the eye are compressed, and the nerve receptors die from lack of oxygen."
   D. "The center of the eye hemorrhages and becomes filled with blood, preventing light from reaching the nerve receptors."

3. Which action by a beta-adrenergic blocking agent controls glaucoma?
   A. Dilation of the pupil, improving aqueous humor flow
   B. Constriction of the pupil, pulling it forward to allow fluid flow
   C. Inhibiting the secretion of aqueous humor from the ciliary bodies
   D. Dilation of the blood vessels in the trabecular meshwork, improving fluid reabsorption

4. Which patient response is most important to check after administering an adrenergic agonist for control of glaucoma?
   A. Heart rate and rhythm
   B. 24-hour urine output
   C. Level of consciousness
   D. Pupil size and shape

5. A patient who has been using travoprost (Travatan) at home for glaucoma of the right eye tells you that the right eye is now brown and the left eye is still hazel. What do you instruct this patient to do?
   A. Nothing; this is an expected response to the drug
   B. Stop using the drug immediately and call the prescriber
   C. Go to the ophthalmologist's office as soon as possible
   D. Instead of instilling the eye drops at night, instill them in the morning

6. Which patient requires the closest observation for an adverse effect after receiving beta blocker eye drops to control glaucoma?
   A. 75-year-old man with severe asthma
   B. 38-year-old woman who is 8 months' pregnant
   C. 75-year-old woman with frequent kidney stones
   D. 12-year-old with diabetes who has developed glaucoma in the left eye after being hit in the eye with a baseball

7. A patient is prescribed latanoprost (Xalatan), 1 gtt per eye twice each day (every 12 hours) for control of glaucoma. The bottle contains 2.5 mL of drug, and 16 gtts = 1 mL. How many days will the bottle of eye drops last if the patient uses the drug exactly as prescribed? _____ days

8. If a patient is to use an eye-drop form of a drug that contains 1.5 mcg/gtt, what dose of the drug does the patient have if the drug is used every 6 hours at 2 drops per eye? _____ mcg/day

## Critical Thinking Activities

Mrs. Lucita Lopez is a 77-year-old woman who has been diagnosed with glaucoma. She also has type 2 diabetes and mild congestive heart failure. She takes a sulfonylurea for diabetes and a diuretic daily for the heart failure. Her insurance will only pay for timolol (Timoptic) as the prescription drug to control her glaucoma. She is to place 1 drop in each eye every 12 hours.

1. What type of drug is timolol?

2. Which of these questions is most important to ask Mrs. Lopez before giving her the first dose of the drug? Provide a rationale for your choice.
   - Do you have an allergy to sulfa drugs?
   - Are you taking a drug that is an MAO inhibitor?
   - Do you ever have asthma or trouble breathing?
   - Do you have difficulty passing urine?

3. Which technique for administering eye drops is most important for Mrs. Lopez? Provide a rationale for your choice.
   - Obtaining two separate bottles, one for the right eye and one for the left
   - Using punctal occlusion immediately after instilling the eye drops
   - Lying down for 15 minutes after using the drug
   - Not applying this drug within 15 minutes of taking the furosemide

4. What specific precautions for preventing diabetic complications should you teach Mrs. Lopez?

# Drugs for Cancer Therapy

evolve

http://evolve.elsevier.com/Workman/pharmacology/

## Objectives

*After studying this chapter you should be able to:*

1. Describe how normal cells become cancer cells.
2. Distinguish the features of normal cells from those of benign tumors and cancer cells.
3. List the common sites of distant metastasis for cancer.
4. Explain the basis for combination chemotherapy for cancer.
5. List the common side effects of cancer chemotherapy.
6. Describe how to manage and document an episode of extravasation.

7. Explain what to teach the patient and family to prevent infection during periods of neutropenia.
8. Explain what to teach the patient and family to prevent injury during periods of thrombocytopenia.
9. Describe life span considerations for cancer chemotherapy.
10. Explain the rationale for hormone manipulation therapy.
11. Discuss the uses of biological response modifiers as supportive therapy in the treatment of cancer.
12. Explain the basis of targeted therapy for cancer.

## Key Terms

**apoptosis** (ă-pŏp-TŌ-sĭs) (p. 485) Programmed cell death (cellular suicide).

**benign tumors** (bē-NĪN TŪ-mŭrz) (p. 482) Types of abnormal cell growth that are usually harmless.

**cancer** (KĂN-sŭr) (p. 482) Abnormal cell growth that serves no useful purpose, is invasive, and without intervention would lead to death. Also known as *malignancy.*

**carcinogen** (kăr-SĬN-ō-jĕn) (p. 486) Any substance or event that can damage the DNA of a normal cell and cause cancer development.

**cyclins** (SĪ-klĭnz) (p. 485) Proteins that promote cells to enter and complete cell division.

**cytotoxic effects** (sī-tō-TŎKS-ĭk ĕf-FĔKTS) (p. 488) Cell-damaging and cell-killing effects.

**emetogenic** (ĕm-ĕ-tō-JĔN-ĭk) (p. 494) Substance that induces vomiting.

**extravasation** (ĕks-trăv-ĕ-SĀ-shŭn) (p. 490) Leakage of an irritating chemotherapy drug into the tissues surrounding the vein used to infuse the drug.

**hyperplasia** (hī-pŭr-PLĀ-zhă) (p. 483) Tissue growth caused by an increased number of cells.

**hypertrophy** (hī-PŬR-trō-fē) (p. 483) Tissue growth caused by an increase in the size of each cell.

**malignant transformation** (mă-LĬG-nĕnt trănz-fŭr-MĀ-shŭn) (p. 486) The many-stepped process by which a normal cell

changes into a cancer cell; also known as *carcinogenesis* and *oncogenesis.*

**metastasis** (mĕ-TĂS-tĕ-sĭs) (p. 486) The spread of cancer cells to other body areas, where they may grow and damage additional tissues and organs, often leading to death.

**mitosis** (mī-TŌ-sĭs) (p. 483) Tissue growth by cell division, whereby one cell divides to form two new cells.

**mucositis** (myū-kō-SĪ-tĭs) (p. 495) Inflammation and ulcers in mucous membranes, especially in the mouth.

**neoplasia** (nē-ō-PLĀ-zhă) (p. 483) New or continued cell growth not needed for normal development or replacement of dead and damaged tissues. It can be benign or cancerous.

**neutropenia** (nū-trō-PĒ-nē-ă) (p. 493) Severe white blood cell suppression with increased risk for life-threatening infections.

**primary tumor** (PRĪ-măr-ē TŪ-mŭr) (p. 486) The original site in which normal cells develop into cancer.

**thrombocytopenia** (thrŏm-bō-sī-tō-PĒ-nē-ă) (p. 493) Reduced numbers of platelets, a problem that increases the risk for bleeding.

**vesicants** (VĔS-ĭ-kănts) (p. 490) Drugs and chemicals that cause tissue damage on direct contact.

---

☉-Learning Activity 27-1 ►

## REVIEW OF RELATED PHYSIOLOGY AND PATHOPHYSIOLOGY

Abnormal cell growth such as a mole or a skin tag is common. These benign tumors are types of abnormal cell growth that are usually harmless unless they compress vital tissues. On the other hand, cancer is abnormal cell growth that serves no useful

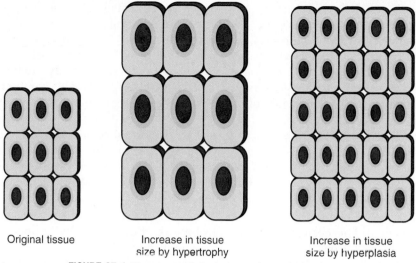

Original tissue          Increase in tissue          Increase in tissue
                         size by hypertrophy          size by hyperplasia

**FIGURE 27-1** Tissue growth by hypertrophy and hyperplasia.

purpose, is invasive, and without intervention would lead to death. Cancer is a common health problem in North America, with more than 1.3 million people being newly diagnosed each year.

Growth of cells and tissues is expected during infancy and childhood, and many body cells continue to grow long after maturation is complete. Mitosis is tissue growth by cell division, whereby one cell divides to form two new cells. Some cells continue to grow by mitosis throughout life. These cells are located in tissues where constant damage or wear is likely and continued cell growth is needed to replace dead tissues. For example, cells of the skin; hair; mucous membranes; bone marrow; and linings of organs such as the lungs, stomach, intestines, bladder, and uterus continue to grow by mitosis even in adults. This growth is well controlled, ensuring that only the right number of cells is always present in any tissue or organ.

Some tissues and organs stop growing by cell division after development is complete. For example, heart muscle cells no longer divide after fetal life; the number of heart muscle cells is fixed at birth. The size of the heart increases as the person grows because each cell becomes larger but the number of heart muscle cells does not increase. Hypertrophy is tissue growth caused by an increase in the size of each cell. Hyperplasia is tissue growth caused by an increased number of cells (Figure 27-1).

Neoplasia is any new or continued cell growth not needed for normal development or replacement of dead and damaged tissues. This cell growth is always abnormal, even if it causes no harm. Whether the new cells are benign or cancerous, neoplastic cells develop from normal cells *(parent cells)*. Thus cancer cells were once normal cells but changed to no longer look, grow, or function normally. The strict processes controlling normal growth and function have been lost. To understand how cancer cells grow, it is helpful to first understand the regulation and function of normal cells.

## FEATURES OF NORMAL CELLS

Normal cells share several important features in the way they grow and function, including limited division, specific morphology, differentiated function, tight adherence, nonmigration, regulated growth, contact inhibition, and apoptosis.

*Limited cell division* occurs because normal cells divide *(undergo mitosis)* for only two reasons: to develop normal tissue or replace lost or damaged tissue. Even when they are capable of mitosis, normal cells divide only when body conditions and nutrition are just right.

 **Did You Know?**

Cancer was first described more than 2000 years ago as a "crab-like" swelling tumor that could spread. The astrologic sign for cancer is a crab.

 **Memory Jogger**

Cancer cells were once normal cells that lost the strict control processes for normal growth and function.

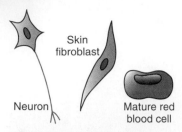

**FIGURE 27-2** Example of the specific shapes of normal cell types.

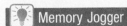

Memory Jogger

Normal tissue cells do not leave one organ and invade another.

*Specific morphology* is the feature in which each normal cell type has a distinct and recognizable appearance, size, and shape. For example, Figure 27-2 shows how the appearances of a red blood cell, a skin cell, and a nerve cell are different.

*Differentiated function* is a feature of normal cells. Every normal cell has at least one special function that it performs to contribute to whole-body function. For example, ovary cells make estrogen, liver cells make bile, muscle cells contract, nerve cells transmit signals, and white blood cells (WBCs) recognize and attack invading bacteria.

*Tight adherence* is the tight binding together of normal cells within one tissue. It occurs because normal cells make a protein *(fibronectin)* that protrudes from the membranes, allowing cells to bind closely and stick together, preventing them from leaving the tissue. Exceptions are red blood cells (RBCs) and WBCs. These cells do not produce fibronectin and do not usually stick together.

*Nonmigration* means that normal cells do not move throughout the body (except for blood cells). This occurs in normal cells because they are tightly bound together, which keeps cells from moving from one tissue into the next.

*Orderly and well-regulated growth* is a strong feature of normal cells. These cells do not divide unless body conditions are optimal for cell division. These conditions include the need for more cells, adequate space, and sufficient nutrients and other resources. Cell division *(mitosis)* occurs in the well-recognized pattern described by the cell cycle. Figure 27-3 shows the phases and activities of the cell cycle, in which one cell divides to form two new cells.

- **$G_1$:** The cell prepares for division by taking on extra nutrients, making more energy, increasing fluid, and growing a larger membrane.
- **S:** Making one cell into two cells requires twice as much of everything, including DNA in the nucleus. In the S phase the cell must double its DNA content through DNA synthesis. (Note that in Figure 27-3, the nucleus is now twice the size it was in $G_1$ phase.)
- **$G_2$:** The cell makes important proteins that will be used in actual cell division and in normal physiologic function after cell division is complete.
- **M:** The single cell splits apart into two cells (actual mitosis). First, the large nucleus (with double the DNA in it) separates into two nuclei. Then the cell is pulled apart into two new cells, each with one nucleus.

Living cells not actively reproducing are in a reproductive resting state called $G_0$. During the $G_0$ period cells actively work and function but do not divide. Normal cells spend most of their lives in the $G_0$ state.

In mitotic cell division one cell divides into two cells. These two cells are identical to each other and to the original cell that started the mitosis. The steps of

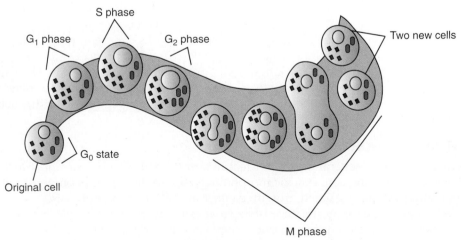

**FIGURE 27-3** Activities inside the cell during different phases of the cell cycle. The yellow circle is the nucleus.

entering and completing the cell cycle are tightly controlled by proteins produced by *suppressor genes*.

Control of whether or not a cell enters the cell cycle and completes the cycle to form two new cells depends on the presence and absence of specific proteins. Proteins that promote cells to enter and complete cell division belong to a group known as **cyclins.** When cyclins are activated, they first allow a cell to leave the $G_0$ state and enter the cycle. These activated cyclins then permit the cell to move through the different phases of the cell cycle and actually divide. The cyclins are the products of *oncogenes*. Proteins produced by suppressor genes regulate the amount of cyclins present in a cell and ensure that cell division occurs only when it is needed. So normal cell division represents a balance between the proteins that promote cell division (cyclins) and those that limit cell division (suppressor gene products).

*Contact inhibition* is the stopping of further rounds of cell division when the dividing cell is completely surrounded and touched (contacted) by other cells. A normal cell divides only when some of its surface is not in direct contact with another cell. Once a normal cell is in direct contact on all surface areas with other cells, its growth is inhibited (contact inhibited).

**Apoptosis** is programmed cell death (cellular suicide). Normal cells have a specific life span. When a signal for apoptosis occurs, the normal cell responds by destroying its own membrane, resulting in cellular suicide. The purpose of apoptosis is to ensure that each organ has an adequate number of cells at their functional peak.

## FEATURES OF CANCER CELLS

Body cells are exposed to internal and external conditions that can damage genes and change how the cells grow or function. When either cell growth or cell function is changed, the cells are abnormal. Table 27-1 compares features of normal cells, benign tumor cells, and cancer cells.

Benign tumor cells are normal cells growing in the wrong place or at the wrong time. Examples include moles, uterine fibroid tumors, skin tags, endometriosis, and nasal polyps. They are not needed for normal function but retain these normal cell features:

- Normal appearance and function
- Tight adherence
- No migration
- Orderly growth pattern, even though their growth is not needed

The most important difference between benign tumors and cancers is that benign tumors grow by enlargement only. They do not invade.

On the other hand, cancer cells are abnormal, serve no useful function, and are harmful to normal body tissues. Cancers commonly have features of rapid or continuous division, anaplasia, lost functions, loose adherence, migration, and no contact inhibition.

- Rapid or continuous cell division occurs because cancer cells reenter the cell cycle for mitosis almost continuously. They also may divide more quickly than normal cells and do not respond to signals for apoptosis. As a result, cancer cells have an unlimited life span (are "immortal").

**Memory Jogger**

Genes that make proteins to promote cell division are oncogenes. Genes that make proteins to control cell division are suppressor genes.

**Memory Jogger**

The most critical feature of normal cells is the careful balance between controlled cell division and appropriate cell death.

**Memory Jogger**

Benign tumors grow by enlargement and do not invade other tissues or organs.

### Table 27-1   Features of Normal and Abnormal Cells

| CHARACTERISTIC | NORMAL CELLS | BENIGN TUMORS | CANCER CELLS |
|---|---|---|---|
| Cell division | None or slow | Continuous or inappropriate | Rapid, continuous |
| Appearance | Specific features | Specific features | Anaplastic |
| Differentiated functions | Many | Many | Some or none |
| Adherence | Tight | Tight | Loose |
| Migratory | No | No | Yes |
| Growth | Well regulated | Expansion | Invasion |

Box **27-1**     Examples of Known Chemical and Physical Carcinogens

- Aflatoxins
- Alcoholic beverages
- Aminobiphenyls
- Arsenic
- Asbestos
- Azothioprine
- Benzene
- Benzidine
- Beryllium
- Cadmium
- Chlorambucil
- Chromium
- Coal tar
- Coke oven emissions
- Cyclophosphamide

- Cyclosporin A
- Diethylstilbestrol
- Dioxin
- Drug mixtures containing phenacetin
- Dyes containing benzidine
- Erionite
- Estrogens
- Ether
- Ethylene oxide
- Melphalan
- Mineral oils
- Myleran
- Naphthylamine
- Nickel

- Nitrogen mustard
- Nitrosoureas
- PUVA
- Radiation (all types)
- Silica
- Soot
- Sulfuric acid
- Tamoxifen
- Thiotepa
- Tobacco smoke (and all other forms)
- Vinyl chloride
- Wood dust

Compiled from National Toxicology Program (2005): *Report on carcinogens* (11th ed.). Available online at http://ntp.niehs. hih.gov/. Accessed June 2009.
*PUVA*, Psoralen plus ultraviolet light of A wavelength.

- *Anaplasia* is the feature in which cancer cells lose the specific appearance of their parent cells. As a cancer cell becomes more malignant, it becomes smaller and rounded. This change in appearance can make identifying a specific cancer type more difficult.
- Specific functions are lost partially or completely in cancer cells. Cancer cells serve no useful purpose.
- Loose adherence is common for cancer cells because they do not make the protein that keeps cells tightly adherent. This change allows cancer cells to easily break off from the main tumor.
- Migration occurs because cancer cells do not bind tightly together and have many enzymes on their cell surfaces. These features allow the cells to slip through blood vessels and tissues, spreading from the main tumor site to many other body sites. **Metastasis** is the spread of cancer cells to other body areas, where these cells grow, invade, and damage important organs, often leading to death. They invade tissues both near and far away from the original tumor. Invasion and persistent growth make untreated cancer deadly.
- Contact inhibition does not occur in cancer cells, even when all sides of these cells are in continuous contact with the surfaces of other cells.

## CANCER DEVELOPMENT

The multistep process of changing a normal cell into a cancer cell is called **malignant transformation**, also known as *carcinogenesis* and *oncogenesis*. The first step in cancer development is damage to the genes controlling cell division (*suppressor genes*) and allowing the genes promoting cell growth (*oncogenes*) to be activated.

**Carcinogens** are substances or events that can damage the DNA of a normal cell and cause cancer development. They may be chemicals, physical agents, or viruses. Box 27-1 lists some common carcinogens.

The original site in which normal cells develop into cancer is called the **primary tumor**. It is identified by the tissue from which it arose (parent tissue) such as breast or lung cancer. When primary tumors are located in vital organs such as the brain or lungs, they grow excessively and damage the vital organ so it cannot perform vital functions; death follows. Metastasis (spread) occurs when cancer cells move from the primary location by breaking off from the original group and establishing new tumors in remote areas.

Tumors that have spread and formed new tumors elsewhere are called *metastatic* or *secondary tumors*. Even though the tumor is now in another organ, it is still a cancer from the original altered tissue. For example, when breast cancer spreads to the lung

 **Memory Jogger**

Cancers spread by:
- Direct extension into nearby tissues and organs.
- Moving through the blood.
- Moving through the lymphatic system.

| Table **27-2** | Usual Sites of Metastasis for Common Cancers | | |
|---|---|---|---|
| **CANCER TYPE** | **SITES OF METASTASIS** | **CANCER TYPE** | **SITES OF METASTASIS** |
| Breast cancer | Bone*<br>Lung*<br>Liver<br>Brain | Melanoma | Gastrointestinal tract<br>Lymph nodes<br>Lung<br>Brain |
| Prostate cancer | Bone (especially spine<br>  and legs)<br>Pelvic nodes<br>Liver | Colorectal | Liver*<br>Lymph nodes<br>Adjacent structures |
| Lung cancer | Brain*<br>Bone<br>Liver<br>Lymph nodes<br>Pancreas | Primary brain<br>  tumors | Central nervous system |

*Most common site of metastasis.

and bone, it is breast cancer in the lung and bone, not lung cancer and not bone cancer. Table 27-2 lists the common sites of metastasis for specific tumor types.

## CANCER CLASSIFICATION

Cancers are first classified by the type of tissue from which they arise (for example, glandular, connective). About 100 different types of cancer arise from various tissues or organs. Cancers are divided into two major categories: solid and hematologic. Solid tumors develop from specific tissues (for example, breast and lung). Hematologic cancers (for example, leukemias and lymphomas) arise from blood cell–forming tissues. Cancers that arise from glandular tissue are *carcinomas* and are more common among adults. Glandular tissues include the linings of the GI tract, the lungs, the ducts of the breast, prostate tissues, and any other glands that secrete substances. Cancers that arise from connective tissue are *sarcomas* and are more common among children. Connective tissues include bone, muscle, fibrous tissue, blood, glial cells of the brain, and other support tissues. Cancer therapy is selected on the basis of cancer type, tumor size, how aggressive the cancer is, and whether the cancer has spread from its original site.

## CANCER CAUSES

Cancer development takes years and depends on several tumor and patient factors. Three interacting factors influence cancer development: exposure to carcinogens, genetic predisposition, and immune function.

*Oncogene activation* is the main mechanism of carcinogenesis, regardless of the specific cause. When activated, these genes produce proteins (cyclins) that promote cell division. Oncogenes are controlled by the products of suppressor genes. When a normal cell is exposed to any carcinogen, the DNA of the normal cell can be damaged or mutated. The mutations damage suppressor genes, preventing them from controlling the activity of oncogenes. As a result the oncogenes are overactive, and excessive growth occurs, causing the cells to change from normal cells to cancer cells. Both external and personal factors can inactivate suppressor genes.

Personal and external factors increase the risk for cancer development. External factors, including environmental exposure, are responsible for about 80% of cancer development. Environmental carcinogens are chemical, physical, or viral agents that cause cancer. Carcinogens can be:

- Chemicals (including those in tobacco).
- Physical agents (radiation and chronic irritation of tissues).
- Certain viruses known as *oncoviruses* (including the human papilloma virus, hepatitis B virus, hepatitis C virus, hepatitis D virus, human immune deficiency virus).

 **Memory Jogger**

Carcinomas grow from glandular tissues, and sarcomas grow from connective tissues.

 **Memory Jogger**

Suppressor gene inactivation leading to oncogene activation is the main mechanism of carcinogenesis.

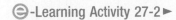-Learning Activity 27-2 ▶

 **Memory Jogger**

Advancing age is the most important risk factor for cancer. Exposure to carcinogens adds up over a lifetime, and immune protection decreases with age.

 **Memory Jogger**

Common cancer therapies include:
- Surgery.
- Radiation.
- Chemotherapy.
- Hormone manipulation.
- Photodynamic therapy.
- Immunotherapy.
- Targeted therapy.

 **Memory Jogger**

Unlike surgery and radiation, which are local therapies, chemotherapy is systemic, circulating to most body areas.

 **Memory Jogger**

The six major chemotherapy drug categories are:
- Antimetabolites.
- Antitumor antibiotics.
- Antimitotics.
- Alkylating agents.
- Topoisomerase inhibitors.
- Miscellaneous drugs.

- Possible dietary factors (high-fat, low-fiber diet; diets containing preservatives or contaminants; preparation methods [smoked, pickled, charcoal grilled]; and additives [dyes, flavorings, and sweeteners]).

Personal factors, including immune function, age, and genetic risk, also affect whether a person is likely to develop cancer. These factors interact with external factors to affect any person's risk for cancer. Cancer is more likely to occur in older people, those whose immune systems are not functioning at optimal levels, and those who have inherited a mutated gene that increases cancer risk.

## TYPES OF CANCER TREATMENT

The purpose of cancer treatment is to prolong survival time or improve quality of life. Although a few spontaneous regressions of cancer have been reported, most patients would die within months of diagnosis without cancer therapy.

Cancer therapies may be used alone or, more commonly, in combination to kill cancer cells. The types of therapy used depend on the specific type of cancer, whether or not the cancer has spread, and the health of the patient. Treatment regimens (*protocols*) have been established for most types of cancer based on experiments with cancer cells and experience with other patients with cancer. This chapter focuses on drugs used for cancer treatment, which include chemotherapy drugs, hormone manipulation, immunotherapy, and targeted therapy.

### CHEMOTHERAPY

*Chemotherapy,* the treatment of cancer with chemical agents, can increase survival time and cure the disease. The killing effect on cancer cells is related to the ability of chemotherapy to damage DNA and interfere with cell division. Thus the tumors most sensitive to chemotherapy are those that grow rapidly.

Patients with metastatic cancer will die unless treatment eliminates the metastatic cancer cells along with the original cancer cells. Chemotherapy is useful because its cytotoxic effects (cell-damaging and cell-killing effects) are systemic and can kill metastatic cancer cells that may have escaped local treatment. Chemotherapy used with surgery or radiation is termed *adjuvant therapy.*

Chemotherapy drugs damage both normal cells and cancer cells. The normal cells most affected by these drugs are those that divide rapidly, including skin, hair, intestinal tissues, and blood-forming cells. The drugs are classified by the types of action they exert in the cancer cell. Table 27-3 lists chemotherapy drugs and their potential to induce nausea and vomiting or damage surrounding tissue.

#### Chemotherapy Drug Categories

There are six categories of cancer chemotherapy drugs. The specific actions of each drug category are different, but the outcomes are the same: failure of cells to divide and cell death. All chemotherapy drugs are *high-alert drugs* that can cause serious harm if given at a dose that is too high or too low, if given to a patient for whom it was *not* prescribed, or if *not* given to a patient for whom it was prescribed. In addition, most of these drugs have a black box warning indicating that they are dangerous drugs and should be prescribed only when absolutely necessary.

*Antimetabolites* are similar to normal metabolites needed for vital cell processes. Most cell reactions require metabolites to begin or continue the reaction. Antimetabolite chemotherapy drugs act like "counterfeit" metabolites that fool cancer cells into using the antimetabolite in cellular reactions instead of the real metabolite. Because these drugs do not function as proper metabolites, their presence impairs cell division.

*Antitumor antibiotics* damage the DNA of the cell and interrupt DNA or RNA synthesis. Exactly how the interruptions occur varies with each agent.

*Antimitotic agents* interfere with the formation of tubules so cells cannot separate during cell division. As a result the cancer cell either does not divide at all or divides only once.

## Table 27-3  Chemotherapy Drug Categories

| DRUG | EMETOGENIC POTENTIAL | TISSUE DAMAGE POTENTIAL | DRUG | EMETOGENIC POTENTIAL | TISSUE DAMAGE POTENTIAL |
|---|---|---|---|---|---|
| **ANTIMETABOLITES** | | | **ALKYLATING AGENTS** | | |
| capecitabine (Xeloda) | Low | None (oral drug) | altretamine (Hexalen) | Moderate | None (oral drug) |
| cladribine (Leustatin) | Moderate | Bruising | busulfan (Busulfex, Myleran) | High | Bruising |
| cytarabine (Ara-C, Cytosar-U) | Moderate | Irritant | carboplatin (Paraplatin, Paraplatin-AQ🍁) | High | Irritant |
| decitabine (Dacogen) | Moderate | Irritant | carmustine (BiCNU) | High | Irritant |
| floxuridine (FUDR) | High | Bruising | chlorambucil (Leukeran) | High | None (oral drug) |
| fludarabine (Beneflur🍁, Fludara, FLAMP) | Low | Bruising | cisplatin (Platinol) | High | Irritant |
| 5-fluorouracil (Adrucil, Carac, Efudex, Fluoroplex) | Moderate | Irritant | cyclophosphamide (Cytoxan, Procytox🍁) | High | Bruising |
| gomcitabine (Gemzar) | Moderate | Bruising | estramustine (Emcyt, Estracyt) | Moderate | Vesicant |
| 6-mercaptopurine (Purinethol) | Low | None (oral drug) | ifosfamide (IFEX) | High | Bruising |
| methotrexate (Apo-Methotrexate🍁, Mexate, Folex) | Low - Moderate | Bruising | lomustine (CCNU, CeeNU) | High | None (oral drug) |
| 6-thioguanine (Lanvis) | Moderate - High | None (oral drug) | mechlorethamine (Mustargen) | High | Vesicant |
| | | | melphalan (Alkeran) | High | None (oral drug) |
| **ANTITUMOR ANTIBIOTICS** | | | oxaliplatin (Eloxatin) | Moderate - High | Vesicant |
| bleomycin (Blenoxane) | Moderate | Irritant | streptozocin (Zanosar) | High | Bruising |
| dactinomycin (Cosmegen) | High | Vesicant | temozolomide (Temodal🍁, Temodar) | Moderate - High | None (oral drug) |
| DAUNOrubicin (Cerubidine, DaunoXome) | High | Vesicant | thiotepa (Thioplex) | Low | Bruising |
| DOXOrubicin (Adriamycin, Caekys🍁, Doxil, Rubex) | High | Vesicant | **TOPOISOMERASE INHIBITORS** | | |
| epirubicin (Ellence, Pharmorubicin🍁) | High | Vesicant | irinotecan (Camptosar) | Moderate | Irritant |
| idarubicin (Idamycin) | Moderate - High | Vesicant | topotecan (Hycamtin) | Moderate | Irritant |
| mitomycin C (Mutamycin) | Moderate | Vesicant | **OTHER AGENTS** | | |
| mitoxantrone (Novantrone) | Low | Irritant | arsenic trioxide (Trisenox) | Moderate | Not Known |
| pentostatin (Nipent) | Moderate - High | Bruising | asparaginase (Elspar, Kidrolase🍁) | Low | Vesicant |
| plicamycin (Mithracin) | High | Irritant | dacarbazine (DTIC🍁) | Moderate - High | Irritant |
| valrubicin (Valstar) | None | None (intravesicular drug) | hydroxyurea (Apo-Hydroxyurea🍁, Droxia, Hydrea) | Low | None (oral drug) |
| | | | pegaspargase (Oncaspar) | Low | Bruising |
| **ANTIMITOTICS** | | | procarbazine (Matulane, Natulan🍁) | High | None (oral drug) |
| docetaxel (Taxotere) | Moderate | Bruising | | | |
| etoposide (Etopophos, Toposar, VP-16, VePesid) | Low | Irritant | | | |
| paclitaxel (Taxol) | Moderate | Irritant | | | |
| vinBLAStine (Velban, Velbe, Velsar) | Low - Moderate | Vesicant | | | |
| vinCRIStine (Oncovin, Vincasar PFS) | Low | Vesicant | | | |
| vinorelbine (Navelbine) | Low | Vesicant | | | |

*Alkylating agents* cross-link DNA, making the two DNA strands bind tightly together. This tight binding prevents proper DNA and RNA synthesis, inhibiting cell division.

*Topoisomerase inhibitors* disrupt an enzyme (topoisomerase) needed for DNA synthesis and cell division. This enzyme nicks and straightens the DNA helix, allowing the DNA to be copied, and then reattaches the DNA together. Topoisomerase inhibitor drugs prevent the actions needed for proper DNA maintenance, causing DNA breakage and cell death.

Other or *miscellaneous chemotherapy drugs* are those with mechanisms of action that are either unknown or do not fit those of other drug categories.

**Combination Chemotherapy.**    Combination chemotherapy is the combination of two or more anticancer drugs given on a specific timed schedule called a *protocol*. These combinations are much more successful at controlling cancer and killing cancer cells than any single drug would be. However, the side effects and damage caused to normal tissues also increase with combination chemotherapy. The selection of drugs is based on known tumor sensitivity to the drugs and the degree of side effects expected.

**Treatment Issues.**    Chemotherapy drugs are given on a regular basis and timed to maximize the number of cancer cells killed and minimize damage to normal cells. The schedule may vary somewhat to accommodate a patient's response to therapy. Most often chemotherapy is scheduled every 3 to 4 weeks for a specified number of times (usually 4 to 12 times). Protocols of giving higher doses of chemotherapy more often, called *dose-dense chemotherapy*, may be used for aggressive cancer treatment, especially for breast cancer. Dose-dense chemotherapy also results in more intense side effects than traditional schedules.

Chemotherapy has many unpleasant side effects. Patients and their families often need a great deal of education to understand why taking chemotherapy and maintaining the schedule are important for managing their cancer. Continuous support is needed to encourage patients to complete treatment protocols even when they feel tired and sick.

Most chemotherapy drugs are given intravenously, although other routes may be used for specific cancers. The standard of care designated by the Oncology Nursing Society (ONS) and supported by the American Society of Clinical Oncologists (ASCO) for safe administration of intravenous (IV) chemotherapy is that administration of these drugs requires special education and competency. This does not mean that only an advanced practice nurse can perform this function; however, it does mean that the individual must be a registered nurse who has completed an approved chemotherapy course.

All health care workers, including all licensed practical nurses/licensed vocational nurses and registered nurses, are responsible for providing care and comfort to patients during chemotherapy administration. Monitoring patient responses to therapy and managing side effects are important parts of nursing care during this period.

A major complication of IV infusion is extravasation, a condition in which a chemotherapy drug leaks into tissues surrounding the infusion site, causing tissue damage. When the drugs given are vesicants (chemicals that cause tissue damage on direct contact), the results of extravasation can include pain, infection, and tissue loss (refer to Figure 6-5, *B* in Chapter 6). Surgical intervention is sometimes needed for severe tissue damage. See Table 27-3 for a list of known vesicant and irritant chemotherapy drugs.

Most chemotherapy drugs are absorbed through the skin and mucous membranes. As a result, health care workers who prepare or give these drugs (especially nurses and pharmacists) are at risk for absorbing them. Anyone preparing, giving, or disposing of chemotherapy drugs or handling the wastes or excretions from patients within 48 hours after receiving IV chemotherapy should use extreme caution

**Memory Jogger**

All chemotherapy drugs affect both normal cells and cancer cells.

**Memory Jogger**

Combination chemotherapy uses multiple drugs from different categories to kill more cancer cells.

**Memory Jogger**

Schedules for chemotherapy administration are timed to maximize the number of cancer cells killed and minimize damage to normal cells.

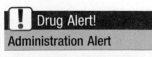

**Administration Alert**

Administration of IV cancer chemotherapy can only be performed by a registered nurse who has completed an approved chemotherapy course.

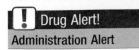

**Administration Alert**

Because chemotherapy drugs are dangerous and can be absorbed through skin and mucous membranes, always use PPE when mixing, handling, and giving these drugs and when handling the wastes and excretions of patients receiving them.

and wear personal protective equipment (PPE), including eye protection, mask, double gloves, and gown.

◀ⓔ-Learning Activity 27-3

### What To Do *Before* Giving Chemotherapy

Most IV chemotherapy is administered in outpatient settings by certified chemotherapy nurses. Because most chemotherapy drugs are highly toxic, precautions are needed to limit the exposure of these drugs to others and ensure patient safety.

Many chemotherapy drugs suppress bone marrow activity, especially white blood cell (WBC) production, increasing the patient's risk for infection. It is important to ensure that the patient's WBC count is high enough before administering chemotherapy. The WBC count is usually performed the day before or the morning of the scheduled treatment. Although there are exceptions, most agencies permit therapy only if the patient's total WBC is above 2000 cells/mm$^3$ or if the *absolute neutrophil count (ANC)*, which includes the segmented neutrophils ("segs," "polys," polymorphonuclear neutrophils [PMNs]) and band neutrophils ("bands"), is at least 1500 cells/mm$^3$. Check the patient's laboratory results for WBCs. Calculate the ANC by adding the number of segmented neutrophils and band neutrophils and multiplying this total by 1000. For example, if the WBC differential shows 1.8 segmented neutrophils and 0.5 band neutrophils, the total is 2.3. Multiply this number by 1000 for an ANC of 2300. Notify the prescriber if either the total WBC count or the ANC is lower than agency policy for chemotherapy.

Because many chemotherapy drugs are vesicants or irritants, make sure that the IV line is in a large vein and has an adequate blood return. Often the patient may have an implanted central catheter access with an internal or external port. These devices reduce the risk for extravasation but increase the risk for infection. Assess these devices before use and follow agency policy for preparing the skin and accessing these devices.

Doses for most chemotherapy drugs are calculated according to the type of cancer and the patient's size. Most commonly calculations are based on milligrams per square meter of total body surface area, which includes the patient's height and weight. So it is important to weigh the patient accurately each day that chemotherapy is to be administered before the dose is calculated. The dose is calculated by the prescriber, and the drugs are prepared by a pharmacist. Check the dose on the label and recalculate it based on the patient's weight or total body surface area. Notify the pharmacist and the prescriber if there is a dose discrepancy.

Each chemotherapy dose is prepared individually for the patient. Use two identifiers to ensure that the correct patient receives the drugs.

Chemotherapy drugs are powerful, and the patient may have a reaction during administration. If he or she has had chemotherapy before, ask whether he or she had any problems or changes during or after the drugs were administered. Take the patient's vital signs (including temperature and blood pressure) and assess mental status before therapy starts. Use these findings as a baseline to determine patient responses to chemotherapy.

Administer any prescribed premedications before starting chemotherapy. Such drugs may include antiemetics to prevent nausea and vomiting, anti-inflammatories, anti-anxiety drugs, and pain medications. (Review information about these premedication drugs in the chapters relating to these types of drug therapy.)

### What To Do *During* Chemotherapy

*Although the actual infusion of chemotherapy drugs is the responsibility of the chemotherapy-certified nurse or oncologist, monitoring the patient during chemotherapy is the responsibility of all health care personnel.* Instruct the patient to alert you immediately if he or she feels different in any way during the infusion.

Stay with the patient during the first 15 minutes of the infusion and retake vital signs. Thereafter check him or her every 15 minutes for any signs or symptoms of an allergic reaction: hives anywhere (especially at the IV site), low blood pressure, rapid and irregular pulse, swelling of the lips or lower face, the sensation of a "lump

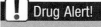

**Drug Alert!**

**Action/Intervention Alert**

Check the patient's WBC count on the morning of scheduled chemotherapy to make sure that it meets agency criteria for adequacy before giving the drugs.

**Clinical Pitfall**

Do not accept the patient's statement of weight or a previously recorded weight. Weigh the patient accurately on the day that he or she is to receive chemotherapy.

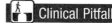

**Drug Alert!**

**Administration Alert**

Administer prescribed premedication on time to reduce unpleasant side effects.

| Box 27-2 | Documentation of Extravasation |
|---|---|

- Document the date and time when extravasation was suspected or identified.
- Document the date and time when the infusion was started.
- Record the time when the infusion was stopped.
- Document the exact contents of the infusion fluid and the volume of fluid infused.
- Document the estimated amount of fluid extravasated.
- Document the needle type and size.
- Diagram the exact insertion site.
- Indicate on the diagram the location and number of venipuncture attempts.
- Record the time between the extravasation and the last full blood return.
- Identify all agents administered in the previous 24 hours through this site (list agent administered, dosage and volume, and order of administration).
- Take and record the patient's vital signs.
- Take a photograph of the site.
- Document the administration of neutralizing or antidote agents.
- Document the application of compresses.
- Document other nursing interventions.
- Record the patient's responses to nursing interventions.
- Document the prescriber notification (including the time).
- Document the written and oral instructions given to the patient about follow-up care.
- Document any consultation request.
- Sign the documentation.

**Drug Alert!**

**Action/Intervention Alert**

When an allergic reaction or adverse event occurs, stop the drug from infusing but keep the IV access. If the drug is infusing high into the IV tubing, change the tubing after stopping the drug and do not let any drug that remains in the tubing run into the patient.

**Drug Alert!**

**Action/Intervention Alert**

Monitor the access site of any vesicant at least every 30 minutes to prevent extravasation or limit damage by preventing leakage of larger volumes.

**Drug Alert!**

**Action/Intervention Alert**

Compare assessment findings after chemotherapy with those obtained before administration.

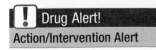

-Learning Activity 27-4 ►

in the throat," or any other type of adverse reaction. If the patient is having an anaphylactic or adverse reaction, your first action is to prevent any more drug from entering him or her. Stop the drug from infusing but keep the IV access. If the drug is infusing high into the IV tubing, change the tubing after stopping the drug and do not let any drug that remains in the tubing run into the patient.

The most important nursing intervention for extravasation is prevention. Assess the IV flow rate and infusion site at least every 30 minutes. Check for swelling or redness at the site, which may indicate extravasation. Determine whether a blood return is present. Ask the patient about any pain or burning at the infusion site. Small extravasations resolve without extensive treatment if less than 0.5 mL of the drug has leaked into the tissues. If a larger amount has leaked, extensive tissue damage occurs, and surgical intervention may be needed. So close monitoring of the access site is critical during chemotherapy administration to prevent leakage of larger volumes. Immediate treatment depends on the specific drug. Coordinate with the oncologist and pharmacist to determine the specific antidote needed for the extravasated drug. Box 27-2 outlines how to document an extravasation event.

Take vital signs and assess mental status according to agency policy during chemotherapy administration. Document all assessments.

### What To Do *After* Giving Chemotherapy

When chemotherapy administration is complete, discontinue the infusion set using PPE. Dispose of the set according to agency policy, usually in a biohazard container. Assess the infusion site and document your findings. If the access site is a temporary peripheral line, discontinue it after all prescribed IV support drugs have been given. If the access is an indwelling central line, care for the access site according to agency policy.

Assess the patient and compare the findings with those obtained before the chemotherapy session. Document all findings and notify the prescriber of any patient changes.

### What To *Teach* Patients About Chemotherapy

Temporary and permanent physical damage can occur to normal tissues from chemotherapy because this treatment is systemic and exerts its effects on both normal and cancer cells. Serious short-term side effects occur with aggressive chemotherapy.

| Box 27-3 | Patient Teaching Tips for Prevention of Infection During Neutropenia |
|---|---|

During the times that your white blood cell counts are low:
- Avoid crowds and other large gatherings of people who might be ill.
- Do not share personal toilet articles such as toothbrushes, toothpaste, washcloths, or deodorant sticks with others.
- If possible, bathe daily with an antimicrobial soap. If total bathing is not possible, wash the armpits, groin, genitals, and anal area twice a day with an antimicrobial soap.
- Clean your toothbrush daily by either running it through the dishwasher or rinsing it in a solution of 1 part liquid laundry bleach to 9 parts water (then rinsing the bleach out of the toothbrush by holding it under hot water for 1 minute).
- Wash your hands thoroughly with an antimicrobial soap before you eat or drink, after touching a pet, after shaking hands with anyone, as soon as you come home from any outing, and after using the toilet.
- Eat a low-bacteria diet and avoid salads, raw fruit and vegetables, pepper, paprika, and undercooked meat, fish, or eggs.
- Wash dishes with hot, sudsy water or use a dishwasher.
- Do not drink water, milk, juice, or other cold liquids that have been standing for longer than an hour.
- Do not reuse cups and glasses without washing first.
- Do not change pet litter boxes.
- Take your temperature at least once a day and whenever you do not feel well.
- Report any of the following signs or symptoms of infection to your prescriber immediately:
  - Temperature greater than 100° F (38° C)
  - Persistent cough (with or without sputum)
  - Pus or foul-smelling drainage from any open skin area or normal body opening
  - Presence of a boil or abscess
  - Urine that is cloudy or foul smelling or that causes burning on urination
- Take all prescribed drugs.
- Do not dig in the garden or work with houseplants.
- Wear a condom (if you are a man) when having sex. If you are a woman having sex with a male partner, ensure that he wears a condom.

Side effects that suppress bone marrow blood cell formation can be life threatening and are the most common reason for changing the dose or schedule. The suppressive effects on the bone marrow cause anemia, neutropenia, and thrombocytopenia. Less serious but common distressing side effects include nausea, vomiting, hair loss (*alopecia*), open sores on mucous membranes (*mucositis*), and changes in cognitive function. These side effects are referred to as cancer therapy *symptom distress*. Teach patients about these effects and actions to prevent complications.

***Neutropenia.***    Neutropenia is severe WBC suppression with increased risk for life-threatening infections. This critical problem is the reason that chemotherapy doses are reduced or delayed and is a common cause of death for patients. Most infections that develop during neutropenia from chemotherapy result from overgrowth of the patient's own normal flora.

Many patients remain at home during periods of neutropenia and are at continuing risk for infection, even though most home environments are likely to have fewer pathogenic organisms than a clinic or hospital setting. The focus remains on keeping the patient's own normal flora under control and preventing transmission of organisms from other people to the patient. Teach patients and family members the precautions used to reduce the risk for infection (Box 27-3).

***Thrombocytopenia.***    Thrombocytopenia is a reduced number of platelets. The normal platelet count ranges between 200,000 and 400,000/mm$^3$ and is important in ensuring that blood can form clots when needed to prevent hemorrhage. Thrombocytopenia increases the risk for excessive bleeding. When the platelet count is less than 50,000/mm$^3$, any small trauma can lead to prolonged bleeding. Patients with fewer than 20,000 platelets/mm$^3$ may have uncontrollable bleeding, requiring

 Memory Jogger

People who have neutropenia are at greater risk for infection but are not an infection hazard to others.

| Box 27-4 | Patient Teaching Tips for Preventing Injury or Bleeding During Thrombocytopenia |
|---|---|

During the time your platelet count is low:
- Use an electric shaver.
- Use a soft-bristled toothbrush and do not floss.
- Do not have dental work performed without consulting your oncologist.
- Do not take aspirin or any aspirin-containing products. Read the labels of over-the-counter drugs to be sure that the product does not contain aspirin or salicylates.
- Do not participate in contact sports or any activity likely to result in your being bumped, scratched, or scraped.
- If you are bumped, apply ice to the site for at least 1 hour.
- Avoid hard foods that would scrape the inside of your mouth.
- Eat warm, cool, or cold foods to avoid burning your mouth.
- Check your skin and mouth daily for bruises, swelling, or areas with small reddish-purple marks (petechiae) that may indicate bleeding.
- Notify your oncologist if you:
  - Are injured and persistent bleeding results.
  - Have excessive menstrual bleeding.
  - See blood in your urine or bowel movement.
- Avoid anal intercourse.
- Take a stool softener to prevent straining during bowel movements.
- Do not use enemas or rectal suppositories.
- Avoid bending over at the waist.
- Do not wear clothing or shoes that are tight or rub.
- Avoid blowing your nose or placing objects in your nose. If you must blow your nose, do so gently without blocking either nasal passage.
- Avoid playing musical instruments such as brass or woodwind instruments that raise the pressure inside your head.

**⓵ Drug Alert!**

**Action/Intervention Alert**

The patient with thrombocytopenia is at greatly increased risk for bleeding. Precautions are needed to prevent an uncontrollable bleeding episode.

transfusions of platelets or other blood products. Drug therapy for thrombocytopenia may include the use of oprelvekin (Neumega). This drug is a growth factor that specifically increases the production of platelets. See Chapter 17 for a more complete discussion of this drug.

Teach patients with thrombocytopenia and their families how to avoid injury and excessive bleeding when they are discharged before the platelet count has returned to normal. Box 27-4 lists tips to teach patients for how to prevent bleeding and what to do if bleeding occurs.

***Anemia.*** *Anemia* (reduced numbers of RBCs) results from the bone marrow suppression caused by some chemotherapy drugs. The normal range for RBCs is 4.2 to 6.1 million/mm$^3$ of blood. When RBC levels are lower than 2 million/mm$^3$ of blood, patients are fatigued and hypoxic. They may be short of breath and need supplemental oxygen. The use of biological response modifiers (BRMs) to stimulate bone marrow production of RBCs is common for some types of cancer. Erythropoiesis-stimulating agents such as darbepoetin alfa (Aranesp) and epoetin alfa (Epogen and Procrit) can prevent or improve anemia associated with chemotherapy and reduce the need for transfusion therapy. See Chapter 17 for a complete discussion of these drugs.

***Chemotherapy-Induced Nausea and Vomiting.*** Nausea and vomiting arise from many local and central nervous system mechanisms. Most chemotherapy drugs are emetogenic (induce vomiting) to some degree, depending on the dose. Most drugs induce nausea and vomiting when given and for 1 to 2 days afterward. Some drugs, such as cisplatin, induce delayed nausea and vomiting that can continue as long as 5 to 7 days after receiving it. Nausea and vomiting often can be controlled well with appropriate drug therapy. One or more antiemetic drugs are usually given before and after chemotherapy. Patient response to antiemetic therapy is highly variable,

| Box 27-5 | Patient Teaching Tips for Managing Mucositis |
|---|---|

- Examine your mouth with a mirror and flashlight twice daily, including the roof, under the tongue, and between the teeth and cheek.
- Check for blisters, sores, or drainage.
- Report to your prescriber any new open areas and those with more drainage.
- Brush your teeth and tongue with a soft-bristled brush or sponges every 8 hours.
- Rinse your mouth with a solution of one half peroxide and one half normal saline every 12 hours.
- Avoid using alcohol or glycerin-based mouthwashes.
- Do not share your toothbrush with anyone.
- Clean your toothbrush daily by either running it through the dishwasher or rinsing it in a solution of 1 part bleach to 9 parts water (then rinsing the bleach out of the toothbrush by holding it under hot running water for 1 minute).
- Drink 3 or more liters of water per day, if possible.
- Take all antibiotics as prescribed.
- Use the topical analgesic drugs as prescribed or as needed.
- "Swish and spit" room-temperature tap water or normal saline as needed.
- Apply petrolatum jelly to your lips after mouth care and as needed.
- Avoid using tobacco or drinking alcoholic beverages.
- Avoid spicy, salty, acidic, dry, rough, or hard foods.
- Cool liquids before drinking or eating to prevent burns or irritation.
- If you wear dentures, use them only during meals.
- When not in place, soak dentures in an antimicrobial solution. Rinse thoroughly before placing dentures in your mouth.
- Perform mouth care before and after every meal.

and the drug combinations should be individualized for best effect. See Chapter 19 for a complete discussion of antiemetic therapy.

Drugs to prevent or reduce nausea and vomiting are most effective when used aggressively and on a scheduled basis. Work with the patient and prescriber to ensure adequate control of nausea and vomiting. Make sure that the patient receives antiemetics before each session of IV chemotherapy. Teach them to continue antiemetic therapy as prescribed, even when the nausea and vomiting appear controlled. If the patient stops taking the drugs, he or she should restart them at the first sign of nausea to prevent this side effect from becoming uncontrollable.

***Mucositis.*** Mucositis (inflammation and ulcers of mucous membranes) often develops in the entire GI tract, especially in the mouth *(stomatitis)*. Mouth sores are painful and interfere with eating. Frequent mouth assessment and oral hygiene are key in managing these sores. Stress the importance of frequent oral hygiene, including teeth cleaning and mouth rinsing. Because most patients with mucositis also have bone marrow suppression and are at risk for bleeding, they must take care to avoid trauma to the oral mucosa. Box 27-5 lists tips for teaching patients how to manage mucositis.

***Alopecia.*** *Alopecia* (hair loss) may occur as whole-body hair loss or be as mild as only a thinning of scalp hair. Reassure patients that hair loss is temporary. Hair regrowth usually begins about 1 month after chemotherapy ends. Inform the patient that the new hair may differ from the original hair in color, texture, and thickness. Assist him or her to cope with this body image change and teach him or her to prevent scalp injury by giving these instructions:

- Avoid direct sunlight on the scalp by using a hat or other head coverings.
- Sunscreen use is essential to prevent sunburn with even minimal sun exposure (many chemotherapy drugs increase sun sensitivity), regardless of skin color.
- Wear some head covering under helmets, headphones, headsets, and other items that rub the head. Also wear a head covering during cold weather to reduce body heat loss and prevent hypothermia.
- Use hats, caps, scarves, and wigs to improve body image during alopecia.

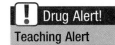

**Drug Alert!**

**Teaching Alert**

Teach patients taking antiemetics to take the drugs as scheduled for as long as prescribed to prevent nausea and vomiting from becoming uncontrollable.

**Memory Jogger**

Scalp hair loss (alopecia) not only alters body image, but it also increases the risk for scalp injury. Teach patients to protect the scalp from sun exposure and from items that rub the head.

*Changes in Cognitive Function.* Some patients have reported changes in cognitive function during cancer treatment and for months to years after treatment, most commonly as a reduced ability to concentrate, loss of memory, and difficulty learning new information. Patients often refer to this problem as "chemobrain." The exact cause of this side effect and personal risk factors for it are unclear. Support the patient who reports it. Listen to the patient's concerns and assure him or her that the problem is likely to resolve with time. Warn patients to avoid other behaviors that could alter cognitive functioning such as excessive alcohol intake, recreational drug use, and taking part in activities that increase the risk for head injury.

### Life Span Considerations for Chemotherapy

*Pediatric Considerations.* Younger children are diagnosed with cancer more often than are older children. Children have the same unpleasant and dangerous side effects from chemotherapy that adults do, and they may not understand why they must undergo this long treatment. Children seem to recover bone marrow function more quickly than adults.

*Considerations for Pregnancy and Breastfeeding.* Most chemotherapy drugs can induce birth defects during the first trimester and can have other adverse effects during the remainder of pregnancy. The use of cancer chemotherapy during pregnancy is not recommended; however, cancer is a potentially lethal disease. Some patients terminate the pregnancy, others delay treatment until after the baby is born, and others start chemotherapy during pregnancy. The decision of whether or when to use chemotherapy during pregnancy is left to the patient. Breastfeeding should be avoided during chemotherapy to avoid infant exposure to these powerful and toxic drugs.

*Considerations for Older Adults.* The side effects of neutropenia, nausea, vomiting, and peripheral neuropathy may have a greater impact on older adults. Immune function, especially the inflammatory response, declines with age. Combined with neutropenia, this age-related change results in a greater loss of immune protection and an increased risk for infection among older adults. Minor infections may be overlooked until the patient becomes severely infected or septic. Stress the importance of avoiding infection (see Box 27-3) and reporting any symptom of infection immediately to his or her prescriber.

Older adults can become dehydrated more quickly if chemotherapy-induced nausea and vomiting are not adequately controlled. Teach these patients to be proactive with taking their prescribed antiemetics and to contact their health care provider if the nausea and vomiting either does not resolve within 12 hours or becomes worse.

**⊖-Learning Activity 27-5 ▶**

## HORMONE MANIPULATION

Hormones are naturally occurring chemicals secreted by endocrine (ductless) glands and picked up by capillaries. Once in the bloodstream, hormones circulate to all body areas but exert their effects only on their specific target tissues. Some hormones make hormone-sensitive cancers grow more rapidly, and some cancers require specific hormones to divide. So decreasing the amount of hormones to hormone-sensitive tumors can slow cancer growth.

Hormone manipulation can control some types of cancer (for example, prostate cancer, breast cancer) for many years. Usually this therapy does not lead to a cure. As shown in Figure 27-4, prostate cancer is a hormone-sensitive cancer that grows faster when the hormone testosterone (an androgen) binds to its receptors. When an anti-androgen is given such as estrogen or flutamide (Eulexin), it binds to the testosterone receptors, preventing the patient's testosterone from binding to those sites. When anti-androgens are present, they block testosterone from enhancing the growth of prostate cancer cells. This action does not kill the cancer cells but just slows their

---

**⊘ Drug Alert!**

**Teaching Alert**

Teach women receiving cancer chemotherapy not to breastfeed until at least 1 month after the therapy is completed.

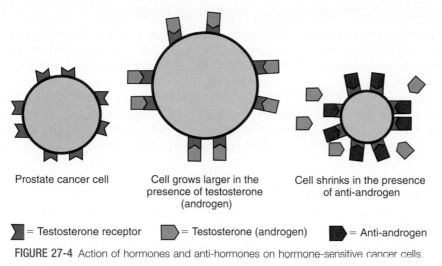

Prostate cancer cell

Cell grows larger in the presence of testosterone (androgen)

Cell shrinks in the presence of anti-androgen

= Testosterone receptor    = Testosterone (androgen)    = Anti-androgen

**FIGURE 27-4** Action of hormones and anti-hormones on hormone-sensitive cancer cells.

| Table 27-4 | Drugs Used for Hormone Manipulation of Cancer | | |
|---|---|---|---|
| **TYPE OF AGENT** | **EXAMPLE** | **TYPE OF AGENT** | **EXAMPLE** |
| **HORMONE AGONISTS** | | **HORMONE ANTAGONISTS** | |
| Androgen | fluoxymesterone (Androxy) methyltestosterone (Android, Methitest) | Anti-androgens | bicalutamide (Casodex) flutamide (Apo-Flutamide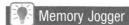, Eulexin, Novo-Flutamide🍁) |
| Estrogen | conjugated equine estrogen (Premarin) ethinyl estradiol (Estinyl) | Anti-estrogens | fulvestrant (Faslodex) tamoxifen (Apo-Tamox🍁, Nolvadex, Nolvadex D🍁, Soltamox, Tamofen🍁) |
| Progestin | medroxyPROGESTERone (Provera) megestrol (Apo-Megestrol🍁, Megace) | | toremifene (Fareston) |
| Luteinizing-hormone releasing hormone | leuprolide (Eligard, Lupron, Viadur) goserelin (Zoladex, Zoladex LA🍁) | **HORMONE INHIBITORS** | anastrozole (Arimidex) exemestane (Aromasin) letrozole (Femara) |

growth. When tumor growth is slowed, survival time increases. Table 27-4 lists drugs commonly used in hormone manipulation for cancer therapy.

Another class of drugs used for hormone therapy is the hormone inhibitors. These drugs inhibit production of specific hormones in the normal hormone-producing organs. For example, the aromatase inhibitor anastrozole (Arimidex) prevents production of estrogen in the adrenal gland and reduces blood estrogen levels. For breast cancer cells that need estrogen to grow, anastrozole limits the total amount of estrogen present and causes slower cancer cell growth.

### Side Effects

Androgens and the anti-estrogen receptor drugs cause masculinizing effects in women. Chest and facial hair may develop, menstrual periods stop, and breast tissue shrinks. Patients may have some fluid retention. For men and women receiving androgens, acne may develop, hypercalcemia is common, and liver dysfunction may occur with prolonged therapy. Women receiving estrogens or progestins have irregular but heavy menses, fluid retention, and breast tenderness. Men and women who take estrogen or progestins are at risk for deep vein thrombosis.

Feminine manifestations often appear in men who take estrogens, progestins, or anti-androgen receptor drugs. Facial hair thins, facial skin becomes smoother, body fat redistributes, and *gynecomastia* (breast development in men) can occur. Testicular and penile size decrease. Although sexual function may continue, achieving an erection is more difficult. Patients may benefit from professional counseling to manage problems with body image and sexual function.

**Memory Jogger**

Hormone manipulation can control the growth of some cancers but usually does not cure the cancer.

## IMMUNOTHERAPY: BIOLOGICAL RESPONSE MODIFIERS

Biological response modifiers (BRMs) modify a patient's biologic responses to tumor cells. The BRMs in current use as cancer therapy are cytokines, which are small protein hormones made by WBCs. Cytokines generally make the immune system work better.

Cytokines and other BRMs work as a cancer treatment by stimulating the immune system to recognize cancer cells and take actions to eliminate or destroy them. Some BRMs are also useful in a supporting role such as colony-stimulating factors that stimulate faster recovery of bone marrow function after treatment-induced suppression.

### BRMs as Cancer Therapy

Two common types of BRMs used as cancer therapy are the interleukins (ILs) and interferons. Some agents can stimulate specific immune system cells to attack and destroy cancer cells; other agents block cancer cell access to an essential function or nutrient.

ILs are a group of substances that the body makes to help regulate inflammation and immune protection. Some are now synthesized as drugs. They help different immune system cells recognize and destroy abnormal body cells. In particular, IL-1, -2, and -6 appear to "charge up" the immune system and enhance attacks on cancer cells by macrophages, natural killer cells, and tumor-infiltrating lymphocytes.

Interferons are cell-produced proteins that can protect noninfected cells from viral infection and replication. Cancer-related functions of some interferons include:

- Slowing tumor cell division.
- Stimulating growth and activation of natural killer cells (which attack cancer cells).
- Helping cancer cells resume a more normal appearance and function.
- Inhibiting the expression of oncogenes.

Interferons have been effective to some degree in the treatment of melanoma, hairy cell leukemia, renal cell carcinoma, ovarian cancer, and cutaneous T-cell lymphoma.

One drug classified as a BRM that has a somewhat different action is thalidomide (Thalomid), which reduces the formation of blood vessels in tumors. When tumor blood vessels are reduced, the tumor is poorly nourished, and cancer cells die. This drug is approved for treating multiple myeloma.

### BRMs as Supportive Therapy

BRMs used for supportive therapy during cancer treatment are the colony-stimulating factors. These factors induce more rapid recovery of the bone marrow after chemotherapy. When bone marrow suppression is shortened or less severe, patients are less at risk for life-threatening infections, anemia, and bleeding. Also, because the colony-stimulating factors allow more rapid bone marrow recovery, patients can receive their chemotherapy on time and may even be able to tolerate higher doses, improving the outcome of chemotherapy.

### Side Effects

Patients receiving interleukins may have generalized and severe inflammatory reactions. Fluid shifts and capillary leak are widespread, with edema forming in most tissues. Tissue swelling affects the function of all organs and can be life threatening. Patients receiving high-dose BRM therapy should receive care in an intensive care or monitoring unit. The effects of BRM therapy are limited to the period of acute drug infusion and resolve when treatment stops.

Many BRMs induce symptoms of mild inflammation during and immediately after receiving the drug, including fever, chills, rigors, and flulike achiness. Problems are worse when higher doses are given and become less severe over time. Fever is treated with acetaminophen. *Rigors* (severe shaking chills) are managed with meperidine (Demerol).

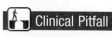 **Clinical Pitfall**

Colony-stimulating factors may stimulate the growth of leukemia cells and are not used with leukemia.

Interferon therapy causes peripheral neuropathy. Some of the problems resulting from neuropathy include decreased sensory perception, visual disturbances, decreased hearing, unsteady balance and gait, and orthostatic hypotension. It is not known whether the neuropathy is temporary or permanent.

Rash and skin dryness, itching, and peeling occur with many types of BRM therapy. The skin problems are more severe at higher doses and when more than one type of BRM is used at the same time. These reactions are temporary but can cause much discomfort and distress to the patient. Advise patients to apply moisturizer (perfume-free) to the skin and to use mild soap to clean the skin. Involved areas should be protected from the sun with clothing or sunscreen. Instruct patients to avoid using topical steroid creams on affected areas.

Thalidomide is a powerful *teratogen* (can cause severe birth defects) and should never be used with pregnant women. Women of childbearing age who are sexually active are advised to use at least two forms of contraception to avoid the possibility of pregnancy.

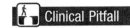

**Clinical Pitfall**

Never give thalidomide to a pregnant woman.

## TARGETED THERAPY

Targeted therapies combine aspects of gene therapy and immunotherapy. These therapies take advantage of one or more differences in cancer cell growth or metabolism that either are not present or are only slightly present in normal cells. These differences result from specific gene activation in cancer cells. Agents used as targeted therapies often are antibodies that work to disrupt cancer cell division in one of several ways. Some of these drugs "target" and block growth factor receptors, especially epithelial growth factor receptors (EGFRs) or vascular endothelial growth factor receptors (VEGFRs). When the growth a cancer cell depends on having the growth factors bind to their specific receptors, blocking the receptors slows or eliminates the growth.

Other agents for targeted therapy may be antibodies directed against a cellular substance needed by the cancer cell for growth or a substance in the signaling pathway of a cell that is important in turning on certain genes for cell growth. Figure 27-5 shows one type of signal transduction pathway in which events outside the cell and pathways inside the cell can be stimulated to turn on cell division.

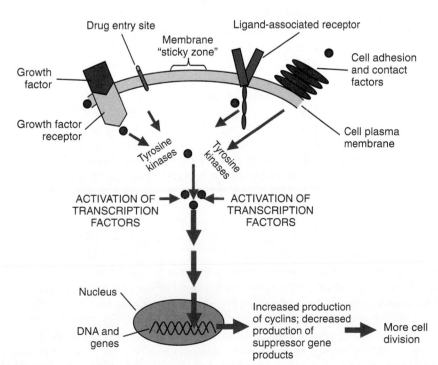

**FIGURE 27-5** Possible cancer cell targets for targeted therapy. The red circles indicate areas for activity of targeted therapies.

| Table 27-5 | Common Agents Used for Targeted Therapy | | |
|---|---|---|---|
| **AGENT** | **MALIGNANCY** | **AGENT** | **MALIGNANCY** |
| alemtuzumab (Campath) | Chronic lymphocytic leukemia | galiximab | Non-Hodgkin's lymphoma |
| azacitidine (Vidaza) | Myelodysplastic syndrome | gefitinib (Iressa) | Head and neck cancer; brain tumors |
| bevacizumab (Avastin) | Colorectal cancer; lung cancer | gemtuzumab (Mylotarg) | Acute myelogenous leukemia |
| bortezomib (Velcade) | Lymphoma; multiple myeloma | imatinib (Gleevec) | Chronic myelogenous leukemia |
| canertinib | Breast cancer (metastatic) | lapatinib (Tykerb) | Breast cancer (metastatic) |
| cetuximab (Erbitux) | Colorectal cancer; head and neck cancer | rituximab (Rituxan) | Non-Hodgkin's lymphoma |
| epratuzumab (LymphoCide) | Non-Hodgkin's lymphoma | sorafenib (Nexavar) | Renal cell carcinoma |
| erlotinib (Tarceva) | Pancreatic cancer; lung cancer | temsirolimus (Torisel) | Renal cell carcinoma |
| | | trastuzumab (Herceptin) | HER2 positive breast cancer |

There are many such pathways, and each pathway has many steps. Targeted therapy drugs can block one or more steps in a pathway so that the signal for turning on cell division genes does not reach the cell nucleus and excessive cell division is stopped. Figure 27-5 provides an overview of places within a cancer cell pathway that can be targeted by different targeted therapy drugs to control or stop cancer cell growth.

It is important to remember that targeted therapy drugs will not work unless the cancer cell overexpresses the actual target substance. So not all patients with the same cancer type would benefit from the use of targeted therapy. Each person's cancer cells must be tested in the laboratory to determine whether or not the cells have enough of a target to be affected by targeted therapy.

An example of a targeted therapy is trastuzumab (Herceptin). This EGFR antibody binds the excessive amounts of a certain type of EGFR produced by breast cancer cells in response to the activation of the HER2/neu gene. Binding this receptor prevents cancer cell division and makes the cells more easily killed by immune system cells. The drug rituximab (Rituxan) has a similar effect in some types of lymphoma. Another example of a targeted therapy drug is imatinib mesylate (Gleevec). This drug is most useful in cancers that overexpress the ABL1 oncogene such as Philadelphia chromosome-positive chronic myeloid leukemia. Table 27-5 lists some agents currently used for targeted therapy.

### Side Effects

Allergic reactions are an issue in patients receiving monoclonal antibodies. Most of these antibodies were developed in animals and may express some animal proteins. More recently much of the animal portion of these antibodies was removed, reducing but not eliminating the risk for allergic reactions. Patients receiving antibodies over time may develop their own antibodies to the drugs, making them less effective and possibly causing severe inflammatory or allergic reactions.

In addition, EGFR and VEGFR antibodies bind to those specific receptors when the receptors are on normal tissue. So side effects can occur in tissues that normally express these receptors such as the skin, mucous membranes, and lining of the GI tract.

**Memory Jogger**

Targeted therapies are effective only if the cancer cell has a target for the drug.

**Memory Jogger**

Because some normal cells have target receptors, targeted therapy drugs may cause side effects in skin and mucous membranes.

ℯ-Learning Activity 27-6 ▶

# Get Ready for Practice!

## Key Points

- Normal cells divide only when needed, and their growth is strictly controlled.
- Transformation of a normal cell into a cancer cell involves mutation of the genes (DNA) of the normal cell.
- Most tumors arise from cells that are capable of cell division.
- Carcinomas are more common in adults, and sarcomas are more common in children.
- The actions of chemotherapy drugs on cancer cells are related to their ability to damage DNA and interfere with cell division.
- The normal cells most affected by these drugs are those that divide rapidly, including skin, hair, intestinal tissues, spermatocytes, and blood-forming cells.
- Regardless of the exact mechanism of action for cancer drugs, the overall results are failure of cancer cells to divide, leading to cancer cell death.
- Although administration of chemotherapy should be performed only by chemotherapy-certified registered nurses, monitoring the patient during chemotherapy administration is a responsibility of all licensed practical nurses/licensed vocational nurses and registered nurses.
- When WBC counts are too low, chemotherapy is delayed until counts rise to acceptable levels.
- Extravasation of vesicants can lead to extensive tissue damage and tissue loss.
- The most important nursing intervention for extravasation is prevention.
- The side effects of chemotherapy that suppresses bone marrow blood cell formation can be life threatening and are the most common reason for changing the dose or schedule.
- The patient with neutropenia is at risk for infections from overgrowth of his or her own microorganisms and from the transfer of microorganisms of others.
- Just like pain medication, drugs for chemotherapy-induced nausea and vomiting are much more effective if given on a schedule rather than PRN.
- Hormone manipulation can help control the growth of hormone-sensitive cancers.
- Not all cancers of the same type have the right "targets" for targeted therapy.

## Additional Learning Resources

Ⓔvolve Go to your Evolve website (http://evolve.elsevier.com/Workman/pharmacology/) for the following FREE learning resources:
- eLearning Activities
- Animations
- Video Clips
- Interactive Review Questions
- Audio Key Points
- Audio Glossary
- Audio Glossary—Spanish-English
- Drug Dosage Calculators
- Patient Teaching Handouts

**SG** Go to your Study Guide for additional learning activities to help you master this chapter content.

## Review Questions

1. Which theory of carcinogenesis has the most support?
   A. DNA damage induces the activation of oncogenes.
   B. Cancer cells are ingested from animal-derived food products.
   C. Auto-antibodies attack specific normal healthy tissues.
   D. Embryonic tissues fail to undergo normal differentiation.

2. A patient asks why cancer cell growth is considered "uncontrolled?" What is your best response?
   A. "Cancer cells always divide more rapidly than normal cells."
   B. "When each cancer cell divides, it usually produces more than two cells."
   C. "As you age, your immune system is less active, which allows cancer cells to grow faster."
   D. "Cancer cells divide almost continuously, and normal cells divide only when they are needed."

3. A patient with prostate cancer reports that he is now having a lot of pain in his lower back and legs. What problem related to this symptom do you suspect this patient may have?
   A. Arthritis from position placement during 6 weeks of radiation therapy
   B. Severe urinary retention from a rapidly enlarging prostate gland
   C. Bone damage from cancer metastasis by direct tumor extension
   D. Muscle spasms from cancer metastasis by lymphatic invasion

4. A patient with breast cancer asks why so many drugs are used together to treat her cancer. What is your best response?
   A. "Each drug works against cancer cells in different ways, and using several increases the likelihood that the cancer will be cured."
   B. "By using several drugs together, we can avoid using radiation therapy, which would cause many more permanent side effects."
   C. "Each drug goes to a separate body area. That way, because your cancer has spread to so many areas, all areas with cancer will receive the right drug."
   D. "The doctors are not sure which drug will work best against the cancer type that you have. Using several at the same time improves the chances that one will work."

5. A patient receiving cancer chemotherapy is experiencing all of the following side effects or problems. Which one must be reported to the prescriber immediately?

   A. Eyebrows have fallen out
   B. Temperature of 101° F (38° C)
   C. Tingling and numbness of the toes
   D. Gums ooze blood after toothbrushing

6. You are monitoring a patient receiving IV chemotherapy that was started by a chemotherapy-certified nurse. After 2 hours the patient reports burning and pain at the IV site. Lowering the IV results in an observable brisk blood return. What is your best first action?

   A. Stop the drug infusion and run at least 100 mL of normal saline into IV access
   B. Notify the chemotherapy-certified nurse who started the infusion
   C. Slow the rate of infusion but continue it since there is a good blood return
   D. Discontinue the infusion, remove the IV, and document the site condition

7. Which intervention is the most important to teach a patient receiving chemotherapy with a drug that causes neutropenia?

   A. Eat a low-bacteria diet.
   B. Take a laxative or stool softener daily.
   C. Use a soft-bristled toothbrush and do not floss.
   D. Avoid using aspirin or aspirin-containing products.

8. Which intervention is the most important to teach a patient receiving chemotherapy with a drug that causes thrombocytopenia?

   A. Eat a low-bacteria diet.
   B. Take your temperature daily.
   C. Use a soft-bristled toothbrush and do not floss.
   D. Avoid using mouthwashes that contain alcohol.

9. Which intervention is the most important to teach an older patient receiving combination chemotherapy for cancer?

   A. Stop taking all other drugs while receiving cancer treatment.
   B. Wear a hat or scarf on your head when using earphones.
   C. Take double doses of vitamins to prevent malnutrition.
   D. Take your drugs for nausea and vomiting as prescribed.

10. A patient receiving tamoxifen (Nolvadex) asks how this therapy helps fight breast cancer. In addition to telling her that the breast cancer cells need estrogen to continue growing, what is your best response?

    A. "This agent decreases your circulating levels of estrogen."
    B. "This agent causes you to secrete testosterone instead of estrogen."
    C. "This agent kills off both the normal estrogen-secreting cells and the cancer cells."
    D. "This agent blocks the receptors for estrogen, reducing its availability to the cancer cells."

11. Which biological response modifier should you be prepared to administer to a patient who has chemotherapy-induced thrombocytopenia?

    A. filgrastim (Neupogen)
    B. oprelvekin (Neumega)
    C. epoetin alfa (Procrit)
    D. sargramostim (Leukine)

12. A patient who has just been diagnosed with lymphoma asks why the treatment plan does not include the new drug rituximab (Rituxan) about which he has read. What is your best response?

    A. "Your immune system is too weak to tolerate Rituxan."
    B. "This drug is experimental and too dangerous for you to take before trying other therapies."
    C. "Your lymphoma cells do not have the protein on which this drug works, so you would not benefit from this therapy."
    D. "You are young and can better tolerate the standard therapies for lymphoma that have been proven effective but have strong side effects."

13. A patient is prescribed tamoxifen (Nolvadex) 20 mg orally twice daily for a total daily dosage of 40 mg. The drug comes in 10-mg tablets. How many tablets does the patient take twice daily? _____ tablet(s)

14. An infant with cancer is to receive vinCRIStine (Oncovin) 0.05 mg/kg intravenously. The infant weighs 16 pounds (1 kg = 2.2 lb). What is the infant's weight in kilograms, and what is the appropriate dose?

    a. _____ kg
    b. _____ mg

## Critical Thinking Activities

The patient is a 15-year-old girl being treated with combination chemotherapy for Hodgkin's lymphoma. This is her second round of chemotherapy, and she is crying. When you ask her what's wrong, she tells you that she does not want to take "chemo" anymore because "this will cause her to be bald forever." Her mother screams that she has to take the chemo or she will die. The girl then says she would rather be dead than never have any hair.

1. Is the patient correct in thinking that her baldness is permanent?

2. Is the mother correct in thinking that her daughter will die if chemotherapy is stopped?

3. How should you intervene in this situation?

# Bibliography

Adamolekun, B. (2008). Seizure disorders. *The Merck Manuals Online Medical Library: Home Edition for Patients and Caregivers.* Available online at http://merck.com/mmhe/sec06/ch085/ch085a.html. Retrieved October 2009.

Amdipharm Plc. (2004). Nausea and vomiting—an introduction. Available online at http://www.nauseaandvomiting.co.uk/NAVRES001-2-NandV-general.htm. Retrieved October 2009.

American Heart Association. (2009). Anticoagulant drugs. Available online at http://www.americanheart.org/presenter.jhtml?identifier=155. Retrieved October 2009.

American Heart Association. (2009). Medications commonly used to treat heart failure. Available online at http://americanheart.org/presenter.jhtml?identifier=118. Retrieved October 2009.

Aschenbrenner, D.S. (2009). Ezetimibe-Simvastatin combination therapy: An update. *American Journal of Nursing, 109*(5), 30-31.

Aungst, H. (2009). Committee weighs in on asthma meds. *RN, 72*(2), 17.

Bademan, E.G. (2007). Act fast against severe hypoglycemia. *American Nurse Today, 2*(3), 32.

Barton-Burke, M., & Wilkes, G. (2006). *Cancer Therapies.* Boston: Jones & Bartlett.

Belavic, J. (2009). Fesoterodine for the treatment of overactive bladder. *The Nurse Practitioner, 34*(8), 14-15.

Boullata, J.I. (2009). Drug administration through an enteral feeding tube. *American Journal of Nursing, 109*(10), 34-42.

Bryant, H. (2007). Anaphylaxis: Recognition, treatment, and education. *Emergency Nurse, 15*(2), 24-28.

Busuttil-Leaver, R. (2008). Benign prostatic hyperplasia. *Practice Nurse, 36*(6), 19-23.

Cain, J.E., Daly, M.L., & Powers, J. (2007). Act fast against anaphylaxis. *American Nurse Today, 2*(2), 30.

Carey, L.P. (2007). Six hot drugs for today and beyond. *American Nurse Today, 2*(3), 12-14.

Centers for Disease Control and Prevention (2010). *HIV/AIDS Fact Sheets.* Available online at http://www.cdc.gov/hiv/resources/factsheets/. Retrieved June 2010.

Centers for Disease Control and Prevention. (2007). National surveillance for asthma—United States, 1980-2004. *MMWR Surveillance Summaries, 56*(8), 1-14; 18-54.

Centers for Disease Control and Prevention. (2008). *Trends in Tuberculosis. 2008.* Available online at www.cdc.gov/tuberculosis. Retrieved June 2010.

Cohen, M.R. (2009). Medication errors. *Nursing2009, 39*(3), 12.

Cohen, S. (2006). Peptic ulcer. *The Merck Manuals Online Medical Library: Home Edition for Patients and Caregivers.* Available online at http://www.merck.com/mmhe/sec09/ch121/ch121c.html. Retrieved October 2009.

Cohen, H., & Shastay, A.D. (2008). Getting to the root of medication errors. *Nursing2008, 38*(12), 39-47.

Consumer Reports. (2006). Evaluating prescription drugs used to treat overactive bladder: Comparing effectiveness, safety, and price. Retrieved July 2010 from www.consumerreports.org/health/resources/pdf/best-buy-drugs/Overactive_Bladder-FINAL.pdf.

Coughlin, R.M. (2007). Recognizing ventricular arrhythmias and preventing sudden cardiac death. *American Nurse Today, 2*(5), 38-44.

Cranwell-Bruce, L.A. (2009). Update in diabetes management. *MEDSURG Nursing, 18*(1), 51-53.

Cranwell-Bruce, L.A. (2007). Anticoagulation therapy: Reinforcing patient education. *MEDSURG Nursing, 16*(1), 55-58.

Czock, D., Markert, C., Hartman, B., & Keller, F. (2009). Pharmacokinetics and pharmacodynamics of antimicrobial drugs. *Expert Opinion on Drug Metabolism & Toxicology, 5*(5), 475-487.

D'Arcy, Y. (2009). *Are* opioids safe for your patient? *Nursing2009, 39*(4), 40-44.

D'Arcy, Y. (2009). Avoid the dangers of opioid therapy. *American Nurse Today, 4*(5), 18-22.

De Clercq, E. (2009). Anti-HIV drugs: 25 compounds approved within 25 years after the discovery of HIV. *International Journal of Antimicrobial Agents, 33*(4), 307-320.

De Clercq, E. (2009). The history of antiretrovirals: Key discoveries over the past 25 years. *Reviews in Medical Virology, 19*(5), 287-299.

Devdhar, M., Ousman, Y.H., & Burman, K.D. (2007). Hypothyroidism. *Endocrinology and Metabolism Clinics of North America, 36*(3), 595-615.

Dörffler-Melly, J., Koopman, M.M., Prins, M.H., & Büller, H.R. (2005). Antiplatelet and anticoagulant drugs for prevention of restenosis/reocclusion following peripheral endovascular treatment. Available online at http://www.cochrane.org/reviews/en/ab002071.html. Retrieved October 2009.

Dubbin, L., & Clock, A. (2009). Reversing neuroleptic malignant syndrome. *American Nurse Today, 4*(1), 33.

Duncan, J., & Corcoran, J. (2007). *Pediatric high-alert medications: Evidence-based safe practices for nursing professionals.* Marblehead, MA: HCPro, Inc.

Edwards, J.L. (2008). Diagnosis and management of benign prostatic hyperplasia. *American Family Physician, 77*(10), 1403-1410.

Eidelberg, D., & Pourfar, M. (2007). Parkinson's disease. *The Merck Manuals Online Medical Library: Home Edition for Patients and Caregivers.* Available online at http://www.merck.com/mmhe/sec06/ch091/ch091d.html. Retrieved January 2009.

Ellis, K.C. (2008). Keeping asthma at bay. *American Nurse Today, 3*(2), 20-25.

Epilepsy Foundation of Western/Central Pennsylvania. (2003). Anti-seizure medication and their side effects. Available online at http://www.efwp.org/programs/side_effects.shtml. Retrieved October 2009.

Ezell, J. (2006). *What* is secondary adrenal insufficiency? *Nursing2006, 36*(5), 12.

Fitzgerald, M.A. (2007). Herbal facts, herbal fallacies. *American Nurse Today*, 2(12), 27-32.

Fitzgerald, M.A. (2006). Managing bronchospasm with short-acting beta$_2$-agonists. *The Nurse Practitioner*, 31(9), 47-53.

Gaither, J.B., & Van Gelder, C.M. (2008). Antidysrhythmic toxicity. *eMedicine*. Available online at http://www.emedicine.medscape.com/article/813046-overview. Retrieved October 2009.

Glass, M., & Spitrey, J. (2009). Heparin-induced thrombocytopenia: Your questions answered. *AACN Advanced Critical Care*, 20(1), 5-9.

Global Initiative for Chronic Obstructive Lung Disease (GOLD). (2008). *Global strategy for the diagnosis, management, and prevention of chronic obstructive pulmonary disease*. Medical Communications Resources, Inc. Available online at www.goldcopd.com/Guidelineitem.asp?l1=2&l2=1&intId=2003. Retrieved October 2009.

Gould, I.M. (2009). Antibiotic resistance: The perfect storm. *International Journal of Antimicrobial Agents*, 34(Suppl 3), S2-S5.

Gould, I.M. (2009). Antibiotics, skin and soft tissue infection and methicillin-resistant *Staphylococcus aureus*: Cause and effect. *International Journal of Antimicrobial Agents*, 34(Suppl 1), S8-S11.

Gould, I.M. (2008). The epidemiology of antibiotic resistance. *International Journal of Antimicrobial Agents*, 32(Suppl 1), S2-S9.

Hadaway, L. (2009). Protect patients from I.V. infiltration. *American Nurse Today*, 4(7), 10-12.

Hain, T.C. (2003). Ototoxic medications. Available online at http://www.tchain.com/otoneurology/disorders/bilat/ototoxins.html. Retrieved October, 2009.

Held, M.L., & Sturtz, M. (2009). Managing acute decompensated heart failure. *American Nurse Today*, 4(2), 18-23.

Heuer, D.K. (2008). The present and future of glaucoma treatment. *Ocular Surgery News*, 10, 10-13.

Holcomb, S.S. (2009). An update on antithrombotic guidelines. *The Nurse Practitioner*, 34(1), 6-10.

Holcomb, S.S. (2009). Common herb-drug interactions: What you should know. *The Nurse Practitioner*, 34(5), 21-29.

Holcomb, S.S. (2008). Easing the anguish of Alzheimer's disease. *American Nurse Today*, 3(12), 18-23.

Holcomb, S. (2007). Dodging the bullae: Stevens-Johnson syndrome. *Nursing2007*, 37(6), 64cc1-64cc3.

Hoogwerf, B.J. (2006). Exenatide and pramlintide: New glucose-lowering agents for treating diabetes mellitus. *Cleveland Clinic Journal of Medicine*, 73(5), 477-484.

Howe, L.A. (2009). Pharmacogenomics and management of cardiovascular disease. *The Nurse Practitioner*, 34(8), 28-35.

Huber, C., & Augustine, A. (2009). IV infusion alarms: Don't wait for the beep. *American Journal of Nursing*, 109(4), 32-33.

Hughes, S. (2009). On the road to better dyslipidemia outcomes. *The Nurse Practitioner*, 34(2), 14-21.

Inott, T.J. (2009). The dark side of SSRIs: Selective serotonin reuptake inhibitors. *Nursing2009*, 39(8), 31-33.

Institute for Safe Medication Practices. (2009). ISMP's list of confused drug names. Available online at www.ismp.org/Tools/confuseddrugnames.pdf. Retrieved October 2009.

Institute for Safe Medication Practices. (2008). ISMP's list of high-alert medications. Available online at www.ismp.org/Tools/highalertmedications.pdf. Retrieved October 2009.

James, S.H. (2009). Hematology pharmacology: Anticoagulant, antiplatelet, and procoagulant agents in practice. *AACN Advanced Critical Care*, 20(2), 177-192.

Klabunde, R.E. (2007). Diuretics. *Cardiovascular Pharmacology Concepts*. Available online at www.cvpharmacology.com/diuretic/diuretics.htm. Retrieved October 2009.

Knowles, M. (1980). *The modern practice of adult education*. New York: Cambridge.

Koski, R.R. (2006). Practical review of oral antihyperglycemic agents for type 2 diabetes mellitus. *The Diabetes Educator*, 32(6), 869-876.

Kudzma, E.C., & Carey, E.T. (2009). *Pharmacogenomics*: Personalizing drug therapy. *American Journal of Nursing*, 109(10), 50-57.

Lawes, R. (2009). Putting the squeeze on asthma. *Nursing2009*, 39(3), 56hn1-56hn3.

Lea, D.H., Feero, G., & Jenkins, J.F. (2008). Warfarin therapy and pharmacogenomics: A step toward personalized medicine. *American Nurse Today*, 3(5), 12-13.

Leibowitz, L.D. (2009). MRSA burden and interventions. *International Journal of Antimicrobial Agents*, 34(Suppl 3), S11-S13.

Lien, Y.H., Shapiro, J.I. (2007). Hyponatremia: Clinical diagnosis and management. *American Journal of Medicine*, 120(8), 653-658.

Lopez, D.P. (2009). Emergency: Acetaminophen poisoning. *American Journal of Nursing*, 109(9), 48-51.

Mayo Clinic Staff. (2009). Alzheimer drugs slow progression of disease. *MayoClinic.com*. Mayo Foundation for Medical Education and Research. Available online at www.mayoclinic.com/health/alzheimers/AZ00015. Retrieved October 2009.

Mayo Clinic Staff. (2009). Constipation. *MayoClinic.com*. Mayo Foundation for Medical Education and Research. Available online at www.mayoclinic.com/health/constipation/DS00063. Retrieved January 2009.

Mayo Clinic Staff. (2009). Generalized anxiety disorder: Treatments and drugs. *MayoClinic.com*. Mayo Foundation for Medical Education and Research. Available online at www.mayoclinic.com/health/generalized-anxiety-disorder/DS00502/DSECTION=treatments%2Dand%2Ddrugs. Retrieved January 2009.

Mayo Clinic Staff. (2009). GERD. *MayoClinic.com*. Mayo Foundation for Medical Education and Research. Available online at www.mayoclinic.com/gerd/DS00967. Retrieved January 2009.

Mayo Clinic Staff. (2008). Depression (major depression). *MayoClinic.com*. Mayo Foundation for Medical Education and Research. Available online at www.mayoclinic.com/health/depression/DS00175. Retrieved October 2009.

Mayo Clinic Staff. (2008). Diarrhea. *MayoClinic.com*. Mayo Foundation for Medical Education and Research. Available online at www.mayoclinic.com/health/diarrhea/DS00292. Retrieved January 2009.

Mayo Clinic Staff. (2008). Heart Failure: Treatments and Drugs. *MayoClinic.com*. Mayo Foundation for Medical Education and Research. Available online at www.mayoclinic.com/health/heart-failure/DS00061/DSECTION=treatments-and-drugs. Retrieved January 2009.

Mayo Clinic Staff. (2008). High blood pressure (hypertension). *MayoClinic.com*. Mayo Foundation for Medical Education and Research. Available online at www.mayoclinic.com/health/high-blood-pressure/DS00100. Retrieved October 2009.

McCance, K., & Huether, S. (2006). *Pathophysiology: The biologic basis for disease in adults and children* (5th ed.). St. Louis: Mosby.

McKennon, S.A., & Campbell, R.K. (2007). The physiology of incretin hormones and the basis for DPP-4 inhibitors. *The Diabetes Educator*, 33(1), 55-66.

MD Consult. Available online at www.mdconsult.com/php/82925233-2/homepage.

Molony, S.L. (2009). Monitoring medication use in older adults. *American Journal of Nursing*, 109(1), 68-78.

National Asthma Education and Prevention Program. (2007). Expert Panel Report 3: Guidelines for the diagnosis and management of asthma—Summary Report 2007. *The Journal of*

*Allergy and Clinical Immunology,* 120(Suppl 5), S94-138.

Nayak, B., & Hodak, S. (2007). Hyperthyroidism. *Endocrinology and Metabolism Clinics of North America,* 36(3), 617-656.

Nursing2009. (2009). Photosensitivity. *Nursing2009,* 39(9), 32.

Nussbaum, R., McInnes, R., & Willard, H. (2007). *Thompson & Thompson: Genetics in medicine* (7th ed.). Philadelphia: Saunders.

Odegard, P.S., Setter, S.M., & Iltz, J.L. (2006). Update in pharmacologic treatment of diabetes mellitus: Focus on pramlintide and exenatide. *The Diabetes Educator,* 32(5), 693-712.

Pagana, K., & Pagana, T. (2006). *Mosby's manual of diagnostic and laboratory tests* (3rd ed.). St. Louis: Mosby.

Parkinson's Disease Foundation. (2009). What is Parkinson's disease: Medications. *Parkinson's Disease Foundation Website.* Available online at http://www.pdf.org/en/meds_ treatments. Retrieved January 2009.

Picazo, J.J., Candel, F.J., & Gonzales-Romo, F. (2008). Update on fungal infections— introduction. *International Journal of Antimicrobial Agents,* 32(Suppl 2), S79-S81.

Pruitt, W.C. (2005). *Teaching* your patient to use a peak flow meter. *Nursing2005,* 35(3), 54-55.

Psych Central. (2006). Medications for schizophrenia and psychosis. *Psych Central Website.* Available online at http://psychcentral.com/library/ meds_schizo.htm. Retrieved October 2009.

Reid, J.R., & Wheeler, S.F. (2005). Hyperthyroidism: Diagnosis and treatment. *American Family Physician,* 72(4), 623-630.

Roman, M. (2007). Asthma. *MEDSURG Nursing,* 16(3), 209-210.

Ross-Flanigan, N. (2002). Anticoagulant and antiplatelet drugs. *Healthline website.* Available online at http://healthline.com/galecontent/anticoagulant-and-antiplatelet-drugs. Retrieved October 2009.

Ross-Flanigan, N., & Uretsky, S. (2004). Antinausea drugs. *Healthline website.* Available online at http://www.healthline.com/galecontent/antinausea-drugs-1. Retrieved January 2009.

Rushing, J. (2007). Administering eyedrops. *Nursing2007,* 37(5), 18.

Safeer, R.S., & Lacivita, C.L. (2000). Choosing drug therapy for patients with hyperlipidemia. *American Family Physician.* Available online at http://www.aafp.org/afp/AFPprinter/20000601/3371.html. Retrieved January 2009.

Scemons, D. (2007). Are you up-to-date on diabetes medications? *Nursing2007,* 37(7), 45-49.

Schulmeister, L. (2009). Vesicant chemotherapy extravasation antidotes and treatments. *Clinical Journal of Oncology Nursing,* 13(4), 395-398.

Soldin, O.P., & Mattison, D.R. (2009). Sex differences in pharmacokinetics and pharmacodynamics. *Clinical Pharmacokinetics,* 48(3), 143-157.

Sucher, A.J., Chahine, E.B., & Balcer, H.E. (2009). Echinocandins: The newest class of antifungals. *The Annals of Pharmacotherapy,* 43(10), 1647-1657.

Theuretzbacher, U. (2009). Future antibiotics scenarios: Is the tide starting to turn? *International Journal of Antimicrobial Agents,* 34(1), 15-20.

Thompson, G.R. 3rd, Cadena, J., & Patterson, T.F. (2009). Overview of antifungal agents. *Clinics in Chest Medicine,* 30(2), 203-215.

Tocco, S. (2009). Phenytoin: Keep patients in the range and out of danger. *American Nurse Today,* 4(1), 12-13.

Tocco, S.B. (2007). Overcoming the fear of tonic-clonic seizures. *American Nurse Today,* 2(5), 10-12.

Todd, B. (2007). Extensively drug-resistant tuberculosis. *American Journal of Nursing,* 107(6), 29-31.

United States Drug Enforcement Administration (DEA) website. Available online at http://www.usdoj.gov/dea/index.htm.

United States Food and Drug Administration (FDA) website. Available online at http://www.fda.gov/.

United States Pharmacopeia (USP) website. Available online at http://www.usp.org/.

Uretsky, S.D. (2002). Antipsychotic drugs. *Healthline website.* Available online at http://www.healthline.com/galecontent/antipsychotic-drugs. Retrieved October 2009.

Urology Channel. (2009). Bladder control problems/overactive bladder. *UrologyChannel website.* http://www.urologychannel.com/bladdercontrol/index.shtml. Retrieved October 2009.

Vacca, V. (2008). Hyperkalemia. *Nursing2008,* 38(7), 72.

WebMD. (2009). Recognizing the symptoms of depression: Drugs to treat depression. WebMD website. Available online at http://www.webmd.com/depression/recognizing-depression-symptoms/antidepressants. Retrieved October 2009.

Weeks, B., & Ficorelli, C.T. (2006). How new drugs help treat erectile dysfunction. *Nursing2006,* 36(1), 18-19.

Workman, L. (2006). The biological basis of cancer. In M. Barton-Burke & G. Wilkes (Eds.), *Cancer Therapies* (pp. 1-20). Boston: Jones & Bartlett.

Workman, M.L. (2010). Care of patients with cancer. In D.D. Ignatavicius & M.L. Workman (Eds.), *Medical-Surgical Nursing: Patient-Centered Collaborative Care* (6th ed.) (pp. 414-439). Philadelphia: Saunders.

World Health Organization (WHO). (2008). *Data and statistics—mental health.* Available online at www.who.int/research/en/. Retrieved January 2009.

Wright, J.M., & Musini, V.M. (2009). First-line drugs for hypertension. *The Cochrane Collaboration: Cochrane Reviews.* Available online at http://www.cochrane.org/reviews/en/ab001841.html. Retrieved January 2009.

Zarowitz, B.J. (2007). Erythropoietic-stimulating agents (ESAs): New safety warning. *Geriatric Nursing,* 28(3), 148-150.

# Illustration Credits

**CHAPTER 2**

**2-1,** From Dewit, S.C. (2009). *Fundamental Concepts and Skills for Nursing* (3rd ed.). Saunders; **2-2,** From Hockenberry, M.J., & Wilson, D. (2006). *Wong's Nursing Care of Infants and Children* (8th ed.). St. Louis: Mosby (**B,** Courtesy Paul Vincent Kuntz, Texas Children's Hospital, Houston); **2-3,** From Perry, A.G., & Potter P. (2009). *Clinical Nursing Skills and Techniques* (7th ed.). St. Louis: Mosby; **2-6 B,** From Harkreader, H., Thobaben, M., & Hogan, M.A. (2007). *Fundamentals of Nursing: Caring and Clinical Judgment* (3rd ed.). Philadelphia: Saunders.

**CHAPTER 6**

**6-3, A,** Courtesy Baxter Healthcare Corporation, Deerfield, IL. In Harkreader, H., Thobaben, M., & Hogan, M.A. (2007). *Fundamentals of Nursing: Caring and Clinical Judgment* (3rd ed.). Philadelphia (Saunders); **B,** From Christensen, B.L., & Kockrow, E. (2006). *Foundations and Adult Health Nursing* (5th ed.). St. Louis: Mosby; **6-4,** Photo from Perry, A., & Potter, P. (2009). *Clinical Nursing Skills & Techniques* (7th ed.). St. Louis: Mosby; **6-5 A,** From Hockenberry, M.J., & Wilson, D. (2006). *Wong's Nursing Care of Infants and Children* (8th ed.). St. Louis: Mosby; **B,** From Weinzweig, J. & Weinzweig, N. (2005). *The Mutilated Hand,* St. Louis: Mosby; **6-6,** From Elkin, M., Perry, A., & Potter, P. (2007). *Nursing Interventions & Clinical Skills* (4th ed.). St. Louis: Mosby.

**CHAPTER 7**

**7-2,** From Wong D.L., Hockenberry-Eaton, M., Wilson, D., Winkelstein, M.L., & Schwartz, P. (2001). *Wong's Essentials of Pediatric Nursing* (6th ed.). St. Louis: Mosby. Copyrighted by Mosby. Reprinted by permission.

**CHAPTER 11**

**11-1,** Photo from Kumar, V., Abbas, A., Fausto, N., & Aster, J. (2009). *Robbins and Cotran Pathologic Basis of Disease* (8th ed.). Philadelphia: Saunders; **11-2,** From Forbes, C.D. (2003). *Color Atlas and Text of Clinical Medicine* (3rd ed.). St. Louis: Mosby.

**CHAPTER 13**

**13-4,** From Goldstein, G.B., & Goldstein, A.O. (1997). *Practical Dermatology* (2nd ed.). St. Louis: Mosby; **13-5,** From Weston, W., Lane, A., & Morelli, J. (2007). *Color Textbook of Pediatric Dermatology* (4th ed.). St. Louis: Mosby.

**CHAPTER 14**

**14-4,** From Goldman, L., & Ausiello, D. (2007). *Cecil Medicine* (23rd ed.). Philadelphia: Saunders.

**CHAPTER 17**

**17-5,** From Hoffman R., et al. (2008). *Hematology: Basic Principles and Practice* (5th ed.). Philadelphia: Churchill Livingstone.

**CHAPTER 18**

**18-5,** From Aehlert, B. (2009). *Paramedic Practice Today: Above and Beyond.* St. Louis: Mosby; **18-6,** From Ignatavicius, D., & Workman, M.L. (2010), *Medical-Surgical Nursing: Patient-Centered Collaborative Care* (6th ed.). St. Louis: Saunders.

**CHAPTER 24**

**24-2, 24-3, 24-5,** From Ignatavicius, D.D., & Workman, M.L. (2010). *Medical-Surgical Nursing: Patient-Centered Collaborative Care* (6th ed.). Philadelphia: Saunders; **24-4,** From Behrman, R.E., Kliegman, R.M., & Jenson, H.B. (2004). *Nelson Textbook of Pediatrics* (17th ed.). Philadelphia: Saunders.

**CHAPTER 25**

**25-6,** From Lilley, L., Harrington, S., & Snyder, J. (2007). *Pharmacology and the Nursing Process* (5th ed.). St. Louis: Mosby; **25-9,** Courtesy Eli Lilly & Company, Indianapolis, and Amylin Pharmaceuticals, San Diego.

**CHAPTER 26**

**26-6,** From Pfizer, Inc., New York; **26-7,** From Yanoff, M., & Duker, J. (2009).*Ophthalmology* (3rd ed.). St. Louis: Mosby.

# Disorders Index

Note: Page numbers followed by *f* indicate figures; *t*, tables; and *b*, boxes.

# General Index

Note: Page numbers followed by *b* indicate boxes; *f*, figures; and *t*, tables.

## The Joint Commission's Official "Do-Not-Use" List*

| DO NOT USE | POTENTIAL PROBLEM | USE INSTEAD |
|---|---|---|
| U (unit) | Mistaken for "0" (zero), the number "4" (four), or "cc" | Write "unit" |
| IU (International Unit) | Mistaken for IV (intravenous) or the number 10 (ten) | Write "International Unit" |
| QD, qd (daily) | Mistaken for each other | Write "daily" |
| QOD, qod (every other day) | Period after the Q mistaken for "I" and the "O" mistaken for "I" | Write "every other day" |
| Trailing zero (X.0 mg)** | Decimal point is missed | Write X mg |
| Lack of leading zero (.X mg) | | Write 0.X mg |
| MS | Can mean morphine sulfate or magnesium sulfate | Write "morphine sulphate" |
| MSO4 and MgSO4 | Confused for one another | Write "magnesium sulphate" |

*Applies to all orders and all medication-related documentation that is handwritten (including free-text computer entry) or on pre-printed forms.
**Exception: A "trailing zero" may be used only where required to demonstrate the level of precision of the value being reported, such as for laboratory results, imaging studies that report size of lesions, or catheter/tube sizes. It may not be used in medication orders or other medication-related documentation.

## Additional Abbreviations, Acronyms, and Symbols
### (For Possible Future Inclusion in the Official "Do-Not-Use" List)

| DO NOT USE | POTENTIAL PROBLEM | USE INSTEAD |
|---|---|---|
| > (greater than)<br>< (less than) | Misinterpreted as the number "7" (seven) or the letter "L"<br>Confused for one another | Write "greater than"<br>Write "less than" |
| Abbreviations for drug names | Misinterpreted due to similar abbreviations for multiple drugs | Write drug names in full |
| Apothecary units | Unfamiliar to many practitioners<br>Confused with metric units | Use metric units |
| @ | Mistaken for the number "2" (two) | Write "at" |
| cc | Mistaken for U (units) when poorly written | Write "mL" or "ml" or "milliliters" ("mL" is preferred) |
| µg | Mistaken for mg (milligrams) resulting in one thousand-fold overdose | Write "mcg" or "micrograms" |

From The Joint Commission, Oakbrook Terrace, IL. May, 2005. Available online at http://www.jointcommission.org/PatientSafety/DoNotUseList/.

# Answer Key

## Chapter 1
1. C
2. A
3. B
4. A
5. C
6. A
7. C
8. B
9. B
10. C
11. B
12. C
13. D
14. C
15. C
16. 25.45 kg

## Chapter 2
1. C
2. B
3. B
4. A, B, D, E
5. A, B, C, E
6. B
7. A, B, D
8. B
9. D

## Chapter 3
1. D
2. C
3. C
4. A, E
5. A
6. B, E, F
7. D

## Chapter 4
1. C
2. A
3. 2 Tbs
4. C
5. C
6. 700 mL
7. 52.3 kg
8. 0.8 mL
9. 0.75 mL

## Chapter 5
1. D
2. C
3. A
4. A
5. B
6. C
7. A
8. C
9. C
10. B
11. A
12. B
13. C
14. D
15. D
16. 2.4 mL

## Chapter 6
1. B
2. A
3. D
4. 56 gtts/mL
5. B, C, D, E, F
6. B
7. C
8. C
9. D
10. A
11. B

## Chapter 7
1. C
2. D
3. A
4. B
5. C
6. A, B, F
7. C
8. A
9. C
10. C
11. C
12. A, E, F, G
13. A
14. D
15. a. 0.8 mL
    b. 3.3 (or 3) mL
16. 0.25 mL

## Chapter 8
1. D
2. C
3. B, C, F
4. A
5. A
6. D
7. B
8. D

9. B
10. A
11. B
12. B
13. D
14. 3.2 mL
15. a. 1.6 mL
    b. 62.5 mL/hr; 15-16 gtts/
       min

## Chapter 9
1. C
2. D
3. D
4. A
5. B
6. C
7. B
8. D, E, F
9. 15 mL
10. 0.5 or ½ tablet

## Chapter 10
1. C
2. A
3. B
4. B
5. C
6. C
7. C
8. C
9. 6 mL
10. 0.5 mL

## Chapter 11
1. A
2. C
3. C
4. C
5. A
6. C
7. B
8. D
9. a. 1500 mg/day
    b. 15 tablets
10. 20 drops/min

## Chapter 12
1. C
2. D
3. D
4. C
5. B
6. A

7. C
8. C
9. 6 mL
10. 2 capsules

## Chapter 13
1. C
2. B
3. D
4. A
5. D
6. B
7. A, D, E, F, G
8. A, C, D, E
9. C
10. 2 tablets
11. 750 mcg
12. 5 mL

## Chapter 14
1. A
2. A, B, D, E
3. D
4. C
5. A
6. A, B, D, E
7. C
8. D
9. 20 mEq/dose
10. 144 mcg/min
11. 0.5 or ½ tablet

## Chapter 15
1. B
2. C
3. C
4. B
5. D
6. A
7. D
8. B
9. B
10. 150 mg
11. 2.1 mg
12. 2 tablets

## Chapter 16
1. B
2. D
3. A, B, D, E
4. C
5. B
6. C
7. D